Evelyn Scott:

A life in letters

Denise Scott Fears

T

The manufacturer's authorised representative in the EU for product safety is Authorised Rep
Compliance Ltd, 71 Lower Baggot Street, Dublin D02 P593 Ireland (www.arccompliance.com)

Troubador Publishing Ltd
Unit E2 Airfield Business Park,
Harrison Road, Market Harborough,
Leicestershire. LE16 7UL
Tel: 0116 2792299
Email: books@troubador.co.uk
Web: www.troubador.co.uk

ISBN 978 1836280 118

British Library Cataloguing in Publication Data.
A catalogue record for this book is available from the British Library.

Typeset by Troubador Publishing Ltd, Leicester, UK

Table of Contents

Part 1: In the beginning . . .

Part 2: London

Part 3: The Benjamin Franklin Hotel

Appendices

Prologue

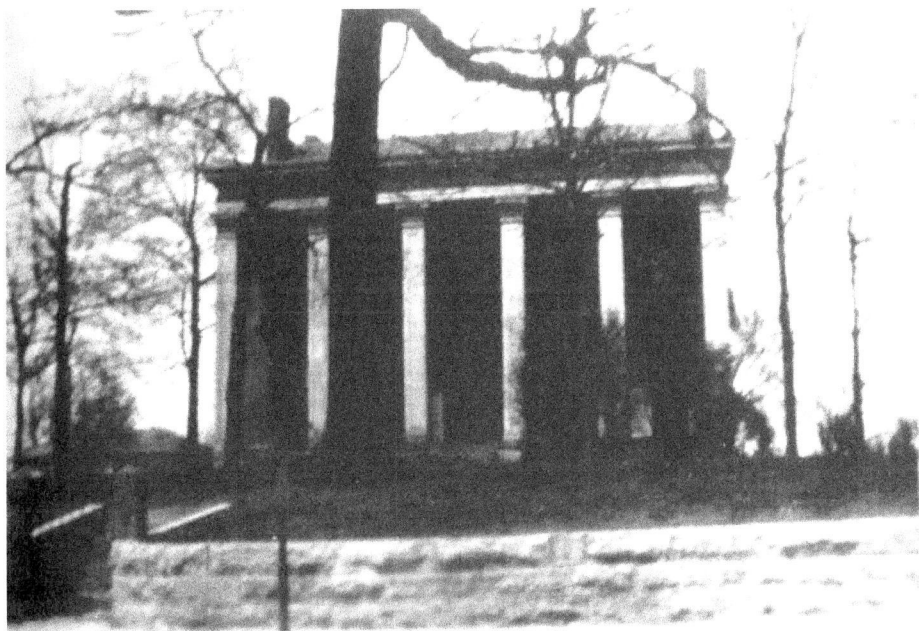

Gracey Mansion, date unknown: *Scott family*

I found the fuzzy photo in a drawer. The house could have come out of *Gone With the Wind*: classical proportions, a white columned portico rising the height of the building, large trees framing the whole. "That", my father said in a tone that discouraged any further questioning, "is the Gracey mansion in Clarksville, in Tennessee where your grandmother grew up". I was perhaps seven or eight years old and transfixed by the idea of a grandmother floating around in hoop skirts sipping mint juleps.

I remember, too, the distinctive typed envelopes that arrived, sometimes several times a week. My mother would go tense,, my father would storm out of the room,, and the envelopes would be put to one side. "Why don't you ever open them?" I would ask. "Who are they from?" My mother would murmur something unintelligible and change the subject. I eventually realised they were from my "Southern" grandmother.

Other children I knew had grandparents who were a part of their lives; I had very little contact with mine. I knew my grandfathers were still alive: we had visited one in North Carolina and the other in upstate New York. I wrote regular childish letters to my maternal grandmother in far-away New Mexico. But my father refused to talk about his mother. He did, however, tell us some things that were part of his own story: that his mother had eloped to Brazil with my grandfather who was 20 years her senior and married with four grown children; that to avoid scandal they had changed their names from Elsie Dunn and Frederick Wellman to Evelyn Scott and Cyril Kay Scott; that my father was born in Brazil where they lived until returning to the United States when he was five; that after their return his parents had had a number of affairs and that he had lived sometimes with one, sometimes the other; that he had spent much of his childhood in Bermuda, the south of France and North Africa; that in his teens, after his parents parted, he spent most of his time with his father in Santa Fe and Denver; that his mother had later married a British writer named Jack Metcalfe, of whom my father was quite fond. But nothing specifically about his mother.

I needed to find out more.

Evelyn Scott was an American author of the 1920s and '30s whose novels sparked controversy and elicited admiration. I discovered that by the time her first novel was published in 1921 when she was 27, she had published 12 poems in the so-called "little magazines", a volume of poetry, eight pieces of criticism, again in the little magazines, and had a play performed. In the following 15 years she published a further 12 novels and an autobiography, as well as three "juveniles"; her last published novel appeared in 1941. Throughout this period and until 1951, she was also publishing numerous poems and critical articles and the occasional short story. She worked on two further novels into the late 1950s, but they were never published. She died in 1963.

I culled this information from a number of sources: Google, biographies and the very sparse details my father shared with me. It is, however, little more than a skeleton much in need of fleshing out. The woman who seemed to haunt my family is hard to discern from these details.

Years passed …

One day in 1985, my husband pointed out a book review in *The Sunday Times*. It was for a volume entitled *Pretty Good For A Woman*, by a journalist and second-hand book dealer from Yorkshire named David Arthur Callard, and the dust-jacket bore a photo of my grandmother aged about 25. It was the first photo I had *ever* seen of her!

I bought the book and devoured it. By this time my father had been dead for 20 years and I was estranged from my mother, who was in any case showing the first signs of the dementia which eventually consumed her. Callard's book contained the same photo of the Gracey mansion I had seen all those years ago. He told the

story of a gifted young woman, a writer whose work was widely acclaimed, who had numerous lovers and loyal friends, who was frustrated by her inability to find the son and grandchildren whom she so wanted to see, and who died in obscure poverty in a shabby residential hotel in New York's Uupper West Side. I was beginning to understand some of the events of my childhood.

More years passed……

I picked Callard's book up again, and realised that there was no real reason not to go to Clarksville to see what I could learn there. I contacted the local museum to say I was thinking of coming to see my grandmother's birthplace, and did they have any information about the Gracey mansion? They did and I would be very welcome.

I flew into Newark airport. I knew from Callard's book that Evelyn was buried in a cemetery very near the airport, and as soon as I had collected my bags and hire car I headed there. The cemetery office was very helpful. "Just follow this man on the little tractor. He will show you where the grave is." The tractor wound round to the far side of the cemetery, and the driver unhooked a shovel from the back. For one horrified moment I wondered if he was going to dig Evelyn up, but he used the shovel to clear grass away from the little metal plaque identifying the plot. Evelyn was buried in an unmarked grave.

The museum at Clarksville made me very welcome. I was given access to all the information they had on Evelyn Scott, I met people who had studied her life and her work, I was taken to see the Evelyn Scott "sights". For me, the saddest of these was the site of the Gracey mansion: long since torn down as derelict, it had been replaced by two very shabby-looking apartment blocks. The maple trees that had graced the front of the house were still there, however, and I picked up some maple wings to bring home and propagate. They never sprouted.

While in Clarksville I was told that a large quantity of Evelyn's personal papers, including letters, were in the library of the University of Tennessee at Knoxville, where they had been deposited by Robert Welker, a former resident of Clarksville whose PhD thesis was about Evelyn's work. It was suggested that I would find it interesting to visit Welker and hear his account of both his friendship with Evelyn and how he came to have so many of her papers, and I was soon on the interstate heading for his home in Alabama. Welker, the personification of a Southern gentleman, made me welcome, gave me lunch and told me about meeting Evelyn, about his friendship with her and about her last days. And about how he came to have her papers. It was clear he had been devoted to her as a writer and as a friend, and she to him.

After that, I really could not leave Tennessee without looking at these papers, and two days later I was in the library of the University of Tennessee in Knoxville, surrounded by piles of boxes and feeling more than a little overwhelmed. I had no real idea what I was looking for, so decided to limit my perusal of the letters to those which mentioned any member of my immediate family by name. I only had a few days before heading back to the UK, and I raced through these boxes, stopping from time to time to read a letter that caught my eye. There was one "a-ha" moment after another as I understood, for the first time, the reasons for so many events of my childhood.

It was a very emotional experience. The collection was mainly carbon copies of letters written during the 1940s and '50s which were unlike any letters I had ever seen before. By far their most striking feature was their appearance. Her typing was erratic, the result of an overused and worn-out typewriter, and she made maximum use of the paper, filling each sheet to the right edge and the very bottom, then turning it 90 degrees and typing or writing across the wide left-hand margin. In addition, many letters contained insertions or annotations in her spidery angular handwriting, the anger and agitation clear in a visual frenzy. I could feel the emotional energy she transferred to the page.

Annotations often recorded the fact that a letter had not been answered. She beseeched my parents to let her know how they and her grandchildren were. She wrote lengthy age-inappropriate letters to me and my two brothers (we were all under six), urging us to urge our parents to write to her. Needless to say, we never saw these. Letters to friends begging them to call on us and report on her family went unanswered. Reading these, I imagined a grieving grandmother craving contact with her grandchildren: as a new grandmother myself, I could share her distress at not seeing them.

I fed piles of dollar bills into the photocopier as I copied what I thought interesting and relevant to bring back to study at leisure.

At home I studied my harvest and began to understand the woman who was my grandmother. I felt, in turn and in varying degrees, sympathy, sadness, anger, irritation and disbelief. My grandmother was clearly unhappy, frustrated because no one would answer her letters, agitated, obsessive, paranoid. I began to understand, too, why the arrival of a letter from her would create the response it did in my parents.

This was the first time, ever, that I had been so close to information about my grandmother. Callard's biography was a portrait of a strong-willed, gifted woman and an account of an unconventional life, but I hadn't been able to relate to it. During my childhood my parents had rarely spoken of her. What they did communicate was an almost subliminal sense that my grandmother was a force for evil. These letters revealed a complex and desperately unhappy woman who was at a loss to know how to connect with her son and her grandchildren.

Because of family and personal pressures, I did nothing more with these letters for several years, but during that time I had at the back of my mind a remark that had been made on my last day in Knoxville: "You know, we have had a number of people here, looking at her papers and writing about her literary development. But nobody has done anything with her family story. It's a fascinating one, and you are the ideal person to tell it. You should consider doing it yourself."

Then, in the summer of 2007, my mother died. I had been estranged from her for some years and I flew to clear her home in Nova Scotia with mixed and very intense emotions. As I went through her papers, I discovered a large collection relating to Evelyn. There were numerous letters from her to my parents (some unopened!) and a lengthy document Evelyn wrote in London in 1951 giving her interpretation of the reasons for their desperate financial straits which I read with horrified fascination. There was also a collection of letters from my father, written a few years before he died in 1965, begging, begging former friends for help in finding employment as he was destitute and unable to get any work, even as the local milkman. It was this last collection which was completely new to me, and it shocked me. It was clear from her earlier letters that Evelyn's constant harassing of her son's employers for information about his whereabouts had affected his reputation to the extent that he had become unemployable. Those letters of my father's were the catalyst to my decision to collect and edit her letters. I was motivated at first, I admit, by a filial impulse to revenge. Revenge is not a pretty emotion, nor a constructive one, but it was the spur I needed to start this project. As I worked, I began to rise above the "family-ness" of their content and to become absorbed in the documentation of the disintegration of a once-gifted mind.

I knew that I was missing letters from the first half of her life, the years spent in Bermuda and France and North Africa. The story would not be complete without them, and so I spent a month at the Harry Ransom Center of the University of Texas at Austin, working my way through collections of her papers and those of her husband Jack Metcalfe and of Cyril, my grandfather. The next year I returned to Knoxville and spent a fortnight in the basement of the university library, photocopying at break-neck speed the large number of letters I had skimmed on my earlier visit. The following year I did the same at Smith College in Massachusetts and at Yale University. Scholars who were interested in Evelyn's work forwarded more letters to me, and my collection grew and became more comprehensive.

The early letters could not have been more different from those I had first seen. During those years she and Cyril had had very little money. Their poverty led them to seek cheap rooms in warm climes where they would not have heating bills, and they ended up in a number of small towns in the south of France and north Africa. Evelyn wrote numerous lengthy letters to her friends back home, describing these places in astonishingly beautiful language. The letters were lyrical and full of detail. Two words could evoke a landscape in vivid colour. She was hugely intolerant of the people amongst whom they found themselves, but that did not prevent her from describing them in vivid, if negative, terms.

These letters were warm and affectionate and full of concern for her friends and their circumstances. She valued artistic integrity above all else, so it was perhaps not surprising that her closest friends were writers. Nor was it surprising that they, like her, struggled to find publishers and earn a living from their work. Letters were filled with commiseration, with practical advice, with serious critiques of work in progress. Few of the letters from these friends have survived, but it is clear from hers to them that these friendships were affectionate and deep, so much so that many survived her gradual deterioration into obsessiveness and paranoia.

None of this matched the impression of her conveyed by my parents. And I would have learned none of this but for the chance spotting of a review in *The Sunday Times*.

I knew what I had to do.

I started by transcribing the material I had collected: it was clear that to do anything further with this enormous amount of material it would be necessary to make electronic copies of everything. I spent months at my computer, typing, sometimes trying hard to decipher the documents, sometimes suffused with anger at Evelyn's harassment of my father, and often distraught at the human tragedy these letters revealed. At the end of this task I had electronic transcriptions of some 2,500 letters, filling 11 large ring binders. Although it was a mighty task, it was very productive as I was forced to pay close attention to the words I was transcribing. And all the while I was trying to identify the best way to present these words to tell Evelyn's tragic story.

Yet more years passed…

I wasn't idle. From time to time I returned to the challenge of presenting Evelyn's story as a coherent narrative, culled entirely from the letters I had collected. It was clear that a large number, perhaps the majority, of these letters had no immediate bearing on this story: these were excluded. A further number were repetitions: these too were excluded. Slowly the enormous archive was whittled down to something more manageable, but still unfocussed. The problem churned around at the back of my mind for some months until the solution suddenly became clear: early in her life and until WWII Evelyn had travelled to or lived in a number of different places, each of which could be the basis of a chapter. After the war, in a relatively settled life with her husband Jack Metcalfe in London, the themes were not the geography of her life but its preoccupations. And finally, in the early 1950s, she and Jack returned to the United States and, after some months in California, returned to New York and a shabby residential hotel where the story was one of Evelyn's declining health and increased mental distress.

And so, after a lengthy gestation, Evelyn's story has emerged.

Denise Scott Fears
Seaford, England
Summer 2023

The story in brief

The story begins on January 17, 1893 in Clarksville, Tennessee when a daughter, Elsie, was born to Maude Thomas Dunn and Seely Dunn. Maude came from a large, wealthy and well-established Southern family and Seely was a railwayman and a Yankee. Elsie grew up in comfort, first in an ante-bellum mansion among Maude's extended family and later in a fashionable part of New Orleans where Seely's work took the family.

Elsie was intelligent and headstrong and, unusually for that time, went to university. She enrolled at Tulane University in New Orleans, where one of her tutors was a Dr Frederick Creighton Wellman. Wellman had met her father some years earlier when they were both in Honduras, Seely on railway business, and Wellman collecting scientific specimens. He had already been married twice, had four grown children, had built a distinguished career as a doctor of tropical medicine, and was planning to travel to Brazil to collect research specimens. His wife had refused to join him and, not wanting to travel alone, he suggested to Elsie, who was clearly infatuated, that she come with him. And so, in December 1913, Elsie one month short of her 21st birthday, they eloped. Their disappearance created a scandal, but they managed to get to Brazil via New York and London without being stopped, changing their names en route to Cyril Kay Scott and Evelyn (Elsie had always hated her birth name) Scott.

They spent five years in Brazil, where their only child, a son, Creighton (known throughout his life as "Jigg" due to an infestation of chigoes, a biting insect sometimes called a chigger, when a baby) was born in 1914. Life was hard and Evelyn's mother, Maude, was sent by Seely to Brazil to help them (and later divorced by Seely on grounds of "desertion"). Cyril never did collect his specimens, but worked at jobs from labourer to the manager of an international mining company. The full account of these years is told by Evelyn in her autobiographical novel *Escapade,* published in 1923. Cyril's account of these years was published twenty years later in his autobiography, *Life Is Too Short.*

The family returned to the United States in the summer of 1919. Maude returned to Clarksville where, as a divorcée, she lived out her days on the charity of her extended family, and Evelyn and Cyril and five-year-old Jigg ended up in Greenwich Village in New

York. There they met and became friends (and sometimes lovers) of many of the literary figures of the day. One, a wealthy lawyer named Hale, saw that the practical skills Cyril had gained during the years of hardship in Brazil could be of great help to him and his family, and invited Cyril and Evelyn to join them at the family estates in Massachusetts and, later, Bermuda. Hale's wife took a liking to the couple, who were trying to live on Evelyn's meagre royalties, and granted them their own house and an income which she pledged would be for life. (She later withdrew these after a quarrel with Evelyn about the way she treated Cyril.)

In Bermuda, Cyril decided to try painting and, as a self-taught watercolourist, enjoyed modest success. There he met a young New Zealander, Owen Merton, the newly-widowed father of two small boys. Merton too was struggling to establish himself as an artist and Cyril took him under his wing. When in the summer of 1923 the Scotts decided to leave Bermuda, Merton came with them. They travelled to Europe looking for somewhere cheap and warm to live and ended up in Collioure, on the French Mediterranean coast not far from Marseille. Collioure proved to be too cold in winter and the family, with Merton, headed south to an oasis in Algeria.

During this period Evelyn and Merton formed a passionate sexual relationship which they carried on under Cyril's roof. It is not clear why he tolerated this relationship, which continued until early in 1925 when Merton ended it. There were a number of pressures on the couple: Merton's poor health (he suffered a number of blackouts caused by the brain tumour which later killed him), poverty, Evelyn's poor relationship with his younger son Tom[1] who stayed with them from time to time, and Evelyn's attempts to reconcile her conflicting loyalties to Merton and to Cyril. The break-up had a devastating effect on Evelyn. She returned to the US where she drove loyal friends to distraction as she wrote lengthy impassioned letters to her friends and to Merton, some of which he never opened, trying to understand what had happened and to renew the relationship. Meanwhile, Cyril took Jigg with him and spent the following year travelling in Algeria and Italy.

Eventually, Evelyn started living with John Metcalfe (Jack), a British author, sometime tutor in mathematics and Latin and Royal Air Force (RAF) reservist whom she had met some years earlier. They travelled to England, living in cheap lodgings and, in the summer of 1926, returned to the south of France to rejoin Cyril and Jigg. The four of them, ever in search of warmer and cheaper accommodation, ended up in Portugal, where they wintered unhappily before again seeking warmth in Algeria. At this point they separated, Jack leaving for England while Evelyn returned to New York with Jigg.

Meanwhile Cyril had moved to Santa Fe, New Mexico, where he established a school of painting. He was not only a talented painter but a gifted teacher, and the school did well. Jigg joined his father there and perhaps for the first time ever, he was able to enjoy

---

1   Thomas Merton, who grew up to become a Trappist monk and wrote the bestselling *The Seven Storey Mountain*.

a stable environment, embracing the outdoor life as well as discovering a talent for drawing and painting. After a year Evelyn and Jack went out to visit them: Evelyn hated the provincial attitudes of the residents but fell in love with the landscape and tried, unsuccessfully, to buy a property there as permanent security for herself and Jigg.

There is no evidence that Cyril ever divorced his second wife, nor did he ever legally marry Evelyn. However, she always insisted that theirs was a "common law" marriage, and perhaps Cyril believed this as well, because in March 1928, in Chihuahua, Mexico, Cyril "divorced" Evelyn. The petition cited "denial of bed and board". Evelyn did not contest this, nor did she attend the hearing. This "divorce" freed Evelyn from the "marriage" that had long since died, and in 1930 she and Jack were married, this time legally, in a small town not far from Santa Fe.

After Jack and Evelyn married, Jigg stayed with his father, first in Santa Fe, and later in Denver, Colorado, where Cyril established what later became the Denver Art Museum. Jigg thrived, enjoying outdoor life and studying painting at Denver University (later the University of Colorado), although he never finished his degree. Instead, at the age of 17 and much to his parents' consternation, he married his father's secretary, seven years his senior, and the couple moved to New York City. After a few months his new wife went off with a man her own age, and the marriage was annulled. Jigg stayed in New York and found work as an artist under President Roosevelt's New Deal.

Jack and Evelyn's early married life was punctuated by trans-Atlantic crossings. Both were trying to sell manuscripts to American publishers, and for Jack there was the additional problem of maintaining his immigrant "quota"[2] status, which meant he had to spend time living in the US. At this point, Yaddo, an artists' retreat in upper New York state, was their salvation. Evelyn had been invited to spend some time there in 1929 after a friend had recommended her, and from 1931 to 1933 she and Jack enjoyed extended stays there. Accommodation and board were very cheap and, most importantly, the other guests were writers and artists whom Evelyn found congenial.

It was not possible for Jack and Evelyn to stay at Yaddo forever. England was cheap and in 1935 Jack used a small inheritance to buy a cottage in the remote seaside village of Walberswick in Suffolk. Evelyn hated the provincial attitudes of the villagers and the bitter winds off the North Sea, but for the first time wrote about feeling settled. However, Jack's poor health from an earlier trip to Africa and their poverty exacerbated his tendency to drink and his fragile mental health. In 1937 he had a breakdown which provoked Evelyn into leaving him and returning to New York to stay with 22-year-old Jigg in Greenwich Village. Her departure shocked Jack and, in what he thought would be the best course of action, he sold the cottage at a loss and followed Evelyn to the US.

---

2   At that time the United States permitted a limited number (quota) of persons who fulfilled the qualifications for residence to apply to live permanently in the US as an alternative to citizenship. Individuals could leave the US for short periods but in order to maintain their qualification for the quota they had to spend the majority of their time in the US.

In 1940 Jigg married Paula Pearson, the niece of their benefactor Swinburne Hale, whose parents Evelyn and Cyril had known many years previously in Santa Fe. Jigg had found work as a news writer and broadcaster and the family, which now included a baby daughter, lived in Greenwich Village before moving to a rented house in the little town of Tappan, New York, from where he commuted to New York City.

When the war started, Jack returned to active duty in the RAF and was posted back to England. Evelyn wanted to join her husband. It was wartime and trans-Atlantic travel was severely restricted but, as the wife of a serving British officer, she was entitled to a passage on a convoy. While she was waiting for this to be arranged, Evelyn went to live with Jigg and his family. Jigg had initially welcomed his mother into their household, but before long she was creating havoc as her behaviour became more and more obsessive, the first signs of the mental illness that was to control her life. Jigg begged Jack to do what he could to hasten her return to England and in May 1943 his wish was granted. Evelyn returned to London to live in the large house Jack had bought which he had converted into flats, planning to rent three of them to provide the income that would support the couple in the fourth.

Evelyn missed her son who, relieved of his mother's presence, had cut off all communication with her. Evelyn could not understand how Jigg could not respond to her letters. Her obsessions were now conflated with a form of paranoia, as she assumed that Jigg's failure to respond was because her letters were being intercepted. This was the beginning of an onslaught which continued until her death in 1963. Evelyn, increasingly frantic, attempted to discover where her son was and why her letters were not being delivered. Jigg begged friends and Paula's family, many of whom also knew Evelyn, not to divulge his whereabouts, and they respected his wishes. These refusals only fuelled Evelyn's paranoia, and her letter writing became more frequent and frenzied as she tried to coax Jigg's whereabouts from his employers as well as anyone else who might possibly divulge it. The effect was catastrophic: Jigg's employers took the view that an employee whose mother wrote such letters was a problem, and he lost more than one job as a result. In the small world of radio news, word spread, and Jigg found it harder and harder to get a job, even though his competence was never questioned.

Eventually Jigg did find another job and he and Paula and their (now three) children lived in a series of rented houses in the New Jersey commuter belt. Somehow Evelyn discovered that one of these addresses was in the town of Rutherford, which also happened to be the home of one of Evelyn's former lovers, William Carlos Williams, both a well-regarded poet and a practising paediatrician. In an example of her willingness to impose on anyone who might possibly track Jigg down, she wrote Williams several long incoherent letters pleading with him to visit the family. Williams did not respond.

Evelyn was also dealing with another personal tragedy during these years. Ever since her return from Brazil in 1919, her precarious finances had meant she often depended on loans (rarely repaid) from her loyal friends, and on her return to London she tried to renew contact with her father. Seely had been prosperous and came from a wealthy family and she was confident that her father intended her to have a generous settlement at his death. Her last contact had been in 1925 and in 1946 she wrote to him at his last known employers, only to have her letter returned with the words "died May 1944" scribbled in pencil on the envelope. This led to another frenzy of letter writing as she desperately tried to learn where he had died, and of what, and what had become of the inheritance she expected and desperately needed. Bit by bit she learnt that after he had divorced Maude, Seely had married Melissa Whitehead, a woman not much older than Evelyn herself. Melissa did not respond to any of Evelyn's numerous pleas for information, but Seely's business contacts did eventually help Evelyn discover that her father had died of cancer in an Army hospital in Mississippi. Evelyn was upset that she had not known her father was ill, let alone that he had died. The Army pointed out that they depended on the next of kin to let them know of other family members to be notified and that his then wife, Melissa, had not told them of any other kin. Another onslaught of letters to courts in every possible jurisdiction failed to reveal any evidence of a will. Evelyn concluded that Melissa had kept the existence of a will (if there had been one) secret and had thus acquired all Seely's not inconsiderable property, including some valuable jewellery which Evelyn's grandparents had led her to believe would be hers.

After the war, Evelyn, isolated in London and unable to make contact with her family, became consumed with a desire to return to the United States where she was convinced she would be warmly welcomed by her son. Jack's large house was becoming a massive financial drain, neither of them was selling books, their only income was from Jack's part-time tutoring at private schools and they were poverty-stricken and in debt. At this point a well-connected and loyal friend in New York came up with the idea of establishing an "Evelyn Scott Fund" to raise enough money to enable them to settle Jack's debts and return to the US. Most of the American literary figures of the day were contacted and many contributed. In the spring of 1953 Evelyn and Jack set sail for New York and travelled on to Los Angeles where they had been offered a residency at a writers' retreat. This was a godsend as it provided them with six months' rent-free accommodation and peace to write.

After their sojourn in California Jack and Evelyn, still impoverished and still no closer to landing book contracts, headed back to New York City. Most of their friends were there, and they hoped that they would be close to Jigg and his family. Jack had planned to buy a small cottage somewhere in the country with the meagre proceeds from the sale of his London house, but found nothing he could afford. Eventually they ended up in a seedy residential hotel on the upper West Side where they lived until Evelyn died. Jack managed to earn a modest living teaching at a succession of private schools, but Evelyn's mental health deteriorated, and her days were spent writing lengthy incoherent letters and keeping track of letters sent and replies not received.

Meanwhile, in 1955, Jigg had landed a job with the US State Department. The post was in Vietnam and involved setting up a news network for the newly-created Radio

Vietnam. It was a politically-sensitive and challenging post, and Jigg embraced it. Again, Evelyn discovered the family's whereabouts, and her letters continued, more frequent and impassioned and bizarre than before. Jigg and Paula had decided that their best defence was to ignore them, which only inspired her to ever more incoherent pleas for information. When she failed to get a response from Jigg she wrote to his superiors in Washington, berating them for preventing contact with her family. A sympathetic personnel officer recognised the problem and prevented Evelyn's letters going beyond her desk, but Evelyn wrote directly to the FBI and to President Eisenhower, demanding that they reunite the family. When asked to explain this correspondence, Jigg tried to defuse it by saying he and his mother could not be more different. This turned out to be an unfortunate assertion: Evelyn's letters were imbued with anti-communist sentiment and in the feverish national paranoia of McCarthyism, this could only mean that her son was a Communist. In fact Jigg's politics were well to the right of centre and he was loyally patriotic, but the damage had been done. Jigg was fired. He and his family returned to the US in 1959, where they lived on the charity of Paula's relatives in California before heading into Canada, ending up in Nova Scotia where Jigg wanted to see a good friend from his youth. A month after arrival the Cuban missile crisis happened, and the family decided not to return to the US. Jigg never worked again. He died of heart failure in 1965.

Meanwhile Evelyn and Jack continued their lives of quiet desperation in New York. The flood of letters continued unabated and, amazingly, loyal friends stood by the couple. Evelyn had smoked all her life, and symptoms of the lung cancer which would contribute to her death began to worry her, as did a heart condition. Jack's health, too, was failing. He developed cataracts which made it impossible for him to continue teaching or writing and had several spells of inpatient treatment for depression, possibly fuelled by his heavy drinking. In 1962 Evelyn had a stroke, from which she partly recovered, and in the summer of 1963 she was hospitalised for "x-ray treatment" of her lungs. She was discharged that August, two days before she died of a heart attack with two close friends by her bed while Jack slept in an alcoholic stupor. She was 70 years old. One of these friends paid for her simple funeral but could not afford a headstone.

Jigg had no quarrel with Jack. During Evelyn's final illness Jack had written daily to Jigg and Paula, describing her treatment, always hopeful that she was getting better in spite of evidence to the contrary. The day after she died, he wrote: "She made my life hell for 37 years, but I cannot live without her". Not long afterwards he was compulsorily hospitalised for depression brought on by grief, and it took the intervention of a life-long British friend to get him released from hospital and to arrange for him to live in London. In July 1965, in London, Jack seemed to rally and to look forward to a new life sharing a flat with two old friends. The night before he was to move in, after a pleasant meal with his friends in a local pub, he tripped on the steps of his hotel and fell. He was taken to hospital but never regained consciousness. He is buried in Mill Hill cemetery in north-west London.

Between 1919 and 1953 Evelyn published 112 works. These included:
1919: her first publication, a critical essay
1921: her first novel, *The Narrow House*
1941: her last novel, *The Shadow of the Hawk*
1953: her final publication, a critical essay

In total she published:
14 novels (including 3 "juveniles")
2 books of poetry
1 play
1 autobiography
38 critical essays
45 poems
13 short stories

About the letters

Sources

I visited a number of libraries in order to compile as complete a dossier as possible of Evelyn's surviving letters As I had decided to concentrate on her relationships with members of her immediate family, material relevant to this collection was found in these five collections:

1. The Special Collections Library, University of Tennessee at Knoxville (UTK) provided the bulk of letters to Evelyn as well as a large number written by her;
2. The Harry Ransom Humanities Research Center, University of Texas at Austin (HRC) contained much material relating to Cyril Kay Scott and to Jack Metcalfe;
3. The Beinecke Rare Book Library at Yale University (BRBL) was the source of much of the correspondence with Lola Ridge as well as with Otto Theis and his wife Louise Morgan;
4. The library at Smith College in Massachusetts (SSC) houses a number of letters between Evelyn and Lola Ridge and Lola's husband Davy Lawson;
5. The Scott family collection (SFC) comprises a large number of letters to and from Evelyn and numerous originals of letters to and from Jack Metcalfe and Cyril Kay Scott.

Each letter is followed by bibliographic information and a code indicating its source.

Appearance

The appearance of the letters matters almost as much as the words on the page: they express her non-verbal state, her agitation, her search for the information that she so craved. This appearance is one of the most striking features of Evelyn Scott's letters, and the hardest to preserve when transcribing to the printed page. The typed letters were often carbon copies, with the imperfections inherent in that, often typed on a machine badly in need of a service, these letters characterised by missing or raised characters and a wide left margin that can only be described as "wonky". Perhaps to save paper, the typing is taken all the way to the right-hand margins, meaning words

you both before, my letters here asking for aid in placing my poems
were never acknowledged by anyone at all, save John Gawsworth --
then of The Poetry Review, and now, pro tem, jobless.

Gawsworth has some real guts, but apparently political "art"
became too much for him at a certain point; and he was accused
of "having lost money" for the magazine. He should have been
backed to carry on. These damn fools who are tin gods today have
got to be obliged to recognize that art is not produced primarily
for a commercial motive. It is something new since the war -- as
far as my awareness goes -- to have stock-holders in a "company"
virtually act as editors of its publications. That is how
this damn fool British Poetry Society is organized; and that is
probably the form of organization that has been imposed on
many publishing houses and distributing centres. This again means
numbers rule where ignorance is NOT bliss. Their votes decide.
Any sleazy rat that wants to can buy a little stock or "subscribe"
and vote even genius out of existence.

So here we stand or sit waiting for any move whatever either in
the States or here toward publishing John Metcalfe Evelyn Scott
and we hope soon again seriously Creighton Scott Cyril Kay Scott.

Naturally to unscramble so many eggs will require years. But
there should be a re-beginning for those of proven distinction, and
this, in turn, will undoubtedly influences policy and improve the
futures of every creator. And in improving their futures the
threats we confront to our civil liberties will also be greatly less-
ened.

You know my mind is as it is, and I must see things in the large,
But the personal problems are inextricable from the general picture
Lasting truth is above the battle; and it merely complicates the
problem of survivals and surviving civilization, to have all the
time thrust on one red-tape that has to do with nationalistic rivalry -- taking money out of Britain, transfering property assets if
any, are examples. Also these damn equators apparanetly argue as
to whether the British "means" test or the American should be
applied -- and BOTH ARE HELL. I dont know to what exent these
same problems recur with you as American temporarily in Germany,
but possibly you too are aware of some.

We arent immortal And we are being compelled to waste years
on futling and fruitless red-tape contention. And there has yet
to be one positive move to publish John Metcalfe here; though at
one moment there is evident stress on native-birth and the next
just the opposite. We want something more sensible as to solutions
for ourselves and yourselves than what we call "just counting Jews.

Love love love love love love
Please you both read my letters -- some people at home wont.
It has led to senseless confusion. Every word I write is pertinent
to our right to resume publishing seriously and yours and Cyril's
and to our right to be at home, instead of stuck here gagged.

Letter dated September 1, 1959 (part): *Scott family*

are sometimes short a letter or two. When a page was completely filled, she often turned the sheet 90 degrees and typed (or handwrote) in the wide left margin. In addition, many of her letters (carbons and originals) have insertions and annotations in her characteristically spiky handwriting, often using a blotchy fountain pen. The overall effect is of a frenetic energy, often conveying as much or more meaning as the words themselves.

A second, and important, feature of these letters is the underlining of words and phrases to denote emphasis, commonly seen in typescripts as the typewriter does not accommodate italic characters and these would conventionally be transcribed to italic font in the printed page. However, their use conveys so much of their emotional potency that I have left these as she wrote them, variously screaming and shrieking her impotency at the forces she felt were keeping her apart from her son and his family.

Evelyn's punctuation was anything but conventional. She was a great fan of the dash, which she used where others might have used commas or parentheses to set off what was often a non sequitur. She consistently omitted the apostrophe in contractions. Exclamation marks also appeared frequently, and could be seen as an indicator of her mental state: multiple exclamation marks were a feature of her more frenetic letters. Capitalisation was generous, if not always according to convention, and there was a period when names of organisations were presented inside quotation marks, almost as though she wanted to convey some doubt as to the existence of these bodies. And, everywhere, commas. All of these are presented as she wrote them. To "correct" them would have been to strip them of much of their psychological importance.

Spelling and other linguistic oddities

Although Evelyn was born and educated in the United States, she spent many years in England and was married to a Briton. Inevitably, her language and spelling are a mixture of British and American usage, and I have preserved this throughout.

She consistently misspells names of members of her family, place names likewise: I have not corrected these. There are a number of other consistent misspellings, which I have left unchanged. Some are minor and are easily understood; others, such as "draught" for "draft" (as in "first draught"), are possible confusions over homophones. All of these I have left as written. Capitalisation is also inconsistent and is preserved as written.

This is not to say that Evelyn was unable to write "correct" English. She was well-educated and literate. Some of her correspondence, especially that to her mother, was also "correct": her grammar and spelling, her descriptions were all "correct" and sometimes elegant. Letters to official bodies (see for example Chapters 21 and 25) were conventional, often formal, in style. It was those letters to her close friends and her family in which she expressed her anguish and rage that were the least "correct" in style.

Editing

These letters are heavily edited. Many of her letters are extremely lengthy (one is 12 single-spaced pages long!) and often wander incoherently among subjects. They typically include a perambulation of ideas and events, not all directly relevant to the focus of this collection: her continuing quest to contact her son and his family.

In order to maintain this focus, I have had to make some difficult and sometimes questionable decisions about what to keep and what to delete. I have tried to retain her development of a theme by excising phrases, complete sentences and, sometimes, whole paragraphs which interrupt the flow of her argument. Normally such excisions would be shown by ellipses [...] but as there are so many of them, I felt that their inclusion would distract the reader. My hope is that the narrative continues without distraction. All the words are Evelyn's: apart from these excisions I have made no changes.

Annotations and insertions

Finally, many of Evelyn's typed letters included handwritten additions. She used annotations to add information that had been left out of a typescript: this was typically an error or information which she felt needed to be included, often "for the record" but sometimes to reflect her own feelings about the subject.

More potent are insertions. Here Evelyn records an often indignant or angry reaction to a letter she has received, often some time earlier. These insertions are typically more "scrawled" than her annotations, larger and "blotchier" as in her distress she pressed harder on her overworked fountain pen, often insulting in tone: in short, the only rebuttal open to her.

Examples of all of these can be seen in a letter from Evelyn to Waldo Frank (image No 13 in Chapter 31). It is a photocopy of a carbon copy from the University of Tennessee collection and, even allowing for the technical inadequacies of the reproduction, it clearly shows Evelyn's use of these devices.

And finally...

Towards the end of her life Evelyn suffered a stroke which badly affected not only the coherence of her letters but the clarity of her handwriting. I decided that, in order to preserve both the message she was trying to convey in some of these letters and the cognitive damage she had suffered, to transcribe these letters, and to record that I had done this in the credit line under the letter.

Acknowledgements

A project like this cannot be completed without the collective effort of those individuals who provided help and support of so many kinds, each in its own way critical. Without their input, this book would not have been possible. My thanks to all of you.

Alex Anderson, Amy Anderson-Rude, Bob and Sally Buchanan,
Ned and Jacqueline Crouch, Bill Eigelsbach, Melody Fears, Phila Hach,
Geoffrey Jury, Karen Kukil, Caroline Maun, Claudia Milstead, Richard Oram,
Julian Peterson, Graça Salgado, Peter Sayers, Elaine Sproat, Cathlyn White,
Eleanor Williams, Shivaun Woolfson

And not forgetting the ever-helpful library staff at the University of Tennessee, the Harry Ransom Center and Smith College whose support made my task so much more enjoyable.

My thanks to all of you.

Dedication

The note below,
written by my then-5-year-old granddaughter,
graced the fridge door for nearly 20 years.

It kept me going.
Thank you, Millie

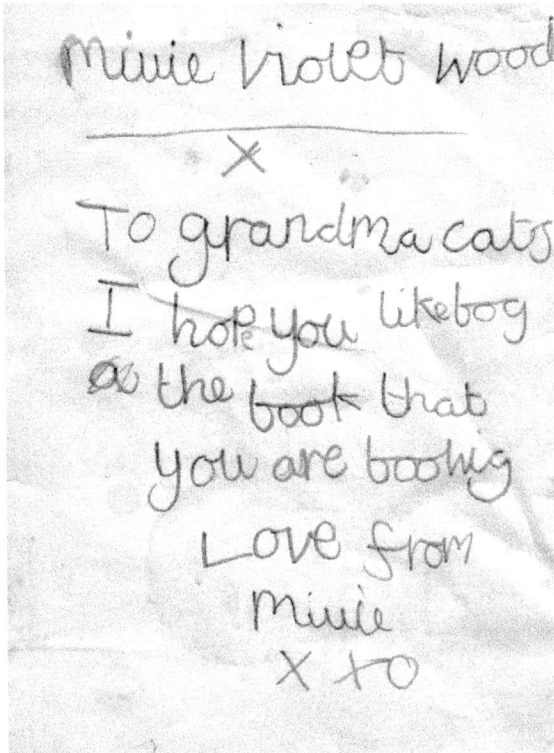

Part 1

In the beginning . . .

The story revealed in this selection of letters follows the progress of the lives of Evelyn and Cyril and later Evelyn and Jack. After an autobiographical account of the the time before Evelyn and Cyril eloped, these chapters record the early years of their life together as they, sometimes with their son Jigg, sometimes not, travelled around the Mediterranean. Evelyn's letters are characterised by vivid word pictures of the places they visited and the people among whom they found themselves.

Chapter 1

Clarksville and New Orleans
1893 - 1912

Evelyn Scott was born Elsie Dunn on January 17, 1883 in Clarksville, Tennessee to Maude Thomas, from an established Southern family, and Seely Dunn, a Yankee railwayman. Some of her earliest years were spent in the home of her mother's Gracey cousins: the photo shows it at its height in the 1870s.

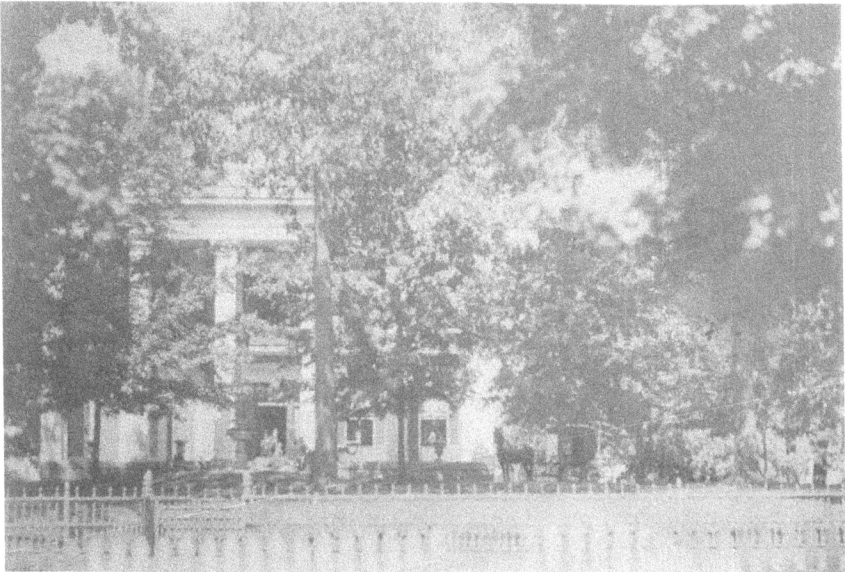

Gracey Mansion circa 1870: *Harry Ransom Center*

In 1956 she prepared a long document, addressed to her son, stipulating that it be preserved with her will and handed to him at her death. This extract is presented here as it summarises, in Evelyn's own words, the years which precede the earliest of the letters which have been preserved. It should be noted, however, that when she prepared this document, her mental health was deteriorating and the style and tone are markedly different from letters written in the 1920s and 1930s.

I was born Elsie Dunn and so baptised at Trinity Episcopal Church, Clarksville, Tennessee, where the parish registry contains both the record of my baptism when an infant, and of the marriage of my father and mother, Maud Thomas and Seely Dunn, then of Clarksville. The date of my birth was Jan 17th, 1893. My father was then twenty-one and was division superintendent of the Louisville and Nashville Railroad, his headquarters Clarksville.

When I was 3 years old, my father was promoted and became division superintendent of the L and NRR at Russellville, Kentucky. I lived in Russellville with my parents until I was nearly 7. We then moved to Evansville, Indiana, where I first attended School, a public school, and my father there, also, was Division Superintendent of the L and N, the job larger than his two previous ones, as Evansville was the office for a larger division. Not long after McKinley's assassination, we moved to St Louis, Missouri, where my mother and I resided while he went to Oklahoma and supervised the building of a new railroad, the Blackwell, Enid and Southwestern,

He had become interested in railway building and promotion, and from Saint Louis, where we were between three and four years, and where I attended the Marquette Public School, earlier the home of my grandparents, Mr and Mrs Oliver Milo Dunn; my grandfather having been Superintendent of the L and NRR in my father's earlier days. My father, while in Memphis in this period, was interested, with several men of greater wealth in building a railroad to be a link between Memphis and Pensacola.

I, with my parents, were in Memphis more than a year, and I went to the Public School there, too, and completed the eighth grade. The school was near a Miss Sally Gentry's where we boarded most of the time, but we were, also, briefly, boarding with a Mrs King. I did not like Memphis and I cannot remember even the name of the street in which we lived.

From Memphis, I moved with my parents to New Orleans, then back to Memphis for a short period, and back to New Orleans, again. My father, I should add, was of Yankee birth, born in Toledo, Ohio, but his parents had come South for the L and NRR when my father was a child.

My grandfather Dunn - Oliver Milo Dunn - was, when we first moved to New Orleans, General Superintendent of the Southern Lines of the Illinois Central Railway; a position his for many, many years - As with the letters, these diary entries are transcribed exactly as written: Jack's with his telegraphic punctuation and Evelyn's in her characteristic scrawl, a chronicle of letters not delivered and of her cleaning of the refrigerator in the communal kitchen.

I lived in New Orleans with my parents continuously, with the exception of the few months of return to Memphis, from the time

I was 12 years old until I lacked three weeks of 21. In New Orleans, my father held several positions connected with railroads and railroad building.

My father, while my mother and I stayed in New Orleans, also went to Spanish Honduras to supervise the building of the railroad from Porto Bello into the interior. I think this was actually after he had been State Head of the Interstate Commerce Commission his office in New Orleans. The Honduras road was a success.

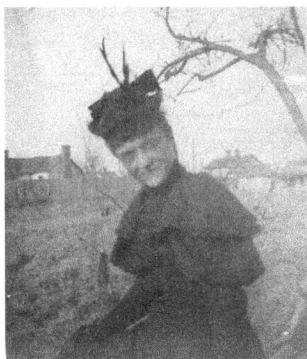

Maude Dunn from family album circa 1885: *Scott family*

It was when my father was living temporarily at Porto Bello that Dr Fredrick Creighton Wellman, then the Dean of the College of Tropical Diseases and Preventative Medicine of Tulane University - the first college of Preventitive[1] Medicine in the USA went, during a vacation to Honduras to diagnose a plant disease that had attacked banana, and met my father. My grandfather Dunn, at that time, was a Director of the United Fruit Company, and as it shipped many bananas, this led to the introduction. My father admired him, and had reason to.

In New Orleans, in my adolescence, my grandfather Dunn was reckoned a millionaire. I may be inexact about my grand-father's railway beginnings. My father attended Tulane University, but he and his mother had never gotten on well, and he left the University before his graduation because he preferred to be entirely on his own, as my grandfather disapproved of his impatience with my grandmother; who was, indeed, a "difficult" woman.

In New Orleans I attended Newcomb Preparatory School, Newcomb Art School, and Newcomb College. I was the youngest student ever to matriculate at the college, having then been fifteen. My father did his best to try to persuade me to be inducted into the formal society of the day, but I developed very early, the typical society misses bored me and aroused a contempt that may have been in part defensive. I could not take everything lightly, as they seemed to. My parents were an ill-matched pair, and I had become aware of their incompatibility when I was seven years old. They did not admit it to me, but it was obvious. I was sometimes, in my teens, taken to Mardi Gras balls at the French Opera House, but my mother had entirely retreated from that social life among the wealthy and would-be wealthy and I soon hated what I saw. I had been writing at intervals since

---

1   This, one of Evelyn's many consistent mis-spellings, recurs repeatedly throughout Evelyn's letters.

I was 7 and was the winner of a prize given by <u>Little Folks'</u>
<u>Magazine</u> for a story entitled "Helen's Wonderful Dream". In New
Orleans, after one unhappy infatuation in Clarksville on visits
during my fifteenth and sixteenth years, I put aside even boys
for books, paintings, Saturdays and Sundays at the French Opera
House, Philharmonic Concerts and every concert I could hear.

I was restless in an unhappy household. My father, when
compelled to realize it, tended, I think, to blame my mother
altogether. I was the Secretary of the Woman Suffrage Party,
already, at seventeen. I had written a number of immature
stories, had sold two - under the pseudonym Hiram Hagenbeck,
the name given by my father to my fox-terrier, and one had
appeared - or maybe two - in the New Orleans <u>Picayune</u>. I had also
sold a story about Creoles to the <u>John Trotwood Moore Magazine</u>
but before its publication the magazine failed. My father was
bewildered by my views, which then included some on philosophy,
and an inclination to become a socialist stemming from reading
Shaw and seeing Shaw first played, and a general conviction that
the world's ways were wrong - as of course they often are and
always will be.

My parents were, I thought, wretched; and my grandfather
Dunn, who had always been a voluntary martyr to an adored and
compassionated wife, was, also, I could see, not happy, after
having voluntarily resigned his position with the Illinois
Central in consequence of a quarrel between my grandmother and Mrs
Stuyvesant Fish, during one of Mrs Fish's visits to New Orleans.
My grandmother could be outrageously arrogant, and she mistook
something Mrs Fish said as insulting. And at this point, my
grandfather, after some years of entirely amiable relations with
the Fishes, took my grandmother's "side" and decided to retire.

My father, thinking me about to be victimized by my
grandfather's devotion to his mother - my grandmother had essayed
to have me at her beck and call - offered to allow me to attend the
Sergeant Dramatic Academy in New York; and I was on the verge of
doing so - as I had stopped college in disgust at the limitations
of the Victorian view of literature - when my father invited Dr
Fredrick Creighton Wellman and his second wife to dinner.

It was in a period when my father's always fluctuating finances
were at a temporary ebb, and we had temporarily dispensed with the
cook; not difficult as my father was seldom at home then, and was
depressed by my mother's presence when he was. I, however, agreed
to cook the dinner for Dr Wellman; whom my father justly said
was the one and only man of real intellectual stature whom he had
encountered since he became an adult and went into business.

The evening has been written of in <u>Life Is Too Short</u>;[2] the

---

2 *Life Is Too Short*, Dr Wellman's autobiography, became the focus of her angry attention some
   30 years later. More on the reasons for this in Chapter 31.

early portions of that fine book having been, apparently, less cut, over-edited, and re-written by someone external to it, than the middle portions.

I was enchanted to discover an adult human being to whom, though I was of the opposite sex, I could really talk about the literature, philosophy, painting and music that were beginning to be my life. His second wife proved a vicious enemy, but I also enjoyed her piano-playing, at that time. She had been a professional and was a pupil of Leschetitzky, her name was Edna Willis. Dr Wellman had met her abroad, after his divorce from his first wife, Lydia Isley, to whom he was married fourteen years, and who had gone to West Africa with him as a missionary, when he had one there as mission doctor to an American mission at Benguella.

Dr Wellman and his first wife and fallen into bitter disagreement as science began, more and more, to affect his religious views. After their divorce, she had refused to permit him to see their four children, and she honestly feared the influence of science on the views of her children.

The second wife was a sophisticated woman; and that Dr Wellman made the mistake he did in respect to their congeniality, is very explicable when one realizes how many are the marriages based on the human predilection for antidotes for unhappiness in an antithesis. She was not shocked by scepticism in religious matters, but she had been disappointed in her worldly ambition for wealth when, after marrying a scientist of international reputation in several fields, she discovered he was almost poor, and that his monetary resources did not extend beyond a good salary and what he received for medical monographs and articles on medical and botanical topics.

Perhaps Elsie Dunn and Fredrick Creighton Wellman fell in love on sight, for I can still remember the comforted and elated feeling with which I went to bed that night, after our guests had partaken of the Sally Lunn mentioned in Life Is Too Short and gone home. I thought continually of Dr Wellman from that time on until we eloped. My father and mother were equally taken with him. Edna Willis Wellman, as she then was, became, eventually, so ruthless an enemy that I could not think of her existence for years without the most bitter and righteous resentment. But it was the first time but one I had ever had the pleasure of listening to a technically fine pianist who played some of the things I myself asked for, and that, too, I enjoyed, with no feeling of rivalry as imminent.

Dr Wellman - or Cyril Kay Scott as he became and is to me - is innately one of the most innocent-minded of men, I think. His character is that I have referred to, one in which emotions felt simply are deep, not easily changing, and intellect, nonetheless, is of the fine type that engenders no inner conflicts.

Before I ever saw him or talked to him alone, along before in
fact, he and his second wife had discussed separation and even
eventual divorce. She had told him she did not love him; but,
as such discussions do in people without his detachment, she had
accused him, in the usual way, of "wrecking" her life, and had
spitefully declared that she would divorce him, not then, but when
it should become "convenient" to her. She had reminded him of his
first divorce, and - knowing the orthodoxy then still prevalent in
New Orleans and among the medical fraternity - she had spitefully
assured him that she had the "whip hand", and would settle the
matter of divorce on her "own terms", at her leisure.

It was not a situation any man with self-respect could have
been expected to endure. I think Dr Wellman would have left her,
and, perhaps, returned to Africa or some other remote place,
even had he not met me. But he was at once interested in me as
a "phenomenon" in that era in the South, a young woman not quite
twenty-one, usually considered pretty, and entirely serious in
outlook.

I was, having left off both college and art school, at loose
ends; and on that first evening had admitted that my education
was scientifically non-existent, as I had recoiled from every
science course offered because these impinged on time given to
imaginative literature, painting and music. Dr Wellman saw my
father sometimes, and my expressed wish to have at least a little
more knowledge of science was mentioned. My father, too, had, by
that time, decided I was too indifferent to science and it would
do me no harm to learn more. The course at the Dramatic Academy
was still pending when Dr Wellman wrote to me the first letter
I ever had from him, and asked me whether I would like to take
a course in laboratory technique in the laboratory where he and
his assistants were engaged in some experiments. I have already
forgotten what they were trying to prove, and remember vividly
only my first look at some beautifully-coloured mosquitoes
through a microscope.

I was almost mawkishly "kind to animals", and I was repelled
by experiments proceeding nearby - some Dr Wellman's own - on
monkeys and small mammals. But this time, once enrolled as Dr
Wellman's student, I had no doubt I had fallen in love.

I was very deeply and grossly insulted on his behalf as well
as my own by the sort of rumour that spread about New Orleans
and Memphis once we had eloped, and which concerned our relations
before our elopement. We took occasional walks together after
"school hours", but we had never so much as kissed until an
afternoon when Dr Wellman asked me to stroll with him in Audubon
Park, and when we were far enough from St Charles Avenue to
be unlikely to encounter other people, told me of his first
marriage, and his second, and said he could not go on as he was
but must get back into some simpler environment where he could

re-assemble a life in emotional wreckage on the basis of the
detachment he felt being shattered by continual friction with
a woman whose animus, apparently, was such as would stop at
nothing.

It was then that he abruptly said at the end of the confession
of unhappiness, that I would probably think him fantastic, or, if
I did not, other people would, but that ever since he had first
met me he had thought of what the primitive surroundings of his
missionary days might be like with a companion such as I was. I
was startled. I had already told him that I was not happy at home,
that my parents loved me, but not each other, although my mother
was impeccably loyal to my father in every outward sense. I thought
later she loved him, but her love was not requited. I had also told
Dr Wellman that my grandmother, as was true, was daily becoming
more eccentric, that my grandfather had given up his career to her,
and that, as a man whose life-long preoccupation had been business,
he was miserable in being idle; and that notwithstanding an
otherwise selfless view of me, his only grandchild, he distressed
himself all the time because I did not love my grandmother as he
did - something that had been beyond my father, too.

Dr Wellman then asked me whether I would like to cut loose
as he would doubtless eventually do from the miseries that beset
us both among people, also, miserable, whose miseries we could
not mend. He said he had thought it all out before mentioning
it, and that we might go to Brazil, where the Portuguese he knew
well, was spoken, and where, among strangers, we could make our
own lives. He said frankly he had little money, and he knew I had
none, but if I agreed I was not to worry for he would take the
responsibility for everything involved. We discussed the Amazon -
for I agreed at once - and other places in Brazil.

Dr Wellman and I exchanged our first kiss at the end of
this conversation at Audubon Park. It was to me, as I think it
was to him, like the sealing of a pact we had made to fight
together for some purer joy in life. We agreed that we could
not meet often, again, until we were ready to elope; as to be
seen together might attract attention to our interest in each
other. It was also decided between us, although this was at his
suggestion, that the most feasible time for leaving New Orleans
would be at Christmas, when college was closed and everyone
was on vacation. He, later, wrote his second wife a letter she
was at liberty to show anyone in which he said whatever was
pertinent to "bear hunting" somewhere in the South. He also
wrote to her as we were leaving telling her he had decided to
cut the Gordian knot, and saying - as was the truth - that he
was taking nothing with him but a suitcase containing a few
clothes, and that 1841 - the money in the bank still untouched
and anything that might accrue as due him was hers, but that
she was not to say anything about what he was doing until he

was far from New Orleans, because once the newspapers got hold
of the facts, there would be scandal; unjust to my parents and
grandparents I add - Dr Wellman did <u>not</u> mention either me or
them.

I was most distressed about my mother, and I tried to confide
in her, thinking to make her see the future as a <u>temporary</u>
separation. But I got no further than saying Dr Wellman and
myself were in love, and I would gladly marry him whenever
this became feasible, and he felt the same; for at that point
my mother rushed for the revolver my father had given me when
wishing me to learn to shoot, and threaten to kill herself.

This experience resulted in a temporary congealing of emotion
toward her. I had thought some revision of our plan might be made
in adaptation to her wishes, as she continually lamented the fact
that I was considered brilliant and had no opportunity to meet any
men fit to "tie my shoestring". I felt, after that, that I must
leave home no matter what, to bring my mother to her normal senses.

Dr Wellman and myself left New Orleans on December 26th, 1913.

Chapter 2

Brazil

December 1913 - August 1919

No letters relating to their time in Brazil have been found. Evelyn did, however, provide a lengthy, if slightly fictionalised, account of those years in her autobiographical novel, Escapade. This work, published in 1923 and still in print, was a literary sensation, attracting opprobrium and praise in equal measure. About 20 years later, Cyril wrote extensively of his time in Brazil in his autobiography, Life Is Too Short.

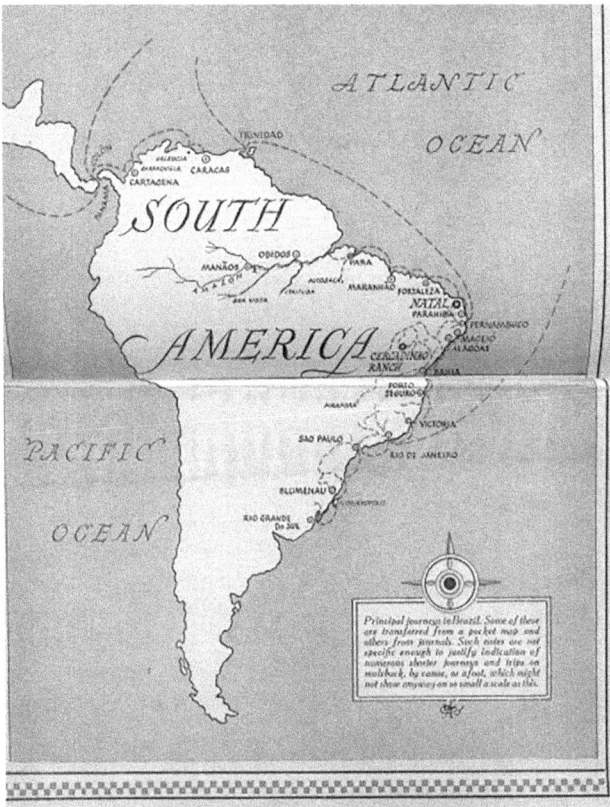

End paper of *Life Is Too Short*

Dr Wellman and myself left New Orleans on December 26th, 1913. But we did not leave together. I told my parents I would like to spend the Christmas holidays at Pass Christian, where I had spent two summers with the maiden ladies, the Misses Sutter. Heart-strings were torn on my side, too, when I said goodbye to my mother. My father took me to the train and bought my ticket to Pass Christian. Dr Wellman - knowing he would be struck from the medical register, as he was, though, later, he was professionally forgiven in several quarters - had taken an earlier train to Gulfport. He boarded my train there, and we both alighted at Pass Christian, and took a streetcar to Biloxi. From Biloxi we went to Mobile, and at Mobile we spent the night, I as literally virginal as ever, and having bought my own ticket, though I had just the money needed for a vacation.

At Mobile we bought tickets for New York, via Washington, DC. All went well as to our arrangements, but one of the Tulane professors, we discovered, at Washington, had been on the train. We changed at Washington, and as we alighted on the platform, we encountered him and I was introduced as Miss Foster, a friend.

We went to New York and were in New York several days; at first at a hotel I think I have since identified as the Prince George, but before we sailed, as we had to begin to count our money, at a rooming-house somewhere in the forties.[3] I wrote to my parents from New York City, telling them what we were doing but saying I could not give our destination as yet, though I would write again soon. We called on my childhood friend, Ruth Whitfield, of Clarksville, Tenn and New Orleans; who was then at a Catholic boarding-house for office-workers on 14th St. She was called to the telephone as we sat in the parlour, and when she returned to us, said she had talked to my father, but had not said we were there and we had just asked her to say nothing until we were aboard our steamer.

I discovered, later, that the second Mrs Wellman had found out that I, too, was not to be located, when a young doctor who was working on mosquitoes under Dr Wellman and who was one of her friends and sometimes took her out, had phoned me at my home to ask whether he could take me to a Christmas dance; my mother had said I was at the Sutters' in Pass Christian; he had phoned Pass Christian and put the Sutters in a flutter. They had phoned my parents. By that time, Edna Willis, as she was at first, had read Dr Wellman's letter, and had decided for herself - as far as we know - that we had eloped. She first insulted my distracted mother by phone, by insulting me; then called in the newspapers.[4] Of the newspaper scandal we knew nothing until we reached Brazil. My grandfather, temperate by nature, and with unusual poise of

---

3   This is a reference to streets in New York City with street names between 40th and 49th
    Street.
4   This article from the New Orleans *Picayune* is reproduced here. Despite considerable
    searching, it has not been possible to find any other press coverage of their elopement.

manner, went to the editor of one of them to try by every means
to put a stop to sensation that was entirely libel except in
respect to the elopement itself.

From New Orleans *Picayune*, January 13, 1914

DR WELLMAN QUITS TULANE MEDICAL
Resigns as Tropical Medicine School Head, Giving Ill Health As Reason
IS STRANGELY ABSENT
Unusual Manner of Withdrawal Starts Rumours, But Regret General

Sickness is given as the cause of Dr Creighton Wellman's resignation, as head of
the School of Hygiene and Tropical Medicine, of the Medical College of Tulane
University, but added to Dr Wellman's sudden resignation is the fact that he is
rather strangely absent from the city, and last night the rumours which had been
whispered in certain circles became loud of voice, and it was said that the eminent
scientist, in leaving, had neglected to settle certain debts owed to gentlemen of this
profession and others.

THE OFFICIAL NOTICE
The official notice of the doctor's departure, given by Tulane University, last night,
read as follows:

"Owing to protracted illness, Dr Creighton Wellman has found it impossible
to continue longer the arduous duties of his position in Tulane University. He has,
accordingly, tendered his resignation, which has been accepted with much regret.

"Dr Wellman has contributed services of great value to the university, through
his aid and counsel in the organization of the school of hygiene and tropical
medicine, in the establishment of an infirmary for sick students and in many other
activities.

"His department will, for the present, be conducted by Dean Dyer of the School
of Medicine. Dr Dyer stated that there would positively be no interruption in the
school and that the lectures and laboratory work would be continued as usual."

RUMORS OF FRICTION
One of the rumours heard was to the effect that Dr Howard King, prominent
because of his work and research in tropical diseases, had resigned from Tulane
because of friction with Dr Wellman, friction which had brought about open
hostility from the medical teaching staff. Dr King was seen after much difficulty
at his residence in St Andrew Street, by a Picayune representative last night and
interrogated as to his connection with Dr Wellman. Dr King very emphatically
refused to throw light upon the affair, and when asked if Dr Wellman had borrowed
any money of him, said, with some show of heat, "That's nobody's business." The
doctor's refusal to say anything further was peremptorily, even surlily, put.

Another rumour that some had heard last night was that Dr Wellman had contracted several debts with personal friends in the profession Christmas Eve day. He told a few acquaintances that he was going for a little rest, and even mentioned that he would visit Covington to hunt bears. As bears are never seen in Covington or its vicinity outside of a circus tent, the statement was taken as being facetiously put. Dr Wellman, it is said, has been in failing health for some time past, and was granted a leave of absence by Tulane shortly before Christmas. He stated at the time he would be in need of a rest, and would be back in a few weeks, ready for the late winter's work preceding preparations for the student examinations in the spring. It was not known that Dr Wellman was in the East until the letter containing his resignation was received.

Dr Wellman and his wife reside at Mrs Gomilla's fashionable apartment house, Prytania and Philip Street, and a call by a newspaper man at the house late last night established the fact that while Dr Wellman was absent from the city, his wife was still here. The lady who answered the summons at the door said, however, that Mrs Wellman was not at home.

WIFE STILL HERE

Dr Wellman is from Kansas City and a graduate of the University of Kansas Medical School. He had two years' valuable experience in Portuguese East Africa, where he studied beri-beri and the sleeping sickness, and returning to the states became well known as an entomologist. He was in charge of the school of tropical medicine at the University of California, and came to Tulane from that university in 1910. He was a brilliant speaker, and with Mrs Wellman, who is an accomplished musician, was popular in society. He was at work on a textbook, took the lead in teaching hygiene in the Normal School, and was very active in every department of medical education.

```
Dr Wellman and I had not yet decided what name to take, though we
had discussed the inadvisability of travelling under the names
ours hitherto, and I had definitely decided to drop Elsie and
become Evelyn, not merely for practical reasons, but because I had
a strong dislike of my baptismal name. At the steam-ship office
we asked first for tickets to Rio, direct, but there was no boat
sailing for sometime; and we were offered, as a bargain, tickets
to Southampton, a stay of seven or eight weeks in England, and the
tickets from Southampton to Rio as one fare; and as Dr Wellman was
fond of England, was a graduate of London University's College of
Tropical Diseases and Preventitive Medicine - he had gone there
when fully trained medically in the USA he was eager to show me
London, and there we went first, en route to Brazil. This was
January 1914.
    No Passports were required in January 1914 either for
England or Brazil. We sailed for Southampton from Hoboken on
the President Grant, of the Hamburg American Line. We had called
```

ourselves, for a few days, in New York, Mr and Mrs Watt; but we
did not like this impromptu name, and when the steamer-tickets
were being signed for in New York, Dr Wellman was drawn aside
by me with the plea not to be Mr and Mrs Watt any longer. I
suggested Scott as better. Cyril came as a matter of association,
though we did not consciously remember Cyril Scott the composer
until it was too late to retract. The Kay was inserted then by
Cyril Kay Scott himself, for ever after our afternoon of decision
in Audubon Park, I had called him Kay, after the Kay of Hans
Anderson's <u>Snow Queen</u>.

The <u>President Grant</u> was more than half empty; such passengers
as there were beside ourselves, mostly German. It impressed me
deeply with the sting of bitter winds, salty rails, etc; for
it was my first crossing. But the deck-space was ample, though
we were second-class. Plymouth, or rather the Cornish coast,
offered me my first view of surf, as there is no surf on the Gulf
Coast. My first glimpse of London was of Trafalgar Square in
rain, as Cyril Kay Scott and Evelyn Dunn Scott emerged from the
tube in coming from the station, where we left our baggage for
collection. We found a bed-sitting-room in Torrington Square, not
far from the boarding-house in which Cyril, before his change of
name, had resided for a time with his first wife and their son
near the College of Tropical and Preventitive Medicine and the
British Museum.

We began to sign our names as above in New York City and
have continued to do so ever since. My twenty-first birthday
was celebrated in mid-ocean; and on ship-board we discussed
alternately possible marriage should the second-wife divorce her
husband, or, if she refused to for some interminable time in
spite, whether or not we could defend our relationship with a
Common Law Marriage in Brazil. We were resolved on a life-long
association as we were, whether we were approved of or not, and
were then of half a mind - indeed it was taken for granted at
first-that we would never return from Brazil to those who had no
sense of real values.

In London, we went to Richmond Park and Cyril Kay Scott carved
the initials CKS and EDS intertwined within a heart on a tree
that may yet be standing. We went to Kew Gardens and on some
pretext asked for the catalogue of their botanical specimens,
and I read with much pride the listing of several <u>Wellmanii</u>. I
had read in New Orleans as much as I could of some two hundred
medical and botanical monographs by Fredrick Creighton Wellman.

In London, we went to Covent Garden to hear <u>Tristan and Isolde</u>
and <u>Siegfried</u>. We saw Granville Barker's production of <u>The Wild
Duck</u> and of <u>The Death of Tintaigille</u> - spelling seems correct! We
ate at very cheap places, and I never had enough, nor did Cyril
Kay Scott probably, though he never said so, in various languages.

We sailed from Southampton for Rio, on the Blucher, of the Hamburg American Line, sometime in March. We had as yet no presage of the approaching war that was to intern this ship but the Germans aboard, unlike the amiable Germans of the President Grant, were an aggressive and unpleasant lot. There were heavy storms, one in the Bay of Biscay, went over the bridge in great waves. I saw Lisbon on a day at shore, even then more the old Lisbon Dr Fredrick Creighton Wellman had known when working for the Portuguese Crown and presented with a decoration - the Order of Jesus, I think it was called, by Queen Amalie, than the Lisbon seen later by my son and his, myself and my present husband William John Metcalfe, when we were travelling together years afterward.

Cyril Kay Scott and myself arrived in Rio with no arrangements for our livelihood beyond one with Janson, the naturalist, behind the British Museum - or in front of it - who had agreed to handle insect specimens for us if we were able to obtain those in demand. Our arrival in Rio, in hot weather, in the season of the temperate zone's spring, is alluded to, and described in part in my Escapade.

Cyril Kay Scott went at once to the American Embassy Consulate and we registered there as Cyril Kay Scott and Evelyn D Scott. We had been told of names changed by documented usage in the USA, and of Common Law Marriages established by consistent agreement between the man and woman to their status as that of man and wife in Common Law. But we were not well-informed as yet and merely did what seemed to us logical in view of our resolve to remain united, and to exact from others respect for our status.[5]

We were in Brazil from the spring of 1914, to August 1919. I think our landing was in April, but it may have been May 1st. We of course signed everything that required signing by the names which were legally becoming ours. Cyril Kay Scott, for instance, was bonded by the Singer Sewing Machine Company, when he went to work for them as an unknown new employee, first a bookkeeper, then travelling auditor. He was with them over two years. In Escapade I tried to telescope events to preserve a story form. Time intervals in it are possibly less exact than here, though the facts in it were actually the facts, and when the war broke we began to be troubled indeed by the fact that we were there without Passports and that the time-period we had gathered to be essential in American Law both for changes of name and Common Law Marriages was possibly far from sufficient yet.

I wrote to my parents from London three or four times, but it was not until my mother was invited by myself and Cyril Kay

---

5   Despite research into common-law marriages, it has not been possible to find any reference to their legal status at that time. Nevertheless, it was widely believed that these relationships had legal validity, and Evelyn clearly believed it to be so.

Scott to visit us in Natal and see Creighton - Seely as yet but
Creighton added when we returned to the USA in 1919 - that we had
the full account of what my parents and grandparents had been put
through in persecution and horror; reporters besieging them, and
when they would not be interviewed, inventing lies defamatory to
our characters

*Evelyn was already pregnant when they arrived in Brazil. The couple had very little money
and they lived first in a poor district of Natal, to the north of Rio. Evelyn sketched their
home in the "baby book" she kept of their child's first year: vivid evidence of their straitened
circumstances.*

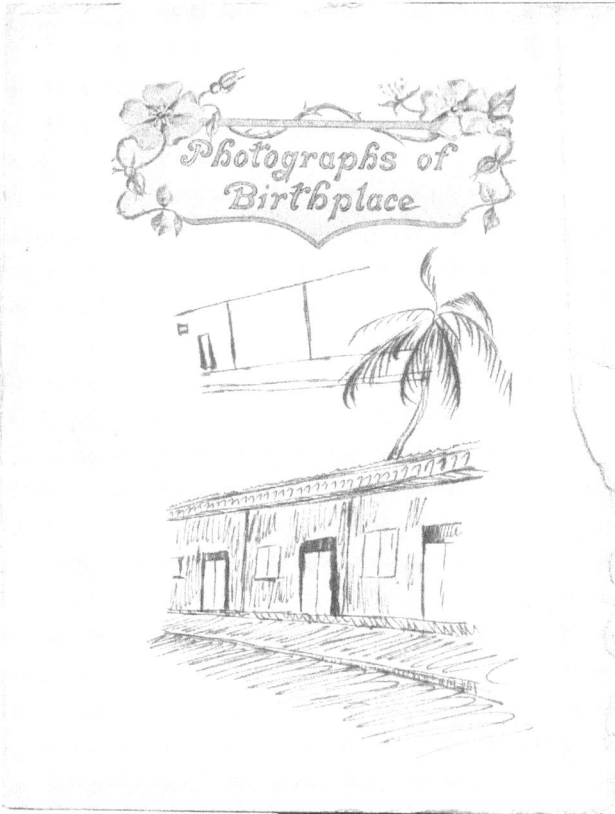

Sketch by Evelyn of birthplace of baby Creighton: *Scott family*

My mother landed in Brazil at Recife, Cyril Kay Scott had gone
there from Natal to meet her, and it was then, when she, too,
registered herself - Mrs Seely Dunn of New Orleans - that the
birth of our son was registered.

Before proceeding North from Rio for the Singer Company, we
had rented a room for a few weeks at the home, in Cascadura,
of two American Vice-Consuls, and as they were decent agreeable
young men, it was the suppressed private wish of us both to be

frank - but of course at that stage we did not dare trust to
comprehension, though we may have had some later.

*The birth of their child was difficult and left Evelyn with gynaecological problems which
troubled her for the rest of her life. The baby boy, however, was healthy. He was named
Creighton (Cyril's original middle name) Seely (after Evelyn's father) Scott. The baby was
soon known as "Jigg": as a baby he played in the garden of their home with the family's
maid-of-all-work and nursemaid, Stephania, and became infested with a locally common
insect: chigger. From this he acquired the nickname "Chiggeroo", often shorted to "Jigg",
and he was known as Jigg for the rest of his life.*

When I did not recover from the aftermath of my son's birth, I went
with my first husband, to the Presbyterian Mission Hospital in
the interior of Pernambuco for a needed repair operation, and was
operated on by the Mission Head, Dr Butler, who had come there from
South Carolina, and was a student of the Mayos. We were, again, of
course, Mr and Mrs Cyril Kay Scott; and our names so registered and
sometimes signed by both must have been scattered over all the North
of Brazil between Rio and Natal. As for Cyril Kay Scott himself, he
was constantly engaged in work that required his signature. When,
even after being operated on, my health remained bad, and he decided
to resign from Singer employment and invest in a ranch he had heard
of in the interior of Bahia, about a hundred miles from Minas
Geraes, he, so that he could be with me and Creighton all the time,
he had the thousand acres of Government land we eventually acquired
to the extent of having it surveyed and paying something down,
registered as his in the name of Cyril Kay Scott.

When the ranch life proved too precarious a livelihood for
a man with a semi-invalid wife, a child and a mother-in-law to
support - for my mother never went back, or rather did not until
we did, return to the USA - Cyril Kay Scott obtained employment
with the E J Lavino Company, owners of manganese and copper mines
in Brazil, who had opened an office at Villa Nova da Rainha; a
town about thirty-five miles from the ranch; and there, again,
he was Cyril Kay Scott, and re-affirmed his change of name with
every business signature.

He was first employed as an office assistant by Mr William
Staver, who directed the mining of Lavino in that part of
Brazil. Mr Staver, already dissatisfied, but liking Mr Scott and
finding him unusually competent - though he was just beginning
to learn the ins and outs of mining - resigned after less than
a year and recommended Cyril Kay Scott as his successor. Cyril
Kay Scott was, in due course, promoted to an office in Sao
Salvador, Bahia's chief and coastal city, and had charge of all
the manganese mined by E J Lavino, which, either just before,
or just after this promotion, merged with W R Grace and became

the International Ore Corporation. As their representative, his
signature of Cyril Kay Scott must have become well-known, not
only in Bahia and Rio, but in the USA, as manganese mining was an
asset in winning the 1914-18 war.

*From Rio the family went to Cercadinho, about six miles from the town of Lamarao, in the
heart of Bahia province to the south-west of Rio. The area was isolated, rural, and poor
and there Cyril tried to establish a ranch which would both provide an income and food for
the family. Evelyn and Cyril describe it in their respective books, and Jigg later referred to
it as "a healed volcanic pustule, the ridge walling it around notched where a river drained
weepings from the surrounding bluffs plushy with hanging forest". The enterprise was not
a success, and the family endured increasing poverty as their crops failed and the livestock
died from disease.*

From the ranch, Cercadinho - a very beautiful place - I had written
to Miss Jane Addams[6] and asked her to help us to ascertain whether
or not Cyril Kay Scott's second wife had divorced him. I had
written to other people the same question, and could get no reply.
My father, in my mother's absence, had divorced her on grounds of
desertion, and she communicated with no one in New Orleans, except
her old friend Mrs Richard Hyams and her daughter. The Hyams did
not know what had been done by the second Mrs Wellman; but Miss
Addams was good enough to have a Hull House lawyer inquire into the
situation; and had written us, or me, that the second Mrs Wellman
had threatened to invoke the Mann Act,[7] to have her former husband
extradited, etc and though it was also said - to quote the lawyer -
that the second Mrs Wellman was, since, herself contemplating a re-
marriage and had sued for divorce, it was, it seemed, in some other
state than Louisiana, and while the facts were uncorroborated, we
were advised to take nothing for granted.
  In 1919, the doctor of the Presbyterian Mission of Sao
Salvador, having agreed with Cyril Kay Scott himself that Evelyn
Dunn Scott was unlikely ever to recover her health in a tropical
climate in a place where medical and surgical facilities were
still very poor, signed a certificate to the effect that she must
go back to the USA for medical reasons. This certificate was
presented by Cyril Kay Scott at the American Embassy Consulate
in Rio, where he was now known as the chief representative of
the International Ore Corporation, and an emergency Passport was
issued to the three original Scotts, Cyril Kay, Evelyn Dunn, and
Seely Scott. We returned to New York in August on a Lamport and
Holt boat, I think it was the Van Dyke - it was not the Vestris.

---

6 Jane Addams founded the first social settlement, Hull House, in Chicago. As both women
   were in public life, it is likely that she and Mrs Wellman shared contacts.
7 The Mann Act of 1910 made it a federal crime to transport a woman over a state line for
   "immoral purposes".

Chapter 3

New York City and Buzzards Bay
August 1919 - September 1921

The Scott family left Brazil in August 1919 and returned to the USA and to New York City. Their passport photo shows Jigg not quite 5, Evelyn aged 26 and Cyril aged 46.

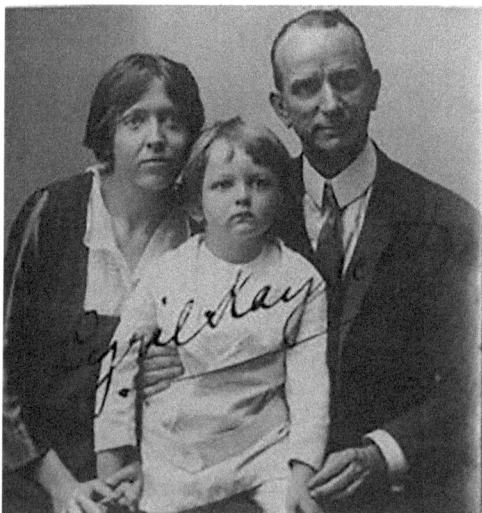

Passport photo of the Scott family in 1919: *Harry Ransom Center*

Very few letters remain from these early years in New York, although a number of empty envelopes were found amongst the various collections: these provide an incomplete record of where the family lived during this period - sometimes together, sometimes with one or other of a series of Evelyn's and Cyril's lovers.

During the years in New York Evelyn and Cyril met Lola Ridge[8] who, with her husband Davy Lawson, became loyal and supportive friends. Lola was a passionate avant-garde feminist and an influential modernist poet. Evelyn's relationship with Lola was hugely important to both of them, and each supported the other in a lengthy correspondence which lasted until Lola's death in 1941.

---

8   Lola's work and correspondence are considered by Terese Svoboda in her book *Anything That Burns You* (Tucson, Schaffner Press, 2015).

To Lola Ridge

[Barrow Street, New York]
[Summer 1920]

Dearest Lola:

Did I write you about our (Cyrils and my) resolution to live apart this winter? It does not grow out of misunderstanding but the contrary, and I think as always that he is the biggest and best and truest person that - well male person anyway - have ever known. I love him so and I will hate to hear the nasty things that will undoubtedly be said by the crass minded individuals who observe the outward change in our way of life. He has a room above Dudleys[9] and I am trying - as yet without success - to discover an unfurnished room for me. I want to get this last months rent off my hands and it is difficult. We have been flat as you may imagine and so many personal readjustments to make that it has depleted our earning capacity.

Do you remember the dark spots on my two front teeth? I have had them sawed off and two spotless false ones - what fate for a poetess put in their place. As a result - it was done without cocaine - my nerves have gone bad and every tooth in my head (I have sixteen cavities, by the way) has ached like fun all week. In spite of that I am writing a novel. I do not know what the immediate expression of toothache will supply to art-but we will see.

I can not think of anything unpardonable I have done lately except that I have bought me a cloth suit for fifteen dollars which makes me look like a poor but honest working girl. My black silk suit with holes worn through it could be described with the first adjective but not the second.

It is now after twelve and I am soaked in the sticky atmosphere of Barrow Street on a hot night. The curtains are dank. The air is thick so that it squeezes my thoughts out in niggardly fashion - no room to flow.

I will go and jump in the new bath tub for my landlady - the one who has bought the house - has built a tantalizing bathroom in the place where I pay to have a dressing room and for a week I can look at it and develop a strong and resigned nature as I contemplate the bathless winter before me.

Well, dearest, write to me and WRITE. We love you. Evelyn

PS Jigeroo is in Greenwich Connecticut where by becoming eternally grateful to a stout lady with a desire to enlarge her personality to the dimensions of her corset he is being boarded at next to nothing on a farm[10] intended to be at the disposal of orphans.

[Typed, typed signature. SSC]

---

9   Dudley Grant, a friend of Evelyn's from early years. He later married another of Evelyn's close friends, Gladys Edgerton.

10   Jigg described this "baby farm" in his unpublished memoir *Confessions of an American Boy*, written in 1960. He wrote: "The unpredictable supperlessness at the farm, the ostracism every Saturday, the fear of being locked up for saying something Portuguese by mistake, and the lunges Mr. Harper made at my pants buttons when he still thought I was a girl because of my bobbed hair, all combined to bring on melancholia... As soon as I came back to Brooklyn... I discovered how keenly I missed the formerly detestable cycle of bacchanalian exhilaration, clammy sentiment and shrill re-awakening from opiates and alcohol... At about the time I would have been dosed if I had still been on the farm, I found myself on fire with thirst for the contents of brown bottles - any brown bottles - then gruesomely depressed, and at last dreamily tranquil for a minute or two as I counterfeited in imagination how consoling it had been to give up fighting against the ghastly taste, resign myself to the necessary interval of nausea, and yield up my will to that of the bottle."

In 1920 Cyril found employment with the Guaranty Trust Company, a large financial institution based in New York City, and through this employment became acquainted with members of the Garland-Hale family, well-established and prosperous members of New York society. While in Brazil, Cyril had acquired a number of practical skills which led to hims being offered a position as general handyman for the Garland-Hales at their property in Buzzards Bay, Massachusetts.

There is very little information about Otto Theis who appears to have been an American of German origin, and was also at one point Cyril's literary agent. Otto later moved to London to become editor of The Outlook, *a popular weekly news sheet. Over the years, Evelyn wrote frequently and at great length to Otto and, later, to his wife Louise Morgan: they both appear to have offered her considerable practical (and financial) support.*

To Otto Theis

[Alpine, New Jersey]
April 21, 1921

Otto, dear:

Cyril really is so much sicker than he shows before anybody. His dislike for the Guaranty is an obsession - he just keeps counting the hours literally before he will have to go back so I dont think he is resting at all. This damn Scott family!

All last night I lay awake planning what I should do if Cyril has a complete breakdown which all the time seems imminent. Otto, you are the only person I talk like this too. Please forgive me.

I wonder if on Monday you will let me have ten dollars extra. I know how it will be - I will be sorry when there is no more etc. I cant help it. Cyril will have to buy a commutation ticket, I have to pay in advance on light and telephone, and of course moving the furniture from Jones Street to 14th Street to be stored. Otto, Im so truly sorry Im not doing better by my loan but I cant help it. We just couldnt let this place get away. Please, please, 'scuse, and come out soon.

Evelyn

[Typed, typed signature. UTK]

To Lola Ridge and Davy Lawson

[Buzzards Bay, Massachusetts]
[April 1921]

Dear Lola and Davy:

We arrived here per schedule on Friday night in the rain (rain not per schedule) and it has been raining almost ever since. The surroundings are beautiful really-poetical, desolate, only we have all been so sick with colds and throats that the poetry is waiting for appreciation. The Garland-Hales have been very lovely to us and after I get used to the unlimited bestowal of favors I shall be really glad. Just now I feel that it is very much more blessed to give than to receive. However as soon as we take root we can begin to imaging that this lovely cottage is really ours and that the charming little water view we have from it is a gift of the gods and demands no gratitude.

We spent the first three days at Mrs Garlands large and very beautiful country house surrounded by automobiles and Arcadian millionaire children who go barefoot and wash their own dishes. Mrs Garland has two picturesque silent sons and one young viking daughter - altogether the most characterful examples of the idle rich I ever saw. I really like them. Though of course things will be nicest when we settle down into our own little rut and write. I think we shall lots.

We love you both terrifically and shall want to know how you are and what you are doing every minute hence. When my tonsils stop demanding my attention I shall write you a letter of more length and I hope more interest. This is only to tell you we are thinking of you as nearly continuously as life allows and that we would like to experience the phenomena, as yet unheard of, of a real letter from Davy and are avid for the consumption of any chirographical enormities Lola is willing to perpetrate. I still insist on hugging Davy even at this distance and we mutually kiss Lola a hundred and eighty times.   Jiggeroo too sends love,

Evelyn

[Typed, signed. SSC]

To Otto Theis

Buzzards Bay, Massachusetts
May 3, 1921

Otto, dear:

Your letter received the day we arrived. Contents appreciated and needed. We have spent three days in over opulence at large country house where millionaires go barefoot and wash the dishes for the good of their souls or the soul of the butler I know not which but are nice and very silent boys and girls very much like Indian princes and princesses. We have large luxurious room and opulent bath in wonderful comfort and a good deal of taste but not enjoyed because of inevitable feeling of poor relation one has in these circumstances. It is as cold as Labrador - no spring whatever yet and has rained every day, but we are at last in own cottage and feel it more possible to take roots.

Mrs Garland and SH[11] have really worked terrifically getting this place fixed up in three days and if I did not appreciate it too much I could enjoy it, but even gratitude will pass and they are really exceedingly nice and kind not to mention lavish. From our veranda we have a charming landscape vignettes of water and pines only slightly obstructed by a neighbors barn. There is lots of milk and automobiles and Sunday we went to Sagamore and could see the surf and I believe Provincetown only twelve or fifteen miles off. I do not like to think of being so close to Boston which is only two

---

11   Swinburne Hale. He was Paula's maternal uncle although that relationship did not feature until after she and Jigg married some 20 years later.

hours because there is something about sandy soil and large cold houses which was too much like Boston must be. Anyhow -

When the weather gets warm this will be a very wonderful place. Mrs Garlands estate is enormous and each member of the family has his or her own little cottage tucked somewhere in the woods. There are several tiny lakes and from all most all the verandas one has some sort of glimpse of black pine trunks against blue water.

Of course Ive been blue (I would be) and of course have worried Cyril (I always do) and waked up at three am to wonder if I was quite mad. Yet I do think coming here was the only sensible thing left and after all readjustments are made may be wonderful. I shall not one moment stop hoping and wishing and willing that you may spend your vacation with us. By that time the Garlands will be in Bermuda and we shall be quite alone and I do believe you would be rested by lovely calm surroundings like these. Also both of us may be better company by then.

Love from all of us,

Evelyn

[Typed, signed. SSC]

Chapter 4

Bermuda

Summer 1921 - April 1923

Not many letters from this period remain; Evelyn's lengthy letter of April 1956 to her son continues with a narrative of the years in Bermuda, and of her relationship with Mary Tudor Garland, Swinburne Hale and the various members of that family. Although she does not mention this in her narrative, Evelyn was busy writing and published numerous critical essays and a large number of poems in the so-called "little magazines" as well as her first three novels: The Narrow House *(1921),* Narcissus *(1922), and* Escapade *(1923).*

It is important to remember that the following account was written in 1956, in a period of increasing agitation and developing paranoia.

In 1921, the Hale-Garland couple went to Bermuda, and the three Scotts were soon asked to proceed there with travelling expenses paid. And though Cyril Kay Scotts duties were lighter in Bermuda than at Buzzards Bay, and his remuneration for these less, the first year in Bermuda could well have been termed a genuine success, as he received enough to rent a small cottage called Greysbank, and to keep his family fed, and in his free hours was not able to write and paint to the extent we had hoped for at Cercadinho, where his acute genre study in the novel, <u>Blind Mice</u>, was written on boards spread on improvised saw-horses, and mostly at night, after farm work, by the dim smoky flare of attacks.

In the summer of 1922, the three Scotts returned to New York City, briefly, but went back to Bermuda; and meanwhile, Mr Hale - uncle of my daughter-in-law, Paula Pearson Scott - had evolved a plan for a cottage to be built on the property he owned called Ely's Lodge, at his expense, to become, with fifteen acres of the ground on which it stood, his gift to Cyril Kay Scott and Evelyn Scott, a capital of fifty thousand dollars, which they would be unable to diminish in their lifetime, but would be the inheritance of their son Creighton Seely Scott - affectionately called Jigg by them, also-on their death, and which, while they lived, would yield them approximately a hundred dollars a month each, and so permit them to sustain independence as creative against all commercial

This combined generosity was to have made come true the dream of every author, writer and composer of integrity. It was, in fact, put into effect to the extent of the building of the cottage of Bermuda's native stone according to an architectural drawing by Cyril Kay Scott, who had practical architectural advice on some details; and of a letter sent to Cyril Kay Scott and Evelyn Scott by Marie Tudor Garland-Hales lawyers, saying that their client, Mrs Hale, was making over to us in permanence fifty thousand dollars on which they were to draw, during their lifetimes, the income its investment then netted of two hundred a month.

We were overcome with gratitude. The cottage, named by Marie Tudor Garland Hale, The Scottage, was completed, and we moved in and found it charming, Ely's land-locked harbour just beyond our windows, a private pool to bathe from, and our good friends as our nearest neighbours, owning the two estates on both sides of the highroad. Creighton Seely Scott, also, was delighted by the sea at this door, and his friend, Thomas Merton,[12] for his daily playmate.

However, a rift had presented itself even before the hundred a month each had materialized; as, while in New York City, the summer before, Charles Garland had quoted his mother to me as having said that she expected to settle this money on us, but was doing so primarily because of Cyril Kay Scott, as I would have amounted to little without him, was "lazy" and "entirely selfish".

I here return to the Hale-Garland rupture, as, during our second year in Bermuda, Swinburne Hale and Marie Garland decided to part; and as I had, in New York City before going back to Bermuda for the winter of 1922-23, insisted on seeing Marie Tudor Garland Cyril Kay Scott present, and telling her exactly what her son had said in quoting her to me. I said I could no longer feel grateful for my share in her part of the benefits we had been about to receive, and I did not want assistance at the expense of self-respect. Cyril Kay Scott assured her he was with me in my candour and that any self-respecting person would feel as I did.

Marie Tudor Garland wept. She said she did, frankly, think Cyril Kay Scott a wonderful man. She did not know, she said, whether she had been unjust to me or not. But as to the money, which had just begun to be sent to us, it would continue ours, as she had given her "promise" and "never went back on her word".

Cyril Kay Scott, when she had left the sublet apartment in Patchin Place in which this interview took place, reiterated to me that I was never to doubt his loyalty, but the situation being what it was, I should take the money already arranged for, and especially for Jigg's sake, put aside a justifiable hurt to pride.

---

12 Thomas Merton's father, Owen, was Evelyn's lover while they were in Bermuda and later in southern France and in north Africa.

In the second and last winter in Bermuda, 1922-23, we still
saw both Marie Tudor Garland and Swinburne Hale; she as cordial
as ever, on the surface to Cyril Kay Scott, but somewhat more
formal with me; and Swinburne Hale the same to both of us. They
were then living apart, he in Ely's Lodge, and she at Parapet.[13]
When we left in either late April or early May, for New York City,
we had our personal belongings crated, hoping to be able to have
them freighted to us once we found an abiding place elsewhere that
would allow us to rent The Scottage in due course when legalities
relating to Bermuda law were sorted out, as the Hale-Garland
divorce decree was imminent, and, for the time, had all but
spoiled the idyllic atmosphere for work The Scottage represented.

To Lola Ridge

Somerset Bridge, Bermuda

[late 1921]

Lola, Darling: There isnt a book shop in Bermuda! The only mildly like one is a store
called The Tower where you can also buy toys, stationery, and a little hardware. Bermuda
consists of about one hundred diminutive islands. The entire population is twenty-
thousand and twelve thousand of these are blacks. At least a quarter - maybe a third
- of the remaining eight thousand are semi-literate Portuguez immigrants. There is no
system of free education, no divorce, no anything later than eighteen twenty. The English
here are the Governor a number of bone head military officials and the people who run
the naval yard. They are scandalized at mixed bathing, at women who smoke etc. Art has
just passed the chrome stage. Among the tourists (and there are about two thousand a
month during January February and March several hundred during other months) there
are mostly rich Jew clothing store families and tired American business men who come
to play golf. The Bermuda public library has Edgeworth, Dickens, Scott, etc etc.

If you could see the excitement and joy of CS and ES when they get your letters youd
know a little bit about how much they love you. Please dont forget to write about your
OWN work and what your new job will do to your time for it. We had our first letter from
dear old Otto since he went to London. I think England has rather got his goat for the
time being. Esther wrote me she had seen you and you looked so pretty - better than she
ever saw you. Youll probably fool people into thinking you are strong. Dont over do it.

Say, dearest, I almost forgot, another lost soul we are sending to you. A little man
called Owen Merton, about thirty I should judge, a Scotch Welshman from New Zealand
who has been for the last year living in Flushing where his wife recently died and left him
two children. He is very hard up, very naive and genuine, and in all respects an interesting
child with real if not stupendous talent. He has been working fiendishly hard at water color
and some of his things are very successful. He is as poor as the rest of us and has been
trying to eke it would with landscape gardening. Not all of Mertons stuff would reproduce

---

13   There were two separate dwellings on the Garland Hale property.

among modern stuff but a few would. We want him to show them to you. Now dont let the personal thing affect your criticism - I mean embarrass you if you dont like the stuff, but it won't help to look, and he is somebody you would like and be liked by I think.

I would give more than I have to be able to have a jaw with you and Davy. Just think - a whole year saved up to talk about! Love and love, Evelyn

[Typed, typed signature. SSC]

To Lola Ridge

[Somerset Bridge, Bermuda]

[late 1921]

Dearest dear:

I havent written anybody Lola, because after I came out of personal pipp I went into late eighteenth century fits. For one month I have been struggling desperately with SOMETHING ABOUT BRAZIL[14], and wept and given it up and made Cyril waste precious energies persuading me to go on AND - at least I really believe I am going to do it right.

Relations between us and HGs seemed yet to be strained as we almost never hear from them, but we are refusing to worry for a while - trying to steal this winter anyway, and get two more novels done. After which let sex and circumstance do its worst. It will be something accomplished at least.

The house is cold but cute. I have done, with Mertons cooperation, the most lurid living room you ever saw. I designed it and he helped me with the planning of a lamp shade, a water color panel on the wall, and the designing of a patchwork hanging which I had conceived but was finding most awfully hard to execute. Merton is as sweet a child as I ever saw. He has absolutely no pretense and damn little capacity for reserve. And I am growing awfully fond of him - but these children, like all of the young, are innocently cruel and dangerous.

Sug and Merton and me speak of you and Davy oftener than anyone else. You know if Davy wanted to come here I believe he could get, in his line, all kinds of work.

I hope by the time I am eighty I shall have learned to live. To accept life completely, to give it everything, and yet to keep something apart from it. There can be a psychological gesture of renunciation and at the same time the fullest participation. But while I see that I haven't become a complete part of my understanding of it.

Today the sea is a blue storm, milking mountains of water all snow. Im going to stop now and go to swim. Im terrified of the coldness and mercilessness of it, but I like to abandon myself to the shock. Characteristic I guess.

Love to Davy and to YOU my dear from me, Jigeroo, and my best blessedly wonderful Sug who every hour he lives gives me more comfort in life.

Evelyn

[Typed, signed. SSC]

---

14   This eventually became *Escapade*, published in 1923.

To Lola Ridge

Somerset Bridge, Bermuda
[January 1922]

Darling girl:

Lola, Im still happy about your liking the book though it taint sold. And I do HOPE you will like what I am writing now. It is an autobiography of myself in Brazil. Not like other autobiographies except in being written in the first person. it is broken in impressionistic bits, a page or so at a time and beings purely objectively in impressions of environment - or rather nearly objectively, becomes more and more subjective to alert free verse self explanation, and is to end with dreams, the final one being a slightly revised shadow play. Shadow play can be used at last and in just the way it ought for it absolutely represents my absolute at that period having been written then. I never went through so many fits writing anything and but for Cyril would have given it up, but he likes it best of anything.

Tell us when you are coming here between now and June. Tell us whether you are writing or not. Id love to see your review of my book.

I love you.

I am just out of bed and Cyril is in bed with bronchitis but we do love you. Happy new year to you and dear old Davy.

Evelyn

[Half typed, half handwritten, signed. SSC]

To Lola Ridge

Somerset Bridge, Bermuda
January 7, 1922

Dear precious Lola:

When I wrote you last we were all in a cottage with Swinburnes parents who are here. They are the sort of people who think that the Dictionary was delivered into the hands of Daniel Webster on Mount Ararat or something like that. Modern art shocks them unless it is in French. They think ladies dont use rouge and have various other illusions about the human race. The time spent there - three weeks in all - was hell. Afterward we went with Marie and Swinburne into their house which was and still is on the build and overrun by workmen. Swinburne has been ill - had a curious partial paralysis of the face, they were both very nervous and full of domestic complexes (so were we, I suppose) and inclined subconsciously to consider the fact that they were helping us as an excuse for superficial lacks of consideration. I nearly blew up. Hell again.

Well, now we are in a cottage which has five - six with kitchen - fair sized rooms in semi tropical style - that is whitewashed inside and out. The floors are bare and unpainted and the modern plumbing is represented by a hole in the ground. But it is - when the weather is warm - very comfortable with a sweet view of an inlet and a tiny far off perspective of seas sweeping a reef. The yard too is graciously green with a red leaved hedge they call match-me-if-you-can and numerous hibiscus bushes. It is as quiet as a deserted grave yard - except for Jigeroo (who has had the croup and still joins me in a consumptive chorus of hacks). Cyril and I write most of the day and usually until about eleven at night and he is accomplishing more than he had time to in years. I am already at page one hundred and two on novel number three, having done most of it at night when somehow the world lets you alone and there ceases to be even the pull of things. Then in that abysmal midnight quiet which seems to be in you you can dive into a quiescent sub-conscious and pull up plums by the handful - psychological plums of the first order.

[Typed, first 4 pages only. SSC]

To Lola Ridge

[Greysbank, Bermuda]

[January 1922]

My precious dear

We are expecting Swinburne on Monday and hope to find out what will happen to the property down here and consequently to us. Bermuda has been very awful since Christmas in some respects. I am ready to move but except to seeing you and two or three others I wish were to some place other than New York. I went to New York with such a romantic feeling of discovering and of course only discovered myself there and that mostly so inappropriate to the environment. Wish we had money to take you and Davy to France. God knows if we will get there. Cyril and I have been thinking that rather than come to Bermuda again we should like Martinique or some other hotter queerer place.

Bermuda is in so many ways exquisite and it scarcely affects me any more. Yesterday though I had a thrill out of it. Mary and I canoed outside the islands and saw those wonderful birds again. I think last year I told you of them - long tails of the full family. They are as large as small hawks with a long forked tail and are snow white with red beaks and black dashed wings and black underscored eyes. They fly low over the green water and their breasts are like translucent jade, while the thin edges of their wings pierced by the glare remain a fiery and immaculate white. The tails are blood rose, like flesh held against a lamp. They have the most beautiful swallow flight. In front of us the waste water of a still Atlantic, no land, green and peacock water darkened with shadows, a hot blue sky smutted a little with clouds, and in this stillness that gull mew, far, high up, like the call of a Valkyrie on a mountain top, and those birds passing each other in the amazing stillness, passing and re-passing with the look of delicate and evil angels, strange eyes, black dashed wings, and jade bodies outlined as with a heavenly flame. Oh, Lola, I wish you and the few other people with lovely insides could have looked at it.

My love to Davy and to You. I love you

Evelyn

[Typed, signed. SSC]

To Otto Theis

[Greysbank, Bermuda]

February 19, 1922

Beloved Otto

I feel like celebrating when your letters come. Because you are so much yourself in such a self responsible way I find you suggest to me the same kind of equilibrium.

Merton maybe I described. Anyway he is five feet seven and slight with a wiry muscular body because for the last five years he has done manual work in order to get enough money to paint periodically. His face doesnt look like anything much until there is emotion in it, and then his eyes which are brown and set under his brows are very warm and kind and alive. He was smooth faced when he came here but is raising a browny blonde moustache which doesnt grow evenly because he has a scar on his lip. When he is estranged from his surroundings he looks like a lonesome monkey. Sometimes he reminds me of Harry Lauder because he chews a pipe in a funny way and thrusts out his rather full under lip. He was born in New Zealand and studied water color in London and Paris and lived in Paris five years with his wife who died of cancer a year and a half ago. She was an American girl and her family live in Douglastown Long Island. He has two kids, boys, and one of them[15] is here with us now. When he was a kid he went in for Tolstoy and it spoiled his paint. He came to New York had no money and has been a gardner for some rich people who patronized him because they thought it was piquant to have an educated man in that capacity. The wife of the household tried to flirt.

He adores Cyril in the most sincere way. And he is himself the most honest to god sincere person I ever saw. Cyril is quite fond of him. He is so emotional that he may talk like a damned fool or he may get off remarks in painting which Cyril says are the most profound he ever heard. He is easily bluffed and the world has put it all over him. I havent any illusions about how long this idylic situation will last and sometimes I want very much to laugh, it is so absurd, and in view of my disgust with Garland messing, so ironic. But Cyril and I know an awful lot about each other and what ever happens to the other two I dont think we are going to lose each other ever.

Goodbye till next encyclopedia from me.

Evelyn

PS We do LOVE to hear from you. Otto, Cyril doesnt know I wrote you all this - he never does. But you will laugh a nice laugh wont you? Please.

[Typed, typed signature. BRBL]

---

15 Merton's son Tom was about the same age as Jigg. The two boys were left to their own devices a good deal of the time and Jigg would later speak of the time in Bermuda as the happiest time in his life.

To Lola Ridge

Ely's Lodge, Bermuda
[Summer 1922]

Beloved dear,

I cant write a decent letter yet a while, for we are camping out in Elys Lodge and in a frightful mess. The hurricane carried off half of the fine cedars on the lawn and a part of the roof so that some of the inside must be done over and many of Maries lovely belongings are injured. Our house had just been finished, but the leaky roof has damaged the walls and floors so that all the labor spent there has gone for nothing. It may be three weeks before we can get into it. I am trying to fight off the restless suggestion of upset surroundings and live out of doors in the brilliant peace, heat, blue water, and an atmosphere of indolence. To counteract the voluptuousness of nothing I shall try tomorrow to start on work on the story for Mr Pitkin.

Cyril has brought a cold with him but he is mentally relaxing and I think we both love to come home to rest in each other after our periodic flirtations with chaos. He is sculpturally perfect and at the same time so warm - finished and yet living, I tried to put in a poem. Cool and warm, white and warm at the same time.

And Jigeroo is maturing so I feel absolutely humble with pride in him. The summer has improved him wonderfully. I sort of feel all at once face to face with a grown-up mind, lacking the defense of facts but quite equal to any I can supply.

Well, as you will see my spirits, considering that I am unwell, are pale rose that may later mount to crimson - this certainly if you come to see us.

Love you. Cyril and Jigeroo do too.

Evelyn

[Typed, typed signature. SSC]

To Evelyn Scott

Clarksville, Tennessee
March 26, 1923

Dear daughter:

Just a note to tell you that I asked J[16] if he would find out if Seely[17] would help me, and relieve him of the job, but he declined to communicate with S, and said I could write to you to do so, as you were the only person who had any influence on him &c. He spoke of my being "on the edge of the brink", and other cheerful things. I never felt more energetic than I do now, and am anxious to get work, or training for something to do, away from here, if I get out of this deadly atmosphere my health with improve,

---

16 Maude's cousin, Julian Gracey, with whom she was sent to live when the family returned to the United States. Maude was dependent on the Graceys as Seely was refusing to support her in any way.

17 Seely Dunn, Evelyn's father. After divorcing Maude, Seely married Melissa Whitehead, about whom much will be written in 1947.

or my nerves, that's where the trouble is. But I can get no assistance from J. It has been made plain that I am not wanted here, except that I have not been told so, and if it is humanly possible I want to leave before I am invited to. I cannot blame J for wanting to free himself. I know that I am a helpless sort of person, and have not taken responsibilities, but you may be sure I will learn to take care of myself, and not worry you if - I can get some financial help, but how can I accomplish any thing without a penny? It tickled my sense of humour when I found I was so near dissolution.

I understand that Seely has built some apartments, in Washington, also his home, and that he has a life job with a fine salary, and that $30,000 worth of gems were found in the big safe in your grandfather's house, which he gave to his wife[18] and the home place is for sale in Nov at $20,000.

With love to you and dear Jigaroo,

Mother

PS Seely's address is "Interstate Commerce Commission Statistical Department, Washington, DC"

J did you the honor to say that you had a "brilliant mind".

[Typed, signed. HRC]

In early 1923 Merton returned to the United States to see his elder son, John Paul, who had been staying with Merton's in-laws on Long Island. He was conscious of being indebted to Cyril and tried to find galleries which would exhibit, and sell, his paintings in order to repay this debt.

To Cyril Kay Scott

~~Owen Merton~~

~~Landscape Designs Color Schemes for Flower Gardens~~

~~57 Hillside Avenue~~

~~Flushing, L I~~

Bay End Farm, Buzzard's Bay,

April 19, 1923

My dear Cyril -

From what Gladys said to me in a note I had yesterday I think Evelyn must have been pretty depressed. I don't know exactly why except that Swinburne's visit must not have turned out well. Look here - I wish I had better news of large sums of money, from here, but I am really doing as well with landscape painting as I had any reason to expect to, this spring - and I did very damned thing I could to try and arrange that sales of pictures will take place. You know you can't rush in somewhere,

---

18   The reference to a "wife" must be to his second wife, Melissa, suspected by Evelyn of having acquired her grandfather's significant wealth which Evelyn assumed would come to her in her grandfather's will. Chapter 26, "An inheritance is lost" goes into considerable detail about Evelyn's search for her legacy.

and simply say "give me 100 dollars for this". By the end of this month I shall have at least 500 dollars - and what I want to say is, "For God's sake take it, and get away as soon as you want to. I know you won't either of you want to stay in New York. If you could borrow a little of the money you could stay quietly in France until I am able to come, and I shall certainly get in some more. I know damned well I can get 2000 dollars if I try hard enough. I have never been licked yet at any special thing I set out to do, and I can certainly do this.

If my failure to get in a lot of money right away is responsible for some of Evelyn's depression - cheer her up - because I have not done every damned thing I can yet - and I am really more vigorous and strong after this, than I have ever been after anything.

It seems feeble to be working for 20 dollars a day - when we need hundreds, but after all it mounts up. I have to date 235 dollars owing to me here - and I have at least 150 in the bank in Flushing as well as good chances of selling some pictures next Saturday when that show opens in Flushing.

I want to come down and meet you, and I hope Tom is not complicating things too much by his disobedience. Damn it, Scott, I will fix things. Don't be disappointed with me, if things are not too hopeful on appearances so far. They really are more hopeful than they seem to be. Bon courage.

from Merton

[Handwritten on personal letterhead (struck out), signed. SFC]

To Cyril Kay Scott

[Buzzards Bay]
May 17, 1923

My dear Cyril,

Marie has just talked to me - Swinburne has an offer from some woman to buy the Lodge and your home or else rent them.

He has written to her as she is concerned in the question of furniture etc - in case he rents the Lodge.

Marie asked me outright - would you accept your home if she bought it - or were you too set against the place now. I said your feeling was only against the way Swinburne had acted I was sure, but that I had always had the feeling that you loved the place and would like to own it. I said I thought you felt there should be no conditions over it, (as I understood) that if you felt later on you would like to change the place for another that you ought to have the right to dispose of it.

Now I hope to God I didn't say the wrong thing. Marie simply said she would not dare to approach you herself, at the time. And she is inclined to act at once.

All you have to say of course is that I didn't know anything about your personal affairs, and had a nerve to discuss them. The thing is if she makes the house your property the deed will be transferred from Swinburne to you, and then you can certainly rent the house for 100 dollars a month.

I said you were in Washington having the details of passports attended to, and I hope you don't mind her knowing that.

I said I needed more money, that I had heavy insurance to pay, and that I would have to get another cheque tonight. So I hope you will get that cheque Saturday morning. I will get 250 dollars if I can and mail you cheque for 200.

In great haste,

Merton

[Handwritten, signed. SFC]

Not long after this letter, the Scott family plus Owen Merton decided that they would be better off in southern Europe which offered not only a warm climate but the opportunity for Cyril and Owen to develop their painting styles in the landscapes surrounding the medieval towns along the Mediterranean coast.

Chapter 5

Collioure

July - September 1923

In the summer of 1923, the relationship with the Garland-Hales had broken down to the extent that Evelyn, with Cyril and Jigg and their new friend Owen Merton, left Bermuda for Europe where they hoped to be able to paint in the cheaper climes of southern France. It has not been possible to find any letters relating to their leaving Bermuda, and so the story resumes when the family are in Collioure, in the foothills of the Pyrenees near Marseille.

Collioure is a medieval fishing port just north of the border with Spain. The harbour is dominated by the church of Notre-Dame-des-Anges with its distinctive bell tower. In the early 1920s, the town nestled by this church and the rented Villa Tine[19] would have been in one of the narrow medieval streets surrounding the church. The soft light, the medieval architecture and the stark countryside attracted a number of painters, and in the 1920s, the town was host to Georges Braque, Henri Matisse, Pablo Picasso, Charles Rennie Mackintosh and André Derain, among others.

Many of Evelyn's letters from this period are in effect travelogues full of colourful descriptions of the equally colourful landscapes and of the local people with whom Evelyn came into contact. Her gift was her ability to convey these impressions in simple language.

To Lola Ridge

Villa Tine,
Collioure, France
July 7, 1923

Precious Lola:

I want to make note of what has happened and I do it in letters to me friends. Is that a cheap economy of invention? I know you want to hear and I simply cant write it twice.

We were docked at Naples at eight oclock and I was too lazy to witness the approach. What I saw when I came on deck was a hot hill of houses with the Castle of Saint Elmo resting rather bleakly on the top of it, and on the other side only a large dim

---

19   This villa, rented by the Scotts, is now the Collioure Museum of Modern Art.

outline of a Vesuvius which the fog had almost obliterated. There was a great stir of people landing. Out of about two hundred second class passengers all but fifteen got off here, and Italian ladies who had luxuriated in soiled matinees for the past fifteen days appeared suddenly in evening dress, the scent of garlic more piquant for the usual perfume of the bottle which accompanied it. Merton had horrible recollections of Naples where he had sunstroke and was often robbed and he awakened in a high key of antagonism which later precipitated itself.

Ellen[20] loves the Italians. Especially when the ship began to be overrun with dark shoddily neat gentlemen who would take us all to Pompeii for the day almost for the pleasure of doing it. Lola, never let any brave man mention in my presence again the materialism of my native land. At least we do our thieving in the grand manner. Naples had an atmosphere of meagre financial desperateness. It isnt the war at all, but these are people who are temperamentally incapable of industry and initiative who are caught in the struggle and cant get out of it. They are like women who have led easy lives, whose soft bodies can not compete and yet they must compete. They must get money somehow in the domesticated wildness of alley cats where they exist.

We had no sooner set our feet on the glaring dock to which we were drawn up when more hungry creatures offered their services, their carriages, their bought advice with a kind of illicit hungriness. We did get a carriage and Ellen, who speaks Italian well, was scheduled to pilot us. We wanted first to see the meanest streets. But driver took us wherever he would - many halts, Ellen rising converses with him volubly. He is agreeable, he wants to take us the longest way - and after the greatest moral exertion we go where we want to and come out right. Mertons eyes ache. He exhibits an evasive tensity. When the driver asks him if he likes Naples he replies baldly that he hates its stinks. The driver looks unabashed and yet abashed. He is agreeable. We must be pleased. He is like a kindly whore who is accustomed to being beat, who steals a little from the gentleman's pockets and is ashamed of it.

Such streets, Lola. Palermo had the same narrowness, the same tortureness, but its filth was new and bright and unsubdued. Old Naples was a decayed body - sharp and strong with people living in it as in maggoty meat - people that ran in and out of dark windowless holes that were meat stalls and butcher shops. In every shop a shrine like a kind of ikon with an electric bulb glaring stodgily in front of it. Such meat shops - harsh pieces of red flesh, dingy tiles, crusts of flies, and always always, visible in the shallow depths as we stared in from the carriage, the worn picture of the saint on the wall above the counter at the back. Such cadaverous women, such anemic children, such an absence of any joy in light or life - nothing anywhere but a rich and crowded hideousness. There were shrines on the outsides of houses too, shrines that were dingy and fly specked, and beneath them also burned and electric light. The vegetables exposed were sold and old

---

20 Ellen Kennan was a friend of both Evelyn and Cyril and was travelling with the Scotts; she had been Cyril's lover a few years earlier.

and there was charcoal dust. Some of the streets climbed endless stairs with the banners of laundered clothes rising tier on tier till they waved at last in the merciless light.

Palermo reminded me of Rio de Janeiro on a smaller scale. It was young. Naples was used as I never saw a city used before. There was not a fresh face, not a fresh house front - nothing that had not come to the end of itself and sprouted again like a tree that is half felled but struggles yet to a little harsh growth. The stinks I had anticipated I didnt find in actuality. It was a visual aroma that I mostly get - black olives, wine jugs, basket makers, chair weavers, cobblers, smithies, wood sellers, all crowded in one street - court yards that had the faint illumination of decay - and people, people in rooms the depth of a wall, people who were crowded helplessly into the street while those in Palermo willingly lived in it.

The fine gardens and drive along the sea are a slightly less impressive counterpart of Rio since the mountains behind the city are further back. There the same bald elegance of expensive passions. We went to a restaurant on the waters edge where we could look directly at Vesuvius which had emerged from its pseudo mystery and looked fine but rather obvious with houses clustering at its gradual feet. Maybe I had seen it too often on the walls on Italian restaurants but it was so exactly what I had anticipated that its actuality did not affect me until that evening when the ship was going out.

The restaurant had a wide veranda and an empty unluxurious appearance but we were very well served with some breaded cutlets, salad, and a kind of short cake with cherries in the middle of it, black bitter cherries that had been steeped in wine so that their acridness was subtilized. The wine was bad here and in Palermo it was excellent. We disgraced ourselves by misunderstanding a charge for services and not leaving any tips. Our vanity was darkened for the day when we discovered it. By this time Merton and Ellen had already disagreed as to Italian charmingness.

I was reckless enough to ask to go to the toilet and a small boy who could speak English escorted me up a torturous spiral staircase above the bar and stood politely outside the Johnny door until I could be admitted. He waved his hands gallantly toward it as the last occupant came out. Such a toilet. A darkness almost complete but animate with smells, a toilet more used than Naples herself and uncleansed by the rains of heaven, a toilet without a chain to pull and with every evidence that the chain had not been pulled that week.

We had another ride in a taxi out the sea way, another past some fine old palaces, and another through some rich and substantial looking squares and business streets. There were huge arcades with rich shops, but the prices were very cheap. How I would have loved to buy presents for all of us. Silk was next to nothing. The dust and heat were terrible. The taxi drivers quarrelled with each other. There is nothing in Naples that can not be bought. Nothing that isnt trying to sell itself.

When we got back to the <u>Patria</u> at half past four, an hour and *[remainder of letter missing]*

[Typed, first four pages only. SSC]

To Otto Theis

Collioure, France
July 9, 1923

Beloved Otto:

I had your letter a couple of days ago. The second class of the Patria was horrible, we almost died of starch poisoning and the general literal putrefication of the grub. Jig had croup and I had a bass cough and a sore chest, and the passengers, Italians going home and a few rotten Americans were the very worst. No lounge only a smoking room very dirty with dirty people and indigestibable babies and gentlemen who could spit farther and louder - much louder - than a southern Colonel in a Bret Harte story. No permanent deck spaces, herding on and off decks partially possessed by the first class. We rented five steamer chairs and spent most of the time looking for them and removing them from Italians who had escaped the property sense except as it related to the belongings of other folks.

However we did have two whole days in brilliant sunshine running a moving picture distance from Moorish castles and Algerian villages on one side, and the slow fatigued landscape of burnt Spain opposite. Also the Azores, very kind hills and funny zig zag cultivation like an infantile insanity. Dutch windmills very calm in the midst of it. Also a day at Palermo which is like Brazil, gaudy, ennuied, and ingenuous. Sicilians seem to like bright irrelevant things, wonderful gay sweetmeats, marvelously naive carts, a new looking city and very old alive hills burning above it. A day in Naples where, thank God, most of the passengers got off, a rapacious Naples rich with filth, and dingier in its richness that I knew a Southern city could be. Everybody wanted to sell something, services, information, taxi cabs, and Pompeii was hawked about like a Coney Island commodity. It did look beautiful though when we were leaving it. Sorrento and Capri were all brittle houses small and white in a kind of winey light, Vesuvius immensely still, and a very dramatic sunset where the sun stood over the water in a huge sphere that had detached itself from the sky and seemed to float.

Marseille was stupe, very bourgeois and middleaged, very commercially cosmopolitan in the population of the streets. The lots of plane trees looked strong and composed and heartily green and there was a quiet color in flower markets and zouave soldiers, but I didnt feel in it any France more subtle than the naturalists.

We had a wild trip to Port Vendres with one parrot and twenty three pieces of small baggage and three unexpected changes of train en route. Port Vendres is one street around a well in port and the ships from Algeria dock under the hotel windows. The Pyrenees are heavy and close above the stodgy houses. There were some sailing ships that on moonlight nights were a labyrinth of stiff frost white ropes against a deep space of dark-lit sky, strangely intimate and close to us. They had sour smelling cargoes that were loaded, unloaded and mysteriously loaded again while we were there (the same black beans sold, docked, resold and returned to the hold to be taken to Barcelona) by strong looking girls and lean strong old women who swung sacks with a rhythmical easiness. We couldn't find a house to rent and as our money was being eaten up in the hotel we came over here to Collioure and took the only place available, still much dearer than we had meant to pay for it.

The Villa Tine is a miracle of perfection, an ugliness that is above reproach. But it is comfortable, has a charming garden in front and back garden of orange and magnolia and is five minutes walk from a swimming place. We have a sternly shy maid who cooks very bearably though she isnt the miracle of efficiency tradition had led me to expect and doesnt do much else. Merton manages the housekeeping and I clean up. If we werent always nervous about money we could settle down to a wonderful year. Merton only has a few hundred dollars and a month was wasted before we even got here (eighteen days on ship, three in Marseille, one traveling, a week in Port Vendres, and two or three days of getting settled in this place). He is a remarkable water colorist Otto. He has wasted six years doing manual labor, gardening, digging, anything, until his wife died last year and left him with two kids, who, fortunately are with their grandparents for the time. We hoped Marie would do something for him, but alas she has the bug that labor in the soil is holy and that he needs it to purify his art. He is pretty blue about the prospect of having to go back. He had a show at the Daniels gallery just before we left but it netted him only about a hundred and fifty dollars and he only got as much more from a little private thing we arranged at Marie's Washington Mews place.

Well, about Collioure. It is on the Midi railway and is about an hour from Perpignan. It is very filthy and very beautiful. It is very near the Spanish border, about seventy-five miles from Barcelona. The Pyrenees have a luxurious severity like the richness of ecclesiastical voluptuousness. The bathing is good. The town is without a WC (our house has one thank god) and there are amorous cats in the streets by the hundreds. There is a fort full of Senegalese. Matisse and some of the pointillists painted here. It is worth seeing and we WANT to see you. I dont know how you would come from Paris but we took the Paris express at Marseilles, then changed at Contrast, at Cette, and at Narbonne. Expresses stop at Port Vendres for the Algerian boats and you could go to Port Vendres and drive about a mile over here or else take a slow train that stops at Collioure. Everybody knows the Villa Tine and already the Anglaise that live in it.

Love to you both. Evelyn

[Typed, typed signature. BRBL]

To Otto Theis

Collioure, France
August 15, 1923

Dearest Otto:

This is the poorest saddest little town but very stark and lovely too. The heat has dried up half the grapes and the fires on the mountains have burnt the cork trees and it just is rich massive flowing lava-like sterility, burnt colors with thick dry shadows in the high hollows and moorish watch towers very bleak on the bleakest heights. It hasnt rained for two months. To recover me from the fatugure of the book we went to Arles Sur Teche for three days. The scenery is absolutely different though only an hour and a half away - mountains covered with greenery that looks young and full like spring and torrents of mountains water rushing to fountains in the streets. All night in the quiet you hear the think cool rush of water going past. The teche is like an Alpine torrent Sug says, white round boulders and cataracts. But it is really a less individualized place than this.

Escapade is out but Im not reading reviews of it until I finish my book.[21] If it does sell it will be - oh, irony - for scandals sake anyway. Wonderful to write with religious solemnity of the most actual thing that ever occurred to you and only repeat the success of a sunday headline in it. I have had no copy yet but will mail you one when I do. The astericks indicate omissions and I imagine look queer but I wanted it to be known that the book was mutilated. Mr Seltzer[22] is indicted by the grand jury on last summers charge. I may be next.

The French are a niggling lot of commercialists and the Americans at least do it in the grand manner. There is nothing but solitude and a few friends. Today is a fete day and Jigeroo has gone with two kids unknown to ride on the merry go round. He is learning French anyway - much more than I am. Merton keeps house and I simply dont speak. Sug is a wonderful and lovely person - the most I ever knew or ever will know - and Merton with a much more limited sweep as he knows himself is absolutely genuine and sensitive and kind thank heaven. Life is complicated but compensating mostly. Money of course still annoys. With Escapade at three dollars I may make something. Marie didnt make the allowance permanent after all.

Our very very most love to you and do come here. We have to get a new place before October but I think it will be in this district. We would always have room for you.

Evelyn

[Typed, typed signature. BRBL]

To Lola Ridge

Collioure, France
September 1923

Darling dear, I tried to write this yesterday when I was out painting with Merton and had to quit because it was giving me a pain to sit in a squidged up position on the hard earth. I wish I could have stayed because I was looking at a funny caravan drawn up below us, a blue caravan with nice little Nottingham curtains very clean in the window and, now that they had unhitched their horse and settled down, two little canary bird cages hung on either side of the front door with little birds singing very at

---

21 *The Golden Door*, published 1925.
22 Thomas Seltzer was a Russian émigré who became a successful translator and academic. In 1919 he founded the publishing house, Thomas Seltzer Inc, which not only published *Escapade* but also works by D H Lawrence.

home on them. Through the open door I saw inside a wonderful dresser with dishes hung in racks and three bunk beds one under the other covered with red spreads and lace coverlids, as clean and cute as anything. A big woman with blond hair and a red face was watering the donkey that belonged to the outfit and another old woman very shriveled and hearty looking was making a fire. If I had sat there longer I could have told you a whole story about them, but as it was I only learned that they came from Normandy. I dont know for why or what.

There was a fete here two weeks ago and the fishing boats were decorated with paper lanterns and the harbour very lovely in the vague night with floating flat-radiance of the candles. We thought about Broadway and how this childish illumination in one key has such a naïve timidity while that other childish illumination is so wonderful bold and varied to such violence. For some funny reason I never thought about America as America, a unit, a country with people in it, not people in a country, as I have since we came here. I suppose I had no sense of America when I left New Orleans and this is really the first time I have felt absolutely removed from it since I felt New York for Bermuda was too close. It is voluptuous like an old ladys memories. I used to feel that way about Brazil but didnt know it would come so quickly about this. I suppose this is the first time I ever indulged romanticism about my native land. Anyway the more I see of other countries, or this one other country, the more magnificently awful my own country appears to be. Not in any way that makes me want to go back. I dont want to go back for a long long time, not until I get all I can out of this distant appreciation.

Cyril and Merton have done marvels in paint. Merton says Cyrils painting has a stark profundity and I think it a wonderfully exact phrase for it. Yes, Lola, we are having a good life now, and when I feel physically well I am awfully happy (when Sug is well, for a time all three of us have been sick). Merton has a weak back he got while day laboring and sometimes when he lifts too many things it upsets him.

The French people are the most quintessence of individualism. The way they do stand back and allow murder and anything else and never interfere with it. Superficially they are the rudest people, or rather fundamentally for it is their real indifference, I ever saw. Might know a popular fallacy would be undone once you looked at it. They butt through crowds, knock you over, never apologise, stare unmercifully at any woman they dont know, and never do the least curtesy for anybody except purely formally for very definite effect. On the other hand their leaving you alone has its advantages. This town is miserably poor and now at the end of summer is haunted by devastated artists who are going to get one picture in the salon before they die or die at once of a starch diet. Some wear Pilgrim Father hair and blue coats, some fence with their palettes, as Sug says, and some trudge to painting armed like Tartarin on his hunting expedition with a meek little wife and three daughters to assist.

You never saw so many awful pictures as are being painted in Collioure at the present moment. We like it though and are in great distress because we have not yet found a house to move to when we give up this. The town is so old and so crowded that there is not but one garden beside ours and ours is THE ONLY HOUSE THAT HAS ANY SORT OF A WC IN IT. Every morning ladies going to market carrying on the left arm the china slop pail with the offering to the all consuming sea in it. Gentlemen trouble themselves less and merely squat. God help me, I shall return to America and light an ikon in the bathroom. The smell of merde is on the breath of the sea and is almost everywhere that a female in a clean dress would like to sit. (I didnt put an h in it Lola, excuse my vulgarity.)

The town is crooked streets that at night are dramatic and abrupt, very badly lit, and old woman in black resting in a crooked doorway, a black cat (there are lots of cats and lots of rats) slinking past her, and a man with a red sash around his waist carrying a sack of charcoal up up into the darkness where a blood and thunder cut throat ought to be hid for some better loot. The Pyrenees really begin here and they are the saddest most austere mountains I ever saw, burnt colored and grassy bleak, with some rocky peaks far off, the peak of the Canigo which is really a very high mountain, just visible sometimes when there is no mist. Over toward Argelesse it begins to flatten and there is that variegated landscape the French make because of cultivating so many things in such small space, vines and olives and little garden plots diminutive in a large plain with a ribbon of blue haze making it perpetually remote like a veiled picture with the sun on it. Please write to me again and say how you and Davy are, and remember we love you both and THINK of you and TALK of you just about every single day, all three of us, and I do hope you are not ill now and are getting on with the book.

Evelyn

[Typed, typed signature. SSC]

Chapter 6

Bou Saada

September 1923 - March 1924

The Scotts were unable to find suitable rented accommodation for the winter months in Collioure, and in the late summer of 1923 they found themselves in Bou Saada, deep in the Algerian desert, about 245 kilometres south of Algiers.

A search on Google Earth shows clearly how very isolated Bou Saada is now; it must have been so much more so in the early 1920s. It was (and is) the central point of a number of trade routes across the northern Sahara. The name Bou Saada translates as "place of happiness". Judging by Evelyn's account of their time there, they found it to be anything but.

Cyril and Owen were, however, able to explore the barren arid landscape with their paints, and these months in the desert produced a number of watercolours, some of which are now in private collections.[23]

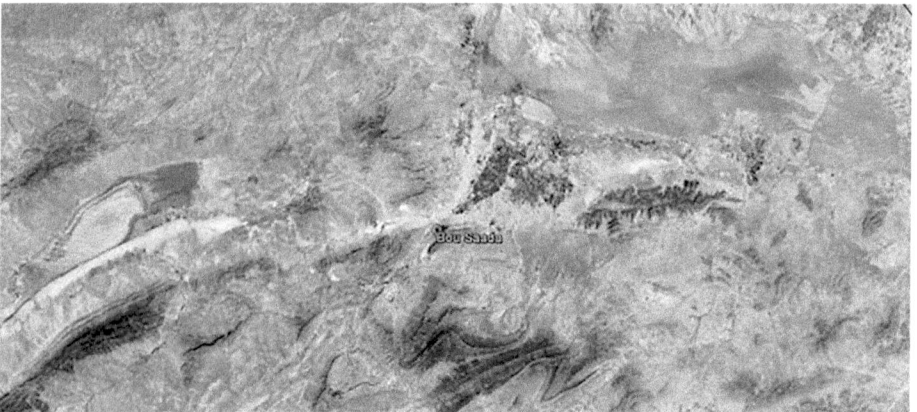

Screen shot of Bou Saada: ©*Google 2020*

---

23   Many of Cyril's paintings are held by the North Carolina Museum of Art; the Thomas Merton Society hold a number of Owen's works..

To Otto Theis

Rue Coumes
Bou-Saada, Algeria
October 11, 1923

Dear Otto:

I havent heard from you in ages and I have the PIPP so I wont write a long letter, but I want you to know our new address which is Rue Coumes, Bou-Saada, Algerie, via Alger.

We couldnt get another house in Collioure, it turned very cold, and we came the twenty-four hours to Alger. But Alger was so damp and expensive that we are trying out here, two hundred and fifty kilometres without a railway. I suppose it is the fatigue of travel but right now I have the worst hump I ever had about a place. There is nothing but sand and mud houses and dirty Arabs and women without faces and I dont think it interesting or picturesque or anything it obviously is, but just dismal. You feel squashed by the inertia of the landscape and the inertia of the people. All the kids have sore eyes and flies on their faces like they were pastries in a window. I dont like it, and more not because I dont think Cyril does and I know Merton doesnt and we havent enough money to move again inside of six months. In fact we had to take the only house there was here for six months. But for Gods sake dont come to Bou Saada except as a wealthy tourist who is going to motor back in two days. This is an oasis and there is very little water but not enough to commit suicide in at that. There are some date palms but they dont excite you.

Lots and lots of love,

Evelyn

PS Marie *[Garland]* took care to mail the snottiest review of <u>Escapade</u> and to write that she has inquired around it wasnt selling. Maybe thats why I dont like Bou Saada. [Typed, typed signature. BRBL]

To Otto Theis

Bou Saada,
October 19, 1923

You are a sweet thing to say what you do about me and writing and things and next to Cyrils faith in me theres nobody I want to live up to more than you, and I am certainly trying damned hard right now to do better than I ever have done, lots. I naturally want <u>Escapade</u> to sell but am scared to trust it will. You see I would like most awfully to get Sug a new suit, and lend Merton some money (he is in an awful fix and deserves a lot) and (Alas, human weakness again) send mother a little, and pay back one seventeenth of all the incredibly awful debts I owe. Well there doesnt seem much immediate chance of that.

I had no mail in three weeks and got it all forwarded today, so I have several letters to answer, but I had to say something to you first. And I will write again more elaborately when we are really in routine. I dont care how many sins of correspondential omissions you are guilty of, I cant keep from writing to you.

Evelyn

[Typed, typed signature. BRBL]

To Lola Ridge

Bou Saada
[October 1923]

My dearest dear Lola:

Well, honey. We are all stuck out here in the middle of nowhere having come in quest of a cheap winter in dry climate. Merton is in an awfully tight box financially and we are trying to invent some way to help him stick it through the year. He has to send money to his kids and that makes it a tight pull. Tom was up at Buzzards Bay but has been returned and that leaves two with Mrs Jenkins so we dont know whether it will be too much for her or not.

I think after we are settled in a place that is liveable we may be able to do a lot of work here, though as a place to paint it presents, once you abandon the obvious picturesque, the most difficult and subtle problem I ever saw. The general neutrality of the landscape makes it about as easy as discerning forms in a white sheet. It is the kind of place that no Anglo Saxon wants to get close to. It repels with its alien quality the most pronounced of which is dirt. Just sand wastes, a few low sand hills, and mud houses so low and flat that they are submerged in the general indefiniteness. Then the people all reduced to a more than conventional uniformity by clothes all white all flowing, or all once white for they are all dirty, the faceless women with their muslin window curtains held up so that only one eye is exposed. I dont feel capable of writing immediately about it yet, but I will later. And so let us know how you are, and have so very much love from all of us, and lots of love to Davy.

Evelyn

[Typed letter and signature; date deduced from contents. SSC]

To Lola Ridge

Bou-Saada
[October 1923]

Precious Lola:

Having unearthed your address from long hiding, I will enjoy a direct communication. I sent you two letters already via Gladys.

Lola about Sug. Well, the promise of fine things in the Bermuda stuff, has been justified and exceeded a dozen times. His last work is exquisite, such a perfect harmonization of sensuous full emotional quality with delicate mental perception I never saw. I dont believe any water color except Cezannes perhaps has ever been as good. The only draw back is his very punk health lately. In fact Bousaada has laid us all out with grippe and bronchitis almost continuous. Merton is doing himself wonderful justice, with very exquisitely realized things, with the most sensitive minute perception which locates emotion in time and space and yet does not remove it from the artists subjective. He is pretty worried about money, but we hope he can stick it out until he has given himself a real chance.

Jigeroo speaks French and goes to an Arab school. He has been ill but happy otherwise. So you see despite inwards this time as you said, darling, is a beautiful time. If money and health permit we will justify it. Our regret is that you and Davy arent here, and oh, again if we COULD get you here.

The arabs are dirty and miserable looking, but there is a fine arid landscape of fleshly hills, a huddle of frail walls of dead dry mud, a hurricane of dark palms against a sky that (when it condescends not to rain) is light. There is the wonderful sinister importance of the women all in red (all the married women of some tribes wear red) shrouded, holding with their palms fan-wise a screen of draperies across their faces. They dont wear veils as in Alger, but are even more concealed. There are the cupolas of marabout tombs that are somehow more voluptuous than one ever imagined plaster, and float above the flat houses like tight bruised lily buds stained with brown and pink. There is on market day always some man from the desert who seats himself in the dust of the Place and recites endless songs that have a slight half-moon rhythm which swings back and back on itself, the choruses accompanied by the hollow agitation of the tambourine drum which he beats as if encouraging himself. Then there are pipes always being played somehow, hollow querulous whistles, equally monotonous. In the evening the muezzin on the roof of the mosque calls, cries out it seems, to Allah. Men along street corners, removing their shoes, make that perfect complete gesture of abasement of which we have no counterpart, laying dust upon their foreheads and bending again three times to place their foreheads in the dust. Then the brazen chanting of the Koran, little boys voices hurrying shrilly, mens voices calling nasally above them. On Thursdays we walk by the synagogue and the Jews in the light of many candles are chanting so differently with a soft vague intonation of breathed solemnity.

However Mohademism is horrible to a western mind. Poverty accepted, slavery of women accepted, disease accepted, and death just the tossing of unconfined bodies into the scratched earth where the rain and the dogs go later to dig it up.

Later I shall maybe get something out of this beside the picturesque. Just now it is the sense of alienation which is satisfying, for one can work in it.

WE LOVE YOU AND DAVY. Please get well

Evelyn

[Typed, typed signature. SSC]

To Lola Ridge

Bou-Saada

[October 1923]

My dearest dear Lola:

HOW ARE YOU? ARE YOU BEING ABLE TO WRITE? Please let us know about your health cause we are worried about it.

Well, honey. We are all stuck out here in the middle of nowhere having come in quest of a cheap winter in dry climate. Merton is in an awfully tight box financially and we are trying to invent some way to help him stick it through the year. He has to send money to his kids and that makes it a tight pull. Tom was up at Buzzards Bay but has been returned and that leaves two with Mrs Jenkins so we dont know whether it will be too much for her or not.

I think after we are settled in a place that is liveable we may be able to do a lot of work here, though as a place to paint it presents, once you abandon the obvious picturesque, the most difficult and subtle problem I ever saw. The general neutrality of the landscape makes it about as easy as discerning forms in a white sheet. It is the kind of place that no Anglo Saxon wants to get close to. It repels with its alien quality the most pronounced of which is dirt. Just sand wastes, a few low sand hills, and mud houses so low and flat that they are submerged in the general indefiniteness. Then the people all reduced to a more than conventional uniformity by clothes all white all flowing, or all once white for they are all dirty, the faceless women with their muslin window curtains held up so that only one eye is exposed. I dont feel capable of writing immediately about it yet, but I will later. And so let us know how you are, and have so very much love from all of us, and lots of love to Davy.

Evelyn

Another note for Lola

Dear Lola, dear. I wrote you yesterday and feel inclined to add this note. I went out with Cyril and Merton when they sketched today and some faithful nuisances in the way of arab kids followed us about half a mile. When I sat down a little distance from the men said arab kids began to cluster around me and chant something that went like ah-ou-ou-aaaaa-ouy-a as loud as they could and to throw stones as close to me as they could without hitting me. Then in French they said if Id give them a cigarette theyd leave me alone, but I wasnt going to offer bribes so, though I had anticipated the request for a cigarette and had intended to bestow one, I didnt. So the au-ooo-auuu stuff went on until Merton came over to rescue me. They are little devils alright.

Yesterday afternoon we saw the dancing at the baptism again and the most charming little girl in a ragged mother hubbard who had unbelievably large eyes bewitchingly biased and painted green underneath. She was only about eleven and with an unhealthy delicacy, a premature sex consciousness mixed with inevitable gaucherie. She did the bird movements with her hands exquisitely and gave a dance du ventre which was to me not the mechanical sex it is supposed to be but a kind of saint vitus dance of the guts. It reminds me of all the stomach aches I ever had. The courtesy in these affairs is for the audience to supply one hundred franc bills to paste with spit on the forehead and turbans of musicians and dancers. Then when the show is over the money is returned. None of the ouled nahils will dance until somebody has put at least two hundred francs in their bonnets. As we werent used to it we watched this weeks board a bit nervously until the show was over, but it came back properly and we had only to buy three bottles of beer for the star performing ladies.

PLEASE WRITE HOW YOU ARE. Evelyn

[Typed, typed signature. SSC]

To Lola Ridge

Bou Saada

[November 1923]

Beloved dear, too funny that the very morning I wrote to know what had happened to you, I got your letter.

My dear, I wish I had really been able to pass on more of my experience here. For the first month I was simply paralyzed by strangeness. I was never anywhere before that every single detail of existence was alien and I couldnt identify myself with it. Then we have all been and still are sick. Sug, Jigeroo, and I were all ill at once and poor Merton got so many responsibilities on him that he had a general nervous blow up and cant paint, but I feel somehow or other that it isnt nearly as serious as it appears but only a kind of accumulated general panic from too much worry about practical things.

It is cold here and the desert is twice bare with the falling of the leaves on the few trees of the oasis and the palms all getting papery and dull. The poor Arabs are dirtier and more miserable looking than ever. Such pathetic creatures, the women all braceleted and veiled in inappropriate accompaniment to the nakedness of poverty that they cant conceal. We live opposite the police station and last night a drunk or a lunatic was shut up there and spent the whole night quavering out something that sounded like ci-ci-moi, in a thick broken voice, pounding and kicking the door, and beginning this curious monotonous song of misery again with an occasional sobbing cry interspersed. The cell they put him in is on the street and I have seen in the stone floor and no furnishing of any kind, but when I began to think how awful it was I had only to recall the home interiors here that are just a muddy darkness, a hearth, a pot, and a rag in a corner to lie on. Only the children of marabouts or priests are rich. There is a big monastery near here which owns many herds and houses etc. The dream of an earthly heaven is gained at the expense of almost all the necessity which the dream promises to supply. As for Arab women, the French schoolmistress says that an Arab boy of twelve will beat his own mother, and women have no authority over their own children after the age of two.

Evelyn

[Typed, typed signature. SSC]

To Otto Theis

Bou-Saada
December 31, 1923

HAPPY NEW YEAR TO BOTH OF YOU.

Dear Otto:

Bou-Saada is a microcosm of society presented with a crudeness and simplicity that a child would get. In looking at arabs you see why and how people arrived at a respectable ideal, at the feeling that it was better to have some decent hypocrisy about yourself than to be simple and blatant in cruelty as the arabs are. They just never need to excuse themselves for doing what other races do under cover, and I find myself anglo-saxon enough to get the hump when I contemplate it. Natural selection functions here without any Christian modification. The biggest most brutal males get the best food and the warmest clothes and look like Jesus Christs of healthy stock, gods all mighty in their own minds without any sickness of the imagination to identify them with their inferiors. They are probably very kind and condescending to the women who are pretty and submissive enough to deserve it, and throw all the best bones to the children that cry the last. But a great many of the children cry most of the time. Every evening you can hear all up and down the streets the little girls sent to ask alms of prosperous relatives. They sit in the doorways sometimes for hours together wailing a stereotyped plea with a monotony and persistence that compliments the nerves of the people indoors who seem to pay no attention to it. The men wear wool burnouses, but I have yet to see any but the Jewish women who have changed their red calico robes for anything more suitable to the winter climate.

It snowed here last week and barefooted girls without any undies (quite visibly) were running around in it. Not that the men dont suffer too in their degree for some of them are the most artistic collections of rags I ever saw, and there are dozens of the nomad variety camping around here in exposed tents with no covering but their skins and no firewood but what they can collect in a place forty kilometres from any woods.

The fact that we live opposite the police station doesnt add to our cheerful impressions. It is a French police station and the arab policemen are too unimaginative to keep up with the New York variety, are really very nice men (honest) - I dont think arabs have any lust for creating suffering like the Spaniards do - but the collects of rags and dejection that are hauled in there every day make we want to make sententious remarks about the failure of a civilization being proven by the populousness of the jails, or something. Theres only one cell (quite as comfortable as an arab home) and quite unfurnished, and men women and children are all stuffed into the same darkness. Just what this proximity does to divert them I dont know, and it may be the kindest method, only sometimes there are crazy men and very crazy drunks who wouldnt be attractive companions for the ladies even in the dark.

Oh, gee, well anyway this is a roundabout way of saying that one winter in a Muhamadon town is enough for a while. We want to go to the Grand Kahyble[24] (cant spell it) April and stay there through May as the scenery is very different from this, mountainous and luxuriant and the Khablye people are not arabs but Burbers (as maybe you know) and have different customs. And then June to go back to France. We'll have to return to Port Vendre and Collioure to collect maroquette[25] if the poor thing isnt dead and then we thought we would go to Brittany and stay two or three months. Merton and Sug then, IF our money is any more than now, want to spend two weeks in Paris. After that the problem of a warm cheap winter somewhere and we have thought of Corsica, the Belleryic islands, or trying Sicily again, whichever lives up to our ideal of prices and weather, and our last spring of freedom we want to go to London for two weeks before we go home.

I wrote the first draft of the kid story[26] and handed it over to Cyril who is helping it out with the addition of a trick dog, helping me to kill a lion the way it should be killed, and translating a whole lot of stuff about arabic customs to put them in the book correctly. He has already put in thirty pages of notes so I shall insist on calling it a collaboration whether he wants to or not. My part of it was the most rapid fire work I ever did, one hundred and seventy four pages in eight days. But dont let that prejudice you agin it, for I think it will be a very amusing little book when it is did, and Mertons illustrations are excellent. It is one of the many little boy lost stories, but this time the little boy lost collects an arab girl and is, because of his ignorance of arabic, tangled up in arab weddings, arab mosques, all kinds of arab customs, walks off with a tame lion, and has two dreams in which camels and desert tribes in rebellion and drums and spahis are all mixed up. The skeleton isnt original. I didnt have it in me to break ground that way for kids, but I think the detail is for kids very fresh and exciting.

Otto, we do wish that your vacations came oftener and that you and Louise Morgan could come here now. If she isnt well London weather is the worst that I can think of for her, and this place, though cold, is mostly so sunny, and really cheap when you get here. It has the best hotel I ever saw in a small town, Hotel Petit Sahara, and when we were there was twenty-five francs apiece a day for all of us, a hundred francs for all, and very good food. The bus ride from Alger here is hellish but only costs thirty-three francs each first class. For a brief stay ANYWAY, even if you didnt love arabs, it is frightfully interesting - a beautiful oasis as far as palm trees go, wonderful desert and low hills around it, and every detail of native life as strange and picturesque

---

24 The Kabyle are ethnic Berber tribes, indigenous to the Atlas mountain region of northern Algeria.
25 Evelyn loved animals and had a number of pets. Her parrot Maroquette came with her from Brazil to Europe.
26 *In the Endless Sands*, published in 1925, fictionalises a week when Jigg went missing in the desert and wasn't missed by his parents until a Berber child brought him home.

as possible in more than obvious ways. Oh, I do wish you could come. If we had beds you could stay with us. We have lots of room but no beds. Tom had to sleep with Jigeroo.

Lots and lots of love from all of us.

Evelyn

[Typed, typed signature. BRBL]

To Lola Ridge

Bou-Saada, Algeria

January 3 1924

Dear DEAR, your letter just five minutes ago, and I shall answer instanta because it happens to be a moment between laps of writing and I like to talk back as your letters come. Thank God, the Garland fund seems to be some use. Merton was saved from the pit of destruction and landscape gardening for the time being, though having to pay two life insurance policies and send monthly money to his kids has made it go almost as fast as yours. The Jewish woman who cooks for us was in a state today with Pyorrhoea and all her teeth falling out and it gave me the hump about what a lack of money does to you. We all need the dentist some and I swore by my pet gods that any money we ever have over living had to go to dentists first. You do too, Lola.

I appreciate your writing that letter when your fingers - or FINGER - had been at it all day. Im afflicted with a wart on my best type finger - the one I had before I went away - which is like a hoof and hurts so I cant use it. When the weather gets warmer Im going to have an operation. It came from typing on that one finger to the exclusion of all others and ought to be photographed to advertise good methods for stenographers.

One thing is disappointing. I do WISH you could come over here for two or three months. If not now later when we are back in France and the weather warmer. You wouldnt be annoyed with company, Lola dear, for I work six hours every day and Sug and Merton are gone all morning and all afternoon until tea at four thirty. We never see a soul and it would be practically the same in France. We live very cheaply and five dollars a week would cover any possible expense for you here, really it would.

Cyril did at last here [sic] from Marie who explained that she didnt write to him because of me, because "on account of Evelyn I cant write frankly". She also said that Swinburne hadnt written because he said I had "made mischief" between him and Sug - made trouble, it was. Thats the incident about the house. I dont feel easy about the money at all but I think it better to leave things as they are, thank your sweet heart for offering.

Did I tell you that Sug and I are writing a childs story together? It is a commercial effort in a sense as we all have no call of inspiration to kids, but I think you will all rather like it. It is laid in Algeria and I have put, with Sugs help at translating data, a lot of native customs etc in it, we have an exciting plot and a fantastic element, all the ingredients which Jigeroo approved. it was read out to him for criticism. Merton is doing some delightful simple drawings for it.

We all love you and if your liver incites you to blue letters why for gods sake write blue letters. We want most of all to hear from you. Bless you and your art, Lola, and may the New Year do more for it what it deserves. Bless your insides and make them behave as they should. Bless Davys health, jobs, and university sources.

And please God, let Lola come to France sometime.

Most, most affectionately from all of us,

Evelyn.

[Typed, signed. SSC]

To Otto Theis

Bou Saada

February 1924

Dear Otto:

This has been a kind of "old home" week, reviving habits and associations of the past. Merton has a lame back gotten while day labouring, and his back went wrong, and the illustrations for the kid book, because he has never done such before and didn't know how to make magazine cover pretty faces, nearly drove him wild, I heard in full about Seltzer turn down of the book, and, after being lavishing praise for not having had the pipp (it was two weeks before that I had the news) had the pipp. then we went over money accounts and I discovered that I had used some of the money Merton was going to send his kids in keeping house here (we run the accounts joint), and that we were in his debt (when he aint got a cent) and that we didnt have enough money to go to Paris as Sug had hoped, and Sug had the worst nervous collapse of a day Ive seen him have in a year - and - were still alive and love each other - but Gosh everybody is tired. We all, even me, behave better than we used to, but then moments of weakness aint entirely overcome.

Sug has suffered a lot lately from severe pains in his bladder and scared me to death, but he recuperates so whenever he does a good picture that Ive decided that he has no ills but mental ills. However their consequence may be as dangerous as any other, and Sugs longevity depends on whether he can put over something, either books or pictures this year. He is nearly destroyed by taking money from Marie as well as afraid it will be cut off, and the only justification to his pride for doing it will be putting over this work. As for his going back to work as he talks of at times, he simply couldnt. He wouldnt last a week. He is acutely neurotic and his heart is worse and worse. He continues to exhibit demoniacal energy by spurts, and if he has any luck he may begin to live more calmly, otherwise not. Mertons being with us which began for me as a doubtful and perhaps selfish experiment, has been entirely justified I think even for Sug, for Merton is sincerely devoted to Sug and admiring of him and appreciative of his qualities and is a perfect angel at helping to remove from Sugs shoulders practical burdens concerned with the details of living.

Im a fiend to make money now. Kid book first commercial job of my life, and we honestly think it is valuable that way. Jigeroo loves it. Mertons pictures go with the book but he wants a flat price and not a high one, they are seven colored drawings and very good and atmospherey of this place, done from Algy models. If this kid book goes Sug and I will write one very two years.

LOTS OF LOVE

evelyn

[Typed, typed signature. BRBL]

To Lola Ridge

Bou Saada

February 24, 1924

[page 1 missing] We agreed to pay half a gardeners wages to get our winter food supply out of this backyard and all we have had so far has been the violets a bowl of salad and a reddish or two. And the old gardener, whose wages are two dollars a month, has every day another child die so he wants about two months in advance. And to show he is worth it he picks me bouquets that are as compact and indestructible as indoor baseballs, and as sedate and defiantly surrounded by prickly foliage as a maiden Victorian with hairpins and frills. If we could find the Arab secret of subsistence on nothing this place would be ideal for us.

But it isnt ideal, and we dont like Arab life a little bit. It snowed today - though all the fruit trees are in bloom, peaches mostly, and only last week were warm and wonderful little shaggy powder puffs on stems in which blood seemed to run instead of sap, and bees and flies crawled and hummed, and the sky was like a blue rock and there were some little snow-foam of cloud right over the trees and it was like snow in the garden of Paradise.

You will wonder then why we dont like Arab life. It is because there is no intensity in it, even of machines, except the depressing intensity of sordid Arab religion? Even if we cant be rich I want to see somebody who is. Never in Bou-Saada have we seen one woman in anything more regal than calico, never one child who wasnt dirty and out at heels. Occasionally a man is impressive by the height of his turban and the whiteness of his linen and the gorgeousness of silver embroidery on his velvet jacket. But you know even he lives in a mud hovel and starves his wife. We were almost swamped last month by trying on a little meagre charity, but it is another grain of sand in all the sand there is, and I dont think the people are very unhappy anyway. They dont protest or want to. And this stupid Koran which is going to take them all to heaven and such a dingy heaven anyway. We think of Romanism as formulated, but that ritual gives much more than this deathly penance of learning parrot wise verse and lines verse and line and droning it morning and night.

Today the administration is trying to make a hit with tourists and has arranged a falcon hunt. Lots of stodgy French and English from Alger down and have gone out thirteen kilometres to see the falcons loosed on some poor hares and pigeons. There is also a dance of the Ouled Nails tonight and if I hadnt got sick we would have gone. But I think the weather will cook that too as it is in a tent. You see the Ouled Nails used to be almost like sexual priestesses but now they live in a licensed house of prostitution and are just a lot of mangy bitches as hard as nails and not much more lovely. A funny thing is that the fact that they are femmes public has not modified certain religious modesties. A Mahomden may sleep with one of the ladies but he may not see her unclothed, nor any women than his wives.

Arabs have this awful puritan license, but it remains puritan for they condemn this world and the flesh and woman as a minister to the flesh. See a ragged ragged old man, a man of fabulous rags, going by with a ragged dirty woman whose slippers are falling to pieces and held on with string, and she has her face as carefully veiled as if most of her anatomy wasnt leaking through the rents and wears. Wish people could see their own conventions in the light of others, but British etc come here, shake their heads, and go back to worship the Virgin Mary and attend balls with ladies nude, so to speak, on the upper level.

Yet Arabs arent a bit mystic. Their God is sensual purely in the sense of external sensational non-subjective. And their music so crass and terrible, their way of singing like brass-the brass city of Solomon in the story - a brazen external impenetrability. Only difference from our puritans is that their contempt for this world is perfect and negative and not a living torturing effort at contempt. And their next world has not such a poetic hell nor such a rapturous and complacent heaven. Heaven you reach by hard work in reciting Koran and prayers, not passion, just rote.

They are so very mental and so naive as well - but it is not emotional naivete, and their conventions have the perfection of fixity. Their shoes which are the only pretty thing the women wear (the few women who wear shoes) of red leather have a touch of green thread a bit of silver embroidery very conventionalized and supplied with a restraint, a mental correctness, which would be westernly impossible to people twice as sophisticate. The jewelry is fine in only a few cases, but mostly quite crude and heavy, of metalled five franc pieces and really made into jewelry as an easy way to preserve wealth among people who have no banks or closets or drawers or trunks to lock thinks in. No furniture in their houses, in poor houses nothing at all but a pile of dry grass to sleep in, in rich houses a rug or two and maybe rugs on the wall, a taboret for coffee, brass trays to carry food in, no knives and forks.

Little girls have a nauseating and unpleasant precociousness and a total unintelligence, just a kind of suspicious cunning and no more concentration than rabbits. They are never, in the country, educated at all, and as most boys learn only the Koran they are as bad. Last week Merton walked out to a small oasis near here and was accompanied home by the son of the caid[27] who was fifteen and had been married three years, and whom in spite of his distinguished lineage, begged old shoes old clothes penknives anything from Merton. All children beg. Even rich peoples children. It is quite convention for a child to beg.

Our house is opposite the filthy jail and the overnight cell opens on the street twenty feet from my bedroom window. So funny and so awful the continuous occupants. First place every morning the French Jew police sergeant goes in to the CELL to pea [sic], there being no toilet in the police station, and comes out arranging his trousers with an entire complacency. Stink ferocious. Most Arab men object to being locked up (they are awful thieves and tricksters but have the self-esteem of red Indians, only the women crassly) and they pound and shake the door all night. Twice recently raids on unlicensed brothels have filled cells with ladies glittering with tinsel and tinkly with necklaces and bracelets. When the door is opened I see inside dark shiny unrelated spots as if there were Christmas trees inside. Then make out a fat woman having a drink of water out of a galvanized scrubbing bucket. Some of the raided ladies insisted on their respectability and emerged to go to magistrate with their faces fully veiled.

Cyril and Merton and me and Jigeroo all love you so very much and so very much want you to be well and to finish the book but not to finish the book until you ARE well. And our dearest love to Davy, please, and, and, and lots of things I dont know how to write…

MY EYES FEEL BETTER FOR HAVING WRITTEN THIS

Evelyn.

[Typed, typed signature. SSC]

To Otto Theis

Bou Saada
March 3, 1924

Dearest Otto;

Gee, you have had a siege from Bou-Saada. The reason I havent written any since you first asked me last year, is that I knew only too well what would be the result. You see I cant write with emotional vividness unless I have an emotional reason for doing it. When you write a book, you always have a mystic belief that somewhere somebody is going to "understand you"- in other words accept your particular affirmations and denials. Well, what you write for a journal that has a definite policy you know this wonderful understanding cant be your object and so you (meaning me) feel cold to start on. I havent any dash at all. When I try to limit my own explorative function I just diminish my work without being able to make

---

27 Evelyn's idiosyncratic phonetic spelling has made it difficult to identify this individual. From the context, it appears he is some form of local dignitary.

the oratorical bridges in which bunk is scarcely perceptible as bunk in which is the talent of the real journalist.

What I feel behind your letter and your constant lovely decency to us, is that you are a damn tired man - lots tireder than you admit - and that we do wish vacation times werent so far away. I think what you say about the crowded house is truly a lovely compliment to a finely satisfactory relation, but I dont care how much you and Louise love each other, London is London and winter and measles and flue are such, and Im sure you are all in deadly need of a change. The cottage in Kent will help I know, but you must take that vacation, and damn it we insist, with us.

This seems to have been contradicted by my last letter which I wrote as a climax of a months fret over money. What we said, or I said, holds good as commonsense, except that it will be probably next to impossible to arrange steamer fares just so, off the bat, so we had as well settle down to leaving in the very late summer or the fall. In the meantime we are quitting Bou-Saada on the seventh and our address until we get a house will be care Mme Catherine Ramone de lHomme, Faubourg, Collioure, Pyrenees Orientales, France.

We hope to get a cheap place at Banyuls where there is fine swimming or if not there Arles or Amelie le Bain. Well let you know at once when we do.

Merton will be in London in May and give us mutual news of each other. Cyril may get as far as Paris but I am going to stay down south.

Of course as a person I think Cyril has the most titanic personality, the most instinctive profoundness of emotion, the most mental stretch of almost anybody living and it will be to me another proof that utter cynicism is the impossible unattainable answer to life if he does not find any sympathetic channel of expression anywhere.

Now if you and Louise will come to see us we will talk of something beside ourselves. And we will find a cheap place for you to stay. And I think we will all have a nice time.

Dont feel my heavy correspondence a burden. We see nobody at all and it is a relief to talk and I do it on paper but with no idea that a busy man ought to respond in kind.

Now, Otto, I aint as dangerous as I seem. Love to you all. Jig is in ecstasies over the stamps and will write to you.

Good luck and blessings,

Evelyn

[Typed, typed signature. BRBL]

Chapter 7

The French Riviera
May 1924 - March 1925

After an isolated winter in the remote Algerian desert, the Scott household returned to France in the spring of 1924. It was clear from Evelyn's letters that she had found it extremely difficult being so far from her dearest friends (Lola in New York City and Otto and his wife Louise in London) and it would have only been a matter of time before they found their way back to Europe.

A large number of empty envelopes, mostly addressed to Lola Ridge and Louise Morgan, were found during the research phase and these have been helpful in establishing the chronology of their lives. The letters that survived describe the return of Evelyn, Cyril and Jigg to the south coast of France, where the Scotts eventually found themselves in Banyuls-sur-Mer, a picturesque little fishing village in the French foothills of the Pyrenees. Merton had returned to London for reasons that are not clear from the correspondence but were probably related to his poor health and to attempts to find a gallery in which to exhibit his paintings.

To Lola Ridge

Banyuls-sur-Mer, France
May 1924

Precious Lola,

I am excited because Merton took the last cash he got and is off today to London on it to try to clinch the interest that has been stirred up there to try to clinch some sales. He is one of the sweetest people alive and with the worry of poor Suggies side should have turned my face to the wall ere now without him. Suggie is just himself, a marvel and lovely, but he certainly has gone through a hell of a lot of pain lately, and as soon as Merton gets back from London Sug will leave for Paris to see a specialist. Im divided between a desire to know the worst and a cowardly horror of the possible seriousness of the diagnosis. I just try for the present not to consider possibilities.

I cant write a letter today because I went to the hospital and had that miserable wart thing taken off my typing finger. I had it last year and didnt do anything and then putting vitriol on it made it worse so finally had to cut way under my nail and take five stitches on my finger and it makes me lame at typing. But gee Im glad to get out of it. Lord, this little operation reminds me most vividly of what you have just been through. Oh, God damn it, there is too MUCH pain in the world.

This is a very decent little flat, funny and dingy and cheap French formality but has a view of the sea and nice gay painted fishing boats and on the roof a lovely terrace that is quite private with a view of piled up mountain and little villages.

When we left Bou-Saada we came back a new way on the train and for four hours saw gorgeous aloof snow mountains like the Alps and June fields of wheat and olives spread out in tired youngness of afternoon light, really wonderful. Alger is beautiful land, but in much of it savagely poverty stricken. Only along the coast the French have made it prosperous. We all arrived ill and Merton again an angel of kindness. If everybody was strong it would be a nice world.

Ill write again when my finger gets more fluent. Please let us know how you are as soon as you can. Im so glad you are seeing that nice place. We all have occasional homesicks for the mermaid water.

Love and love and love and to Davy please when you write,

Evelyn

PS Banyuls is ten miles from Collioure where we were last year, is a larger town and cleaner but less picturesque.

[Typed, typed signature. SSC]

To Louise Morgan

Banyuls-sur-Mer
June 6, 1924

Dear Louise:

Dr Bennett carried Mutt to London to put him in a sanatorium and have him examined by a nerve specialist. Hell probably stay a month. It is supposed to be a secret that he is there and Dr B has promised to tell no one and let no one come near him, but if you will telephone and ask how he is Ill be much obliged. Phone is Langham 1190. He went off doped.

Dear Louise, you are sweet to have written so nice a letter in such a nasty place and to cheer me up about the awful end of your so-called rest, and I could hug you for what you say of Suggie, who I do think with all my heart is one of the greatest men that ever lived and a very great artist. *Just as great an artist as a man, emphatically.* I am convinced that it will some day be recognized, because the proof is so indestructible and beyond contention, but I love you for seeing it now when it hasnt become a fashionable thing to see. Warm genuine appreciation like yours is a great help, and Sug has had to stand alone in every way more than anybody ought to.

I am so all in I can scarcely write, Im ashamed to say that before doctor B had got out of the house I collapsed and behaved like a regular Victorian. I think I cried for eight hours at a stretch and would have graced the pages of Dickens, though I had the grace to do it in my own room. Today I have my monthly visitor and am generally so low that a mere boo frightens me.

I wish you could have stayed to see the circus that was perpetrated the night you left and every night since, a wonderful little two by four show right under the window. They had a caravan in which they carried a pig, five chicks, and a dwarf, and there was a poor tiberculor lady with a baby who did bareback riding in a lachrymose way, a plump and sprightly lady who was a tight rope walker, and a papa who could turn somersalts and juggle barrels on his feet. The dwarf was the clown. One joke was to select five small boys from the audience, offer to take their pictures, and pose them thus *[series of stick figures drawn here]*. First little boy is holding his nose. Second boy has his head in the air very proud and his fingers in the armholes of his vest and is watching the sky. Third little boy is pointing disdainfully. Fourth little boy squats on his hams. Says boy one, Mon Dieu, what a smell. Says boy two, It wasnt I. Says boy three, there he is. Boy four says nothing. How is that for French rural wit to be exhibited at Collioure.

As for our part of the visit, we loved you and having you. I wish it could have been for a long, long time *you are writing.*

Our love to Otto. Im going to write decently when I recuperate.

Evelyn

[Typed, signed. Handwritten insertions. BRBL]

To Otto Theis

Banyuls-sur-Mer
June 8, 1924

Dear Otto:

I have made a mess of my affairs again. My private opinion is that Mertons collapse is due as much and more to the artificialities that have hedged in his personal life as it was due to worries about money. He simply can not be anything but spontaneous and obviously honest.

I am enclosing a letter to him[28] which I want you to deliver simply because you will be able to judge whether or not he is in anything like a condition for serious discussion, which I can not judge at this distance. I cant take any of his friends into my confidence. I want you to read the letter, however boring and annoying the process, for Merton knows that you are the only person with whom I have always been quite frank and it may be a relief to him to talk to you. I shall write him that, as soon as he is well enough to be about, he will please go to see you to talk over some plans, and you can go somewhere to lunch or tea and have the letter presented. If you dont want to do this, Otto, it will be alright. But I am asking it knowing I impose a difficult thing on

---

28 This letter has not survived.

you. Judging by what happened to Merton physically, this is really a matter of life and death. I think it best he should not have come back here with an emotional elan and have a shock. It might produce the same result as before. I think it would be better to get the edge of the shock over while he is among doctors and friends. If you disagree please tell me.

I can trace a great deal of the depression and overkeying of last winter to incidents relative to myself and him. I hadnt considered enough what it was doing to Sug, but now I see the whole thing, in spite of Mertons protests, is a physiological and psychological impossibility for Merton too.

If you will read the letter you will have something of an idea of how things stand. I really love Merton very much, but I love Sug more I know or I could not dream of hurting Merton this much. But I wont discuss it for I am in an utter inward mess - almost as bad as four years ago - and worse because its all happened before with no solution. Merton is as thoroughly sweet and genuine a person as ever lived and I have three years, nearly, of knowing him to test my opinion by. He really has been a constant pleasure to me. Sug, of course, remains the man with the most titanic pride, the greatest moral and mental strength, and the most infinite capacity for tenderness and self-immolation without bunk I ever saw, also the most wonderful theoretic foresight based on sensitive intuitions. But - My defect is that I had too much of an analytic bent to accept the usual self-deceptions, but nothing wherewith to conquer my most ordinary of human nature. Anyway Merton will get over it.

If you dont want, when Merton is better, to deliver this letter, or if you prefer to mail it to him, alright, only please be sure he is better. But if you will let him talk to you I think it might do him good. He is really very self-respecting and self-responsible - not an artistic monster - and I dont think he will impose on you very much. He may regard this quite sensibly or he may want to rush down here, but anyway it will, it seems to me, be good that he has some forewarning of what Sug and I have discussed.

Affectionately

evelyn

Just say no flat if you want to keep entirely out and mail the letter back, but there wont really be a mess.

PS An hour later: perhaps it isnt fair to you as Sugs friend to ask you to do this, so will you keep up on Mertons health and mail him the letter when he is much better? That neednt envolve you. I wish youd read the letter though. Merton will never be nasty to Sug and he might need a friend very much who was also our friend.
[Typed, typed signature. BRBL]

There is a period during the summer of 1924 during which no letters appear to have survived, although undoubtedly many were written. Evelyn writes again in October from Beziers, a short distance along the coast from Banyuls; these letters focus on the deteriorating relationship between Evelyn and Owen Merton, due largely to the additional pressure put on him by his late wife's parents to return to Long Island and take responsibility for his children, Tom and John Paul.

To Louise Morgan

23 Place Emile Zola

Beziers, Herault

October 1924

Dear Louise:

This was what happened in Paris (of course). Jig and I had only been there three days when Jig acquired one of his old bronchial colds. The dampness of that place is simply poisonous to us. He was sick for a couple of days, too sick to go anywhere and then I came down with the same germs and an attack of grippe that gave me fever and made me so ghastly if unimportantly ill that I imagined Id have to go to a hospital or something to get out of the hotel. As a matter of fact I was only really ill a little longer than Jigeroo, but as we had planned a week in Paris you can see how our time was chiefly occupied. I was so all-in and discouraged I didnt budge except to go out and get my meals and two expeditions in those first two days when we went to the Louvre and to Les Invalides. Then as the devil would have it, I hit town the same day as Roger Fry[29] and Sug was seeing a lot of him and not at our hotel either and we only saw Sug for dinner.

Then Merton came up to take me back - youll hardly believe me if I go on with this tale of woe, but its all true - (AND THIS IS A SECRET WHICH WOULD RUIN Merton IF KNOWN. NOBODY HERE OR New York TO KNOW HE WENT TO Paris) - Merton came up after a week with his aunt and uncle seeing the Midi, took leave of them and came on the same route on another train, to go back down south with me because traveling distances makes me ill and I cant risk them alone.

Well Merton is still in miserable health and aunt and uncle, who travel well when alone, are so afraid he will come at them for money that they travel cheapest when with him. He was sightseeing on his feet and had to stand on several crowded train trips, did their errands, and missed some of his meals and his heart gave out, so he reached Paris sick too. He had to lie down most of the time between packing and was really ill when he got on the train with me. For cheapness in seeing France and with the idea of avoiding fatigue we came via Dijon, spent the night there, were misinformed about trains, and even at the station (which we went to with our lunch only started because the train left an hour earlier than time table said) had a practical joke played on us by some railway employees who told us our train was in and about to leave when it hadnt even come (was a half hour late) so that as a result my trunk

---

29   Fry was a British artist, influential critic and member of the Bloomsbury Group. Evelyn later maintained that he had praised Cyril's painting.

was left behind to be shipped petit vitesse by a hotel employee (it has all the clean clothes in it).

Aboard the train there wasnt a seat in the second class (the PLM[30] is a hellish rich mans road, only one second class car in a long train) so we bought first class on the train (if we had bought first class before we left we could have caught a later express and saved half the journey). All of us had colds and were fagged without lunch. Arrived at Avignon at eight-thirty that night (trip one thirty to eight thirty) the town had three hundred pilgrims in it and no hotel room, so we all had to go in one room (something discretion disapproves) and the beds were impossible for two, so, Jig and Merton getting to sleep first, I spent the night coughing on a chaise lounge. Well Avignon was charming to see and we sight-saw the whole day, but left at five that evening expecting to get a dining car dinner. Diner was taken off and we bought ham sandwiches, after eating them had to wait a half hour at Cette where we might have had dinner anyway, and did try, but I was so tired it made me lose it.

Arrived at Beziers at nine and I was unwell and so sick I could hardly get to the hotel. Spent the next day in bed and Merton rushing around to try and get some kind of servant to help out in this flat. Yesterday I revived and here we are. (It wasnt time for me to be unwell either, moving did it, so not imprudence.)

You will understand I am in no state to judge of the beauties of Beziers, which Merton picked out because it was the only big town in a hot climate in which he was able to find a flat for three hundred francs a month. Place Emile Zola is appropriately surrounded by wagon yards, wood yards and alcohol manufactures. Otherwise the flat is a shrunken edition of Banyuls, very decently furnished in an impossible style, and has running water and a two burner gas stove. This place is like a mixture of Spain and my own dear southland. It is a big and rather ugly middle-sized city where bullfighting is the chief interest of the population. The leading citizens look like retired planters and never seemed to wear clean collars, but there are a great many of them, a place de theatre, innumerable newly decorated movies, and lots of cafes. Its amusing really, but I havent yet seen the wonderful subjects which Merton promises to disclose for painting.

Sug was lovelier an ever and I wish you had been able to come over. Just now Merton has an extra hard row to hoe because of the trouble in getting back enough health to get any work done but it hasnt hurt his sense of humour or his disposition, and I guess we are all going to be rich and famous yet. Only damn mortal flesh.

I wish you would feel sometimes later that a trip to France was what you needed. Youd like to see this funny place anyhow.

More and more love to you and Otto.

evelyn

[Typed, typed signature. BRBL]

---

30   *The Chemins de fer de Paris à Lyon et à la Méditerrané*, estabished in 1857, was one of the main French railway companies at the time.

To Lola Ridge

Beziers
October 15, 1924

Darling Lola:

Gladys must have told you all our news, the wonderful hit Sugs pictures made in Paris etc. Several critics used the strongest terms of praise and in a discriminating way, for Parisians are at least mentally sensitive to the new experience if not themselves very richly creative. And Roger Fry is such a staunch believer in him that it does your heart good in a day when nobody in power ever seems to bet on anything but the safe thing. Sug wrote that the gallery has been crowded straight along and the show will be extended for a few days. As we didnt know any newspaper people we have been quite surprised at all the press attention too. Merton thinks such a thing never happened at a first show before.

This brings me to the bullfight I went to see. This beastly town is half Spanish and has Spanish matadors and things. I saw six bulls killed - there were two more to be - and four horses, and never saw anything so ghastly as the CROWD. I think the Spanish are drunk of drama and the dramatic element in appreciation is aesthetically non-valid. I think Spanish art and life goes to pot in drama - even El Greco is tainted - and in the mass its a mess. Picassos real aesthetic sense is limited and utterly lost in the grand gesture though that gesture is concealed under the prose nicety of cubism-naturalism of the arts. The ultra cubists are utter if sincere fakes.

Well, back to Beziers which is like a little Toledo on a high hill, very beautiful from a plain and canals bordered by huge hundred year old cedars formally planted. But OH what swinish people. The dregs of French peasant winegrowing commercialism without any picturesque much less aesthetic elements. Rich wine growers and wholesale grocery men. Its a nasty place, even after Paris which I found absolutely vacant and formal over a commercialism less romantic and titanically grotesque and even more cruel than New York. Notre Dame is a banal tradition, but the only beauty in the place is there in a however inferior gothic remnant. The only art I like is gothic art and Chinese classic and Egyptian. We were too bust to see theatres and things, but I went a lot to the Louvre which is inhabited by American ladies sewing circles and culture clubs, and to the Luxembourg which is the rottenest piffling gallery I ever saw, except for one room with two Cezannes and a few impressionists. And we saw the modern show in some board barracks uptown, and it was a mess of conflicting formulas - not three pictures that had any relation to immediate seeing. The French have forgot that the living eye is the basis of the visual experience and are more literary than the Academicians, only Academic literaryness is at least sometimes amusing as anecdote and these things are charts.

Sug and Merton simply rose to the gods after such a sight. Sugs things are really beautiful enough to make you cry, Lola, the best, and Merton had evolved from that youngness and fresh virile color into an infinitely greater complexity of organization without losing the powerfulness of a youthful experience. He will always be of a more lyric bent than Sug, but it is wonderful to note the fine point of divergence - Sugs toward an exquisite mental balance evolved from hair-trigger emotion and full of emotion, and Merton always clinging to the emotional vision with the mental subtlest intimated but not stated in such exquisite fullness. Well Ive had fun out of seeing them.

Mertons rather ill yet, in fact damn wobbly, but I think a year will see him his old self. *[remainder of letter missing]*

[Typed, not signed. SSC]

To Louise Morgan

Beziers
March 12, 1925

Dear Louise:

I am in trouble again, as Otto would expect, and this time I dont see any cure. Merton has left here in a condition that looked near insane and is bound more or less for London, but I don't know whether he is desperately ill on route, has committed suicide, or has breathed a first sigh of relief in freedom.

Our mutual problems have worried him unbearably. They are these:

--The Jenkins[31] have his kids.

--He has no money to support his kids.

If the Jenkins learned of our relation even respectably as marriage they are so jealous of him and devoted to the memory of their daughter, they might likely prevent him from seeing his kids at all.

It is made harder in that he is fond of the Jenkinses, and they of him, he owes them money and they have been lavish in solicitude since he was ill.

II If he was known to be married to me or living with me his aunt and uncle in London would withdraw the help they give such as financing his show etc. They may help substantially if he is tactful but he would have to pay them long visits and jolly them.

III His health and emotions combine so that to give up painting for a job would finish him - at it alone would me to have him.

IV I wont live with anybody unless I can see and be with Sug frequently, leaving Sug free to form his own alliances but with the same proviso. This is Sugs wish as well as mine. Constant difficulties in manners make this difficult. Jig calling Sug father and me living with Merton make servants etc difficult to both Sug and Merton.

V If Merton gets his own kid with him and he broods all the time because the kid loves him and is away from him, the kid will get wise. The kid incidentally showed a wild jealousy of me in Bermuda - Merton adores this kid.

---

31 The Jenkins were the parents of Owen's late wife and, since her death from cancer, had objected to his having care of his elder son Thomas. While with the Scotts, Thomas had not been well-behaved towards Evelyn.

V My health is horrible and I am a physical coward beside. I cant be left entirely alone while Merton either goes to America to see his kids or to England to stay with relatives.

VI Merton has to provide for his kids and he can not do so thru his earnings. Anything complicating diplomacy complicates this.

VII Merton is unconsciously respectable and resents an equivocal relation. He adores Sug but is jealous of him - I dont wonder.

VII My bad health and depressions are a strain on anybody. Merton has worked hard taking care of me when he wasnt well himself.

IX Ill health hampers sex the original basis of our alliance. I am getting fogged out and prematurely old. I am an awful pessimist. I am no worldly help.

Thus, Merton finally decided he wanted to quit. Except for a completely insoluble sexual miss I would try hard to make all with Sug. But we dont get over the mess. I want him to be free in that way. He is less able than Merton to see after a semi-invalid. I love Merton very much, only less than Sug, and as a sex mate he makes me very happy. Id give all but very beautiful demi-semi non sexual socalled free relation with Sug to have Merton. But I cant kidnap him and if he doesnt want me I gotta accept it.

I wont bother or pressure but I shall be dotty if I don't know he is alright. I am here alone. Oh Louise I will be so grateful. I do love him very much - [*illeg*] will cure me -[*illeg*] thats the awful nothing lasts with me.

Love Evelyn

[Handwritten, signed. BRBL]

To Louise Morgan

Beziers, France
March 16, 1925

Dearest Louise:

Can you convey this letter[32] to Merton by hand? Is that asking too much of you? We did have such an awful explosion I cant bear quitting or not quitting to finish in excitement. I want to be calmer and more decent about it. I will be so grateful to you if you can convey this letter. I know where Merton[33] is because the postman was confused about the mail address and showed me a telegram Merton had sent him.

Probably you and Otto have a nausea of these perpetual seances, and I hope someday I can give you a kind of apologia por vita mia which will make them less revolting as a spectacle? Sug is the greatest man that ever lived, and I love Merton very dearly, and I cant change these two feelings. Well you are a kind and beautiful and generous friend, and thank you dear dear Louise.

[Typed, not signed. BRBL]

---

32 This has not survived.
33 The implication is that Merton is in London.

To Louise Morgan

Beziers, France
March 17 [1925]

Dearest Louise:

Thank you thank you thank you for your telegram.[34] I am still a little lightheaded with worry as I havent had any word as to what happened after the departure and I still cant believe that my invariable messes prove me all wrong, but it is a pretty sickly feeling to have got to this again.

Poor Merton has about as hard a practical problem as could exist. In the letter I sent you I told him to wait six months to settle it, if he emotionally wanted to. But anyhow there is the chance. Of course what is making fatigue now is simply not knowing whether Merton is ill or well or glad or sorry or how much in need of practical looking after. I judge he aint dead or Id have heard of it. Im amused at my own suc [sic], as last night I woke up with the absolute conviction that Merton was alright and everything would be adjusted, and then suddenly realized how when you are too tired to think any further your mechanism makes you believe what you want to believe.

But anyway if I am not running up too big a bill for telegrams, will you wire me again if ever you do have any news? Or if you should actually see Merton too write me your opinion of how he is. Maybe he is fine and anxiety wasted, but until you know you cant keep your imagination quite under. This is six days of silence.

The postman showed me a wire from Montpellier last Thursday and yesterday I tried to follow that up by wiring to some friends Merton has who were at Montpellier and had expected to come over here on friday last, but didnt show up so he must have stopped there to head them off, which looks as if he was all there on thursday last anyway. I wired the friends that I had lost Mertons mail address and could they supply it, a very diligent telegrams, signed Scott only, and they know who we are. I also paid a reply, but no answer came so I guess they had left town. they were only transients.

I also wired to Merton himself care of Francoise at Coullioure as he had intended going there to pack up his things, and asked him in wire to acknowledge the message, but there was no answer to that either. I dont dare wire anybody in Paris for fear of making a scandal. So there is nothing to do but wait and see what happens. I guess I am a pretty thorough idiot alright, trying to make life square with things nobody else can, and thinking all the time next year next year when everything is settled everybody will be happy again.

[Typed, not signed. BRBL]

---

34   This has not survived.

To Louise Morgan

Beziers

March 18, 1925

Dearest dear Louise:

Day before yesterday I wired Mertons English friends to know if they had his address, said we had lost it and had important mail. Yesterday noon an answer from Merton said, leaving for London address care Bennett. So he had been in Montpellier all the time I was reading the newspapers to see if any suicide or accident had happened to a foreignor. Well the fact he did something awful is nothing in my life if the reasons for doing it were the obvious ones. I have done too many awful things myself to judge without corroboration.

It all began when Merton first showed uncertainty about our future and his capacity to adapt himself to it. He went to Cette to collect himself, and I would not have minded his going if he had not gone leaving me so many suggestions that his worries connected with me were too much for him. When he came back without telling him I drank a whole bottle of codeine and took twenty-four heart depressing pills. I had worked myself into a state that I thought I was killing Merton and Sug both. Im ashamed of having done it since it didnt work and only gave me pains in the heart and Merton the worst scare he ever had in his life. Then his assurances that things would work out right bucked me up again. I guess he never got over the suicide scare and subconsciously turned against me from that moment, for almost ever since everything he has said about our future has been unhopeful and uncertain. I guess he has been trying to break ever since and couldnt bring himself to it.

Please dont ever tell about the suicide thing because Sug doesnt know of it and I never want him to. It would only give him another trauma, and as far as I can tell about myself I never want to do any such again. That the third real time in my life I ever did. Once Otto knows. Twice was three years ago in NY when Marie butted in and this time. And I am heartily ashamed of things like that that go no further.

When Merton said he was going to break for good I went clean stark mad, not that I didnt know what I was doing, but I was frantic to keep him, and I cant do tricks to charm, so I took it out by saying I hated him (when I love him) that he was a fiend from hell or something equally polite (when he is a fuddled, oppressed, perplexed and in many ways lovely person) that I felt like murdering him (that was almost true) that I hoped he would go thru as much hell as he was causing me that moment (and as soon as he left I wrote to the Garland fund to see if I could get him any money and I havent an ounce of revenge in me overnight) and then I struck him (something I never even wanted to do to anybody but mother when she and Sug quarrelled, then sometime both) and in trying to keep me from hitting me in the face I mean me hitting him, he pushed me back with so much force that I fell on the floor (it just happened to be slick tiles) and my hip and back have been all over bruises. After which he rushed out of the house like a lunatic and I heard trucks going out tho there is no train at that hour to Paris, but must have been one for Montpellier. Jig was sent to call him as he left the house, and he came back and said I was "beautiful" - god knows why - and offered to kiss me goodbye - which I wouldnt accept.

Well, that is the whole nasty story, except that I spent all night praying he would come back, and all the next night imagining the doorbell had rung and he was there, and got so superstitious that I looked in the Bible every day to see if it prophecied that he was coming back.

Louise nothing has ever altered my feeling for Sug, who is the most beautiful and noblest and strongest person I ever saw and a wonderful artist as well. But I cant help the sex sidetrack. It is very complex - and i cant help at the present moment loving merton just unreasonably, and, of course, hoping he wants to reconsider things, tho if he doesnt being thru with me is simple. it always has been. but i am on a good deal of a helpless strain, waiting to know whether all the expressions of love just were contradicted in a couple of hours of argument or not. Of course the kids have nothing to do with it. The competition is between me and mertons desire to succeed as a painter, and i am a handicap to that. I offered six months to decide this and will probably get turned down which serves me right for being a fool. But darling please tell me how sick you are and how wicked i am to pile confidences now? and let me know what you see and think. I love you and otto and lots because you love sug.

I thank you with all my heart for your GOODNESS. i will never never forget it. and for your being able to love the beauty of cyril and yet find affection for merton. i thank otto same because he always does see tolerantly.

[Typed, not signed. BRBL]

To Louise Morgan

Beziers

March 19, 1925

Dearest dear kid, the daily bulletin in which you can trace conditions of mind evoluting, but with a good deal of conscience for having made a sick wimmins telephone all over town, tend to be telegrams etc. Dear Louise, please forgive it, but I simply didnt know what else to do.

I guess I want now to win you over to my state of mind about Merton. Please dont blame him. If it is true and it seems that he doesnt love me that is hardly a matter for condemnation on any grounds but taste, and if he took a long time to find it out and did so inconveniently, I guess there is no propitious moment for doing exactly the opposite of what the other fellow wants you to. As to the way it was done, taking into account that Merton never is clearheaded when he is confronted by a lot of unanswerable problems, and very few people are, with the other fact that I went wild at once he suggested that he felt he had to quit to save himself from assuming something he couldnt carry thru - will those things combined, always accepting his temperament and not criticising it by an ideal, explain to me pretty thoroughly his taking the worst way to do it. Any way would have seemed bad to me.

I still want him and I still offer the six months to find ways, but the answer to that is so simply does or doesnt he want me and will pretty soon be answered I guess. Naturally all my reason tells me it is in the negative, tho I hope differently. We werent unhappy except during the last month when he was stirred up by the Jenkins about his kids and by the faint hope of money on this show. Then every day there were arguments as to how this could be settled, and as the arguments never got anywhere it was like taking fifteen minutes a day for both of us to butt our heads against a stone wall as hard as we could. The result was a bruised brain a piece and absolutely no capacity for anything but negative measures.

Yes, Sug, is here and as always as near perfect in understanding and exquisite in tolerance and a gently ironic benevolence as any human being could be. Its up to me to make my selection, which I still must in confessing I want Merton, but nothing can ever break down my love for Sug or mar his beautiful attitude toward me, and Merton never wanted that no matter how hard things were I know. being calmer only makes me clearer in knowing how much I do want Merton and how very unlikely it is that he will care to resume anything he has made such a struggle to break from.

Merton was always very frank in saying he could not bring idealism into any relation without sex, and maybe my being ill just killed his feeling for me of which sex was a symbol. evelyn

[Typed, typed signature. BRBL]

To Louise Morgan

chez Mme Francoise Bernardi
Faubourg, Collioure
April 4 [1925]

Precious old dear, dont feel a hundred because I think you make yourself so lovely to everybody you look about twentyeight at most instead of ninetyeight. Thank you for note when in such a scramble of things. Im glad Mr E whoever came out alright, and I know you helped him same as me.

Please you and merton open letter which is money for two months for jig and me but I am borrowing on sug at present and I want merton to get an overcoat and I want you all to see if I can make this check over to him, please ask otto, if I cant just keep it, but I want merton to take out the necessary on me.

Well there are some sweet people in the world, you and otto and mutts and sug for one. I feel rather sick from moving but pretty happy. I hope you can come to paris. listen, honey, say again can you stand having me on you when you have all them companies. I am so scared of putting too much on you? Please be brutal if necessary. Sug is going up with me and try to find a place for jig near him. we have no fire in this house and are frizz but collioure looks damn fine after beziers flats. Seeing my poor old polly parrot[35] today. I think he knows me. Love you and bless you and thank you for UNDERSTANDING people I love - all best two so completely. I want to know more about this here novel. evelyn

[Typed, typed signature. BRBL]

To Louise Morgan

Collioure
April 5, 1925

Dearest Louise:

Merton probably hasnt told you but he had got down to five shillings when he wrote me. He must have some money and he must be made to take what came in that bank envelope because I will have more next month. Please ask otto how I can turn this money over to merton quickest from this distance. My future as much as his depends on what he does now and he has GOT to have it.

I wont write any more but get this in the mail and please see that something is done about this so i can bless you again, you are so damned good to us. Thank you dear dear louise and good luck

evelyn

[Typed, typed signature. BRBL]

---

35 Evelyn had a pet parrot which she brought from Brazil and which followed her around, although it is not clear who took care of the parrot in the intervals when he was not with Evelyn.

Chapter 8

Merton

March - August 1925

The letters in this chapter cover the period from March 1925, when Owen Merton sent a telegram to Evelyn to tell her he was leaving, until the end of August that year when Gladys Grant wrote to Otto Theis to describe, in harrowing detail, the effect that Evelyn was having on her friends as she tried to come to terms with Merton's departure.

These letters, written to close friends, are very personal expressions of emotional turmoil. They are self-indulgent and self-pitying in equal measure while betraying little thought of the sensibilities of the recipient. Given her reputation as a novelist and essayist, they are astonishingly verbose and incoherent. Portions refer to Evelyn's previous relationships, and how they compare to her relationship with Merton, and display little sensitivity to the possible feelings of her correspondents who also knew Merton and had shown themselves to be his friend. The letters also include lengthy passages about her relationship with Cyril and, irrespective of her reputation as a novelist, poet and essayist, there are numerous long, confused passages relating to her feelings about both Merton and Cyril which have not been included as they repeat the sentiments Evelyn expresses in other letters.

To Evelyn Scott

EVELYN SCOTT
23 PLACE EMILEZOLA BEZIERS 22 MARCH 1925 PARIS
LOVE YOU PLEASE TRUST ME LEAVING MUTT
[Telegram. SFC]

To Owen Merton

OWEN MERTON CHEZ MICHEL BERAUDI
FAUBOURGCOLLIOURE MARCH 29 1925 BEZIERS
UNLESS BREAK FOR YOUR PERMANENT HAPPINESS PLEASE RECONSIDER
AND COME BACK TO MAKE PLANS WITH CYRIL ME LOVE YOU DONT BELIEVE

THIS NEEDED WIRE NO IF DECISION MAKE *[sic]* IS FINAL ALSO YOUR HEALTH
[Telegram. SFC]

In June 1925, Evelyn and Merton returned to New York on board SS Roussillon. *Once in the United States, she stayed for varying periods with loyal friends in New York City, while Merton went to stay with his in-laws, the Jenkins, at their home in Long Island. Evelyn spent her time during these few months writing long and anguished letters about the relationship with Merton.*

To Lola Ridge

c/o Gladys Grant
31 West 14th Street
July 7, 1925

Darling darling Lola:

I hope you are better. I wish you were in the country. I am just as obsessed as ever and will be until I hear from or at least of Owen. It is as I told you impossible to for to mentally reject by hatred three years of the closest identity I ever had with any living creature. Owen is in me as a part of myself. One thing must be clear to him. If it is the sign of me in pain that has made him feel any escape from the present good for me, that is not true. Any compromise for me, provided it is not a sheer act of sacrifice for him, provided he wants me still, is good for me and will save me from this deterioration of will and health that I dont seem able to stop. If he cant live with me I will live by myself, but is it necessary to kill everything in us in order to save the best for him. Isnt he killing himself inwardly too.

I dont know how mad I am, but I must pretend to hope for the present to save myself from literal almost physiological insanity. My depression has been the secret fear of losing him. His depression has probably been largely the spectacle of my depression. The reason I have been afraid is that I recalled the kind of brutal insanity which possessed him after Ruths death[36] and I was afraid that trouble would, as it has, drive him into the same state again. If he has been afraid of my dying like Ruth that is nonsense. I shall be quite well with time and something to start with. And if he is too ill to bear me as a practical responsibility I will handle myself, given his psychic cooperation in doing it. Dont threaten him with disaster for Gods sake, yet make him see that which I know, that his own sensitivity can not survive sanely the present method. I want to help him anyway on earth. If he really hates me then of course the help must be for me to disappear for him. I must find out.

Dont worry about me because it is quiet here and the last thing that can be done isnt far off. *[Remainder of letter missing?]*

[Typed, not signed. Possibly incomplete. SSC]

---

36 Merton's wife Ruth had died of cancer.

In the beginning . . .

To Owen Merton

31 West 14th Street
July 10 [1925]

Dearest love:

Please remember nothing is changed. I am going up to Ellens to Nantucket Saturday. I hope you will feel like telling me how you are. I feel so calm somehow and as if I knew this gesture was only a phase though I suppose you will do your best to convince me it is a fact, and it does hurt very much, and I shall accept your gesture if I finally must. But sweet my heart why should I be made to suffer if the very knowledge of why and how you are. You dont want that, you are too good, and it must be your own pain that blinds you to the unnecessary agony you cause me. But I love you and trust you so much under and I only live to somehow somewhere know your great troubles are solved.

You have always exaggerated my health. My weaknesses that are habitual are slight when after all I can dance and swim and ride a bicycle. If you will remember my health began to go down with doubt and it will go up again if I can ever be sure that you have enough faith left to try. The tragedy we have felt has been so much chimeric fears preying on us and so little tangible trouble.

The Jenkins would come around too if you took the bull by the horns and married me and that is the only reason I have wanted you to. I have learned by experience that the world sure can cock you up if you are outside the pale. Well by marrying you get inside. I wouldnt try to keep you if you turned agin me, but I would be in such a position I couldnt be kept from seeing you if you were ill etc. I have always known this, and when I spoke of deception I really uttered timidly my terror of just exactly what has occurred and what could not occur if things were so convention could not exclude me.

But lovey you are as free as the air if you want, so dont insult me before others by hiding like a pursued animal. If I didnt know your beautiful mind and heart inside out I couldnt stand it, but I know the pain and confusion that forced you again to make this gesture. You may convince me that I am a liability in your life, but not this way. You hurt me and yet leave everything obscure, and you do not kill my love for your exquisite natural sensitivity and gentleness. You have been so tried God knows I dont wonder at anything you may do even to em, but it aint necessary dearest love and I do believe time will tell you that this was your mistake for Tom and you and all of them. Am I bad for you, dearest? I dont truly think so. And I dont think I make the money worse. I love you. Wont you be a little more civilized even about telling me to give you up. Well hurrah for love because I had rather love you under these circumstances than not at all. And if I ever can be allowed to help you, Muttsie beloved, it is all the same, for you.

Bless you and let me kiss you forever because it is until death do us part for me. I cant give myself utterly and change.

Goodbye dearest Muttsie, but I hope you will write.

[Typed carbon copy, not signed. SSC]

To Louise Morgan

31 W 14th Street
July 11, 1925

Dearest Louise:

I have been very ill. Owen is ill and in anguish of mind. The Jenkins have landed on him with threats and reproaches and rubbing in of obligations and he has been told how the children cry for him, little John does. The Jenkins have now set out to separate Owen and me and may succeed. They won't allow me to speak, write, or even indirectly communicate with him. They won't let me know of his health and God knows what they tell him of me, and I have no legal recourse.

I have been under drugs myself and am pretty ill. If we had had money and had defied them it wouldn't have happened. I feel as if my world had smashed - but most a perfect agony of anxiety about him. Forgive him you two he has a terrible lot. I'll have to tell Suggie, but must think out how to make it easiest for him about me. I am pretty ill and bust for cash.

Evelyn

[Handwritten, signed. BRBL]

To Louise Morgan

Westport, Connecticut[37]
July 17, 1925

Dearest Louise:

I have been through hell since I saw you. Owen was an angel all the way here, but as we neared New York he sank into the most morbid state I ever saw, looking at me in a kind of anguished way and repeating, Yes, you are beautiful. Yes, I love you. I love you very much, and so on, so irrevelantly and with so little joy in making love I had the horrors again. I asked him if he was anticipating trouble with the Jenkins and he would not answer. When we were on deck he used to look at me and walk away, and seemed trying to hide some horrible depression he didnt dare express. He wasnt ever away from my side for a moment. I was seasick and he seemed to think I was going to die. Just before we arrived he insisted on repacking all the bags, gave me in mine all the letters I have written him, and some letters he wrote to his mother when he was a boy that I had asked to see. Then he put the ring I had given him in my bag too. Valid excuses of precaution were given for all of this.

On the morning we left the boat he made me stay on board while he did my bags for me in the customs. Mr Jenkins had come to meet him and was frankly mad because he was delayed by Owens attentions to me. When I spoke to him he was rather rude. That gave me a premonitory fear. As Owen said remember we are going to be separated but we are very close and together. And I said, yes, forever.

---

37   These letters from Westport were headed "c/o Goggins". Although there is no information about the identity of Goggins, it is very likely that Evelyn had found lodgings there.

Then Owen said, Those steady eyes, as if he were trying to remember something, and about to break down.

I didnt see him until the next day. Hell had broken loose. Little Tom crying all day when his father spoke of France, Mrs Jenkins telling him she had guessed this and he was sacrificing his children for a wicked woman. Pa Jenkins had a bad something and would go off if he knew Owen had committed adultery, and so on. In short it was me or the kids. Take your bloody kids and go to hell - if we dont stop you by interfering legally for your own good - or but that low down whore ruiner of homes in her place. Owen went off his head in the interview I wrote you about. With no money he couldnt move and kids with their rejoicing over him had broken him down anyway. He took the step he threatened in Beziers, for ever since I tried to commit suicide the conviction of the hopelessness of money has become a mania with him. He left me, by telegram, not a word to say where he was. Just - to Gladys - I dont think Evelyn and I should meet again, schemes wont work, please dont write.

Then he disappeared. The Jenkins put a block on communication and he concurred. He couldnt stick it otherwise. Today Harold Jenkins sent me a note he had written by Owen saying, I am sorry you have been made to feel responsible for my affairs, for of course the break in my relation with Evelyn Scott was my own decision. I did it to avert a worse calamity later as no possible plan could be made to work. I have behaved inhumanly again but it was because there was no way out, etc.

Result of this experience I have been in bed two weeks taking the stuff they give to DT patients, and with the doctor threatening to put me in an asylum where I could be watched. But I guess Im coming thru. I dont know quite. I love Owen just as much, and understand the terror that has been growing in his mind because it was what did make me take poison and made me so anguished in London - there really is no cure to the money and children with the Jenkins attitude of stop at nothing to kill me confronting us. So I quit and start somewhere else for the present. If Owen pulls out and wants me later and I aint took I am his because I never loved sug more nor anybody else as much, and with money to relieve worry we had everything in common to make us happy and the happiest sex I ever knew. But so it goes.

I dont want to scare you, but I have to break this thing to Cyril gradually and if I should decide to come over to London to work later would you help me to find a place to stay, perhaps outside the city, till I got myself together? I cant afford to stay in New York all the time and this has given me the horrors about it. Beside, if I get Owen again it wont be here. It will be abroad at some point when the Jenkins have become impossible and made him give up his determination to stick by the kids.

May I come and get a place and not see you too often and maybe talk things over with the Bennetts and decide for myself where how and for what I am going to live.

Ive gotta come to London. You wont be scared of me will you. I wont stay stuck with you forever, but you and Otto are sweeter and bigger than anybody here and being in the same town with you will help me, and relieve darling Cyril who shouldnt be hard hit too.

Love and au revoir, I hope

Evelyn

[Typed, typed signature. BRBL]

To Lola Ridge

Westport, Connecticut

July 17, 1925

Dearest Lola:

The letter you enclosed was a note from Owen to Harold Jenkins, relieving them for responsibility for the situation and telling them to tell me that he did it to prevent a worse tragedy later. I dont know what that means and mad as you may think me I will not accept the note any more than the first gesture. Owen says in the note he can not receive either letters or messages from me.

Owen is trying to kill my love for him but it is not dead yet. Not until I know he is happy in what he is doing, for I have seen every stage of his desperation and I think the money problem with the children has made him a little mad. I do not demand anything of him except some kind of fidelity to our mutual love and trust which I know exists in his heart as well as mine unless despair has changed it to hatred. Perhaps I shall live after this. God knows. But my belief in the possibility of beauty being in a human contact between men and women dies with this I think if this dies.

The important thing to make him know is that I DO NOT REPROACH HIM. I understand that he believes he is acting for the best. I understand that he thinks he is saving all

I want something to live for. I shall have to live alone anyway. Why cant I live for him, unless his last word to me that he wanted me most, his last words, oh my darling, ejaculated in anguish, were false. They werent. Let him go off anywhere to any occupation he wants, but surely he wont deny the merest rite of friendship.

You must believe he has been good to me or I would not love him so. To me even this horrible struggle he is making to give me up for his children is a proof of the qualities in him which I love, at least because they resemble my own. Let him know there will not be pain in our future relation if he will accept it in any form. I have exhausted pain. Either pain or me will soon die.

I cant write further, but he must know I love him, as the conviction that he has made me hate him is strengthening his despair to this point.

I love him. I love him. He cant kill my love this way. It cant be done. What kills love happens from an inside necessity and not from the outside. Torture wont kill my love for him because the torture is not expressing him.

I am trying hard to find him money.

I feel saner and calmer because I did have that letter[38] which Owen found so hard to write. I am sorry for him for I know how it hurt him to write it. Please make him know I feel saner and calmer.

The sight of his handwriting reassured me of him even tho the note was such a hard one.

[Typed, not signed. SSC]

Evelyn wrote a series of lengthy self-obsessed letters to her close friends and to Merton: the following is a typical dissertation of the emotional and sexual bonds between them. As Merton's parents-in-law had forbidden communication between Owen and Evelyn, she wrote to him care of Otto and/or Louise, sealing these letters in inner envelopes which were to be passed on to Owen. It is not clear whether Owen received these, or whether he received them and failed to open them; some were not opened until the 1980s by Otto's son Michael.

To Owen Merton

c/o Crawford
86 West 11th Street
August 7, 1925

Muttsie dear, the one thing you ask is to leave off writing until you are whole, and my dear dear the one thing I want to do is to help you to be yourself and that certainly at the expense of any pampering of my own feelings. And I wonder if you can forgive and answer this one more letter? I pray pray pray that you will forgive my writing it and that you will answer it. Im afraid John was convinced that you would do neither.

But Muttsie, I will still believe in all your beautiful honesty and knowledge of me if you can bring yourself to be a little more exact if your dear tired struggling to be yourself can manage it. You see you are making the decisions, and in that you have the advantage of me. You know I am here and will be no matter whether you decide never to see me or something different. I know nothing except that, according to your letter, you will not be brutal and hateful again.

But are you escaping from conditions that made you ill and me ill, or, in spite of a belief in one another that I know wont go, are you escaping from me, concretely, because, no matter what the conditions of freedom given you or the leeway to do all possible for your kids without practical thought of me, you simply no longer want me? Dont find it too hard to say if it is true, Muttsie, because I will not think of you unjustly if you do. All I said before holds good. Only do not also say something brutal merely because brutality is easy for the moment and you know my love for you would survive even that.

I think you must truly know whether my existence in the world for you is something you had either do without even it leaves you footloose in other relations.

---

38 This letter has not survived.

I have come out of my London trauma. I see plainly what drove you away from the emotional key of that despair. But having once despaired that much. I am like a person after a long illness ready to compromise with happiness and still find good in living.

Now I am ready for the blow if it is the truth, but wont you be sure it is and tell me. I could live apart from you wherever you are going to be. I could give up Jigeroo, as I must anyhow for a time, for various periods. I could make our practical life as if you were a lover with your own family ties, and I a mistress with an independent life. And this would be no sacrifice, because as it is anyway I have to live alone, only if love of me and all possible future happiness in being with me when you can is not gone, then my life alone would point toward something, and I would feel strong and purposeful about it.

But in any case the practical details of your life need scarcely be influenced by me, and I would take entire responsibility for myself and my health. I have to anyway, Muttsie, and dont you suppose I wouldnt joyfully if it made you any happier or gave you anything to consider me yours quite irresponsibly.

Oh dear I hope this wont make you angry with me. Im even more undefended than you are Mutts, because you can salve your hurts by withdrawing, and suspense only increases mine and the relief is not in my hands. Dont run away because you have this, it aint no compulsion.

PS Id live here in New York with you on Long Island. Id live somewhere abroad near you and not with you. Id be separate from Jig half of every year if need be. Id go indefinite times and never see Cyril or Jig. Id do my own moving and railway trips. Id fib beautifully.

[Typed, not signed. BRBL]

To Lola Ridge

Long Island
August 16, 1925

Dear Lola

When Evelyn has so much to forgive me will you please not be too hard on me for not opening letters from you or for not replying to them. It is hopeless to try and explain why one feels one must do certain things to anyone else - and I have the worst conscience in the world anyway now, only may I say that in doing a great wrong - I am avoiding doing a much greater one. I wish I could have seen you - only now that everything is changed I don't feel I should see anyone.

I can't say anything Lola, that is why I did not write to you before.

Yours truly,
Merton

[Handwritten, signed. SSC]

To Louise Morgan

c/o Crawford,
286 West 11th Street
August 21, 1925

Precious Louise, I am coming to you in about a fortnight and then maybe you can help me find some cheap place near London to spend the winter.

Owen is sailing with Tom tomorrow on the <u>Majestic</u> and will be in London soon. I judge he will be willing to talk to me when I arrive. Dear, I want above all for my own pride to talk to Owen and establish it with him that I am and always will be his friend, and I want you to give him this letter. He is to be blessed for nothing, but I am really crushed by the letter I have from him today[39] which states the one irreparable condition, more final than anything practical or external, and still the least one for which he can be blamed. He is out of love with me, sexually I mean, and of course being still intensely in love with him, this is terrible and painful. He doesnt know why. He thinks an idealistic friendship is to grow naturally out of this happening. And it will. I mean that my idealism is sufficient to make me desire terribly to be the poor childs friend. But he doesnt realize the essential commonplace of his own growing out of love with me.

Darling I can scarcely wait for your understanding. I have almost gone mad these two months, and of course Owens leaving without me is pretty crushing tho he did it on the assumption that we would meet in London as John told him I was going there.

Well be kind to him. Life is hell alright for all of us. And as a last kindness persuade him to wait over and talk.

I know too well where love is ardent enough there are no difficulties that are insurmountable and where it aint there is no hope. Only I long for a little decency and clarity.

Bless you and keep you precious things. I will maybe get the Leviathan but I will wire you the boat when I sail, maybe send you a wireless.

dear lovely things god bless you

evelyn

Please be good to poor Owen, misguided in everything except knowing his own heart and when love is dead in it. Dont try to give my letter to him until he comes to you. He has promised he will go to see you when he gets there.

[Typed, typed signature. BRBL]

To Otto Theis

31 West 14th Street
August 27, 1925

Dear Otto:

For Evelyn - and you and Louise, too - I'm so afraid! If she gets another shock and

---

39   This letter has not survived.

goes to pieces as she did here, I don't know how she is going to stand it. At the same time it is terrifically hard on anyone and everyone around here. She has no thought for or mercy for anyone else. Please don't think by saying this that I mean it as harsh criticism. Evelyn was in an abnormal state and could not be held responsible. Also we could not blame her for anything in such a terrible situation, except perhaps for her use of Lola who is in just as bad, or worse, health.

I am not outlining the facts as you undoubtedly know them and I dont want to be an alarmist. At the same time Evelyn's mind still harps on the one thing - Merton, Merton, money for Merton, letters to Merton, etc. If that string breaks, I'm afraid she'll break too. And both Merton and she are so twisted up with resentments, complexes, emotional difficulties, in their relations with each other that I am in serious doubt if it can ever be patched up. Intellectually Evelyn see this, too. but she won't and dare not realize it emotionally. Tom, who is with Merton, is one difficulty, Cyril another. Merton has come out with jealous resentment and hatred of him and God knows whether Merton can even stand Evelyn's remaining Cyril's friend. This is understandable after the situation in southern France and Algeria which Ellen Kennan sketched to us. Ellen has little in common with Merton but she said he bore almost more than any man could - responsibilities for all the practical things to the minutest details, constant encouragement and patient criticism for Cyril's painting, acknowledged love of Evelyn but never daring to show affection and Evelyn sleeping in the room with Cyril every night, etc, etc. Cyril accepting everything and doing nothing - (I can't blame him either after what he has been through. The whole thing was too awful for everybody.) Of course this last is entirely confidential. Even Evelyn doesn't know I know it.

Evelyn is with John Crawford and Becky Edelson now. She is there because they have an extra room and she simply can not stay alone. She was with us, as you know, for the first two weeks. That time was a nightmare for all of us. Merton's interview and abrupt leave taking - futile attempts to reach him by telephone - his brutal telegram to me for Evelyn[40] - her complete hysteria complicated by her taking all the sleeping tablets in a bottle - (This was not a suicidal attempt. I had given her a large dose and it had not taken effect at once, so when I was out of the room she took the rest. The result was almost like a stroke. She lost control of her limbs, her mouth, etc. Her legs, arms, everything gave way and she could talk only with guttural swollen syllables.) Then literally she nearly went mad. She tried to dress and go to Douglaston and had to be restrained by force. She begged piteously for something to kill herself with. Later, when strong, she beat her head on the piano and took the dull grape fruit knife to bed with her. (Fortunately I had hidden all the other sharp knives.) She had to be watched every minute and was quiet only when given dope at night (until about 4 AM or when planning some way to reach Merton). The minutes she had started something, she wanted results and started something else. She would not wait and her various

---

40   This telegram has not survived.

plans marred each other. She turned against her various friends and a few times grew suspicious that we were not mailing her letters, sending her telegrams, telephoning her messages, etc. That worried me more than anything as I was afraid of persecution mania. The doctor, May Mayers, a friend of Dudley's, was a marvel. She held Evelyn's confidence until just before we had to leave. Then Evelyn turned against her, too. But during the worst item the doctor was the one person who could calm her and reason with her. And May was a wonder about coming whenever I grew desperate. She even went out to Douglaston and spent three hours talking to Mrs Jenkins. Lola, too, did everything in the world to help, and Martin Lewis went out to Douglaston although he disapproved of the whole thing.

All this happened in our one back room. Evelyn's bed was right there and she was crying or moaning most of the time. It took time to get her quieted at night even when she was given medicine. Then she woke about four and began crying or smoking. The result was that Dudley nearly broke down, too. He was worn out to start with and we were to start on vacation the Friday after Evelyn arrived. It was utterly impossible to leave her, then, so he managed to put off his vacation one week. But that finished him. By Friday of the following week he got the worst attack of nervous indigestion I ever saw. I had to send for the doctor for him and had two patients on my hands in the same room. All this time I was supposed to be feeding Evelyn egg nogs, cooked cereals and cream, vegetables, etc - all on one gas burner and with practically no cooking experience! You can imagine that I was ready for a vacation, too. (Fortunately I was extremely well to start with.)

I had made up my mind, selfishly and cruelly perhaps, that even if Evelyn had to go to a sanatorium, we had to get away! It was literally a choice, for me, between sacrificing ourselves futilely for Evelyn, and saving Dudley's health and perhaps our future. Evelyn was better and realizing how hard it was for us. She was beginning to get response to her telegrams. Her father came up from Washington[41] and she made him take her to a hotel - where however she didn't stay. Saturday morning we heard Evelyn was going to Lola's who was in no fit state to nurse her. Dudley got up, sick as he was, and went to interview Mr Dunn who promised to get Evelyn an apartment. Then, in spite of everything and to our utter amazement, we actually found ourselves on the boat for New Bedford. We went to Sconset on Nantucket Island where we stayed with a good friend, Ellen Kennan. Dudley was all in and I was nearly as bad. It took us ten days or so to recover and I managed to persuade Dudley to take an extra week. It is a marvellous place to rest and build up. We came back much better to find Evelyn better, too. She had her tonsils out and recovered marvellously. Becky and John have taken good care of her and John actually succeeded in getting the first word through to Merton. The rest, and probably this, you know or Evelyn will tell you. I don't know

---

41   This is almost certainly the last time Evelyn saw her father; this meeting is repeatedly referred to in her later search for information about her father's death and his will (see Chapter 25).

why I have bothered you with all these past troubles unless to justify myself to you. I don't want you to think that I ran off leaving Evelyn in the lurch too cruelly or that she and I have had any falling out. We are better friends than ever, if possible.

Please forgive this letter and writing.

Very sincerely yours

Gladys

[Handwritten, signed. BRBL]

In the autumn of 1925, Owen, accompanied by Tom, returned to Europe for the last time. He built a house in Saint-Antonin, in south-western France, and travelled and painted widely in southern France. He also played the piano in the Saint-Antonin cinema and was president of the local rugby club. He died in January 1931 of a brain tumour.

Chapter 9

The Scilly Isles
September 1925 - Spring 1926

After the break-up with Merton, Evelyn and Cyril continued their separate ways. No correspondence relating to Cyril's return to North Africa survives, nor of his later journey to Europe with Jigg and Elsa Pfenniger, his Swiss mistress of whom Jigg was extremely fond.

In 1925, shortly before her break with Merton, Evelyn and Jack Metcalfe had met at the home of mutual friends. Jack recorded this meeting briefly in a diary entry which gave no clue as to its future importance. After the parting of the ways with Merton, she and Jack began living together; again, no surviving letters refer to the development of this relationship. Nor do any surviving letters clarify the decision Evelyn and Jack made at some time during late 1925 to go to England, where Jack had family connections, rather than return to the United States. Eventually they found themselves in the Scilly Isles, a popular holiday destination in the English Channel, living out of season in a boarding house.

As Evelyn travelled around Britain with Jack, her letters reverted to the vivid travelogue style of her early travels through North Africa and the French Riviera. Gone were her introspective essays on the nature of love.

A few words about Jack, full name William John Metcalfe. He was born into a prosperous family (Evelyn often claimed they were "minor nobility") in Heacham, Norfolk, and privately educated before studying at the University of London. He wrote a number of works of science fiction (what might be called "fantasy" today) and was called to the Royal Navy Air Force during WW1. After the war, he remained a reservist in the Royal Air Force and supplemented his meagre royalties by teaching Latin and mathematics at a series of private schools ("crammers").

To Maude Dunn

c/o Theis, London
September 17, 1925

Dear Mother:

Again I have held off writing in the hope of having money to send but I must wait until next month again. You see we have no fixed source of income of any kind, just depending on what sells and what doesn't, so one month we have some money and the next we don't. I have been interested in all your letters and all the Clarksville news, but I get blue when I can't send money and don't feel it worth while for me to write.

I have had my tonsils out and that cost something, but it is a great relief. I have been suspected of having TB and floroscoped and x-rayed and found a little doubtful but not a real case. So it is a relief to know anyhow. I've stayed in London in order to be doctored but it is much too like New York in expensiveness for a permanent residence and to make things cheaper Jigeroo and Cyril went back to Italy. Cyril sends some pictures but exhibitions have to be about two years apart in order to accumulate work of the best quality and you have to live in between. He is not at all strong any more.[42] Of course I miss them terrifically. London always seems like a city of the drowned after New York and the English are so impersonal and their desire to keep everything on a purely formal plane is almost an insanity. Sport and politics have to take the place of everything personal, though of course underneath they are the most sentimental race on earth. I don't really like them or feel drawn to them. In some ways even the French are much closer, though they lack a subtle kind of imagination and are too diagrammatic on a mental plane.

The weather here makes seven kinds of a day in one. It is balmy spring at ten am, winter at twelve, a dreary rainy autumn at three and at six before the sun goes it may be spring again. Not as disagreeable as it sounds really. But oh the types, the stony blue-eyed wooden well bred usual men, so good looking and so uninteresting. And the women with heavy chins, slab sided figures, lovely skins, and perfectly vacant personalities. Naturally that isn't all, but it is the average. The shops are dreadful. You don't mind having no money for what you don't want to buy. Ready made clothes *[missing page(s)]*

Jigeroo isn't going to school now, but he has been to French, Italian and Arab schools, French spoken in the Arab school. I don't know where he will go this winter. If I get rich ever I'll put him in a boarding school in Switzerland. He looks very much like me everybody says. He is way above my shoulder, about to my chin, pretty solid, and has a fine color. His eyes are not as blue as they were, and his teeth need straightening some. Otherwise except for size he looks about as you remember him. He speaks slowly and has a lazy walk except when he plays very hard. His sense of humour is superb and he is chocked full of temperament. His appreciation of pictures and books is five years in advance of his age. In school he is no good at all, won't concentrate and seems to think education a joke, partly because he is always changing schools and they are all different. He draws astonishingly. Almost everybody likes him and certainly he is a handsome kid, but I've got to get enough money to give him a more practical education so if he is ever up against it he won't be at such a disadvantage.

---

42   Cyril was then 54 years old.

Lots of love and hopes for your health, and do forgive the hard time about money. We are still gamblers and paupers about that. Only there are bound to be streaks of luck.

elsie[43]

[Typed, typed signature. UTK]

To Otto Theis

c/o Mrs Clark

Tresco, Scilly Isles

January 24, 1926

Dear Otto:

I don't want to wear you out with correspondence, but you were so good about the check and medicine and so on as you are about every damn thing you get axed when anybody gets in a hole, big or little. I do think you are pretty gran', Otto, and so do John, and there aint no good way to tell you about it. It must be the bloodiest nuisance in the world to have all the endless perpetual things on you, and this week there will be another, as by the beginning of next week I will want the check for five guineas (guineas,[44] not pounds - and I will make him wait a bit longer for the next payment), and at the same time ten pounds more for myself as we pay board in advance. Will you please send the money cash registered but not in 5 lb[45] notes as one pound is all they can cash here. If it gets here next Mon or even Wed will do.

I never saw such a tiny place that gave such impression of variety. Down where we were today there was a waste looking flat, faintly blooming, with moss on the sandy earth. It had the suggestion, where the sea was hidden, of a vast desolateness like the Campagna at Rome, and over toward the water long rolling hummocks were covered with a yellow grass, shining as blond hairs, dry but unseeded, and bristly-stiff, but growing thick as the fur of an animal. When we climbed the summit of the last point of land, we could see a rocky nudity of beach exposed and on one upstanding boulder a very large gull, very still and alone, presiding over the reflections in the brackish puddles that the sea had left.

We made a detour around the governor's bloody "abbey" which looks like the ancestral castle of a Long Island millionaire, and passed a large pond or small lake, according to your temperament from which a pair of wild ducks darted with their nasal cries. And when we had got back on the more trodden road that would take us home it was nearly dark and what is called the Round Island Light, that John is very fond of and will put in a story, was making a pale ember in the ash of the [*illeg*]. Then all at once it swelled like a window into the lovliest rosiest depth of hell, and was the most beautiful red red red menace I have seen in a long time.

---

43   Evelyn continued to use the name she was christened with when writing to her mother.
44   The guinea, a monetary unit no longer in use, was 21 shillings or one pound, one shilling.
45   The unit of English currency, the pound, is written as "£", but Evelyn is writing as it sounds. The correct representation of this amount would have been "£5".

Well - here we are again. The food is per usual and one grows used to it - though I do miss coffee of which I have not had a drop, and the missing of which makes me think much of you. I would also appreciate one of Louise's most divine salads as but for fresh meat and the oranges we have got ourselves we would sure have scurvey.

Well, I do wish this was a lesser run from London. The great bird life in the spring and the feathered population now is limited (no personal reference meant). But I have had great pleasure from the cormorants, who have necks as long as baby swans but not sinuous. Their black feathers are usually so wet they seem like eels in a dripping fleshiness. They swim with their bodies mainly submerged, and when they dive it is in the neat pointing attitude of a human swimmer, for they leap an inch or two out of the water, and spring with a half somersault on the fish theyve sight. They look so like pogy sly old men in wet bathing suits, but with a sinister agility.

Maybe birds won't interest you, but the surf yesterday in the storm would have. We were on the rolling moor that is at this end and on a pinnacle the wind almost took me off. The harbours all around are full of small mountains like miniatures of Rio and on these a perfect fury of lashing vapour at a gigantic height. Thank Pete we brought books tho work goes fine, but stops at noon, tho John does another batch of typing by the shades of night. His book seems to me to be doing well.

Love to Louise Evelyn.
John sends love too.

[Handwritten, signed. BRBL]

To Evelyn Scott

Clarksville, Tennessee
[February 1926]

Dear Elsie:

I am enclosing two little Valentines for Jigaroo - he is still young enough for Valentines, and I hope he will be pleased with them. If he does not know about St Valentine, you can explain it to him. Very likely he doesn't, living in foreign countries so much. But to me the day was full of thrills and St Valentine was a very real person, and you celebrated it with enthusiasm too, and always received such numbers of elaborate Valentines. They are not near so fancy now, and the lace paper ones seem to have disappeared.

I can't thank you enough for that money you sent, it is such a help, I've only spent a little for "foolishness" and the rest I'll have to use of necessities, pay the Dentist and other things. It's difficult to get money from J[46] - and medical treatment costs so much, that I have to do with old clothes. I don't know what I would have done without your check. I don't want J to know about it, if it can be helped, or anybody else.

---

46   Maude's cousin Julian Gracey.

Do write to me,
Worlds of love to you and dear Jigaroo,
Mother

I have a little ring, with a blue set, the first ring I ever had - that I have long wanted
Jigaroo to have, but I don't know how to get it to him - and two other trinkets that I
wish I could send them, that he admired, and liked to play with. Tell him I still have
his little tin man, and rooster.

[Typed, signed. HRC]

To Louise Morgan

Tresco, Scilly Isles
[April 2, 1926]

Dearest Louise;

John and I have equal joy in hearing from you, but I have the most time now to write. I
have just finished the last draft of the novel and nothing to do but revise it for which I need
johns help after his own writing is over as you know I can not spell anything.

Its grey here and chilly but not really bitter. Now I have my book done I shouldnt
care when I went to france, but to save paying another fare to england, john is trying to
get his air force[47] time changed to may, and then, naturally, wants to get more done on
his book.

Hes an awful sweet person, honey, and I think providence should be
acknowledged for once that he happens to be, considering I was in such a mood of
irresponsibility that i might have got myself in for almost anything. Johns particular
kind of straightforwardness is sometimes as amusing and exciting a shock as the
immediacy we are so intrigues with. Anyway, the more I am with him, the more,
thank god, I find I like to be. I think he is a quaker with a temperament, contradicting
sounding since the Quakerism itself is a species of temperament which the other
seems to contradict. But he is by nature, and without any sacrifice of self-respect and
self-assertion when the core is touched, the most constitutionally tolerant, not to say
indifferent, human being i ever saw. With that does a kind of melodramatic voluptuous
play-acting (that is somehow also real) about morbid themes. He is a toothgritter, but
on principle, for beyond personal pride, he has no more principles than a nanny goat.
But the whole melange is somehow very lovable.

I like to think of our relations going on a long time, but god knows if they will. Not
that John shows any inclination to the contrary, but he is thirty-four and while a year
older than me, a lot younger, being a man, and I think I have to keep before me the
possibility that he may some time when least anticipated by either of us be successfully
vamped by some young lady who is like my daughter. However, I hope I am learning
to enjoy whats good in the present and not destroy it by anticipating the unanticipable.

---

47   John was in the Royal Air Force reserves.

IMPORTANT: I have written the bank to cable Otto one hundred and fifty dollars in pounds that I want for my trip. Otto please excuse the liberty without asking him, but I wanted to catch the mail, and I had it cabled and to him to provide for any unexpected changes in plans. It is to be cabled in his name, and, because you are moving and I didnt know cliffords[48] address, I asked them to send the notice to the Outlook office. I trouble Otto with cashing it because, if possible, I dont want to touch a cent of it before I go to France, and if it came here with difficulties I might be tempted to. I am going to ask him to please hold it for me until I am ready to take the boat when I will draw it out, as it will take more than that to put me and john in Marseilles with a place to spend the summer. I guess Ive lost sight of poor Owen now. My conscience is in a mess that theres no use attempting financial loyalties to everybody at once. This month I have to send more to that accursed Haire[49] too.

Or if Otto will please take care of it. It may get to him in a fortnight, but perhaps longer as easter holidays have upset the boats from here and i just sent off the notice.

Here endeth the fortyninth chapter, and the collect for the day is bless you both with the most extravagant blessings, but very real, of both of us.

evelyn

john per evelyn

ps I BOBBED my landladys hair this am and her whole family is quarreling with her about it. She is fifty-two so it is a great defiance, but it looks quite well and there was sadistic pleasure in whacking it.

[Typed, typed signature. BRBL]

To Louise Morgan

Tresco, Scilly Isles

April 7, 1926

Louise, darling, you can not hope to keep quantitive pace with my corresponding. Until I get hold of a History of the Civil War to begin book two[50] on, I have all my mornings for letters. John is helping me correct spelling and punctuation in the afternoons. He has laid off his novel for a bit and is beginning a short story which has a very spirited opening and promises to be both good and saleable. We are still in the air about plans, for the air ministry had an Easter holiday and has not answered his inquiry about training camp.

As for having the specific things altered, I am afraid everything is past altering but the green dress Whitehead[51] made, and that I am having let out here as it is a very simple matter. The skirts are being ripped but they miss three or four inches in the belt

---

48   Clifford Street London, Otto's work address.

49   Dr Haire, the gynaecologist who attended Evelyn when Jigg was born.

50   Evelyn was at this time working on the book which would be published in 1929 as *The Wave*.

51   Whitehead appears to have been a seamstress. At the time it was not uncommon for women to have their clothes "run up" from commercial patterns (including Butterick) by seamstresses.

and I dont think the seams will do it and there is no more to do to them. That leaves the green dress and the grey coat (which, by the way, has lost somewhat by having the buttons moved to their last extremity) to travel in, which would do except that it is going to be hot in may when we hit Marseille. I have that old black crepe de chine of Phyllis Crawfords which it may be can be ripped to make a skirt. Do you think it would go with a green crepe de chine jumper? I got some samples from Peter Jones[52] and figured out the cost of a cape dress (they are very a la mode again) - short cape, plain skirt with one pleat in front, and tailored silk jumper - with, possibly, as it only takes three eighths of a yard and the pattern comes with the dress, a soft hat of same stuff as the skirt, and it came to a little over five pounds, figuring on Miss Whiteheads possible price. If I had the money here I might have tackled asking her, but I dont know yet whether we can get thru month (I begin to see Ottos troubles).[53]

John had another income tax, and had to gibe three pounds for a contribution for a grave stone for his uncle Reggie (just departed). Also another payment to Haire, and we must have two hundred dollars clear just to reach Marseille. John will get some and me some next month and we can do it, but five or six pounds on a dress is a plenty so I thought of writing to Miss Whitehead just before I leave and asking her if she could cut over black crepe de chine and make a blouse.

Oh, well I could talk on all day. Ill spare you. Thank you for the Butterick address, and Im glad - or hope - it sounded so - that you are feeling a bit more chipper. I want to hear any news from the kids. Give Otto a hug, beloved, and for yourself all my lesbian outpourings which, by the way, John has by no means overcome. John says to give you both a handsome lot of love from him.

We had a wonderful scrap last night, of the only kind we have had since we came, about the bedclothes, and me turning over in bed when John cant sleep. I wish I had had a dictaphone. John accused me of "sighing" and keeping him awake. Its a species of tyranny that must proceed from his subconscious as he has never showed it except when half asleep. Then he says I have all the sheet, when I have three eighths of an inch and so on. It is screamingly funny, and shows the subconscious of a bachelor I think with thirty four years of managing his own bedcovers.

I bobbed the daughter in law of my landlady and am now being solicited by a neighbour, it having gone abroad, John says that before I married him I worked in a beauty shop.

agin, love,
evelyn

[Typed, typed signature. BRBL]

---

52   Peter Jones was (and still is) a fashionable London department store.
53   As John's agent, Otto had a role in ensuring his tax affairs were up to date.

To Louise Morgan

Tresco, Scilly Isles
April 19, 1926

Dearest Louise, from the pit the screeching of microbes and another request.

I let the female here attack the hopeless skirts. She has made them some larger but if anything hopelesser than ever. Would it be an outrage after all to have Staples[54] two days when I get there. You see this female works on the inspiration basis, and is a laundress and has a baby and wont try things on, so she sends them back with the damage done. She has "altered" my white Arab skirt, and the skirt to my green suit, and the whitehead Green dress. I think Miss Staples, by pinning them on me, could make them look less like sugar sacks. Also, perhaps, perhaps, something could be done to that black silk dress with the white loose panels, the jabot, and high collar, by using the loose panels to set in on the hips and so widen the skirt. I dont think theres be time to make anything new but those would help a lot. Also that green skirt (dark green) Miss Staples did something or other to, might be let out somewhere. Could you stick this?

We are leaving here on the fourth, if the money comes, and - also if second money comes, wont stay in London much above a week - from the fifth to the twelfth or fourteenth. Could you, oh could you, be burdened with mrs staples two days in that time? I am going to see Haire afternoon of eighth. I dont know what hour, but that wont take long. Then dentist some day, and passport people, other time free.

John and me are so germy we cant see two dollars ahead, but Id rather have a cold now than moving day. John is writing a fine somewhat Conradish short story, and has just finished one called "The Funeral March of a Marionette" that I like terribly - based on thing I saw of those kids with an idiot guy falks[55] in an invalids chair. Maybe hell sell em. Hes awful sweet and being heroic about writing against germs.

LOTS OF LOVE and John says to give you special and tell you how you are lovely girl and he wants to see you and otto and we both do LOTS evelyn

[Typed, typed signature. BRBL]

To Otto Theis

Tresco, Scilly Isles
April 19, 1926

Dear Otto:

This besieging is not an attack but an apology. John is so sensitive on the money question that he slurred our difficulties and I did not realize that when the board was

---

54 Miss Staples appears to have been another seamstress.

55 This is a reference to Guy Fawkes, a Catholic who in 1605 was involved in a conspiracy to blow up King James I and the Houses of Parliament. For this he was executed. Children now celebrate Guy Fawkes' Day by dressing effigies and parading them in wheelbarrows or similar to solicit money ("a penny for the Guy") from passers by.

payed this am we wouldnt have anything to buy matches, cigarettes, or oil for the stove - which last is serious as we are both laid up more or less with flu. So Im writing this because I axed for money for the end of this week and now, want to let you know the boats are changed and to get it here Friday it must reach Penzance in time for a sailing at 9 Friday morning.

Otto, when I get to France I wont devil you no long. I wrote to the bank on the thirty-first about cabling that money. Oh damn money, it do make the future look uncertain. But Im letting off steam to you, it cant be done before John, as he already has a COMPLEX and wonders what Cyril will think of him, and so on. I trust Cyrils understanding but am by no means sure John and me and Jig, half time Jig, can subsist very comfortably on our twenty five a week. However theres always hope. Otto its no longer a question of a grand gesture about this money, but that I owe you in plain cash just for electricity and gas and youve never said how much. Sometimes when you think pisin (I dont mean that) poison is so cheap and life is so dear you wonder why you do it. But it is and you do, and if I try to "wish I was dead" I aint sure I mean it.

I hope my groans dont hit you at a hard time. If they do throw a brick at me. I cant mention money in any ordinary tone of voice.

Lots of love from both of us to yawl.

evelyn

[Typed, typed signature. BRBL]

To Lola Ridge

Tresco, Scilly Isles

April 23, 1926

Beloved dear, I had such a vivid dream about you last night and yet I havent the faintest idea this morning what it was about - just the strong impression of you that held over until morning and made me feel like writing to you. I sent a letter through Glad and hope you get it, but I dont know that she has your address, so this through Ellen who, last letter, mentioned having heard from you.

I hope spring is there. March gave here fallacious hints, and April has been one succession of hair and wind storms, of chill unimpassioned moodiness. Scilly is such a Noahs ark of a place, but with most of the animals left out. Just a few human breeds in twos and twos in squat little stone cottages, neat like ships at seas, but as plainly adorned.

Youd be amused with the interior of the room we have to work in. It is very tiny, very low ceilinged, and, like all Scilly houses, with a window not much bigger than a porthole. The furniture (it is a dining room) is broad striped plush and ornate machine carved backs - three chairs, two arm chairs for head and foot of table, and a chaise lounge about big enough for one of Snow Whites seven dwarfs. On the chaise lounge is a red sofa pillow covered with a Nottingham lace tidy. The sideboard is red, imitation mahogany. On it reposes a cracked Sunday teaset of royal blue and gild, mended with liquid cement and non-usable; two "hand painted" bowls (non used) and a huge imitation cut glass bottled revolving silver-plated canister. All the bottles except the mustard pot are empty but everyday it is put on the table for every meal, presumably, because it is so heavy, to keep the tablecloth from blowing off. On one wall are three hunting prints, pink coats, hounds etc, one without a glass, and two with glasses cracked. One the sideboard wall is another chromo of Highland Cattle in a Turneresque debauch of sunset and water. On either side the sideboard hang two green plush mats triangular in shape framing small round mirrors. Again, on the third wall, is an enlarged photograph of my landladys father-in-law and mother-in-law- an old lady like a mild and Christian monkey, a cocky obstinate looking little white haired man who obviously takes to himself full credit for his wifes faithfulness. There is, too, an enlarged and colored photo of the landlord and landlady - she, wearing a knit jersey and pince nez (all highly tinted) and he, with his moustache bright gold, standing beside her and looking a bit of a beau. On the mantel shelf are three vases decorated with Watteau figures, all the vases as tall as funeral urns, with huge gilt urns, the one in the center mounted high above the others on a base of china that is like a tower. Mingled with this adornment are crowds of adenoidal family photographs, some framed, some unframed, some passepartoured,[56] and the mantel shelf has an embroidered linen lambrequin. The highly polished brass fire set adds the last note. Through the window, Tresco harbour looks like a pan full of blue water with some funny paper sailing boats on it.

By the time we leave we will have been here almost four months, so we know it well.

John and I are only waiting for enough cash to move. I dont want to crush Cyril with responsibilities, and I hope to Pete to get something soon from the advance on novel - if there is any. And then - oh, it will be joy to see Sug and Jig again and Elsa, too - but especially Jig. I think, I hope, John will like them and they him. Now I still wish that you, dearest honey, were coming to spend the summer with us. Therell always be a place if you get enough just for fare. I truly think youd like John. I dont know anyone just the same type - a little like Cyril, a little like Martin,[57] more callow than Cyril, and less hardened thru bitter experience than Martin. But he has been good to me, Lola, very, very, very.

This is just little more than gossip. I dont know what I want to talk to you about, further than I want to talk. I wish we could all see you. Darling, your transparent alabaster red-hot furnace fire warms a lot of space over the chill Atlantic. I wish I knew how to send warm back. And I do long to see the poems. If you cant write please delegate somebody to tell me how you are, something about practical happenings, your health, and so on.

---

56   Passepartout is a black paper tape used to bind the edges of pictures as a cheap alternative to framing.

57   There is no information about Martin's identity – or perhaps this was a mis-typing of "Merton".

Love and love and love. This year in general counts up a good number 1926 = 18 = 9. Good year for your book. I am trying to arrange to go to a spiritualist seance in London. Ill write you about it.

evelyn

[Typed, typed signature. SSC]

To Louise Morgan

Tresco, Scilly Isles

April 28, 1926

Dearest kid, you are sweet to bother about Staples. It is alright, for my worry is not about wearing something smart, but wearing anything. I had the female here alter two skirts and the green dress and they are awful!!!. Green dress not so bad, only a little uneven and needs cleaning - but skirts!!! What I fear is that it will be downright hot in Marseille in May. I have literally no garment for such. So if you do hear of any other woman Id be glad.

I hope the weather changes. Wonder what you all think of the coal strike. Scilly is coalless, but fortunately not very cold. People here cheerfully suggest we wont get to France. John can't leave till after the 11th. What is the rumour there?

However I'll ax that in person. We leave Monday am.

Au revoir and [*illeg*]- just like!!! from John and me.

Tuesday I'll be in Lunnon! Wish I loved Lunnon more! But it will be fun to see you.

Evelyn

[Handwritten, signed. BRBL]

This is the last surviving letter from the Scilly Isles. There is no record of the decisions that led to Evelyn and John ending up in Cassis-sur-Mer not far from Marseille on the south coast of France, nor of their journey there. Nor is there any account of how it was that Jigg, then 12 years old, came to join them from Tunisia, where he had been living with Cyril and his then mistress Elsa Pfenniger.

Chapter 10

France, Lisbon and Algeria
June 1926 - April 1927

These months were typified by the continuing search for places to live which would be warmer during the coming winter months and within their meagre budget. Evelyn's letters as they travelled around the Riviera were more like the travelogues that had characterised her letters in previous years. Her descriptions of the places they visited and in which they lived invoked comparisons with the letters she wrote from North Africa: vivid descriptions of their surroundings and (sometimes not so positive) accounts of local customs.

None of the surviving letters contain accounts of the departure of Evelyn and Jack from the Scilly Isles and the decisions which led to them ending up in Cassis-sur-Mer, on the Riviera not far from Marseille. While there, Evelyn and Jack were reunited with Cyril and Jigg and all four made their way from Cassis to Cintra, near Lisbon; it is possible they chose Portugal as they were already familiar with the Portuguese language from their years in Brazil. There they spent the winter in a cheap hotel before returning to Algeria.

To Lola Ridge

5 rue Victor Hugo,
Cassis-sur-Mer, France
June, 1926

Beloved Lola:

John, Jig and myself are at Cassis, a village one hour from Marseille. Cyril and Elsa are at l'Estaque, two hours away.

If you can get the fare, wont you come stay with us. Our flat has only two rooms, but we can get you another outside where you can have breakfast in bed and bigger meals with us - only walking a step so to speak.

It is warm, but there is the sea and calm, and we love you so - John and Elsa both want to know you so. Jig sends his dearest love to you and Davy. So do I.

Blessed, you could take a boat to Marseille, wireless us the day before you get in, and Cyril, John, Elsa, me and Jig all meet you easily at Marseille. You need a change beloved as well as you need many other things. The boat fare, second class, is about

$145, but you must have fruit or something of your own. In summer the journey is not rough. You could see Gibraltar, Paloma, Naples en route as we did and wd bring you right here. If I get anything on my novel you won't need any money here. I doubt living with us wont cost you with room, more than a dollar a day. Please we all want it.

Evelyn

[Handwritten, signed. SSC]

To Otto Theis

Cassis-sur-Mer
June 11, 1926

Dearest Otto:

My personal news (Strictly confidential, for which again I guess I go against Johns inclination to confess) is as follows: Cyril took John to a first rate diagnostician in Marseilles yesterday. He (MD) coined the word physisthenique to apply to him as opposed to neurasthenic. Says Johns vital energy is absolutely depleted and must have been so for some time. My private opinion is that he suspects John of TB that I will not say so to John and heaven grant it is sensation. Anyway, John is to stay out of doors all day, to write out of doors if he will write, to recline while writing, to go up on the terrace and assume as much nudity in the sun as propriety will allow, and to take two kinds of injections of something which it would need Cyril to elucidate. Also to weigh himself daily and to take his temperature morning and evening. To exercise little. Blood and urine are still at the laboratory and John goes in tomorrow to get the results. Im glad he has been. All the time he was in Scilly his constant tendancy to extreme exhaustion worried me, especially as we had few pipps and there was no mental explanation (usually sufficient cause). Cyril thought he might have TB too, but now hopes he hasnt. He ate little at Scilly, tho bucked up in London, but here eats less.

He is going to the air force mid July, doctor or no doctor, and it may do him good. Anyhow he adores the airforce and psychology demands he doesnt resign from it. I think one reason he loves it is it is the only out of door life he has led in years and he feels better there. Hell be leaving about the 12th and be in London a day or so before going to camp, so he will see you.

Wish Louise could come down for the three or four weeks John is gone, bedroom and swimming all ready for her. Also tennis with Cyril and Elsa twice a week Cant it be done, en route to America or not? She has only to wire me and I will meet her at Marseille, Cyril ditto and well bring her out here.

Had a nasty shock this month. I wrote to have maries money sent to me at marseille, Bank just replied that the cheque which comes for mr scott which he has asked to be divided between you did not arrive this month (May). I am writing Walter Nelles to see if he is still the one who attends to it and has maybe forgotten, and hoping to god the crisis is only momentary. Surely it must be but it is damned upsetting and I do need that advance Zelma talked about. So again will feel most humble gratitude if you find it possible to see her and say a word in general which will incline her more to see I get it.

Large quantities of the mush that embarrasses you are here about to overflow the page so, with our most affectionate and largest love for Louise and yourself, I will quit before the page grows too dewy or syrupy for your perusal.

Evelyn

[Typed, typed signature. BRBL]

To Otto Theis and Louise Morgan

Cassis-sur-Mer

June 24, 1926

Dearest kids:

Wreck. Found a house but rent half again Beziers. Everything twice price last year. Still, better than England. Submerged in effort to run house with fool woman and people sticking on prices for les anglaises. Cassis rather fine to look at but too picturesque. John like a polar bear in the heat. Needs an ice cake to lie on. Jig lovely, with us at present, crazy about John. Don't worry Louisa, ain't no difference and Jig had complexes too. It wont change affection anyway. Sug looks well and his oils are gorgeous - some fine water colors as before but oils and the triptych he is working on astound me. He is a beautiful and wonderful, and only Sug. Which doesn't keep me from loving John, but Sug is graven on me like this....

He and John like each other, Elsa being a dear, but given Jig a good dose of Romanism along with kindness. She is fine to him, tho.

Love from all five
Evelyn

[Handwritten, signed. BRBL]

To David Lawson

Car-sickness, France

August 7, 1926

Very dear Davy: I was happy to get your letter, even though it did not contain the best of news. I think about you both constantly, and it does me so MUCH good even to see your handwriting again and get a direct word that, if things aint much better, they aint much worse either.

We dont think we are going to stay in France. Our reasons are this - first John isnt well and French food habits and climate dont agree with him particularly. Secondly, the fluctuation in the franc has made us lose about half of such money as we have gotten over here, as, by the time I write to America (or even John to England) when we happen to have notice that there is any money due us, by the time it gets here the franc, bought at the exchange of the original date, has again depreciated, the cost of living here has advanced, and the fifty or hundred dollars

97

we started with arrives here, three weeks later, worth just half what it was. We have managed to get along anyhow, but it is not a cheering experience to people who are being economical, and there is the prospect, if Poincares cabinet does not survive the extreme odds against it, that something more drastic and generally disastrous may occur.

Consequently, we are considering what are the few cheap places left in the world to live in. North Africa is the cheapest, but politics here will affect there. Austria and Italy are the only two places where exchange is cheap and Vienna is very very cold in the winter. There remains Rome, which is raw but not so bad, and not so hard to get to from here, and would be very little less effort for Lola to reach if she comes over in a Fabro boat which stops at Naples. From there it is four hours to Rome, but if we go there and Lola comes, we would go to Naples to meet her.

You must not be prejudiced against meeting John by last summers experience. I think hes a dear, but just judged for himself without regard to me, I think you two would like him. Hes very reserved and very English, in a nice sense, and, if that helps you to be prepared for the best, as unlike Owen as two people could be. He and Cyril get on grand. John wants to meet you all, and I wish sometime in the next year or so we could go to America. But as usual cash.

Dear Davy, again, my best and most love to you and to her.

Evelyn

[Typed, signed. SSC]

To Louise Morgan

Hotel Europa
Cintra, Portugal
October 15, 1926

Louise, old darling, whats matter. Its been months since weve heard from you. wont you drop us a line and let us tell you how I got ill - I would - in Spain - our money almost but disappeared - and I got ill again of mild flu precipitated by rage and have been in bed strafing. And about how despite every known discomfort the landscape of Spain was worth suffering for once, less granite than Africa, but rick and forever looking earth near Fraga, the finest tents and plateaus of red, orange, purple, rockless treeless soil I ever saw - the most enormousness. And again, near Guadaloupe, plush look of clay hills in the finest barren purples, wine pinks, or bright gilt sallowness of trampled what. How Spain is bigger and stiller, save for magpies, than any country but the desert. The people all have a pride so envolved it must keep them from progress, for indifference they must feign in all but the passionate ceremonial of dancing or bull fighting and perhaps the feigning has become real - an arrogant torpor, shot with suspicion-their most fiery trait. They are courteous exceeding, but not warmly, more to exhibit their superiority to the petty, than from any outgoing to a stranger. I dont want to go thru equal discomfort again, but glad we did it.

Portugal is in proportion to Spain on the scale of the map - nothing grand, not even Cintra - but a modest lovliness, grandeur in little, with minute crags and wild woods confined in the acreage of the former kings domain. His palace, in execrable taste, never the less is a miniaturise of Byronic gloom and dominance, standing on the tip top of a hill above us, and piercing the sky with a fretted tower. Near it another Saracen ruin. It is not as cheap as we hoped, dearer than France, but too dear getting here to move away again. Cintra is smart, for the Portuguez, but the season is ending, the villas look shady and blind with closed shutters, and a pretentious casino displays yawning waiters and other employees staring in perpetual idleness thru a grand entrance up with nobody approaches. Ive forgotten all the Portuguez I ever knew. It was unutterable folly to try this, considering money.

Wish you could come over and work with us. We have a proposition from this hotel if we cant find a house. It is practically closed in the winter and man says he will give us five rooms and board all four of us for a hundred escudos a day, making about one hundred and fifty a month. Of course there will be extras so we have to think. And Jig has to have a school. Still, if we do, think how easy - always have another room rented for you if youd take the notion. Food not wonderful but fair - his usual price thirty five escudos a day for a person is a little under two dollars a day, there are boats direct from England, no train fare, and we could meet you. Dont you want a change again? We all work so youd have to. The isolation is fine for that. Its only when bits of bad luck seem to be the result of being off the business field that I wish we had money to break the isolation oftener - but I spent far more on me alone going to America last year than on all of us crossing Spain.

Mustnt forget to add an impression of Guadaloupe where we stayed overnight - way up in hills a sudden very white little town houses built low with moorish arches over the street, and, in the early morning, a market conclave of peasants in the doorway of a very old grey and gigantic church attached to an elderly monastary. The men uniformly in shirts of a sombre piercing blue, tight trousers, velvet braided waistcoats or jackets black sashes, and broad steeple crowned hats like the pilgrim fathers. The women shawled. It is a convent popular with fashionably religious Madrid that goes there to repent and retreat, but the obscure geography of its location leaves the peasants as authentically out of date as tho they werent perfectly picturesque. We liked an overnight in Toledo, too - a perfect little medieval background to an El Greco painting. And the Prado was a wonderful museum.

Madrid is like a raft, city complete up to the minute, yet old fashionedly stylist with many liveries and carriages and gardens and set things to do, it floats on a sea of what, among villages not much more substantial than the mud huts of the Arabs. There is no colour of the literal sort in the northern Spanish town - the dwellings are of mud brick unplastered, the floors are earth or dirty brick, the people are vigerous with a kind of slovenly energy - but there was no gaiety in dress except in Fraga where, for some reason, alone, the women are as elegant as Velasqueth princesses in wide

flowered skirts, tight neat bodices, and vivid demure shawls crossed like kerchiefs.
In Garonna we heard a fine Catalan band and saw the same dancing we encountered
in that end of France. It is Catalonia until Barcelona, but it was only after Zaragossa
that we heard pure Castillian, very easy to recognize even when not understood.
Altogether, we feel we were fools, considering Jig needs an overcoat and I cant get it
and some other things, but cant regret another folly which I hope has only temporary
bad results.

Lots and lots of love to both of you - and think about a visit

evelyn

[Typed, typed signature. BRBL]

Louise Morgan

Cintra, Portugal
November 19, 1926

Dearest Louise:

Of course I know you are too busy to write a length. Im wondering if you got
your passport straight and hope yes. I went to see a very cautious and patriotic gent
here who objected strongly to my having a bad photograph on my old one but finally
decided that I might possibly say you all like I was born in Tennessee. You know - got
in here with my passport expired. Ran out in Madrid and the consul couldnt give me
a new one in a hurry so I came on. It was gravely stamped by two sets of officials who
could read the visa but not the English part.

Its too wet here anyway. Cintra is where the English come for a change because it is
just like Scotland, and you should see the inside of the Palace of Pena that perches with
such specious confidence of the highest crag over us. All the court reception rooms are
done in IMITATION marble, with IMITATION woodwork - really paint and plaster - so
on. Queen Amalie slept in a bedroom where the furniture is decorated with something
as near like the strings of black beads worn by respectable widows as you could get in
carving. The triumph is the billiard room - one half size billiard table in a cubistic ocean
of marquetry, and all up and down the place settees which, in their rears, culminate
in mirrors exactly like cheap café ornament with huge overhangings of oak carvings.
Presiding over the scene, and the nineteen ten journals dramatically left where Manoel
had scanned them after his last royal high ball, are huge black nigger[58] figures bearing
lamps and torches. Its the most genteel sporting design I ever struck. But the view would
be wasted on almost any monarch. Unfortunately it is a view - that is to say there is
almost too much of it - but it is very lovely. And there was a swan in the park that was
the original one Hans Anderson dreamed about - enough to make rape voluptuous for
a thousand Jupiters - or was he the swan or was lada. Well, anyhow, I forget. Only we are
going to leave here as soon as we can get to Africa again where it is CHEAP.

58   This term was in common usage in the 1920s when Evelyn was writing.

I am dying to pea, hence a certain hecticness. So I will stop, as the saying is.

Lots of love, evelyn

[Typed, typed signature. BRBL]

To David Lawson

Mme Metcalfe[59]
Cintra, Portugal
[late 1926]

Dear ol Davy:

I guess Glad will have told about our reckless attempt to see Spain in a week - for which we had nearly three what with break downs in the borrowed car and getting ill. It was fun and no fun. Spain provided a barrenness more gorgeous than any I ever imagined at times - others sheer depressing monotony. But there were high spots that top everything in visual experience. It was autumn, so the rather uninteresting green had appropriately disappeared for a general tawnyness richer and more suitable to such harsh indifferent stretches. The conservatism of the Spaniards struck me forcibly - I think their ritualistic pleasures - dance and bull fights - are a bit of a Freudian outlet for their violent repression. Cautious and more so than the English - they make no mystic explanation of this. They lack subtlety. The English are so subtle emotionally - so disunited there with their deliberately commonsensical minds. The French with such subtle machines and no emotional data worth looking for. The Spaniards, in a birdseyes, tho I am not quite assuming myself an interpreter after one glance, are neither mystical at heart nor subtle of mind - but are primitives with their crudity congealed, and so somewhat concealed, by the formalism of the orient. Catalonia is non Moorish Spain - and its music, the only escape from a cheap modernity, is barbaric - a voodoo challenge to sex.

Southerly Spaniards really are moors with an underlying thing more naive and less refinedly brutal than the real north African product - I think. None of that goes does it with my other sense of a landscape as pure in color as snow is white. Its enormousness was its most constant quality - and Spanish grandiosity is like a simplification by an inadequate mind of grandeur, too untouched for bombast. Spaniards, en passant, seemed neither nervous like the French, nor emotional like the Italians, nor exalted by moral self mystification like the rest of us. But sensual - Puritans in temper as I always thought the Arabs were - the constant quality of the puritan being a mental view of sensation which is the product of his inferior but persistent intellectualization of himself.

Well I wont go on for days and weeks. Portuguese are nearer slave bred negros than is any other race. Their racial self respect has been vitiated. They have the wistfulness of their lack of confidence. Are gentle, treacherous, and easily influenced

---

59 Although not married to Jack at the time, it appears that Evelyn was passing herself off as his wife to avoid comment.

to generosity - I think. But it is not as cheap as we had hoped and we cant stay all winter.

Lisbon is very old and lovely. Cintra is only fifty minutes away. It is an anglicized summer resort abandoned in the winter. We have rooms in a hotel which is empty so that for nothing he gave us empty bedrooms to work in. The board is thirty five escudos a day, a small tax and a few extras. It would come out at about fifty dollars a month. Elsa is in Swiss with her mother who is ill. Cyril is here for a while. Cintra is a Byronic relic of the old court of Portugal with fussy palaces and so on but a very charming miniature wildness, sea in the distance, trees, and constant milky fogs in the soft green of dripping evergreens. There are lots of forests, somewhat artificial but very pretty. It is chilly but no shakes on New York.

Again LOVE. Please let us know how you all are. Please.

Cyrils VERY best love too,

evelyn

[Typed, typed signature. SSC]

To Otto Theis

Mme John Metcalfe[60]

Cottage Jean

Kouba, Algeria

January 16, 1927

Dear Otto, will you believe I was just settling down to write to you and Louise a letter with no requests in it? But you as only possible court of appeal in present distress is unfortunately suggested by everybody. it is thus: We have had a month of much endurance and some pleasure getting here) but the advent of plague in Oran which stopped the boat sailings and sent us around the longest way thru Morocco has played hell in other ways. Thomas Cook of Lisbon being a Portuguese Thomas Cook did not freight our luggage we now find until two weeks after we left Lisbon. He also freighted it to Oran via Gibraltar. So there sits the luggage containing all our reference books, and for me the entire guts historically of the Civil War novel. I was very distressed by being obliged to leave Lisbon just when I had reached the most ticklish point in the first draft, for tho it is easy to rewrite from the first to polish it is most difficult to retrieve the rhythm of a whole when it is broken just as its momentum is gathering.

Because of Cyrils show and Johns need to return to England, Algeria ends on April 15th. I can unpack textbooks in a Paris hotel with Jig, and if Cyril can sell sufficient pictures to pay fair we are going to NY to consider a school or something for Jig who has had a very unsatisfactory year and is beginning to feel the peculiar isolation of his situation. Imagine pipp, added to perhaps by the fact that we have with us only the clothes on our backs and no housekeeping linen, and that John lessly but also needs some of his books on Scilly for his next novel.

---

60 It may be that Evelyn felt it necessary to appear married in a conservative Muslim country.

Well, I would have cabled you what I am gonna ask but that our check from America was in Paris and we have to wait until it is mailed to Paris and sent back before we collect, and tho we have found an apartment we cant leave the hotel because we cant pay our bill until the money comes. So - I couldnt cable and cant send you any money until I have it.

Alger is very warm compared to Cintra. That is to say one wears wool undies and sweaters in the house and is comfortable. In Cintra one did so and writhed just the same. France is just a little better than Portugal, but my dream of Algerie as the cheapest place in the world dates back I am afraid, and is no longer appropriate. Then there are all these here new taxes on foreignors which we may or may not escape. I think I know how the Russian emigrants feel in America. Its a sensation very inhospitable to be taxed hard for living in a place, and the justice of the move doesn't modify the impression.

Cyril is beastly unwell with a heavy cold he has had up and down since we left Cintra. It worries me somewhat but I hope it will wear out here. All of us were ill on our way here and in bed at various places and stages. Im glad Louise didnt come to such a heaven for grippe as Cintra turned out. The Portuguese are SCUM-SCUUUUUUUUM. The country is nice in a spring gardeny way. Ill write Louise of our I am afraid futile wish she could be with us to finish some more work.

My humble love. I feel just like a drunkard that promised mother and then misbehaved again, for I did think I would NOT ask you to buy anything else for me. From all of us godspeed, happy new year, and our devotions. evelyn

Do Foils[61] possess any volumes of a book called Annals of Our Times by Irving, being a collected excerpts from the newspapers of England during the years dating from about eighteen thirty nine to eighteen eighty. It is in three volumes, also in trunk, and John bought them in a junk shop for a penny each. They are invaluable reference and have suggested to me using satire on newspaper style in parts of the book where events are merely referred to. This book is less necessary than the other two, but Cyril wants to own a copy anyhow, so if you do send a note maybe it wouldnt hurt to add an inquiry re this. Foils might look it up for later. On the other two speed am more requisite.

Again LOVE. Please let us know how you all are. Please.

Cyrils VERY best love too,

evelyn

[Typed, typed signature. BRBL]

---

61   Foyle's bookshop on the Charing Cross Road in London. Foyle's was then the world's biggest
      bookshop in both size and the number and range of titles stocked.

To Louise Morgan

Kouba, Algeria

January 17, 1927

Dear Louise: I wish you were coming to Alger for their narration and lots of other things. I wish you could - sometime. Especially as, after Cyrils show, IF he makes enough, it is our intention to go to USA while Jack goes back to England for a bit. We are losing too many contacts and Jig needs a school or something. He is very lonesome this winter and not very happy. In Portugal he did not make a single acquaintance. I am very much worried about Cyril, who left Portugal with a bronchitis and has it still and just can I think pull himself about, though his grit and pride exceed many admissions of the fact. Jack is a very very sweet and comprehending thing and I shall always be glad of my misdemeanors that gave me the opportunity of knowing him so well.

Tuesday: Since beginning this Cyril has cajoled the bank into giving him money before it comes from Paris and we have occupied Cottage Jean. Kouba is about six miles out but has a tram nearby. Our suite is very swell in that it has a real bath room and johnny, almost an American bath room, tho the hot water heater requires a wood fire under it. We have two bedrooms a kitchen a sala and sal-a-manger. They are the first floor of a country home of one of the legal profession who is now in town. Nobody but ourselves is in the house. There is a terrace at our disposal and last night, feeling very tired and gloomy, I retired there to meditate and saw all Alger in very delicate emerald due on the black hills under clouds all startling from an invisible moon. The ghost light expanded away from town and I could see all the scallops of beaches and surf quite plainly. It really is a lovely location, but beastly inconvenient as the shops are miles off and nothing, not even milk, delivered, and we have no present prospect of a servant. It took Jack until a quarter to twelve to do the marketing. Also it is raining profusely daily, and we miss our belongings which, as I wrote Otto, are somewhere, presumably, between Gibraltar and heaven.

We had a mild month of it, honey. The mysterious motor car in which we toured Europe I reveal to you privately as a used Renault of seven horse power which Cyril learned to run via Elsas brother when in Switzerland. Such a vehicle has never been known to do even as much as a Ford and was the first manufactured that ever crossed from France to Portugal. Cyril had it on a triptych which allowed him to keep it in Portugal three months, and before we left Cintra the time limit ended. Since then feats of bluff have been in order. First bluffing the officials at Vila Rial not to detain him on an expired license, and then - Well I will narrate in order. Cooks[62] told us Vila Rial was the best place to cross the border on. We got there and found a large river and no bridge. Were ferried over in a specially hired barge which consumed much of our wherewithal. Cyril was ill with bronchitis and has been for a month. Yesterday on

---

62 Thomas Cook; the travel agent had agents in numerous locations.

arriving here he at last went to bed with thermogene[63] iodine hot water bottles and all he has needed and hasnt cotton. He is there now and I hope hell stay some time.

At Sevilla I acquired the cold and not having his character and being blind with streaming eyes I laid down at once. Saw Sevilla mostly from the window in the few days there. It is a very cheery place despite colds, sunny, orange trees on the sidewalks, very new except for the vastly gloomy relic of the cathedral with a chaotic and occasionally impressive architecture and a very large bull ring also presumably dedicated to Christ.

We had intended to get a boat at Gib to Oran and from there to Alger, fairly short and inexpensive. At Sevilla received word that sailing was cancelled because of plague at Oran. Could only get our money back promptly by applying at Gib. We needed it so went on, via Jerez and some real sherry. Andalusia in its extreme south is all sterility, sun, prickly pear corrals and brilliant sea. Algiceras received our expiring bodies and John came down with tonsillitis. We went to Gib Xmas Even and found the garrison thinking of merrie England and rum punch. Sad English ladies with blond hair growing grey bought wild narcissus and berries to make things look like home tomorrow. It must be a queer exile under that overweight of fortification with Spain seeping in.

We had to choose between traversing the north to Port Vendres in snow and an open car and trying Morocco. No tryptichs issued for war zone. But we tried it, going to Ceuta on Xmas and eating cold lunch for Jigs plum pudding. We landed safely but it took a long chat with commanding colonel or sumpin he was to get a letter to let us thru. We were put under promise not to travel before nine or after five. Soldiers looking statuesque and important on all the heights by road. Bristley blockhouses - pickets in cocked hats and cloaks flapping dramatically in an icy wind. Mountains all snow. Tetuan is a motley hubbub of races. From there to Alcazarquiver over a pontoon at Larache where this week there has been more ado with Rifs. But once over the border we were in something more civilized than Spain. Good hotel at Kenitra where Jack was sick and we ran out of money and had to wait around until we could see the first of the month near and a wire possible. Reached Fez New Years even and got our money there. Saw all the French as drunk as the English at Xmas. Had champagne gratis at the hotel and all got sick on it - it being gratis. Saw wonderful walls and amethyst and jade gates (mosaics but fine) and an Araby Douglas Fairbanks never dreamed about.

After that Telemeen[64] en route went up mountains at dusk, motor lamps wouldnt work, ran into clouds, night fell, couldnt see where the cats cradle road went. Had

---

63 Thermogene was a proprietary medicated wadding which purported to ease the pain of rheumatism and similar ailments.

64 Despite extensive research it has not been possible to identify this location; however, the other places mentioned in this account are in a sparsely-populated part of the Algerian desert and it is likely Telemeen was in a similar area.

to get out and light matches to find mile stones. Road leaped over precipices, but we didnt. Bumped into Tolemeen walls about eight pm with our nerves in ribbons. Next day saw Cascades hanging in spun sugar over hundreds of feet of red and orange granite. (And I forget desert around Guercif, camels again, mountains steely and snow dashed, nearer like a milky night). Went to Mascarra where Jig was ill. On to Orleanville which is like a dump yard inside a jail. Reached Alger a week ago in a sleet storm that cracked the wind shield. All dead tired, no clothes, no linen for housekeeping, no books for reference, more or less ill yet, and Cyril a good deal.

Conclusion that it was worth while but not for often. Also that we are a good deal embarrassed for money. But once having made the fool essay of Portugal we had to get out with the car. Portugal is farther off than Mars.

My eyes wont let me go on. Cooking and house took too much of day. But do write when you feel like it, if for letters one ever does.

evelyn

[Typed, typed signature. BRBL]

The following two letters refer to the years Cyril and Evelyn spent in Bermuda with the wealthy Garland-Hale family (Chapter 3). Even though Cyril went to be their estate manager, a friendship developed between the Scotts and the Garland-Hales, who built a cottage ("The Scottage") for their continued occupation: this offer was later withdrawn. In addition, Marie Tudor Garland pledged them an income of $50 a month each for the rest of their lives, to be paid on her behalf by her solicitor, Walter Nelles, also withdrawn. The financial impact of this withdrawal would clearly have had major implications for Evelyn and Jack.

To Louise Morgan

Kouba, Algeria

February 8, 1927

Louise, old darling, Well, a very heavy blow has just descended upon our solar plexus, and I want to quote to you and Otto, in moderate confidence of course, the following letter received yesterday from Marie:

"Dear Evelyn:

"This is not an easy letter to write. Chiefly because in the past you have misunderstood me and quarreled with me.

"I find that it is impossible for me to continue as a patron of the arts! (Exclamation hers) I have come to the point where I am not only earning my own living, but am earning yours too. I am telling you this because I think you may wish to earn your own.

"I am finding it increasingly hard since I gave half of what I had to Swinburne to make a living off an income dwindled to almost nothing. Each year, to meet my obligations to you and to others, I have drawn upon my capital until that has almost disappeared. As I have a sense of humour I suddenly realized that I was trying to earn enough to take care of everyone but myself.

"I am in business, apart from everything else, and I may make good, but at present I am not making enough to go on with my annuities and I have to cut them out. I wish to reduce yours to half this year and pay nothing next year. This will give you a chance to look around and provide for yourself.

"I shall ask Walter to send you six hundred dollars this next year. I think you know without my telling you how sorry I am to have to do this.

Your friend,

Marie T Garland"

Which leaves us where we were five years ago except that Cyril has a chronic pulse of about a hundred and thirty and we are in Africa instead of New York.

Cyril is in Bousaad so I cant consult him yet. The joke is that all the checks have gone to him for over three years but I guess she couldnt forego a direct one at me knowing I was still getting my share. Of course in winter I was with you I was able to hold off thanks to you and Franks, but Cyril did not use it all for him anyway and it was what he had kept out that he called mine that went on this unfortunately expensive journey from Portugal. It has taken Jack all year to finish his novel so, tho he is working hard trying to get some short stories off to Peters, he has nothing ahead at present. Africa is a fine place to spend a small income but a poor one to find a supplement for no income at all. And even to get to Paris on fifty dollars a month doesnt look optimistic. If Migrations sells I may get a little from it next fall. I

In the meantime - Well, here we am. Of course Ive got to get back to America tho just how aint very exact. Im going to collect all the good clippings I ever had of my work and try to put it up to somebody or other to give me another hand out for a few years. Of course Cyril cant support me as of yore (even not counting his own affairs and the sacrifice of great painting) with a heart at a hundred and thirty all the time and a bronchial tendency getting worse - tho I know him and expect him to be as prodigally inclined re me and Jig as he always was, bless him. Nor do I see Jack, who is really very inexperienced in jobs and worldly things, very certain to contend successful with USA EVEN, which makes it a sickening thought, at the complete sacrifice of his imminent success.

Poor old Jig hears we are hard up and is a darling wanting to sell stamps and so on. But I want him to be EDUCATED since obviously he is to receive no inheritance. So its back where it was when Otto first knew us and Gladys took me to the general electric for a job I didnt get. of course if I get no help Ill have to go to work, which seems sillier now than it did then after having got as the publication of seven books and the acceptance of eight (EVEN tho they aint sold miraculously).

I am still choking in the implacable fact - but there it is - and the funny thing is I have expected it in nightmares for four years at least. And I still feel that it just couldnt be true that I have to give up writing, and, maybe, from what I guess anyhow, Cyril painting too. Of course the immediate problem is framing for Sugs show, and the getting of all of us away from here and to America. I have written asking Walter to try and get me the six hundred more of a lump instead of fifty per month, but he probably wont. We have just enough on hand to carry us thru the rest of time here with economy. Cyril of course can sell the Renault but it was worth so little to start on it so wont be no fortune. Otto was right, they aint no quiet life for this crowd.

But something in my gizzard is so mad I dont feel half as despairing as commonsense tells me I should.

We LOVE YOU TOO, YOU BET.

evelyn

[Typed, typed signature. BRBL]

To Marie Tudor Garland

Chez Mme Kay Boyle
Monte-Carlo, Monaco[65]
February 19, 1927

Dear Marie:

I have just received your letter of December 5th which has been forwarded to me.

Of course I am terribly surprised since you said at Bermuda "I have done this so you needn't ever have to worry again about your actual bread and butter". It simply never occurred to me after this that it was a contingent gift, otherwise I should never have come to Europe but should have made other plans.

I am very grateful for what I have received and am sorry to hear that your own resources have diminished.

During these years I have always hoped that some day we might come to a renewed understanding and friendship.

I shall get back to America as soon as I can, and try to make my belated plans for my future.

Again I thank you, and please know that I have always wished you happiness and good and always shall.

Very sincerely,

[Typed carbon copy, not signed. UTK]

---

65   There is no evidence that Evelyn left Kouba to travel to Monaco at this time and this return address appears to be a way of concealing their whereabouts from Marie. Evelyn and Cyril had been giving Marie the Theis' London address, and their dealings with her had been largely through her lawyer, Walter Nellis.

Chapter 11

Montreal
August 1927 - Summer 1928

The first indication that Jack and Evelyn were in Montreal is this letter from Jack to Louise Morgan. It is clear from the empty envelopes found at the Beinecke Rare Book Library that there had been a quantity of earlier correspondence, with Evelyn writing to Jack from Paris and later from Staten Island in New York, and Jack writing from Chislehurst in Kent where he would have been staying with his friend John Gawsworth, and from Bosham in Sussex, where his elderly relatives lived. No correspondence from these months survives.

To Louise Morgan

1206 Mackay Street
Montreal, Canada
September 7, 1927

My Dear Louise,

Here I am, and really fixed up at last. There was no word from Antigonish[66] and funds were getting low so I accepted a non-resident school job here in Montreal for the winter, till I'm on the quota. The above address is that of my digs. I'm not actually in them yet but shall be in a few days. The school begins on the 12th. It's quite a good one, - fair salary of $1600 but very, very light hours and Friday to Monday free each week.

Evelyn has just returned to N York after spending six days with me here in a hotel. She's looking very fit and sends love and things to all three of you, - so do I.

I'll see her again at Xmas vacation and after that she may come up here and live with me until Easter, - ca depend… Anyhow, I'm v bucked to have a nice job all settled and it won't be so intolerably long to May or June and the quota.

How are you all?. . I'll see you all again in May when I return to England. What fun if you came back for your visit to USA with me then!

No more just now. I'll write again soon.

---

66   Jack had applied for a teaching post at Mount Saint Bernard College, in Antigonish, Nova Scotia. Although he did eventually find employment at another college in Montreal, the surviving letters do not identify it.

Love to you all three,[67]

from

John

[Handwritten, signed. BRBL]

To Louise Morgan

1206 Mackay Street

September 13, 1927

Louise, beloved kid:

I dont know who owes a letter, but I must regale you with Montreal. It has made a patriot of me. All the most brutal part of France become American! A large flat city with more miles of double two story houses than ever existed even in London, and dingy shops from which skyscrapers spring like dreary aspirations. There is a big mountain quite alone and butt on the town. You gaze upward at it and think there midst natures solitudes will be escape from the eleven thousand rubber neck wagons taking the eleven million boozed Americans on tours which respectably excuse their presence above the line. You climb through seedy suburbs and seedy intimations of a park, and the world lives before you - as wide as it looked at Bezier, with the Saint Lawrence broken up in bits of canal like looking glasses, and smoke from factories adding something sumptuous to the general magnificence of distance. But beside you, to support you in your Byronic contemplation, have appeared miraculously all the eleven million Americans, appropriately, interested in nature, and buying birch canoes and moccasins to take home to the little ones.

There is a tourist tram, so called, in which, for twenty five cents, you can make a belt tour of the city. All the buildings not two story tenements, are orphanages, catholic day schools, or hospitals. For every twenty houses there is some barracks like institution. And for every institution there is a brand new baroque catholic church, than which there is nothing worse. Everything exists except libraries. Cheap department stores are almost as numerous as Woolworths, grands, and shops in which to buy pious tinsel religious junk. The place is in the spittoon age. The most delicate gesture any landlord or landlady can make to a guest is to present a cuspidor to him.

But Jack was darling, and while low when I sent the postal, has a job at last and is bucking up. Jig and I may go to stay for a while at Xmas.

Always our ardentest affection to Otto, and to you armful.

evelyn

[Typed, typed signature. BRBL]

---

67 Louise and Otto had had a son, Michael.

To Louise Morgan and Otto Theis

1206 Mackay Street
October 27,1927

Dear Louisan Otto:

Thought you might be interested in this (its Jigs birthday) - just had a letter from Marie in which she says that as my marriage to Jack[68] making "easier" for her, she is permanently discontinuing all assistance (it is indicated she means Cyril too) after December. So Ill have to be hiking back to USA December 1st whether jack goes or not.

Why didnt I learn to cuss in Hindustani.

love

evelyn

[Typed letter, typed signature. UTK]

To Louise Morgan

1206 Mackay Street
November 8, 1927

My Dear Louise

Why don't you write to a bloke? I've been expecting to hear from you for ages, so buck up. I'm so on my own here that a letter from you will do me good. Damn the bloody Canadians! Anemic, smug dilutions of USA with a pale reflection of its approved vices and still paler, sicklier reflection of its unacknowledged virtues. Oh, God, for some good smutty stories to shock these Montrealers! Perhaps the Quebec lumberjacks have guts, I don't know. These folk haven't enough seminal fluid between them to stick a diatom on to a glass slip. Their flavour is that of the bland belchings of a Congregationalist minister who's been eating lentil soup and has to fart at the wrong end. These people are a suburbia without a metropolis, the most perfect apotheosis of parochialism, small-townism, I ever saw. And simply greasy with virtue. They've nothing really of their own, make no unique contribution to anything whatever. I loathe them.

Apart from Canadians life ain't so bad. Only six more weeks and I go on vacation to New York and return here in January plus Evelyn and Jig. Fortunately I get paid enough at this school to make this a feasible proposition. Then, I suppose, I'll return to England whenever that cable comes, some time in the Spring, after which I get on the quota[69] and sail back to USA.

---

68   Evelyn and Jack were not married at the time, even though she had been styling herself "Mrs Metcalfe".

69   The National Origins Quota system required that a person wishing to register to reside in the United States had to return to his home country and apply from there to be included in the quota for that country before re-entry. Jack's immigration status was to become a constant theme throughout the remainder of his life.

How are you all? How's Michael and how's the paper? Especially, how's the novel? Have you any time for working at it? Please do write and tell me all your news.

Well, this is most of my news for the present. Do be a sport and write.

Heaps of love to you all three.

Yrs ever

John.

[Typed, signed. BRBL]

To Louise Morgan

Apt 12, The Hollywood
800 Dorchester Street West
January 22,1928

Louise, dear

I think I wrote you from the much upholstered boarding house in which we first landed amidst Pekinese dogs, radios, and Nottingham lace. But we are moved now into a comparative privacy that seems luxurious. As our flat is smaller than seventeen Cliffords Inn[70] I rather dreaded the accommodation of three people to it. But somehow, despite its being in Montreal, it embraces so much more convenience than weve dreamt of in the last years that we dont get in each others way - not very much. It is warm. The double windows open when it is desired and the sealing away of the winter is not final and exclusion of fresh air. And the water for baths is almost always hot. And one can pea at leisure, without having to wait until some of the other boarders aint doing it. And there is a kitchenette for breakfasts, though for the other meals we still go out.

I write from nine to one and from two to four. Jack gets up - me with him - at half past five, and writes from breakfast after six thirty until school time at eight-fifteen, and for a couple of hours at night, from seven to nine oclock, and on Saturday and Sunday. Jig going to a tiny English school and has a gymnasium twice a week and ice hockey. And somehow our schedules are so neatly joined that even the fact that Jack and I sleep in the living room makes no crowdedness. And its only now and then that I get fretful with not making money for more. partly because the older I grow the more I like indulgence of the flesh, and partly because, as usual, Cyril is the one person who can make anything. He lectured at Amherst last week most frightfully successfully, and tomorrow morning he is starting west. Of course there will be more show for the rest of us when this quota business is settled, but salaries in Montreal for anything are most economical.

As usual in this perpetual foreignness of environment, I get most of my dramatic effects from the weather, and I am still as much enraptured with the coldness as I dreaded it. It snows every day, a little. I dont care for the insipid brilliance of what is

---

70   The Theis' London address.

called the best weather, when the streets look like the careful blue and white and lilac of Academicians who are just beginning to realize that Renoir lived. But I do love the warm, secret, indoors feeling of the greyest days. And a kind of delicious insipidity in the white ornaments of trees and bushes, and the especially private look of yards and gardens, while the sky is such a lurid darkness, and I think that the little lambs are gambolling somewhere down in hell. The icicles on the eaves make all the roofs like pantry shelves in frilled paper. And when even the inside of your nose has a medicated sanitary feeling as any little drop of moisture you are breathing freezes. There is a sweet bitterness over everything like a very innocent perfumery. You dont get cold, because everytime you poke your nose out of the house, you get such a slap from the elements that you can walk about for an hour or two quite numbed and peaceable. Then suddenly you are reminded because your ears begin to ache.

Lots and lots of love, darling kiddie, from all of us

evelyn

[Typed, typed signature. BRBL]

To Otto Theis and Louise Morgan

800 Dorchester Street West

February 17, 1928

Dear Peoples,

We're very cozy here in our minute flat of about 1 9/16 rooms. One real room for E and self, half a room for Jig, and the remaining 1/16 divided between kitchenette and bathroom. Evelyn likes the cold and wishes it were colder! At the moment it's thawing and raining and very muggy. Everyone says there never was weather so abnormal - but that happens to us everywhere we go.

Jig is fit, and has got skis, and is enjoying his school. Evelyn's hard at it as always, and so am I.We shall probably be here until my school ends in June (unless I happen to get a cable re quota before that) - and then I shall come over to England and see you all. Mind you let us know of any changes of address if you leave No 17 as you think of doing.

No more just now. Write soon. God bless you and good luck, and love and hugs from

us both.

John

[Handwritten, signed. BRBL]

At around this time Cyril had moved to Santa Fe, New Mexico. His motive appeared to be, at least in part, to establish a school of painting while at the same time taking advantage of the opportunity to paint more of the desert landscapes he had successfully painted in Algeria and the south of France.

Meanwhile, and apparently without Evelyn knowing anything about it, he had taken steps to end his "marriage" to Evelyn. He crossed into Juarez, in the state of Chihuahua just over the border in Mexico and, supported by a lawyer recognised by the court as "Attorney-in-fact", succeeded in achieving this. Evelyn and Cyril had never been legally married, even though Evelyn consistently referred to their union as a "common-law marriage", an institution which was not recognised in the state of Louisiana where Evelyn had been living before their "elopement". Cyril may have been able to make this claim as common-law marriage was, and is still, recognised in Kansas, were he had been (and still was) legally married. Perhaps the Mexican judge should have done some research before hearing this case. Or perhaps he was persuaded that Evelyn was "acquainted with the laws" in force at the time.

Below is an excerpt from a certified translation into English of the Mexican document granting Cyril a divorce. It is not clear whether Evelyn knew about this-the certified copy of the judgment refers to Cyril's lawyer having "power of attorney". The statements made to the court do not appear to be accurate statements of the circumstances surrounding their marriage, but the court nonetheless accepted them and granted the decree.

CIVIL COURT

C.JUAREZ-CHIH.

CERTIFIED COPY of the judgment pronounced
in the ordinary civil suit for necessary
divorce instituted by Mr Cyril Kay Scott
against his wife, Mrs Evelyn Dunn Scott
City of Juarez, Chih. March 16, 1928

Attorney José Amador y Trias, Judge of the Civil Court of First Instance, of the Bravos District, acting with the Secretary in legal form, CERTIFIES: That there appears in the ordinary civil suit for necessary divorce instituted by Mr Cyril Kay Scott against Mrs Evelyn Dunn Scott, a judgment which word for word is as follows:

JUDGMENT

City of Juarez, March 14, 1928. After hearing this ordinary suit for divorce instituted by Mr Cyril Kay Scott against his wife, Mrs Evelyn Dunn Scott, and

(1) WHEREAS, by petition dated March 1st, Mr Cyril Kay Scott presented a suit for divorce to this court against his wife, Mrs Evelyn Dunn Scott, based on the causes enumerated in Fraction V of Article 76 of the Law of Domestic Relations which is equivalent to Fraction VI of Article 235 of the Civil Code, that is to say - for unjustifiable abandonment of the home by his wife resolving not to return thereto. In this petition Mr Scott shows that his marriage with Mrs Evelyn Dunn Scott was celebrated in the United States and was a common law marriage perfectly valid and recognized by the laws of the country wherein it was celebrated, and gave this as the reason why he could not produce a marriage certificate of any kind, as none existed;

(2) WHEREAS, Mrs Evelyn Dunn Scott filed answer in this cause acknowledging same in its entirety and showing therein that it was a fact that she was united in matrimony with plaintiff on December 26, 1913, by common consent, and the free will of both parties, in accordance with the common law which is in force in the United States; that she is acquainted with the laws of said country, and that the statements made in the complaints in reference to the laws of the United States, as well as in reference to the laws of Mexico, are entirely correct; and she concluded her answer by asking that notice be waived, that she confessed the complaint in its entirety, and that the suit be terminated by citing the parties for judgment, and issuing order declaring the marriage bond existing between the plaintiff and defendant, dissolved;

THE UNDERSIGNED JUDGE DECREES:

(1) Mr Cyril Kay Scott proved the action for necessary divorce in this suit, and Mrs Evelyn Dunn Scott did not present exemptions thereto;

(2) THEREFORE, a decree of divorce is hereby granted with dissolution of the bond of matrimony by both parties hereto for the reasons contained in Fraction V of Article 76 of the Law of Domestic Relations and Fraction VI of Article 235 of the Civil Code, that is to say - the unjustified abandonment of the home by the defendant, the said parties being free to conduct matrimony.

Thus it was adjudged and signed by the Honorable Judge by the Civil Court of First Instance of the Bravos District, Attorney José Amador y Trias

(Signed) - J AMADOR Y TRIAS

A R CORRAL, Secy

[Typed translation of original Mexican legal document, signed, sealed, with cover. SFC]

To Louise Morgan

1206 Mackay Street

May 2, 1928

Dearest Louise:

Well, my dear, if wishes were - not horses (why horses anyhow) - but could produce the hard cash. Jig and I would come over with Jack next month, rent a flat with Mrs Dewey, and give ourselves ample opportunity for witnessing the reunion. Hang it, of course it is the usual thing. Jack sails on June twenty-eighth. We are all hung up until after the quota and might as well, in theory anyway, spend the interim in economy comparative in England, as dwell in New York. Only the lump sum for the fare over is lacking.

Did you know blessed Cyril has gone and went and got married again John Crawfords sister Phyllis.[71] Phyllis is really matured into a complete and lovely

---

71   Phyllis Crawford was the sister of John Crawford, the friend with whom Evelyn sometimes stayed in New York. She became Cyril's fourth wife.

astonishment. She had her hair bobbed a few years ago and suddenly seemed to reveal her personality at the same time, has grown awfully pretty I think, and is as quick as a whip and as detached as most of us aspire to be. I think she has always adored Cyril, and the more ardent turn of affairs was in the air when the 'orrid quarrel about Jig[72] precipitated my departure from John and Beckys establishment last fall. And then she went down to Santa Fe with Cyril and they got married.

I dont really believe any tragedys will result from this. Phyllis is sincere, honest, has a lovely sense of humour, can earn her own living if she has to - has done so for a long time and is an expert in library work, is in good health, is irreligious, is only thirty years old, just, and has had enough troubles of her own to have come comprehension of other peoples. So thats that again.

Now we have resumed the old plan of settling temporarily anyhow in the same vicinity, with Jig to have the right of way with both. Where that will be the lord yet probably doesnt know. Cyril got started on his western lecture tour, but his dates were so inconvenient with breaks in between that, having to halt and spend money in the intervals, it was not turning out as well as he had hoped. He arranged for a show in the State Museum at Santa Fe, and went to fix it up and discovered there was a very good opening for a class there. So at last accounts he was trying to get the lecture bureau to transfer the dates they had made for next fall, in the hope they could make an intinery that would keep him busy steadily for a short time instead of sporadically for a longer time. If it pans out he will spend the summer teaching painting at Santa Fe which will allow him to paint - he has hardly touched a brush for one year - the very type of country he most loves. Then about October try the lecture game again. I think this is much better than the original - because of the paint - and hope it pans out. But in the meanwhile none of us know where we are at. As soon as Cyril gets enough ahead he offers to pay the fares of all of us out west, but that aint yet, and anyway would be wasteful until he himself is certain he will find it worthwhile to stay at least a year.

Jack is sailing for your shores June twenty-eight, and hasnt the faintest idea whether the quota will let him out in three weeks or six months. Jig and I are hung up. What we plan vaguely is to spend July in NY with the dentist, then find a place out of town. But places out of town near New York and economical are sure scarce. Also to find a two room flat to sublet for July, and find it before we leave here. For petes sake tell us if you hear of any.

By the way, Jig is a man - puberty and all. He has a moustache. Next yet at the limit he will have to shave it. He is a little over five foot seven how, with a bass voice. I dont know what to do. And so nice, and so lonesome, and no exercise at all now the skiing

---

72   There is no information about the reasons for this quarrel. Jigg would have been 12 at the time, and in his unpublished memoir *Confessions of an American Boy*, writes in scathing detail about his treatment at the hands of his parents' friends as well as his opinions about Phyllis.

has stopped - Margaret[73] gave him skis and a ski suit which touched me like hell. He looks far more like Cyril than he does like me.

Evelyn

[Typed, typed signature. BRBL]

To David Lawson

800 Dorchester Street
June 16, 1928

Dear Davy:

As I go over your letter it is such a succession of generosities that the proper answer to it would be on large THANKS down all the page. I am arriving in New York about nine thirty in the morning and fortunately Ruth Whitfield is going to meet me and help with luggage and so on; so that beyond seeing you there would be no use anyway. And as for that, I shall call on 793 Broadway[74] the minute I get my belongings settled - on the afternoon of the twenty-eighth, or evening - unless I have to wait for my trunks or some similar uninteresting impediment exists. And what blessed fun it will be for me to see you both again!

Honey aint you all got this quota thing in your bean yet! Poor old jack, far from coming to NY for me, is due in england for his quota number. He can not enter on the english quota except when sailing from an english port. If he went in from canada he would need to reapply here after a years residence; and then perhaps wait. As we still want to avoid any backdoor complications if we can, he goes back now with the hope that his number will come up by September. If there is a hitch, we will have to again make other plans. Im to hang around NY until the government verdict becomes definite. Then if the gods are good - we will settle down for next winter near Cyril and Phyllis.

So he and Phyllis settled in Santa Fe for the summer to take stock. In the meantime he has had no trouble in getting a fair sized class in painting; but he says a lot of them are vacation pupils and he has no idea whether there is an income in that which will be year around. He has three shows being arranged for but none at once. However, what really pleases me is that he has done some of his best things just recently of the New Mexico desert, which he thinks very wonderful country - less subtle than Algeria, but with a gorgeous austerity none the less. Well, you know what I think of dearest Cyril, and I sure am praying that it turns out so that he will be relieved of strain and just left to feel free for painting first. He is not strong enough to go on forever gambling for Jigs future and so one, in the practical... *[remainder of letter missing]*

[Typed, two pages only. SSC]

---

73 Margaret DeSilver, wealthy New York socialite and loyal friend of Evelyn and Jack. She gave them significant material aid in a number of ways on more than one occasion.

74 David Lawson's New York address.

Cyril had been in Santa Fe for some months when in June 1928 Evelyn and Jigg returned to New York, leaving Jack, whose teaching appointment had come to an end, in Montreal pending his return to London. Meanwhile, Evelyn, with Jigg, took lodgings in Woodstock, a small town on the Hudson River about 100 miles north of New York City.

To Lola Ridge

Woodstock, New York

August 9,1928

Lovely girl: I can telephone on a party line from out here; but there are twenty-one phones on the same line and the connection is terrible - and costs eighty-five cents. That is why I have requested the aid of various unknown aides, who may annoy Davy with their telephone calls from town; but I am sure he will forgive me if he realizes what a relief it is to establish even that approximation of direct connection with what is going on.

My eyes are still wabbly; and if I ever get settled near an occulist I can trust, Im going to take desperate measures. As long as I dont write Im splendid; but Im afraid that, even aside from economic pressure, I have forgotten how to enjoy literal idleness.

Cyril writes that he has Jigs fare to Santa Fe - or will have it in a few weeks. And when it appears I will have to come to town to send him off. As he cant prolong his treatments at the dentist anyway, I expect to bring him in a day or two ahead to pack and have the bridges off. Hazel may be able to find some place for me to stay, but if she doesnt maybe I will call on Davys charity again, if you are feeling better then. Im afraid I would have to allow at least three days for dentistry and packing. Then, in the interval of uncertain plans, I guess Ill come up here again.

Anyway - I love you (the only platitude I cant withhold) dear, dear, dear, dear lovely thing.

evelyn

[Typed, typed signature. SSC]

To David Lawson

Woodstock, New York

August 16, 1928

Dear absolute brick Davy: I was very much touched by all your generous alarm on my behalf. You are a sweetie. But it would not do much good for me to run away in a fashion that would prevent my knowing what happened. You see my denial of mother is an intellectual matter, and while to have her with me permanently in one menage would, as I know from past experience, end work and happiness; I have that subconscious affiliation with her than can not be eliminated by the mandates of reason. When Cyril took charge of her letters he was doing his reasonable best for me; but it didnt work. I had subconscious horrors about her all the time. To give you an example, while I adore Cyril so completely as a human that I could never resent his interference on my behalf, I never forgave Alfred Kreymborg for being rude to mother.[75] This will show you that my personal pride as well as infantile affection is still identified with mother.

I wrote Margaret DeSilver about the last news - which is that the Graceys[76] are going to begin an action against my father. If it works some money may be gotten for mother, tho I doubt it will be enough to solve things. Anyway I believe they wont ship her here until that is settled. This gives me a few months leeway, I gather. In the meantime, if there looms up, as I fear, the alarming possibility of me being involved as witness in the lawsuit against my father, Margaret says she will pay my fare to England, which would be a more effectual escape than hiding in New York. But I am also waiting to find out what comes of that.

However, the immediate favor I would like to ask is this.

Dear Davy, again thank you from me heart for the real and beautiful friendship you so constantly show. I will be in town in September when I bring Jig in, as I said, and will be very humbly receptive to advice. I have been so worried and upset that I have done almost no writing, and would like to concentrate on finishing something before I bike off to England or somewhere else.

If I sent a small check by Jig - ten or fifteen dollars - could you cash it? It is hard to cash checks here.

Best love of Jig to me and to you and her,

evelyn

[Typed, typed signature. SSC]

To Lola Ridge

Woodstock, New York

August 28, 1928

Beloved:

Jack telephoned from Montreal last night and said he had got no job yet and his money was getting so low he thought he would have to return to England while he had the fare. He was evidently pretty overwrought, and I have decided to leave for Montreal tomorrow night so that I can at least see him before he goes - or maybe we can fix a plan between us about coming here.

with apologies - no I wont keep this up - and so much love

from evelyn

[Typed, typed signature. SSC]

---

75 Alfred Kreymborg was an American poet, novelist, playwright, literary editor, and anthologist. The letters do not record any information about this incident.

76 The Graceys were cousins of Maude Dunn, with whom she had been staying ever since her return from Brazil. The action against her husband, Seely Dunn, was presumably for financial support for Maude to relieve the Graceys of their financial responsibility towards her.

Chapter 12

Felixstowe

September 1928 - Spring 1929

At some time between late September and early October 1928, Evelyn and Jack returned to England while Jigg joined his father in Santa Fe. At first they stayed with Jack's long-time friend C Thompson-Walker at his home not far from London in suburban Kent, leaving after a few weeks to travel to Felixstowe, on the North Sea coast of Suffolk to find lodgings near what had been Jack's childhood home.

To David Lawson

care C F Thompson-Walker
Chislehurst, Kent
September 25, 1928

Dearest Davy:

My time since arrival has been spent mostly in bed - throat chest eyes (due to unheated houses). It is quite cold.

Dear Davy. this has been an odd experience (the visit) which I will narrate for you and Lolas delection some day. It is seeing England for sure.

And no friends in the world were ever what you and Lola are and have always been to me. I just relapse into weeping mistiness when I try to express it. I love you both very deeply (and Pete knows I ought). But you both know all that.

Darn if you are so good to me. Wish I could ever be half.

England. my England

Of cold meat pie

Of raddled cheek

And haughty eye,

Of Indian Colonel,

Roman dame,

I sometimes wonder why I came!

(But I don't - Jack is a good reason.) Love, blessings, thanks to you and Lola from both)

[Handwritten, not signed. SSC]

To David Lawson

Chislehurst, Kent
October 8, 1928

Dear Davy:

Lola spoke of it being possible to call on somebody for small sum of money if we were in straits. I don't trust her not to make exaggerated sacrifice, so I write you stating case, dear Davy. and ask you to use your judgement.

Jack, as you know, has quota, it will require being in US by Xmas. We thought to leave soon but he lacked fare. Constable says that if he will finish an appreciable part of new novel before sailing they will give him a portion of his advance - enough. I think - to pay fare.

But he lacks $500 needed in pocket to show customs before quota landing is permitted. Margaret, when I asked her before leaving, said she would send it. She called today she was broke and did not have it.

It is not a loan in the usual sense, since it is not to be touched by us even with the idea of paying back. It is merely like a wad of fake bills to flash at the government and return to owners when we land. I have written to Glad and to Ellen asking if they could manage to contribute to the fake. I would not do so if I believed there were any risk, but the money seems to me absolutely safe, except that it will be withdrawn from circulation elsewhere until we land with it.

You know the true conditions under which Lola made the offer, and so I'm axin you to decide whether or not this situation can be passed on to her without tempting her to self-sacrifice.

Can you suggest anyone to whom I could apply? I'm passing the hat only people must understand it is not a loan in the usual sense.

Rather worn out with this stewin', yet know your worries are worse than mine.

The gods bless and keep you both. love you me and Jack,

Evelyn
Jack doesnt know yet I am writing this.

[Handwritten, signed. SSC]

To David Lawson

Chislehurst, Kent
October 9, 1928

Dear Davy:

If Jack and I can raise the $500 to flash at the government we will sail Dec 14 or a little earlier - say 7th if Jacks writing allows. Will your 2nd studio be occupied or could you let it to us for four or five days? We hope to be able to go to NO[77] by freight boat almost at once but could find no sailings from her to NO that fitted in. Anyhow if we get to NY Jack is in.

---

77   New Orleans.

If that happens and you can take us in. I would ask you to leave your key with Lola and we could go from boat by her place, if she is well enough to give it us.

I'm kind of homesick and longing for you all. I enclose a note to Lola *[below]* as I don't know whether she is using Cox or house.

With very much love always
Evelyn

[Handwritten, signed. SSC]

To Lola Ridge

Chislehurst, Kent
October 9, 1928

Beloved:

How I wish I could break down the doubt unplanted now of ever finding an ear for what gives me the word of poetry. It makes my pen halt and refuse to write it. If it were not for that. I could give you an adequate sense of a scene meant for you when, yesterday, walking over Westminster Bridge just as rain came over sun and sun burst faintly or the shivered rain again, we looked East along the solid low enormous ramparts of Somerset House. and below them to the embankment, faintly with scurrying red busses and then further to some grey shape of commerce that was probably a Brewery between us and London Bridge; and the gulls were whirling - like little rotating white machines - children's inventions, I thought, and the barges at the South Bank - the dingy bank - lay stranded in a bramble bus of schooner masts and the soiled Thames water tuned murkily a half-blue, as if peace had shone upon it an instant in passing on.

The other way the Houses of Parliament and Westminster Spire took that sonorous contour that fog and evening gives to everything here - and there was the intimation of sunset too reserved to flame forth.

Afterward Jack and I walked up the Strand and down to Temple Gardens where the flowers do credit - as in old English gardens - to that timid poetry too doubtfully expressed in other places. The dahlias were a whole city up and down the wall - sulphur pale end of a red that I wanted to call Charlotte Corday, if allowed to give them a name.

There was a little sunken garden, a nursery for baby asters, with a minute pool like a fairys sea. and a minute bronze cherub riding on top of it.

All of London I get thru the eyes. I love its bulk, which is orchestral, and is always softened and liquefied by the gentle darkness of mists in sun.

Of the people I have a mood of weariness, due to meeting too many relatives.78 They make me like better to think of raucous New York and all our screaming rather ugly youth, where this is a at least no dry-rot niceness yet.

Love, Beloved, and anxious hopes to hear good of you,

---

78 Probably a reference to Jack's maiden aunts, who lived about 60 miles away in Sussex.

Love from Jack too to you and Davy,
Evelyn

[Handwritten, signed. SSC]

To Lola Ridge

Chislehurst, Kent[79]

October 18, 1928

Sweetheart. I know you will be glad that I have recovered the use of a typewriter. It at least eliminates for the time one of the lesser tests of our friendship for me. As for the other way round, however. I am really so improving in capacity to decipher that it is a sort of a pleasure of sanity to peruse one of your distinguished flourishes.[80]

Jack and I hope to reach New York by mid December, depending on possession of the five hundred needed to show customs. His passage has been advanced on condition he has three quarters of his new novel done before we sail. I have mine.

Cyril has hopes of a job in west by Jan 1st. There the remains problem of a week in New York. For Gawds sake dont let Davy re-rent that place even if he can, but will you both inquire when it comes up if there is any place available to rent for a week at that time? Im leery of landing there with no place decided on if I can help it. Shall write to the Waverly Hotel in Waverly Place if there is no other way. Scarcely heard from anybody.

And. oh. I forgot to tell you we have lodging at Felixstowe in a house where Jack lived in childhood - it was then his home not lodgings. This is where the German Empress used to summer but nothing remains but a mouldy dwelling, modestly regal, now hotel. We face the North Sea and empty atrocities occupied by summer trippers but now abandoned to the gales. It is like a locust shell that has been shed. this town in winter-all new and a perfect husk, but lifeless after summer. Except that the sea stays cold and alive and yesterday was stormy with the sun brazening sulphur brown clouds and the gulls mewing, and a few nursemaids with prams running to escape the rain on the elegant promenade beach where nobody walks after Sept 1st. It is all new here, with an after war newness that makes England the lame counterpart of Douglas, Long Island,[81] but it is very cheap at this season. Love and love to you from us and to dear Davy

[Typed, not signed. SSC]

---

79 It is clear from this letter that while Evelyn and Jack have moved to Felixstowe in Suffolk, they are continuing to use Chislehurst as a forwarding address.

80 A reference to Lola's distinctive handwriting.

81 Douglas is the home of the Jenkins, Merton's parents-in-law.

To Lola Ridge

c/o Chislehurst, Kent
November 5, 1928

My Dear Lola,

This place where we are now is a seaside town where I went to school as a boy.
and strange to say we are lodging in what used to be my old home! - (By the way, this
is Felixstowe. Suffolk but I have put the Chislehurst address at the top of this letter as
being more sure to find us as long as we remained in England).

Evelyn sends you both her love. Please remember me very warmly to Davy.

Love, and all good wishes, - and again, thanks,

from

Jack

[Handwritten, signed. SSC]

To Lola Ridge

Leopold Road
Felixstowe, Suffolk
November 7, 1928

Now my heart and light. i would take your money at once - naturally - having asked
for it - but i have already got the five hundred collected. I did not know i could do
it so easily or i would never have troubled my poverty stricken angel (or poor but
unstricken angel.) So I wont need it. tho i am afraid this comes too late to prevent the
bother. Anyway. that will relieve me of arguing with you about who has it. You raised
cane about money from unknown sources, so why in hell should you expect me not
to? HUH!

Marie has cut off everybody now - cyril included - and it strictly depends on us.
Jack is unbusinesslike - and me you know, gawd save the day. I have been meditating
on taking a trained nurses training - provided I can, wearing a belt, keep on my feet
that much. It would be interesting of course and not so bad on the eyes as a job where.
instead of working as i do now by careful lighting and with days of rest to save them, I
would have to use them eight hours in any sort of light. But really we are a blank until
we reach new york.

However with every appreciation we accept the studio until we can look around
- a few days - to it is hard on you i realize. I thought of asking ellen to let me use her
place for a rendezvous day of arrival as i dont see any taxi man mounting davys stairs
with trunks. Ill wire both of you when date is fixed.

Am giving up smoking for time. Feel very heroic but with heroism in danger of
toppling.

I still have to write you someday about the countryside in Sussex with Aunt Mary
- the geniality of it was lovely, and the safe, safeness of realizing that nobody would
ever be disagreeable or mention a disagreeable topic. People loved their gardens,

gossip, tea - a sunny, dreaming kind of backwater where the intrusion now and then of a tragic hint was scarcely credible. It made me feel as when a child before i began to think for myself and trusted my parents. They still do - in God the Father.

Lovely, lovely, lovely, to you and to davy, always,

your grateful evelina (as aunt mary insists because she once had a small sister, died in

1862, named evelina)

[Typed, typed signature. SSC]

To David Lawson

Felixstowe, Suffolk

December 4, 1928

Dearest Davy:

Guess we all seem worlds worst pills in making so many demands on friendship and. technically standpoint of letters returning to little. Virtue counts very little. I only know because I have seen it what Cyril puts into starting these new enterprises that are to save us all from starvation - and thats what his art school idea is intended for. Just one year ago and the specialist Cyril had in new York said that his nerves were in a condition, with his heart, that would either kill him or land him in invalidism for life (this is confidential) and yet he is still going and having persuaded the unutterably hyde bound citizens of El Paso to send at least a fair number of their daughters to him, besides bucking the troubles that came when he and Phyllis went away from NY. So, dear Davy, while there aint a leg to stand on in one way, please be forgiving. Indeed I see you are.

Jig has no such excuse, except that he is a bum letter writer. However it appears that he did not receive your sweet present or anything, as I just had a letter from him written November 12th in which he says he has had no word from you, no clothes, no magazines nor nothink.

To add to my misdemeanors, I am enclosing a check on me for ten dollars plus one dollar - eleven dollars. to cover so much of my debt to you as you have admitted (and Im honestly grateful you have been that measly little frank dear Davy) plus ten dollars which I ask you to send to mother, What a sentence. I mean one dollar to you and ten to mother. It is my Xmas present and i am very anxious to get it there and dont know how else.

Mrs Maude T Dunn. 611 Madison St. Clarksville.

Fear she is pestering Cyrils soul away. Yes, things have gone right to the extent of having Jacks fare and mine and the 500, which last is a great responsibility and i shall be glad to get it back in the very nice owners hands on landing.

Believe I wrote you last week that we are sailing on Dec 14 on the American Banker - due in with luck Xmas Eve. Then to decide whether we go to El Paso or get jobs in New York.

Jesus bless you both as he would and do lots for you if he had more power on Olympus.

Jacks dearest love. Hope to see you and Lola Xmas day. We will go from the boat to Hazels for that night and perhaps stay on there if it is convenient to her. I dont want you to have to sleep with Lola. She aint well enough. But I still have your downstairs key and if you can fix it so i can get in upstairs maybe youd let me get meals on your stove now and again, as we cant afford any restaurant eating this time, and hazel may want to use hers.

blessings again, evelyn

[Typed, typed signature. SSC]

To Otto Theis and Louise Morgan

c/o Abrams, 66 Perry Street
January 16, 1929

Sweet Peoples,

Evelyn maybe has told you I got job as captain of a coal-barge in East River, held the job 10 days and then got run-into by a tug or something one night.[82] Three of us barges tied up abreast. Tug hit outer boat and shock caused my lines to the dock to part, so we were all three carried upstream to Hellgate. Were picked off by police launch just in time, 2 minutes later the barges hit rock and sank. I lost my clothes and bedding but saved the novel. Got back same night to E in Hudson St to find her ill with flue. Now much worse, so she's in hospital at New York Infirmary. Don't know what next. Am using spare time in writing but may get another barge job if vacancy occurs.

How are you all then? Write to us. Forgive haste. E sends bestest love and hugs to you both. So do I.

Yrs ever,
John

Lots of nice free publicity for John Metcalfe in all the papers as result of barge mix-up. Headlines "Two Saved from Hellgate" etc etc

[Handwritten, signed. BRBL]

To Louise Morgan

c/o Sommers
449½ Hudson Street
February 10, 1929

Dear Kiddie:

Lord deliver us, dont reproach yourself about writing. As a matter of strict etiquette I should have written. But life has been exhaustingly full since we got here and my inclinations. if I had the temperament would be to pass out like Merton in some sort of collapse

---

82 Hell's Gate is a narrow tidal stretch in New York City's East River and is known to be dangerous to navigation. A search of online archives for New York City newspapers on this date has not yielded any information about this incident.

First there was the barge. Today Jack is in bed with flu. I had flu and went to hospital as you know. but which it was revealed that I have a tumour in the uterus (a small and tame one they say however) inflammation of the uterus (not due to tumour but to a hurt acquired in Montreal) diabetes (not advanced) an inflamed appendix, and a derangement of the liver probably due to the sluggish effects of my general prolapsis. Also anaemia. Im taking iron injections and diabetic diet. but the real cure would be total irresponsibility - and for Jack as well. You know all about it.

Cheerio and lots of em. in other words as true but less nostalgic of Blighty - our best beloved love to you and Mickey and very much adored Otto. Evelyn
[Typed letter, typed signature. UTK]

To Otto Theis and Louise Morgan

c/o Sommers
449½ Hudson Street
April 7, 1929

Dear Peoples,

Excuse scrawl and great haste. Evelyn now in hospital after operation (successful) and therefore unable to answer your nice, nice letters, - says she sends bushels and oceans of love, and will write when able. Expects to be out of hospital in 10 days. Then we hope spend a month in country - but this address will always find us.

E's operation consisted in a complete remodelling of the vaginal landscape, general refitting and spring cleaning. Involved great pain for a week afterwards, catheterizing only every 6 hours and of course, in rebellion, she wet her sheets all the time. And more even than that. Formidable and tumultuous movement of bowels while I was visiting her - also in sheets. Nurses dashing around with pallid smirks. But enough of this--

Love and hugs to you all three,
Yrs ever,
John

[Handwritten, signed. BRBL]

Chapter 13

Yaddo and Santa Fe

July 1929 - August 1930

Very few letters written between the spring of 1929 when Evelyn was living in Greenwich Village with Jack and July 1929 have survived, so we know little of the events that took Evelyn to Yaddo, just outside Saratoga Springs, New York, for the first time.

Yaddo was first opened as an artists' colony in 1926. The house belonged to venture capitalist Spencer Trask and his writer wife Katrina. The couple wished to give something to society and, after the deaths of their four children, it was Katrina Trask's wish to create a haven where artists could work and flourish. It still flourishes, albeit in a slightly different form, today.[83]

It is hard to overstate the importance of Yaddo to both Evelyn and Jack. It provided them with generous board and accommodation at a very reasonable price but, more importantly, the other guests were a cross-section of American intellectual life. They included artists, writers and critics and Evelyn found their company supportive and stimulating. Yaddo's executive director, Elizabeth Ames, provided Evelyn and Jack with much-needed artistic support and financial succour on several occasions.

This chapter opens with Evelyn's account of her first visit to Yaddo: shortly after her arrival she left for Santa Fe, leaving Jack at Yaddo. Meanwhile Cyril and Phyllis had left El Paso for Santa Fe, where he had established the Cyril Kay Scott School of Painting. As she travelled west, she wrote extensively to her friends; her descriptions lyrical and vivid, much as they were of Bou Saada.

To Maude Dunn

"Yaddo"
Saratoga Springs, New York
July 2, 1929

Yes, dearest mother, you are very beautiful in your patience about money. If I could ever get through with doctors and dentists I would be enormously nearer being of proper

---

83   In 2009 the New York Public Library mounted an exhibition entitled *Yaddo: Making American Culture* and a volume of the same name was published [McGee, M (2010): New York, Columbia University Press] celebrating Yaddo, its guests and their achievement. Yaddo welcomed its first guests in 1926 and continues today as a successful centre and retreat for artists of all disciplines.

help to you. I shall have to go again in Santa Fe for I have infected philopean[84] tubes and it takes a long time to treat. Also there is proud flesh growing outside where the stitches came out and that will sometime have to be cut off. Still I think I am better as we made a very difficult journey up here in a terribly crowded train, stood most of the way. I had to help carry baggage, and still seem to have no very bad effects. I knock on wood however. I couldn't have done that before the operation.

In a money sense our trip up here was unfortunate. We just made it. The round trip for us both was ten dollars each. That was bad enough. But breaking up Perry Street we had to take so many things with us, typewriters etc, and had to have porters. We also missed the bus from Yaddo and had to take a taxi there. That made five dollars extra just for luggage. But as I told you this place once arrived is extraordinary. It was left by some people named Trask to be used as a summer home for people doing work in arts and sciences, and of course the board is nominal and doesn't half pay the expense. You have to be recommended by the trustees and there is always a long waiting list. And you can only come once. I hope Jack can stay on after I go.

It is a beautiful estate of five hundred and seventy acres. Part is public gardens, the rest meadows and farm. The main building is a kind of imitation of a baronial hall, very much on the grand scale. The reception rooms are tapestries, paintings, a fountain, impressive draperies, old Italian furniture. For our seven a week each, the cheapest imaginable board, Jack and I were escorted to a huge double bedroom with a view of miles of lush country and the Green Mountains of Vermont like blue clouds that never move behind. We have a private bath. I am writing in a room as big as Perry Street and mine for work while I am here. Jack has a studio of a rustic type about a quarter of a mile from the house. There are fifteen artists as guests, some for a fortnight, some for all summer. We were asked for long, but account of Jig could not accept. Breakfast is served on trays in bedrooms. Lunch is optional - upstairs or down. Tea downstairs. Dinner downstairs. Plenty of servants all very quiet and English trained. The hostess is a Mrs Ames[85] whom I like very much. No dressing to match surroundings, fortunately, as most guests are supposed to be poor.

Dearest love and more soon as able. I hope for better news on money later.

elsie

[Typed, typed signature. UTK]

---

84   Fallopian. Evelyn continued to experience gynaecological problems following Jigg's birth.
85   Elizabeth Ames, the administrator at Yaddo, was very supportive of Evelyn and Jack in a number of ways over the years.

To Otto Theis

care Mrs Cyril Kay-Scott[86]
415 San Francisco Street
Santa Fe, New Mexico
July 3, 1929

Otto, dear:

Your letter written while Louise was in Paris was a treat to friendship. I didnt answer it the same day as I felt like doing, only because I can not write perfunctorily to my dearest beloveds. Now we are up at "Yaddo" there is breath.

Otto, this "Yaddo" place is to all intents and present purposes paradise. Lola is here for one thing, but there are permanent reasons as well. The estate is five hundred and seventy acres. Jack and I have a huge double room which makes you feel should hold levees. We have a private bath and a studio each. All this costs seven dollars a week. And I can only stay a fortnight, having decided to make a bee line to Santa Fe while the money was good. It is a test of maternal feeling that I can. From an acre of window, I now look down a terrace lacking powdered hair and peacocks, to a fountain that would delight a proper marquise, and then to meadows of hay, and then to hills lavish as they only grow in America, and then to the Green Mountains of Vermont - chalk blue and stern and invitingly aloof. Rain clouds are swelling dark on the sky. The pine trees converse in aromatic threats. The bird songs pepp up and die away like the freshest of small musical water. The bees behave as bees should. It is so still my typewriter sounds like a blasting machine. We have breakfast in bed. What, what more can you ask. And none of the people so far are unpleasant.

After the 15th I go to Santa Fe. Hope Jack can stay here until his book is done. I have 22 letters to write. Literally. Love and love and love, evelyn
[Typed, typed signature. BRBL]

To David Lawson

124 Park Street
Santa Fe, New Mexico
July 28, 1929

Davy, dear:

I called you up Thursday morning several times, but nothing doing. Did you leave early after all I wonder. From what Jack said from Yaddo you didnt seem to be there yet.

I feel the altitude here. It makes my head ache a lot, but they say you get used to it. If I can get in shape physically, I shall enjoy every minute - first in work, and second in looking at an old land of the gods which somehow got into this western world.

---

86 Evelyn gave as her forwarding address that of Cyril and Phyllis. Despite this Santa Fe address, this letter was written from Yaddo.

Burnt and bitter and lovely and colossal - the half desert with its little green flows to plateaus dead of everything but more vivid than life. The Indians are suspiciously affable - rather broken winged birds, but they still belong in their clothes that mingle their civilization with Mexico. Mary G is here on visit and asked us to her hotel to see Indian dance. Sun dance - great fat man leading had sun made of eagle feather around a white plaque, wonderful bonnet - not much else. Stamping and hopping very agile, while chorus chanted monotonously and drum thumped. Then Eagle Dance by two men who wore huge wings, and headdresses and tail feathers. It was very fine in a plastic way.

Havent written a line yet and so MUCH mail. I wont write often and I suppose you never. Yet I do so long to hear how Lola and that magnificent poem go and how you are and the gamble of the examination. Wont you sometime tell me?

Very deepest love to you and her, Davy dear,

evelyn

If you ever can vacation here - gee. I think youd love it, Davy. And Lola would make the world ring with what she saw. Gee, gee.

[Typed, typed signature, SSC]

To Lola Ridge

124 Park Street,
[late July] 1929

Lola, lovely and dear:

I was sorry to hear through Jack[87] that you had been having more hard times, my precious.

Until we got to the Kansas prairies all was America as I have known it too well. You have seen them doubtless, so know how that more rugged sea of the earth seemed to hurl itself on the train, more capaciously than any waters. I went to bed in the lake of grass and grain on Thursday and at three am Friday morning looked thru my window and felt that the tide has suddenly been arrested. That great rocks had been startled out of the night to meet us. That was Colorado which I didnt half see. It wasnt till reaching Lamy at ten and being met by Cyril and Phyllis (Phyllis is far finer than any of us conceived, Lola. She is a beautiful, staunch person, humanly clear and sound straight thru) and Jig, that I began to realize yet another world - mountains blazing with white cloud wreaths, and a solemnity of no pioneer remembrance merely, but of the only eternal our senses can approach.

The Indians I dont hope to "understand". But I felt their sulky pride of children under the affability of broken spirit. It is as if inside they had retreated from man like the land - gone inward to die, not quite beautifully, but with unimpaired dignity, but with something alive and hatefully protected against the rest of us.

---

87   Jack was at Yaddo with Lola while Evelyn was in Santa Fe with Cyril and Jigg.

Jig is a delight. Sends his love to you. Cyril wants to have a permanent school here. El Paso was hell.[88] To that end if I can I shall help buy a plot of ground and a three room adobe house for a beginning (dont tell). It is what I can do if at all for Jig who feels free and happy here and released from the east, no place for youth. Nobody has any luxuries and Cyril cant paint, but it is being alive and somehow sanely and more comfortingly.

Cyril is recognised as distinguished as a teacher and there is hope, but it takes capital and a long time.

Bless my dear and her work. Give my love to Davy. Cyril sends his to you two.

evelyn

[Typed, typed. signature. SSC]

To Otto Theis

415 San Francisco Street

August 9, 1929

Otto, me dear, you were a sweetie to keep me posted about england, reviews, etc. Jack is still at Saratoga[89] about to finish book and making useful alliances. Im here until Oct 1st and longer if he decides to come out later. Cyril is superb as always, without the opportunity to paint or write a stroke, making everybody think that all he ever wanted to do in his life was teaching painting for six hours a day. I have heard numbers of artists here say that they have never seen better work done by the classes in any school in the world. However these pupils are for the summer and phyllis and cyril do not want to return to el paso if they can help it, so to try to organize for a winter class here will be another job. Phyllis is sense and humour and the most gorgeous simplicity (not stupidity) in accepting our complex family I ever saw.

Jig looks like his own grandfather he is so huge - five ten and a half. Its rather fun to look up to him. He doesn't want to return to the east with me and he is so unhappy in ny[90]. Here he has found three or four real friends for the first time since tom merton - they are painters sons too mostly and intelligent and decently imaginative without conventional warnings. Besides there is all the state of new mexico to play about in. So what I want to do is to help make this place a home for Jig here. When able i should like to invest in a bit of land and an adobe house. Wish Jack and I spend winters here and summers in england, but god knows when fares will be so plentiful as to account for that.

Otto the country really is astounding. I never saw better. Spain perhaps a little and parts of NA[91] as good, but no better anywhere. Saw an Indian Corn Dance at Santa

---

88 Cyril had opened his first school of art in El Paso the previous year. It was not a commercial success.
89 That is, Yaddo, located just outside Saratoga Springs.
90 New York City
91 North Africa.

Domingo Pueblo on Sunday which i couldnt digest in years. Mud walls in tiers lined with spectators with indian faces, colors of clothing violent as a sunset on the arid orange - hills behind them turning purple dusty with rain storm lightning. Indians in dance stamping long monotonous lines, women sculptural, sedate, with cedar wands waving to keep time - men are nearly naked, women uniformly dressed in black and red with high green headdresses. Old men about drums chant and enact some dramatized petition for rain. Drums have never stopped since daylight. One set of dancers take place of others. Sitting by me Mabel Dodges Indian husband like kind old lady with fine face. Beside him an Indian granny with hair like an iron grey stallion, and long yellow nails crusted with dirt.

Mexicans almost as pronounced as Indians. Lots of modified but genuine cowboys.

Made myself very ill but worth it by driving to Taos on operation stitches. What a gorgeous upper land. Lawrences[92] ranch in the garden of eden tho not worth a sou commercially. But God what a situation. Olatuea much higher than santa fe is willow green with chamita bushes, behind this never-never of plain are the Taos mountains that look like the faceless gods of a universe. Taos pueblo built like an arab village in tiers, women on the roofs at work.

Could go on forever. Disadvantage is that altitude has so far played hell with me. Love from Cyril and jig and ME and of course jack would but he is so many miles off.

evelyn

[Typed, typed signature. UTK]

To Lola Ridge

124 Park Street

August 11, 1929

Darling one: I am in a panic. My mother has written that relatives are turning her out and that my cousin Elizabeth, past insulter of all I love, who lives in Tarrytown, has my address and is coming out here to get the low down on me and find means of sending mother to me. It makes me feel suicidal, but in a nightmare way, as the literal result of mothers descent on me is too awful to be believed in, so that truly I dont believe in it. I have written post haste to Sophie about an old ladies home - the kind to which you pay an entrance fee and are recommended socially. Of course I believe that mother would have to be taken to it in a straight jacket. Mother says the Graceys simply do not believe that I cant afford to keep her - my trips to Europe and all that. Mother is in agonies herself. She affects me as a rabbit!

[Typed, not signed. SSC]

---

92   D H and Frieda Lawrence had a ranch just outside Taos.

To Otto Theis

124 Park Street
September 5, 1929

Dearest Otto:

Well, Cyril has given up El Paso as too much of a hell hole of mediocrity for a life residence, and the school is being reorganized up here. I think it is going to make a smashing hit. All the big bugs on the new board, and town giving studio. But it is, very privately, the usual strain to get through the preparations financially. There will be nothing coming in until the new school is actually under way, and they are buying a house and a bit of property and there is the removal of all the property portable from El Paso. Its the first home Jig has ever had except the Bermuda fake. And thank god for once in my life Im being able to do at least a ninetieth as much for them as they have for me (qt).

Cyril has worked on it a long time but now has the town by the ears and the artists here quite frankly are unanimously for him and his teaching and work. All the good ones are on his board, including John Sloan and so on. So I think it ought to go. Of course he wont be able to paint for another couple of years, but I still pray hell get the chance for that in the end.

Jig is the joy of me life. I enclose a notice[93] of the hanging of his picture in the school exhibition at the museum. He has the goods as an artist, but has a poverty complex from watching his parents sweat.

Darling old Jack has spent a productive, but I hope to some degree lonely summer at Yaddo, and has finished his book. He is now dickering with publishers in NY, and expects to come down here the middle of the month where, as living is cheaper than in NY, we hope to stay until January.

Love from everybody here to you all, and from me from the 'eart, always, old dears,

evelyn

PS Otto dont tell but I have put my eyes out on a nursery story.[94] Hate it. Never do another. Began it before knew <u>The Wave</u> would go. Isnt quite done yet. Hell hell hell to write, dont dare let anybody know I did it, nom de plume.

[Typed, typed signature. UTK]

There is little information about Evelyn's changes of address. The letters suggest that the address on San Francisco Street may have been the address Evelyn shared with Cyril on her arrival in Santa Fe and from which she and Jigg moved to the Park Street address. They also imply that at some time during the autumn of 1929, Cyril and Phyllis left Santa Fe for Denver, taking Jigg with them. There is no indication of what took Evelyn to a third address in Camino del Monte Sol. She also refers in one letter to having lost

---

93 This has not survived.
94 Evelyn is referring to *Blue Rum*, published in 1930 under the pseudonym Ernest Souza.

money on a house she was trying to purchase as a permanent home for herself and Jigg.
It is not clear which house it was.

To Lola Ridge

586½ Camino del Monte Sol
Santa Fe, New Mexico
December 27, 1929

Sweet, sweet, sweet:

To think I have left your letters unanswered over two weeks. To think I sent you no message for Xmas - or Davy - and not even one to Cyril, Jig or Jack. I was ill for all of three weeks after I got here, and am still unwell, but this is not important, being no more than altitude and a state of mind. I am so full of disgust for Santa Fe I cannot express myself even in profanity. No use going into it, but the divorce between Phyllis and Cyril, my return here without Jack, Jigs love affair with a girl older than himself[95] and the fate of the Art School have unleashed that almost impersonal malice of a small town, and I have been through many of the same things I did when Cyril and I first separated. Current assertions: I came here last time to break up Cyrils home. I succeeded. I am back because I am in love with him. (If I try to defend Cyril against the most scurrilous falsehoods that is the answer. You see his leaving here for Denver infuriated those who had profited by the Art School boom here.) Cyril only went to Denver because he had played fast and loose with art school funds. (There werent any.) And the whole rigmaroles about Jig and Selma.

Oh, to have some real escape into this country whose vastness at present seems to exist only to emphasize the picayune nature of humans. I look at the very mountains as if they had betrayed me by being gorgeous and aloof. My weakness is such a profound aloneness among my kind that when I am literally living alone I lack the fibre to bear it. If I have one human who is mine, to whom I can turn for re-affirmation of everything of which the crowd is unmindful I can be as contemptuous of crowds as the pride of my mind would have. But this has happened to me before, and when there is not a human being to turn to for complete trust it seems beyond me to keep going at all.

From your nostalgic and loving,

evelyn

[Typed, typed signature. SSC]

---

95   Selma Hite was 7 years older than Jigg, who was then 15. They eloped the following year and moved to Greenwich Village, where Selma later ran off with a man her own age. Evelyn and Cyril managed to get the marriage annulled.

To Lola Ridge

586½ Camino del Monte Sol

[early 1930]

Sweet, sweet Lola: I think about you and your affairs so much. Are you weller? How is the book going? But dont answer - only sometime or other.

I feel sort of emotional today over decision I am making, if lawyer can get me out, to lose what I paid on the mud Mexican cottage and give up the idea of living in Santa Fe. It isnt the Phyllis Cyril problem, as so many people thought it would be, but another nest of complexes uncovered all relating to small towns and N Orleans. I have an obsession to the effect that I am being looked askance at morally and that people are trying to cut me. Its quite horrible to have this infantile throw back come on like an attack of measles. I couldnt understand myself until, after much analysis, I harkened back to New Orleans, my mothers idea of being cut after my father got broke and my grandmother got crazier. Only cure for morbid reflex is, apparently, to accept the invitations and go in for social life - and that spoils writing. Didnt you ever hear of anything so nearly batty! Living remotely superior, and suddenly here I feel as if people were being deliberately nasty to me, when my intellect tells me that is impossible. However, I have just about decided that I can not settle down in a small southern town. It only hurts because of spoiling nice plans for Jig.

And it does look so pretty here!

love and love, evelyn

[Typed, typed signature. SSC]

To Lola Ridge

Santa Fe, New Mexico

[February 1930]

Beautiful love;

What I feel pretty awful is that I have run through my own prosperous year and have nothing to show for it. Misfortunes seem to be with Cyril forever as far as money goes and as it is I let the piece of property go and - was a fool, I dont know - lost outright what I had put into it. Because to have gone on would have meant borrowing at eight to ten per cent from money lenders who had to be pain in the year. So that idea of making Jiggys future safe is certainly a fluke. Cyril still has three thousand dollars to get paid up on his part, and seems pretty sure to have no income at all here during the winter months, as the attendance at art school is for summer only. I dont want this to go beyond you and Davy and Glad, however, as bluff as usual is still the thing. But what actually scares me is the idea of leaving here and leaving Jig with them when they may be reduced to ten dollars in the world as they were last week. And then if they dont pay up on the house they lose the whole thing, which is several thousand of investment already. Cyrils too old[96] to ever get back into any business, and if this

---

96   Cyril was 59 at the time.

dont work I dont know what will. Makes me sort of sore that the people who profess to like him and admire him never have made any effort to sell his work.

The mother thing is another crisis. No Home will admit her in any state but Tennessee and that is the one place she hates to go, and as I slumped from sending her a hundred a month for a little while down to twenty-five and the relatives had to take on things again, they are again after me. They write that I have sold a hundred thousand copies of my book and must be rich. That makes me angry, but at the same time it is sentimental vanity still and I ought to be more honest about the home arrangement and brutal. I suppose its loving Jig so makes this mother stuff get me so much.

But in between such tiresome consequences occasional time to remember what really important, eh! Such as the white fog of perpetual snow in the pines on the mountains-the spirit look of fresh snow-falls when I look out the kitchen door at night and see a silken back yard and silver and silver drifting faintly down. I really love snow now. Then I can think of "wash his pale hands in the milk of the light" and things like

CERTIFIED COPY OF RECORD OF MARRIAGE NO. 807

Marriage Certificate

STATE OF NEW MEXICO   COUNTY OF RIO ARRIBA. SS.

Holy Bonds of Matrimony

Copy of Marriage Certificate of Evelyn Scott and Jack Metcalfe: *Scott family*

that. Also that acceptance to the scheme of life which is mostly hell brings some sort of immediate unwordable compensation which adds a dimension to living - only I only achieve it sporadically - it seems nearer a perfect surmounting of all the limitations of literal action when you realize it.

Blessings and love forever. evelyn

[Typed, typed signature. SSC]

On March 17, 1930 Evelyn and Jack got married in Tierra Amarillo, New Mexico, about 90 miles north of Santa Fe. There are no letters extant referring to the decision to do so, nor to their choice of that town (although Evelyn says in a letter dated November 23, 1953 that they chose such a remote place to avoid any chance of being pursued by the sensationalist press). Nor do any of the letters they sent their friends in the weeks after the ceremony refer to the fact of their now being formally married: as they had been posing as married for some time, they may not have felt the need to emphasise their new status.

Not long after this ceremony, Jack returned to New York to stay with friends for a few weeks before returning to London to await notification that his quota application had been approved, leaving Evelyn in Santa Fe with Cyril and Jigg.

To Lola Ridge

449½ Hudson Street

August 5, 1930

Dearest Lola,

What do you mean, I should like to know, by signing yourself my "friend if I want you"?! Don't talk so! You should know I want you as a friend!

Poor Evelyn was thinking of packing up to leave Santa Fe when she fell ill, - bad tonsillitis and also a broken tooth-bridge. So that means delay. She hopes to have the bridge fixed and be well enough to travel by about the 14th or 15th of this month - and will first go to Clarksville for this awful family pow-wow about her mother. I am hoping to be able to meet her when she arrives at Clarksville and see her through the unpleasant business. Golly, how glad I'll be when we're together again. I have been missing her terribly, Lola, so badly, finally, that I get too restless to settle down to good work. But it won't be long now I hope.

Drop me a line whenever you can, and good luck, dear Lola, with health and work.

Very much love, and kisses from

Jack.

PS Please remember me affectionately to Mrs Ames.

[Handwritten, signed. SSC]

To Otto Theis and Louise Morgan

Care Mrs M T Dunn
Clarksville, Tennessee
August 24, 1930

Dear Peoples,

Here we both are in Clarksville savouring the dilapidated South in company of our mother and mother-in-law respectively. A hearty breakfast of bacon and eggs and much much coffee is found useful, and sustains us through the day. However, all good things must come to an end eventually and we are probably leaving here this week. Then about 3 weeks in N York and then England. We shall probably be in London for a few days round about end of September or early October. Oh what fun to see you people again! Blessings to you, and hugs and kisses from us both.

Jack ("John")
and Evelyn

[Handwritten, signed. BRBL]

This letter marks the end of Evelyn's time in New Mexico, although she did continue contact with Cyril and Jigg. At some time in the autumn (and again, no letters relating to their decision to travel have been found) Evelyn and Jack sailed again to England and to the start of a new chapter in their lives.

Chapter 14

Falmouth and Salisbury
October 1930 - June 1931

In the autumn of 1930 Evelyn and Jack sailed to England; no letters about their decision to return to England have survived. After a short stay with Jack's friend, C F Thompson-Walker in Kent (about whom we know very little other than that he and Jack were at university together), they spent a few weeks in Falmouth in Cornwall, before leaving for Salisbury in Wiltshire. None of the letters gives any insight into the choice of either Falmouth or Salisbury: they stayed in lodgings in both towns. No letters from their stay in Cornwall have survived, but the letters from Salisbury evoke pre-war England with the same vividness as her earlier descriptions of Algeria and France.

To Lola Ridge

c/o C F Thompson-Walker

Chislehurst, Kent

October 17, 1930

Sweet one:

I wonder whether or not you have returned from "Yaddo" and what great poetry has come out of your stay? And how are you in health, my dear?

We leave for Falmouth in Cornwall tomorrow, darling, thank God! Jack wrote his last line on July 20th and I mine on August 8th. The frittering away of time and shrinking cash on travels and diplomatic errands puts fear into one. Anyhow next week begins the building up.

The boat trip was ten days instead of eight, and part of it was very rough and left us ennuied of this world and squeamish. I haven't really got my bearings yet. We had a week in London (last) and this week an ordeal at Bosham with the aunt, returning here last night, and tomorrow to Falmouth. I'll send our permanent address as soon as I get it. Darling, I have 56 letters to write. That leaves only dregs of expression for my dearest ones. A note from Cyril says nothing and no letter from Phyllis or Jig.

London is all wet wool enveloping the spirit. Only sometimes toward evening the lights burn in tearful drama on a chiaroscuro that excites one mystically, as though life in this cockney region where our hotel is were some great ceremonial of the people in a medieval church. Barrows of fish glitter like salty carnage. The cake shops drape sticky offerings. The flower stand smells of violets and chrysanthemums acrid and flaunting. Then the bold signs: Ladies Lavatory; Gentlemens Lavatory, Hot and Cold Water, out of the street and people scurrying in and out of tiled caves, seem as lively and peculiarly London as the fish barrow and the flower sellers.

There is misery everywhere. Bedraggled dames of unfathomable age nodding over match boxes and pencils, drunks abandoned in doorways, sidewalk artists announcing their peculiarly stark observations on life in impermanent mediums of charcoal and chalk.

Jack and I frequent pubs, upstairs the pub dining room with flowered paper and great domestic-looking sideboards suggest French provincial hotels. Downstairs it is all beer and chatter, but up there family life reigns. There is no place more sacred to the memory of Queen Victoria than a pub dinning room. Choice of "veggies"! That means cabbage or sprouts! Twice since I came I have had spinach. This was a triumph. There are French restaurants where they speak of salad, but meals there are too expensive for us. We have to stick to British standard and there are filling viands for 2 bob.[97] But oh this queer, mystical unimaginativeness! This thought that is thoughtless! This instructive meditation on the past! This solidarity that equals natures own. I marvel at Jack's comparative elasticity. He's done great things, really, in even half adapting himself to me. What an over-subtle race, the English. A savage waste. An Englishman self-deprecates. That is the sign.

Love love love and hope of all the best for you my angel and anxiety for news of health and work. I'm writing Davy. Do you think Miss Ames really means to have us again next year?

Always and always,
Evelyn

[Handwritten, signed. SSC]

To Maude Dunn

c/o Mrs M Sweet
7 Glenmore Road
Salisbury, Wiltshire
February 16, 1931

Dearest Mother:

At last we are in our new lodgings, as advertised before we left Falmouth and had several answers but this one the only endurable one. Unfortunately we could not get into it until today which made five days in hotel and though we went to cheapest here our bill for room and board was forty dollars. We had not enough money on hand to pay it, not having calculated on that but my advance came and saved us. Wasn't that luck?

---

97 Colloquially, two shillings.

Falmouth was so low and wet it made Jack ill, and while I am more used to low levels I found it enervating. Salisbury is colder but we feel much peppier here so far. Our rooms are very plain and there are inconveniences re bath etc, but we are buying our own coal so as to have good fires and it is apparently not going to be any dearer than Falmouth. Also while at Falmouth we did have a sweet view of the harbour our rooms faced the street and we had no privacy. Here we have no view but overlook a cute little garden and it is very quiet, though there is one child - two children, but one at school.

The hotel we stayed at which so nearly proved our undoing was The Old George, built in 1320. It has housed Cromwell and Samuel Pepys and Dickens etc. Salisbury is so stodgy that Falmouth in retrospect seems as gay as Paris; but it makes up for that by its archaeological interest. The cathedral, while not so fine as Chartres, is very beautiful - built in the eleventh century, and with romantically ancient tombs. There are many very old houses in town. Lots of Tudor fronts and overhanging first stories. Meandering through the streets are four small rivers which give a Holland like appearance to certain spots. The cathedral close is a very fine green faced with Tudor and Queen Anne houses occupied by clergy. The close had a fortification surrounding it.

But far more exciting than town or cathedral was the expedition to Stonehenge on Saturday. We took a bus to Amesbury and walked the two miles to our destination. Those Egyptian looking ruins, more like a crude Karnac or Phylae than anything English or even European, standing out against the desolation of Salisbury Plains (a slightly rolling plateau like that on which Madrid is built) gave me a real thrill. Of course they arent as large as a modern dwelling house of good size, but the individual measure of the stones raised by hand is as incredible as the pyramids. Three hundred burial barrows have been excavated in the immediate surroundings, and crude implements, jewelry and funeral urns brought to light. We saw some of the barrows but the things they contained are in the museum we have not yet visited. I always thought Stonehenge was druidical but the guide says it is pre-druid, about four thousand years old. They were sun worshipers at any rate and the great stunt is to see sunrise on midsummers day when it strikes the entrance stone before the temple and thus is the longest day of the year marked. Under each of the small stones that made the outer circle lay a charred skeleton indicating propitiatory sacrifices made during the building. The big stones - twenty-five or thirty foot each - were local, but smaller ones seem to have been brought from Wales - a job at the time.

The rest of Salisbury Plain[98] is given over to army depots and airplane hangers and it is an exciting incongruity to see this other thing.

The country around here has fine aspects but on the whole is much less picturesque than Cornwall. However, except for expense, I am very glad of the move. It's nice to have seen it and Jack can go up to London from here cheaply.

---

98   Salisbury Plain was then, and still is, a major training area for the British army.

Just as would happen - the day I arrived my elbow went through my coat and I split my hat trying to pull it over my growing hair. Then I tried to buy another hat and found none in town I could get on my head.

elsie

PS yes Lady Metcalfe is a relative tho not a close one. Jack's dad's first cousin was the earl of pawsomething Kintaw (can't spell it) and he has various other titles[99] on that line. Also his mother was Irish nobility on one side. Speaking of that, I have discovered titled Dunns in London. Never would have believed it as Mr J Gracey's early teasing gave me a complex about the name.

[Typewritten, typed signature. UTK]

To Louise Morgan

7 Glenmore Road
February 25, 1931

Jack will be seeing you in a little over two weeks. I wish you could come stay with me while hes up there. Not that the attraction when Im working constantly and must be very boring as society would be so great, but this place, so like a two dimensional landscape - worn tapestry with only a few bright threads supplied by the sky at sunset - it gives me a worse pipp than Cornwall. Its beautiful at times but too much like a bloody gawddamned grave. Theres the cathedral, not for use - a huge monument to things all dead. The town has that cemetery in its heart. I cant see any life in it.

We walked to Stonehenge there again real antiquity so much more rooted than aerodromes around. I feel as if Im not seeing this, but millions of dead eyes are using me to see it. there are lovely sallow downs around us and four little quiet rivers, and we walked over to Old Sarum[100] and saw the Roman city with the grass on it. English people so nice but I could stay here twenty years and be swallowed in this vast, formal indifference and lose all hope. I hate being like this - I mean not fully appreciating after vulgar, hideous screaming America but there is also warmhearted young America. This country seems to me rotten with moral cowardice - and feeble with caution. maybe its working much too long and hard.

Anyhow, I shall look back on it with certain aesthetic thrills but not wish to repeat them for a very long time, not until I feel very powerful myself - if I ever do. London seems much more friendly because there is a slothful current from outside. But here its all so stagnant, so gorgeously miasmic.

Ill write again soon because I want to hear from you. Blessings. Love and much from us both. Good luck. Thanks for book.

Eveline

---

99 It does indeed appear that Jack had illustrious ancestors. One, Charles Theophilus Metcalfe, 1st Baron Metcalfe, had a distinguished career in the colonial governments of Canada and India during the 19th century.

100 The ancient centre of modern Salisbury.

PS Our digs are incredible. Jack will tell you. Landlady asked me if American accent came from the pilgrim fathers.

[Typed, typed signature. UTK]

To Maude Dunn

[Fragments of an undated letter from Evelyn to her mother, probably written while she and Jack were living in Salisbury in 1931]

I went out to Winterslow Rectory[101] and stayed two days. There was so much sociability I couldn't write. Still it was a help. England is the most dismal country on earth when you're alone in it. There have been two days of sun in the two weeks Jack has been gone. I had a lovely room at the Rectory. It looked out on fields and had fine old fashioned furniture that suited the country surrounding. Tall elms outside the window were inhabited by rooks that kept up such a din I thought more of them than my book. The country had the grave, resigned look I haven referred to. No bright colors, but a very subtle sobriety. The church next door is fourteenth century. The Rector and I don't get on well; and I soon found myself arguing with everybody there- my great failing. Of course they were all polite but I landed one bomb after another. They are hidebound reactionaries - dyed in the wool Tories. First it was Gandhi I defended, then Einstein, then the Germans, then modern art, etc etc.

Jack's near relatives are only moderately well off. The forty room house "goes with the living". All those things are bequests of the church for the use of incumbent. At Winterslow are Jack's Cousin Gertrude (the old lady who came through Santa Fe last summer from California) her husband, Cousin Edward, and her unmarried daughter, also Gertrude, besides the rector and his wife. The two Gertrudes are very discontented as a country rectory seems to them gloomy after California where they lived nine years. It is very stuffy and over proper, though pretty, the little church dating from thirteen hundred.

I am also suffering from a hurt to my operated innards again, so we are very topsy turvy. Hope all better next Sunday and a better letter. Very very much love.

hug and kiss, elsie

I'll have to cut this short. Never saw anything except the outer site of Old Sarum - a moat surrounded hill with the fragment of a church and a couple of towers on it. The castle on the second hill we have never yet visited. Hope we have time before we leave.

[Typed fragment, typed signature. UTK]

To Lola Ridge

7 Glenmore Road
March 4, 1931

Precious own:

I have an abscessed tooth which gives me for today a kind of germy passivity. I feel

---

101 The home of Jack's elderly relatives near Bosham.

as if I were lying on my back in hot grass looking at clouds that went by ever so slowly and thinking about you, as if it would be too much trouble to move for a cyclone. I wouldnt care. But at the same time caring a lot about everything nice.

Salisbury is the greyest place I ever visited. Theres no actual death here - but a dream that is much deadlier. The country is all pale sad grass and sombre ploughed earth and very old too sturdy trees. Nothing could move the trees, they are so rooted in the deathliness of the landscape. There is the cathedral spire dominating the houses and it is exquisite, but it looks through the mist like somebody elses dream, that of some poet who never knew of us or even guessed that we could be. The sky is the only alive thing over these old houses, muffled in their thatch, and these little rivers that are so indifferent to the sea. There are all sorts of heroic dramas every day between sunrise and sunset, between rain, snow, sleep and abrupt pallid sun. Sometimes the downs across the railroad cut looked as if the soil in them was powdered coral, it shines so rosy though the yellowed grass under the sunset that is blue and rose. The little rivers are sown into everything with threads of red. Last night it snowed under a new moon - thin snow that showed the garden through.

But I dont like England this year. Its too discouraging. I feel so sharply having been cut away from this two hundred years ago and left with the crude earth of such an unenglish world. And never can go back.

Workpeople in England look whipped, belly driven. They lack the pride in economy of the French, and dont seem to feel in their hearts that they have a right to anything better - so they have no right. And the stupidly privileged, with their biological instincts so keep and their minds so mazed, and the thoroughly nice english who are liberal but have clammy hands, afraid of taking hold on anything for fear it maynt be nice.

Jacks a dear but he isnt well and his country seems to make him too sadly his own. I dont think hes any happier over here.

Sometimes I absolutely hate this place.

Love you and davy, love and love. Jacks too.

Shall return US instant book done. Money situation bad and shall be hard put to know what to do there. Get my advance but that settles nothing and must see Jig. He is so lonesome with the world hes just discovering isnt his as he thought. Loves his dad but his own generation surprises him by its unlikeness to himself. He blames Denver for the world as I once Clarksville Tennessee.

love again, evelyn

PS shall let you know first minute I do when arriving NY. Jack goes to london for two weeks soon. His book coming out - short stories only.[102] Done in last several years. Hope better money than last time.

[Typed, typed signature. SSC]

---

102 *Judas and Other Stories*, published by Constable in 1931.

To Maude Dunn

7 Glenmore Road
March 7, [1931]

Dearest Mother:

Just had your sweet letter and thank you for your compliments. You make me feel uncomfy saying you want to imitate my example; but I think it is good in part in a purely practical sense, for you do let inferior people make you suffer a lot more than they ought, and as they can't be altered or made any bigger in their outlook it would save you a great deal if you could will yourself into a certain amount of indifference to them. I hope you will for our sake and for my own for it is painful to see you constantly upset by folk inferior to you.

I wrote you how Stonehenge thrilled us. And of the beauty of the Cathedral. I also believe I spoke of Old Sarum which antedated the present Salisbury and was built in Roman times - a double moated town on an eminence of which nothing remains but a fragment of the church and the foundation of the castle and a tower or two. But even that is enough to reconstruct a picture with; and I imagined very easily rude armies besieging it. The outer moat has an earthen parapet about eighty or ninety feet - maybe a hundred - high - so it must have been a job to get into it against archer on the towers on the top. When we were there on the other occasion, the castle had the gate locked so we only saw the outside; but this week we will take Phil over and try to get in so next time I can describe it more accurately.

Yesterday evening (first social do we have had since October) we went to see Jacks relatives at the country parsonage five miles from here. A nice old Georgian house with FORTY rooms. Some of them are cold and unusable, but the central portion of the house has radiators as well as fireplaces and the rooms have huge windows triple glasses looking on big old fir trees and a garden. The parsons study has sixteenth century carvings on mantle and dado that are very interesting. But he is a study - about six feet two and very good looking, with a lined Roman senator sort of face, he dresses like a clerical fashion plate and wears a monocle. He is very suave and the last thing one thinks of as a preacher from the circuit riding fundamentalist point of view.

Am interrupted so no more now. March check enclosed.

Dearest love

elsie

PS My throat infection is trench mouth and not cold - hard to treat.

[Typed, typed signature. UTK]

To Maude Dunn

7 Glenmore Road
March 10, 1931

Dearest Mother:

Sunday is my Jonah day as well as my letter day. This week I have an abscessed

146

tonsil and may have to go to the doctor to have it lanced. So again my correspondents get the worst of it. I shall at least answer your questions, my dear.

Delay about money was my bank's misunderstanding. They mailed it instead of cabled it but it came OK.

I cried with cold in London when I was first there with Cyril and again when I stayed with the Theises in the Temple about six years ago. I didn't happen to have a very heavy coat and hit a particularly damp and bitter spell.

Did I write you that my landlady asked me if I got my accent from the Pilgrim Fathers?

There were twenty one unsolved murders in England last year and eleven were attacks on women. I really am nervous when I go out alone. Two months ago a servant girl was found dead and horribly mutilated on Blackheath near London and about same time a middle aged woman in Lincolnshire and a girl was burned in her car and died when she was rescued though she told of attack by man beforehand up in Scotland and a woman was attacked in a railway carriage and decapitated. None of this is anything compared to the wholesale murders in USA but they do affect the imagination.

It's very sober around here - what with the town full of parsons and the landscape a monument of antiquity. We have a lunatic asylum nearby and there is another at the other end of town.

Lots of love, elsie

[Typed, typed signature. UTK]

To Maude Dunn

7 Glenmore Road
April 12, 1931

Dear mother:

Jack has been sick a bed, with, I think worry. The combined effort of job and teaching in Montreal almost did him up.

I've had a bad time with me innards again, but that is getting run down from fatigue and worry and is improving. I suppose I always will have such lapses. Yes, I wish my tonsils were out, but you remember trench mouth as well as your advice discouraged me.

The streams around Salisbury are just natural water - four little rivers that break and join around several midget islands

I do need clothes altered and can't seem to find a decent sewing woman in Salisbury. And the ready-mades are a fright. It's getting warm and I can't get out of a jersey and skirt. Almost as bad as in Bezier. I couldn't buy anything there. French winegrowers wives dress like mutes at a funeral. Heaps love, elsie check enclosed

[Typed, typed signature. UTK]

To Maude Dunn

7 Glenmore Road

May 3, 1931

Dearest Mother:

Thank you for all your sweet letters. Jack and I are still fagged and not too well but I think we are recuperating gradually. It isn't that Jack needs to be in England specifically for the writing of his books, but to follow up contacts that will be valuable in making a success of its publication. We could have stayed nearer London this winter if we hadn't been fools and assumed that Jack was bound to get a Guggenheim.

I am very concerned about being nearer Jig,[103] but of course will have to spend next winter wherever Jack finds a job. Meanwhile I am consulting with Cyril re schools and all the expense of having Jig stay with me somewhere either part of this summer or next winter.

It has been raining here for three solid weeks without four good days in all. But I don't think it's much worse than Clarksville from what you say.

Perhaps we will have a few days free before we leave here. I don't know. I would like to investigate that castle and write you about it. Jack mailed you the views and you can get some idea of the place at its best. The newer part is hideously commonplace but the old landmarks are very lovely. Also the downs[104] around delight me. All green with crops, they are less subtle than they were last winter but very sort of virginal and untrodden upon. Then the hawthorn is in leaf and will be out next month and there is a huge quantity of it. The garden here is very seedy but forget-me-nots still survive and wall flowers are blooming profusely, as well as primroses. Primroses are everywhere. Boys on bicycles have primroses fixed on their handle bars. The English express their whole sense of poetry in love of flowers. The chestnuts are in leaf and bud, everything looks tender and lavish, if only it were not so wet. Swallows have arrived and thrill me as always with their scissor winged darts between earth and sky and the violent blue that flashes from their throats and under wings.

Did you get delayed April check? Time to send another and I want to be sure. Maybe you acknowledged it and I have just forgotten as I can't keep all your letters, but I don't remember.

Dearest love,

elsie

PS after June 1st, write me care Miss Abrams, 66 Perry Street, NYC, as I hope by then to have started to New York.

[Typed, typed signature. UTK]

---

103 Jigg was then aged 17 and living with his father in Denver, Colorado.
104 Salisbury is on the edge of the Wiltshire downs, a chalk habitat characterised by rolling hills and grazing sheep.

Chapter 15

Return to Yaddo

Spring 1931 - Autumn 1932

Not long after their return from England, and after a short stay with friends in New York City, Jack and Evelyn returned to Yaddo. It was not long before they left Yaddo to go their separate ways, Evelyn to Denver to join Cyril and Jack to England to stay with his friend John Gawsworth. Not many letters from this period have survived, and those that remain provide a sketchy account of these months.

To Maude Dunn

66 Perry Street
June 22, 1931

Darling Mother:

When I landed two years ago I let Jack go on ahead in a taxi and came behind with remainder of luggage. When I gave the porter a bill and asked him to change it he RAN OFF with the bill. I suppose nothing is done because in the first place the real foreigners don't know what to do and in the second people are afraid. I thought of writing a letter to the Times and then got scared of revenge. The police are too crooked to appeal to and most people would rather have a small sum stolen and let it go than go into court in a hopeless attempt to arrest. There are no policemen near any of the piers, which makes it seem an absolutely put up job.

My dear, I don't know whether Jig ever got your parcels or not. I have been three months trying to find out if he got a cable I sent him to General Delivery in March. Jig is in love[105] and he seems as hard hit as I was with Tyler Miller and perfectly irresponsible for the time as regards anything else.

Jack is pretty sick and heat and job hunting anxiety don't help. I am glad Yaddo will give us a chance to turn around. As yet no decision on my book. It is a strain. If Jack finds no job here he will have to return to England. I shan't go with him but lord knows what I will do. However I'm not trying to decide yet.

---

105 The object of Jigg's affections was Selma Hite, seven years his senior and his father's secretary. They eloped shortly after this letter was written.

I forgot to say that Lady Alexandra Metcalfe did marry a distant cousin of Jack's. Her husband was aide to Prince of Wales for years. Either his father or his grandfather was aide to Queen Victoria. Aunt Mary has a picture of this cousin whatever his name was in the uniform as Queen Vic's aide. Jack is what is called "highly connected" but the hell of a lot of good it does us! However, if he had money and ran where his cousins do I would not have met him. It's usually the poor branch of a family that turns out the most interesting people.

Sunday Jack and I went out to see Gladys Edgerton Grant and Dudley Grant in Jersey. They are near Cranford[106] and drove me over to see the house my paw lives in. It is a fairly nice apartment but nothing wonderful so I expect the panic and all has hit him too. Dudley, for a joke, took a picture of me looking at the house. I'll send you one. Cranford is a hyper respectable and stodgy suburb place with pretty trees. To our great astonishment we found Seely Dunn unconcealed in the telephone book. I looked at all the visible kids but don't know that I saw my half b*[rother]*.

Love and love and love,

elsie

[Typed, typed signature. UTK]

To Otto Theis and Louise Morgan

Yaddo

Saratoga Springs, New York

September 14, 1931

Dear Peoples,

I trust the old address will find you. How is life? Bless you all three, and I hope the news is good.

Having failed to get any sort of possible job in this country, I am returning to England in November. I hope to get a small sum from the Royal Lit Soc Fund,[107] and to supplement this by occasional reviewing. I must get cheap digs, somewhere, and, if I have rather more money than I now expect, join the Savile.[108] Evelyn wants to see Jigaroo again, so she will go to Santa Fe for a few months and then come over to England and join me in London. I imagine shell come over in Feb or March.

The news of Merton's death has rather laid her out for the time being and I, of course, have had to pretend to be as surprised at it as she. That is to say, I have not told her that I already knew of it from you, and it is rather important that she should not

---

106 Cranford is only a few miles from Scotch Plains and is located on the route of the Central Railroad of New Jersey. It is entirely possible that at this time Seely was employed by them.

107 The Royal Society of Literature describes itself as "the senior literary organisation in Britain." Among other activities it awards grants to writers.

108 The Savile Club was one of London's "gentlemen's clubs". Jack would have wanted to belong to a club: male members of his family would have joined clubs as a matter of course. The Savile Club was particularly favoured by literary figures and Jack would have seen membership as a valuable opportunity for networking.

know that I did know of it all this time. So will you please remember this in any letters to either of us?

This place, "Yaddo", is excellent for work and I've written lots. Evelyn's book <u>A Calendar of Sin</u>, comes out with Cape-Smith in October over here. We stay here at Yaddo till end of October, then go to New York for a week or two while I'm arranging my passage to England and my re-entry permit, etc, etc. I fancy I'll be in London in the latter half of November.

Well, much love to you all three, and I'm looking forward enormously to seeing lots of you in town. Evelyn, if she knew I was writing, would of course send love hugs and kisses.

Yours ever,
John

[Typed on Yaddo letterhead, signed. UTK]

To Lola Ridge

Yaddo
October 4, 1931

My dear lovely little big guiding flame: I wonder where you are. I had your letter from Nice a week ago and three days ago Jack heard from Otto who said you had written him from Corsica. Will you be back in Nice and will the Poste Restante be called on? I wont ask you what is going to happen next, but I suppose even you dont know. So I had as well turn to our news. It reads rather like a railway guide.

Next Wed, Oct 7, Jack goes to NY for his sailing permit. He will stay two days at Margaret De Silvers. Then he returns here. On the 12th, I go down to have a party at Lenore Marshalls. I dont know whether the social strategy envolved will net anything or not but I feel I cant refuse it. That will be for two days, also, and I will come back to "Yaddo". On the 28th Yaddo closes and we return to NY, to stay with Margaret until Jacks boat leaves and I am off for Santa Fe. Unless <u>Calendar of Sin</u> sells - at five dollars - I will only be able to remain in Santa Fe a few weeks, but during that time Jig has got to come down to see me. He is feeling, Im afraid, a little neglected. His love affair is a lyric and thank god has absorbed emotions that might have indigested, but just the same he isnt quite able to envisage financial pressure and he thinks I am staying away a mighty long time.

Yes, its rotten in one way to have Jack return to London; but it is his only hope if he is ever to get on. Constancy to me has made a real failure of his prospects up to date and I learned from Merton what the threat to ones art can do to ones emotions. So while it is a risk in the personal, sexual sense, everything is a risk and from the choice of evils this seems to be preferred. I think we will survive it. Other men exist in my horizon and maybe other women will appear on Jacks. Maybe they will occupy the whole space. Theres no way of saying. But we have got our deep affection and there is Jacks British devotion to the established to match with my growing and ever growing fear of fresh beginnings. Anyhow, it has to be gone through with and left to the gods.

Yaddo has been a heavenly interlude, how heavenly I realize afresh as the time for making ends meet again draws near. There have been nice people here. Mrs Ames has been very fine to us. I feel such complex things in my gratitude for it that I would rather talk them than write them.

Did I write you that merton died in June of a tumor on the brain? It explains many things, Lola dear. I was awfully broken up for a few days because when you love people completely once you love them always and this is not incompatible with resignation and a real preference for not being with them in the flesh any more. He left Cyril forty pictures and Cyril is preparing a Denver show for them. Poor merton. All the purity that fumbled and compromised in life remained true in his work and I wish he had lived to reap the reward I think someone will have from it.

> Bless my lovely and may I hear more and the happiest of her soon.
>
> With all the love of me and Jack, evelyn

[Typed, typed signature. SSC]

To Lola Ridge

> care The Denver Art Museum
> 1300 Logan Street
> Denver Colorado
> [January 1932]

Very dear:

Perhaps you have been too ill or too harassed or too deep in work (which I hope) to miss letters; but I have felt for months my own perpetual urge toward you stifled by worries and involvements, and it seems horrible when I think of the time that has passed since I wrote.

Cyril ill and in California, Jig and Selma married (and theres so much to that I shant attempt to tell it until I see you) and harder work than I ever did unless last winter, and three moves since November, not to mention an operation and an illness, the winter has gone by like a jumbled nightmare.

Could it conceivably be that I or Jack and I might see you this spring? I leave for New York in Mch unless there are more tragedies or near ones here. If I get the gug[109], ok, and if I dont get it I dont quite know what, because I must get over to Jack who is worrying as usual. If I could be sure of the cyance[110] I would suggest going over to Paris to see you.

I am simply dead dog tired, honey. Selma has been quite ill and Im still worried about her, and poor sleep and so on.

---

109 Evelyn had applied for a fellowship from the Guggenheim Foundation who awarded these to authors who had been published.

110 It is hard to know what Evelyn meant. Perhaps a mis-typing of "finance"?

Dont feel desperate. Just tired. I hope to heaven you have had what you wanted most from your intricate experience of europe. God you are missed.

your very and always evelyn

[Typed, typed signature. SSC]

To David Lawson

1300 Logan Street
January 19, 1932

Beloved Davy:

Well, Davy, my dear, the flu and all kept me abed until mid December, and I had just got my stride in work and settled to it when Jig, arriving for Xmas, told me (I asked him outright for it was stated in Santa Fe) that he and Selma had run away and gotten married last June. This, for the present, is confidential with you and Lola (and I shall tell Gladys) though of course it will soon be out. Jig had not told his father or me; but Selma had appendicitis soon after and wanted to see Jig, and she told the nuns, who told her aunt, and her aunt, of course, told the town. And these infants believed they were keeping a secret. Selma was 23 and Jig 16 so the marriage could be annulled if anything were to be gained by that. We talked it over, and as Cyril was coming to Santa Fe in February, I decided to have the family conclave then when we could all be together.

Jig returned here after Xmas, but on Jan 7th first Selma then Jig long distanced and in quavering voices told me Cyril had been in bed a week with flu, had developed pneumonia and the doctor believed that his heart would not last out the ordeal. I had just rented my house, paid in advance, and I would have come up here in a car and left my duds behind if there had been a car available; but the round trip is fifty dollars, so there was nothing for it but to pull up stakes. I did and came here on the 10th. Cyril has rallied a little, but the doctor still doesnt guarantee a recovery and insists that Cyril must go to sea level as soon as he can travel to rest his heart (this is 5000 ft, Santa Fe 7100).

I hadnt wanted to spring problems at this point but before knew of the illness I had written Cyril how important it was for him to get to Santa Fe as soon as possible for a serious discussion of Jigs affairs. So he immediately asked what I meant. I then told him.

Anyhow, Cyril has just weathered publicity given his divorce[111] before this hundred per cent public, and nobody knows how the elopement and secret marriage of his young son and his secretary will be regarded by the mammas and papas whose sons go to the University of Denver. There is a possibility, though I still hope not a probability, that the announcement may cost Cyril his job.

In his state, with Jigs inexperience and ill-preparedness to make a living, and Selma (though I think she can hold down minor office jobs and she wants to work) everything is in the air; and of course anxiety as to Cyrils recovery is the most serious problem. He has gotten a good foothold here - just got 10,000 grant for the school from Carnegie institute,

---

111 Cyril had by this time divorced his fifth wife, Phyllis Crawford.

etc - and it will be rather too horrible if he gets knocked out by this. Its all ironical, as usual. The family romanticism, always conflicting with the need to make a living.

Of course I hate seeing it happen because I judge from many opinions unaffected as mine might be by a maternal bias, that Jig has a very definite and extraordinary painters talent; and it is all he is interested in or shows a real aptitude for. And how the hell can he, at seventeen, support a wife and make a career, or even support himself with a wife. But theres no use crying about it and one simply has to wait on fate. As soon as Cyril is strong enough for company, well make the announcement. Selma is a sweet and attractive girl, though the degree of her practicality is Im afraid, exampled in her marrying a kid of this age. Arent we all brilliant that way!

The dearest love of all of us.
With heaps of love from
evelyn

[Typed, typed signature. SSC]

To Lola Ridge

62 Westbourne Road
Forest Hill, London
April 24, 1932

Lola, sweet and dear,

I found Jack in poor shape as HE had spent most of his money to join the Savile Club on the advice of several as to the political value of doing so. The I think rather foolish dear had made all HIS economies on food and such things and grown very lethargic and unable to work - done frighteningly little for the five months time he has been here. I set in to cure this state of mind with beefsteak and fresh vegetables, and three days has made some improvement already.

Now Im wondering if Jig is behaving himself, though, I am glad to say, Selma seems to have a valuable sense of practical values and I believe I can trust her to see he doesnt mope and starve without reason. And I trust somebody or other will be doing the same for Cyril. I feel Ive grown very hard-boiled and untemperamental compared with what I used to be. But the people I care for most dont seem scared enough of what they may do to themselves.

England looked pretty in a blurred dream of the usual rain (which has continued sporadically) and the flat out here isnt bad. Two fair sized rooms, a small kitchen and an antique bath. It will be the first time I have done my own work in England and may be no economy as my sense of values when buying has not been developed on this side. However the privacy is more grateful than the advantage of lodgings for the present. It takes an hour and a quarter to get practically anywhere, so we havent yet investigated friends and relatives. A trip to Bosham and Aunt Mary may come very soon.

Jig and Selma are, I think, at 127 East 34th, though I forgot to write it down and am sending my letter to them care of Margaret. Would Davy, being good to us in so many ways already, be further good and let the kids have the blankets out of the trunk I left on his hands? I forgot to tell them they could and fear they may have bought blankets already.

I love you, I love Davy, Jack loves you both. Dear, dear, dear

evelyn

PS Im keeping the irish sweeps ticket preciously In the fantastic event of winning anything, Davy and me are going to divide it. Why mightnt a miracle like that happen now and then!

[Typed, typed signature. SSC]

To Lola Ridge

62 Westbourne Road
May 20, 1932

Lola, blessed,

Thank you for having jig and selma. I do think jig is a real painter, though, as Cyril says, in the making yet. Selma has a lot of good qualities and I certainly dont complain about her as a daughter in law in most ways. Anyhow, as long as she and jig are OK by each other what the hell.

Im writing soon and loving you all the time. Jack too. Hes pretty low mostly. I think its money and lack of success. Disappointing year over here. Snobbery in england makes a hopeless case for the little known and impecunious. He hurts himself so much some times its hard to stand. But I have acquired either fatalism or optimism I dont know which and am confident about everybody as long as starvation and death are held off.

devotions of us, darling

evelyn

[Typed, typed signature. SSC]

To Lola Ridge

62 Westbourne Road
June 19, 1932

Beloved dear:

Jack and I have just returned from four days at Bosham, with Aunt Mary, who, poor soul, seems to me to be really failing in health, and thus, by foreshadowing her actual demise, rebuking us somewhat for our hard-hearted thoughts. Preliminary to each visit there I get in a state of rebellion and animosity against the hypocrisy of keeping my opinions and habits under my hat. However, I realise, too, there would be no possibility of Aunt Marys comprehending even the least significant of ones opinions. Eighteen-eighty was her last date and is going to remain so, and any more said merely fuddles her poor old head and without registering anything more definite than fear.

She was very nice to us and the beauty of the weather, with a temperature of eighty and the fields full of buttercups, obliterated to some extent my usual impression of life in a mausoleum. Bosham always upsets digestion with too much starch and too frequent tea, but even that could be taken lightly because of the flowers. Aunt Mary bestowed upon me a very old locket worn by her mother in memory of four dead daughters - all died in childhood. One of them, Eveline, being confused with me. Aunt Mary, instead of calling me Eve-lyn, in proper British style, invariably addressing me as E-vie-line. The locket, which looks old and thin, contains a braided design of the intermingled locks of the four little girls: In mo[112] of Clara, Flora, Eveline, Rosa is graven on the back. It was worn by Aunt Marys mother, one Charlotte Brindley, whose portrait, in a voluminous costume of wide stripes, with a phenomenal brooch and a cap with strings, hangs in the bedroom we occupy.

On the return journey we were advised at Chichester to take the wrong train and found ourselves en route to Brighton, instead of London, via Horsham. As we had to wait at Brighton to re-establish ourselves on the correct route, we decided to skip a train and see the town where Jack used to live as a youth and where his mother died. It was a gorgeous day, and the front with the elaborate parade and glinting glass and tin roofed pier and the plethora of humanity on the beaches, made the most colourful cockney England I have yet seen. Under the arches of the parade terraces are numberless shops - souvenirs, fish, balloons, bars etc. There is a miniature electric railway, covering the shore to a place called Black Rock, and we took a ride in it, and had a peep into numerous bathing huts where people were dressing or undressing or having tea. At the station at which we descended a cockney adventurer with a banjo had set up his hat for pennies, and four girls, probably from factories in the White Chapel neighbourhood.[113] Got out of the train and danced together in the street in a heavy but hilarious manner, joining in the chorus of the gentleman with the banjo. It is the first time I ever saw Londoners dance in the street as the French do, though Jack says I would see it frequently if I had any habit of the East End.

We also saw a wonderful newly caught sea monster, very slashed about and bloody, exposed on a block of wood for the populace to guess what it was. I couldnt and am still wondering. It was bulky like a porpoise but longer, with very little eyes set far back from its snout. Would Davy know what it was?

Sweet dear, I have gone through life looking for people with pride, as the people I could best love; and I have met but four people - no five - with the pride that must be in a whole person. You know who they are. This is a lonesome world. It is an ugly world, and I would be for any species of revolution which would not rob me of art. Without art, I think all of us would wither and die.

Darling, darling, darling,

evelyn

[Typed, typed signature, SSC]

---

112 "...in memory of..."

113 Whitechapel, a district in east London, then characterised by numerous small workshops. Brighton was then (and still is) a popular destination for days out.

To Louise Morgan

[62 Westbourne Road]

August 7, 1932

Darling kid: I have been in bed ever since I got back, sweetie. In Paris all my insides got on a rampage and I had systemic poisoning and inflammation of the bladder. The French doctor scared me to death - its part of their business I think - and when I got back here still very low we had a specialist, one Mr Palmer out, and he charged five guineas damn him, but it was worth it to relieve our minds. None of those dumb bunnies said what poisoned me, but I have made my own diagnosis from familiar symptoms and decided the trench mouth germs I have carried in my system ever since Algeria (as I gathered from Santa Fe diagnosis two years ago) had got all through me. However palmer said whatever pisined me, got the upper hand of me because I was suffering from complete nervous exhaustion. Exhaustion had produced a slight recurrence of prolapsis here and there. I was to stay in bed two weeks and do nothing at all.

Scuse such a long dissertation of innards. I think its ghastly you dont have no holiday.

Very lovingly from us both,

evelyn

[Typed, typed signature. UTK]

To Lola Ridge

62 Westbourne Road

September 10, 1932

Sweet: We have had a middling summer. I was ill through most of July, with nervous breakdown from overwork, and with some sort of systemic poisoning, not diagnosed which affected my innards various ways.

Confidentially, Im worried about Jig, who doesnt seem to be happy; and waiting for further data before definitely deciding whether I should return to NY to look over his and Selmas affairs in the capacity of a detached (if possible) advisor. There have been rifts, though please never mention, for they may be made up by now, and I dont want to anticipate. I never had a chance to talk it all over with you fully, as I do most of my affairs. It seemed to me a mistake on both sides, but a mistake I wouldnt interfere with. Selmas role at twenty-four as the wife of a seventeen year old child as unlike her as possible, with no money and no future assured, and nothing much to flatter her where she need flattery or to secure her in life, demands a nobility of her I never could quite believe in. However, I am saying nothing yet to anyone. Jig would not like to have anyone suspect unless, of course, the time comes when things have to be said openly; and the present unhappiness may be transient.

Jacks and my devotions, dear one, and may your health be strong again as your art always will be.

evelyn

[Typed, typed signature. SSC]

To Lola Ridge

care Gilbert F Wright, Authors Agent

37 Museum Street, London WC1

October 6, 1932

Lola, precious, I dont write oftener because I keep waiting to have something nicer to write; and things dont get better so I just send this to let you know I am thinking of you all the time anyhow.

Mrs Ames said you werent very well at Yaddo, and referred to your bronchial trouble; so I am afraid your dear and blessed chest is acting up again. I wonder if you have gotten any work done, and ever so much else.

For you and Davy alone to know until more do, Jig and Selma have busted up and Jig is back in Denver.

Jack and I are leaving Forest Hill next week, and above is temporary address. I expect to be back in NY in January, completely broke as usual. The gods never willed a peaceful time to any of us, did they!

Anyhow, we love you and Davy, and it will always comfort us to know you are, and I shall always wish I had more than words with which to prove how much.

I think we will move to the seaside town of Lowestoft[114] which may be cheaper than London in the winter.

With love and love from us to you two,

always, evelyn

[Typed, typed signature. SSC]

---

114 Lowestoft, a Suffolk fishing port, is on England's North Sea coast.

Chapter 16

Lowestoft
October 1932 - April 1933

In October 1932 Evelyn and Jack left the south of England and found lodgings in Lowestoft on the North Sea coast of Suffolk, exposed to the biting winds. Lowestoft was (and still is) a fishing port, and Suffolk would have been familiar to Jack, who grew up in neighbouring Norfolk, but to Evelyn it offered yet more opportunities for her insightful and sometimes biting descriptions of her new surroundings. This first part of their Suffolk sojourn was not to last: in early 1933 Elizabeth Ames, the administrator at Yaddo, invited Jack to return, and in March 1933, he and Evelyn once again set sail for New York and Yaddo.

Evelyn had been busy writing and publishing over the years and although this book is primarily about her family story, we cannot forget that she was enjoying some success as a novelist, with a generally favourable critical response and modest sales. In 1925 she and Cyril jointly published In the Endless Sands, *the fictionalised story of Jigg's Algerian desert adventure; this was soon followed by* The Golden Door. *Two years later saw the publication of two more novels:* Ideals *and* Migrations. *Perhaps her most ambitious work,* The Wave, *about the Civil War, was published in 1929 to considerable acclaim. Two more "juveniles" followed:* Witch Perkins *in 1929 and* Blue Rum *(under the pseudonym Ernest Souza) in 1930. In the same year she published* The Winter Alone *and a year later* A Calendar of Sin. *During the time in Lowestoft Evelyn was working on* Breathe Upon These Slain *and shortly after their return to Yaddo, her last book of this period,* Eva Gay, *was published. During these years she was also publishing a number of poems and critical essays. This prodigious output, combined with the volume of letters she was writing to her numerous friends, is impressive by any standards.*

To Louise Morgan

"Lyndhurst"
Alexandra Road, Pakefield
Lowestoft, Suffolk
October 19 [1932]

Very dear Louisa, havent we got AN address? We are in a bungalow which gives us two charming peeps of sea about half a block away, is as quiet as a grave, and has accessible from it about a mile of cliff and little frequented natural beach. Those are the assets. The liabilities are a north sea that is extremely northerly at times and no heat but one fireplace (small) and the kitchen stove. Also one utterly mad landlady who is convinced that we are secret emissaries for Al Capone and put even the gas meter[115] and the bathroom fixtures on her inventory! I dont know in which column to set down our eight potties, one commode, one bed pan (besides the lavatory) which are the lavish equipment for this establishment. Jack writes in the settin' room and me in the kitchen. My labours are presided over by Kitchener as the patron saint, a large photographic group of an unknown family (presumably the landladys) and oleograph called: "Missed! A Bengal Lancer at the game of Tentpegging - Facsimile of a water colour sketch by Miss E Thompson". And another oleograph entitled: Cock Robins Funeral, well calculated to bring tears to the most reluctant eyes.

The settin room is adorned with etchings and a piano inhabited by the warring souls of all the lost Lowestoft mariners. There is also a real oil painting of (conjectured) Juliet and her nurse; and a chromo of a strange interior which contains a spinning wheel, a Turkish coffee set, and two blunderbusses, besides several chickens rooting on the rafters. To contradict the homely atmosphere created by the presence of the fowls, is a very grand lady. She is being told dreadful news by a deformed maiden of the servant class, while on the floor sleeps a man in a Roman toga who hugs another blunderbuss in one arm and, with the other, protects a naked child (either asleep or dead - we are uncertain).

The bric a brac was rather out of key in its simplicity and modernity, and comprised about ten plain coloured vases for flowers. But since the landlady set down the three cracked and handleless cups in the pantry we are afraid to trust ourselves with the vases and have put them away.

Last night after having chattering teeth all day, we took a walk on the beach and heard the water and the stars, so to speak, and didnt feel cold at all. The Suffolk country people talk like Swedish Americans with their baints etc. Lowestoft is certainly the last place to find excitement but it is infinitely more attractive than Felixstowe and if we had money to invest this would be a good, cheap unfashionable neighbourhood for a house. Sunday we bussed to Oulton Broad and while its not much from the road, we could see fine melancholy marshes in the distance which ought to be romantically bleak and full of hants.

I am very nearly laid up with a mashed big toe nail which is painfully being shed. That takes my mind off heaps of things.

Love and lots, from Jack and me, to you both,

evelyn

[Typed, typed signature. UTK]

---

115 It was common at the time for landlords to install "shilling" gas meters in lodgings. This meter was linked to the main gas supply for the house and the tenant fed it with shilling coins to purchase (often at a premium) gas for heat and sometimes for a small gas ring for a kettle.

To Lola Ridge

Lowestoft, Suffolk
October 31, 1932

Dear lovely:

Selma left Jig, darling; but I think you may be right in subtler ways. I dont think Selma was in love with Jig even last winter. But she wanted to be married to him and she wanted to please him. And Jig, of course, even when most infatuated, was gauche and brusque while she was smoothly voluble. But I also fancy there was a kink in his psychology even at the time the marriage was accepted, last winter. And perhaps resentment by the time you saw them. Anyhow, Selma while Jig was away, got her another boy friend, Jig suspected, she denied, and Jig caught them in his room, when he returned to town suddenly. I think he could have been won back if he hadnt had an unadmitted desire to be free anyhow. But of course he was shocked, hurt, excited. He was with the Grants, but suddenly found he could bear New York no more and took train for Denver. The marriage is being annulled, I think. Im unhappy as his mental state is reported not too good, and as heaven knows now when another meeting can be afforded; but I am thankful the break came before the relation has grown too complex with time. Theres loads about it I never told last year. There was no time. Besides, I was trying to make myself accept it. And now, naturally, this is between you and me and Davy. (dont smile for I am more discreet than I used to be. I dont mean the break is a secret, but opinions and causes left out of general public reckoning.)

We were mad with depression in London. The English are cold, Lola. I was thinking recently that never once has any English person made a gesture of real friendship toward me or an imaginative one to ease the foreignness. Sensitive and cold together. Cold in utter indifference to the fate of everything not touching them immediately, just in theory, the sensitive and mystical regarding what is at the inner core of their lives. They are, therefore, satisfactory in a love relation, but in friendship only after a long, long time and when special occasions break the ice.

Up here better than misfit in suburbia. It is gloomy in a Wuthering Heights way. Bleak coast, the sea from our windows. Gulls, fishing boats, and perpetually troubled weather. Fine natural beach, miles of sand. No "scenery" as all flat. But Lowestoft old fashioned and unpopular. Herring industry supports it. Wonderful humid-coloured ocean, only massive with storm - other times I see from window silver poplars and a faint neutral blue water just being born. Very cheap living compared to city. We have little bungalow. Only sprouts to eat! dont grow anything. But lots of herring roe.

Glad Davy is fine, god bless him. Hug him. Jacks, in this instance, unenglish love, and,

to both of you, the heart youve always had,

evelyn

[Typed, typed signature. SSC]

To David Lawson

Lowestoft, Suffolk
November 22, 1932

Davy, dear:

Jig is still in a state of melancholia, I gather. Cyril is so worried by big things hes hopeless about any minor ones. And were all, like your blessed selves, with noses above water and no more.

We are freezing here, but it would be good for work if I could get in a proper frame of mind. Concern for Jig has been eating into my resources despite every bit of will I have to fight it. I am writing a childrens book but it doesnt go as it should so far.

Im in my usual way of sending self-centred news because in this complete isolation, there aint no other; but feelings arent all on ego, and love and longing for those who mean most to us are present just the same.

Bless you both and forgive me, dear Davy,

evelyn

PS I had the first mild quarrel of my life with Cyril because of slow and no communication re Jig. Cyril, poor darling, is quite literally pathological about letter writing. I have to realize that and put up with suspense, since he still is saving Jigs life by taking material responsibility.

[Typed, typed signature. SSC]

To Lola Ridge and David Lawson

Lowestoft, Suffolk
March 2, 1933

Dearest two:

Jack and I (Thanks to Mrs Ames who by cable - so perhaps best not mention it yet - asks Jack anyhow to Yaddo for a short time) leave on the <u>Bremen</u> on March 24th. I dont know that Davy remembers it but the last time we landed in June 1931 we were held up at the dock by a gang of thugs who got five dollars from us as blood money for releasing our baggage which they had simply taken away from the Cunard porter. If Davys forgotten I shall explain later, but it was quite serious. They thought Jack foreign and when they became obstreperous and offered to beat him up he offered to beat them up, whereupon I sailed in with an American voice and threatened them with the police - that helped. Anyhow I wanted to really get to the police, but Hazel, to whose place the baggage was taken, thought if I did the West Street gangsters would damage her property. So we did nothing. But I am genuinely terrified of landing alone.

I dont know what time the <u>Bremen</u> takes going west but I suppose five days. Jack is in bed again with gastric hangover from flu so I expect he will arrive very frail. Mag DeSilver says we may come there again and I hadnt wanted to but Ive written all over the place about cheap rooms so I think well have to (Ive had no responses) until we can get bearings.

Love and love and love and dont forget, I shall write Ellen at once. But I might as well let this go because I 'avent time for more today and I want you to know when we get there anyhow. All ze love going, evelyn.

PS Tourist Third, <u>Bremen</u>

[Typed, typed signature. UTK]

Chapter 17

Farewell to Yaddo
May 1933 - February 1934

The invitation to return to Yaddo was too welcome to refuse. Evelyn had always been very productive during previous visits, partly due to the excellent facilities and, perhaps more importantly, to the company of like-minded artists and writers. For a woman who placed immense importance on the pursuit of artistic and literary talents, Yaddo was a place of sustenance, and these letters convey the atmosphere of life in this closed community.

To Lola Ridge and David Lawson

Yaddo
Saratoga Springs, New York
May 15, 1933

Lola and Davy:

Mrs Ames, Eloise and Jack send love. And I do so very much. Mrs A asked about Lolas coming here and I said it was no use unless she improved. Hope thats ok. I think about you over and over and over, and there seems little use as things are speaking my wishes for you. You know them too well and their feeble expression has been too much repeated.

Its rather sad here this year. The economy of regime, though all comfort within reason still exists, suggests too much an end. Spring doesnt belong - or else we dont in spring. Mrs Trasks ghost no longer seems in opposition to other presences. Its ghosts meeting ghosts.

Or do I think so because I am as I am?

Mildly pleasant crowd here: Philip and Penina Reisman, painters, rather sweet enfants terrible. Ruth Suckow and her husband Ferner Nuhn. A plaintive sycophant with a resourceful wit and a bruised self-respect named Charles Yale Harrison. A tall sea-going boy, intriguingly shy and to himself, who writes Conradish stories, Floyd or Lloyd Collins. Grace Lumpkin, an elderly little girl, straightforward to bluntness and rather engaging. Albert Halper, who is so completely an average American that hes rather wonderful: as if at last one had actually met - what! A real cowboy, after the movies. Or a real Englishman. Or, or. But hes naively frank and all his mentality covers he regards from his own for him authentic angle. Carl Carmer, who is kinder and more sensitively aware of social obligations than anyone else, with qualifications as an artist that remain ambiguous. Louis Adamic lusting for revenge on capital.

Eloise[116] is very pregnant and refreshes with her own interest in the experience. EA has been very kind and suggests we stay on in the farmhouse down the road.

For you two I hope and hope. We love you so.

e

[Typed, typed signature. SSC]

To Maude Dunn

Yaddo
June 8, 1933

Dearest Mother:

I think it too bad you have all that annoyance about the house. And those family quarrels. Looks as tho they never fail to occur when there is any disposition of property.

Thank you again about the money. I'll wait, unless you have pressing need, until I get the Santa Fe trip paid for. You have to go via Chicago, and change to another road, and even some shortest way, it is three days and two nights. There is a round trip slightly less but not much - I mean less in that it is a hundred and fifty for going and coming instead of eighty-five each way, but I don't know that I can pay that out now. Sure wish they lived somewhere else.

I gave the name of the donors of this place wrongly. It was Trask. Big portraits of them hang in the reception hall, and Mrs Trask's grave is a lovely spot, the highest on the property, with a Keltic cross to mark it and very lovely pine trees. She died in 1921. "Yaddo" is a corporation now, but for the purpose of managing the estate only. The name comes from Mrs Trask's child's mispronunciation of "shadow". The child, now dead, heard her mother (who had just lost another child) say she had a shadow on her life. Child called it Yaddo. It really is gorgeous. I wish I could write a whole book here. The country is superb, and Saratoga such a funny nineties looking place. The races begin there next month.

I get very funny letters from strangers about my book. Perfect cranks write to one just because of seeing ones name in print. Some sound like lunatics, tho occasionally a really appreciative letter. And people here are autograph mad.

We do want to hear more about the cemetery. I am letting my hair grow, my dear. And it looks much better than you'd think. Being straight I rather like. It is more distinguished than the curly. Besides, it waves a little when the weather is damp.

---

116 One of the maids at Yaddo.

Well, lots love. I have a frantic week ahead. Leave here a week from Monday. Have more interviews to give in New York. Lots of errands and things to see. Will be there three days. I'll send Santa Fe address as soon as it is exact. I won't stay with Cyril and Phyllis for fear of gossip.

Love again. elsie

[Typed, typed signature. UTK]

To Lola Ridge

Yaddo

July 1933

Lola darling:

I misplaced Davy's letter with the Mount Sinai[117] address so I have to keep on bothering him! We felt very happy hearing you had gained eight pounds, so I do hope Davy will let me know if you and the doctor manage the country sanatorium because that really might do a lot to set you up.

I sympathize with Davy about your darling squiggly handwriting! I adore the sight of it, but Im rarely absolutely certain as to the content of that inimitable calligraphy. Still - I gathered you were up on the roof in the sun and that, as a general indication, sounded good.

Jack god-blesses you and wishes he had been able to look in. He saw May who declares his liver a little worse than last time, but insists it is because he had to knock off the medicine and promises something better when it is resumed after a few months. His general health does seem improved.

This will sound like a clinical report, for my foot is giving me the deuce. I went to Schenectady to a specialist and he said I had a bone broken and wanted to operate. I balked, called in another man here, and he said what nonsense merely a strain and gave me ice packs and icythyol.[118]. Im a little bewildered between them and may surreptitiously call in a third opinion to arbitrate sub rosa on the others. Anyhow Im quite crippled for the present. Am disturbed by fear of being an inconvenience to Yaddo, tho Mrs A has kindly let me use garden studio temporarily so I wont have to walk.

Did I write you Jig and Cyril were in Mexico? Seventy five cents a day room and meals! Nothing in particular happens. An increasing overdose of communism versus art.[119]

Love all around and around you and Davy both,

evelyn

[Typed, typed signature. SSC]

---

117 Mount Sinai is one of the larger New York hospitals: it appears Lola was once again in hospital.

118 Icthyol was the brand name of ammonium bituminosulfonate, distilled from shale oil and used for the relief of skin conditions including eczema and psoriasis.

119 There was an active and continuing debate at Yaddo during the 1930s about Communism. There is an account of this in McGee's book about Yaddo.

To Lola Ridge

Yaddo
July 3, 1933

Beloved dear:

I hope the heat lifted a little in New York, as I know how one feels the weather when in bed.

This morning Ferner Nuhn[120] is in my studio doing a cartoon of me which he thinks wont be any good. So my letter writing day combining with posing has not yielded the crop it should. However, and however uninspired my communications while I am assuming this dual role, I had to drop you a line. Mrs Ames is much distressed to hear of your illness and Eloise even more so.

I havent any news except that the snowballs are blooming outside my window and look very New England cool in their green white. I guess I told you of work: four short stories and four articles and a longish poem and four chapters on final draft of kid book. As for sales, quien sabe!

Sunday dinner is approaching my sweet so… And dont feel I ever need answering. Just hope things go better. Just wish and wish I wasnt as always a useless friend. And just bless you with my heart as you breathe because your existence is such a happiness to we who love you.

Jack is no better much, but May says couldnt be expected for months to improve.

His dear love to you all with mine.

evelyn

[Typed, typed signature. SSC]

To Lola Ridge

Yaddo
July 12, 1933

Lovey, I had a note from Davy who says youre gaining, which is something for us to be a little happier over though there probably doesnt seem much for you in bed.

I wish I could walk in in visitors hour, and so does Jack who is going to NY in an hour to stay for the day and see May Mayers about the liver, again, and would so love to see you if he could stay longer. He sends heaps love.

As a coincidence I am also doctorwards bound. I sprained my foot on the tennis court ten days after I came, and, as I foolishly went on using it, it has grown persistently worse. So Ferner Nuhn and Ruth Suckow are driving us to Schenectady today to see an orthopedic specialist. I dont look for anything very grave but am annoyed, as I was making up for past years by pretending to lead an athletic life. Were a bit alike in one respect, darling - sort of willing to ignore the

---

120 American writer and editor. While at Yaddo he made numerous oil sketches of the other guests, including Evelyn.

obvious in health. Though its heroism in your case and hardly that in the stance of a bad foot.

Mrs Ames and especially and so warmly Eloise are concerned over you, but I think it a good thing you had foresight of yourself and didnt try to come here, as I think Mrs Ames, with any encouragement, would have planned, because Yaddo isnt a good place to be very sick in, and even mildly sick does inevitably make one feel ones self a cog in the communal machinery as I have discovered lately, though all are as nice as possible about it.

There is the usual ebb and flow of guests, and quite an exodus July 1st, with a new lot now installed. On some days I feel the company as a mild pleasure, and, on others, face them and meals with nausea prepared. Not that it is any especial fault in the gathering, but that communal life steals the need ineradicable in my nature, as in yours, for solitude. We are still gratefully accepting an extension of our stay here.

Yaddo exhausts all ones pence of small talk. I sometimes marvel that, after more than two months, words come out of my mouth to say nothing at the dinner table. Its sort of depressing to meet so many people and, always, with each one, feel the pit which separates ones self from the mass of mortals dug a little deeper. Thats why I return again and again to you and Davy and Cyril and Jig and Jack and such very few.

Bless you, my lovey, bless you, bless you. Im so tired of the invisibility of my world to those here and so thankful to remember how much of it walks about in your flesh, which must get well.

Lovingly,

[Typed, not signed. SSC]

To Lola Ridge

Yaddo

August 27, 1933

My angel-one, Im getting better at it and there werent more than six words of your heavenly scribble I missed this time! And its no spindly scribble either, but has the look now of the power they wont let you put into writing.

Then there are the things you realize of crowds, which Jack, poor darling, feels as acutely as a physical pain. They simply wont let you get back in and down into yourself where the poetry lies. Its all got to go forth in extroversion and polite adaption to matters that dont interest or move you or to combating tendencies you actually dislike. The habit of being alone and depending on that for ones strength, once its acquired, is certainly incurable.

Jack goes on on his nerves and with period discouragement and impulses to chuck his book (full of splendid writing) because of bad pages due to bad days. Im working in bed very comfortably and dont quite know how I got into this short book (for me) on England, which I began in Lowestoft and is like a sort of <u>Narrow House</u> got cosmic, and I have no idea what it will be like in the end. Jack loves its being English so that rules him out as a critic. Also swatting when I can on the French revolution for the next one, but should like to write it in France which would appear impossible.

And so the days go. So still now the pine trees give an occasional twitch just to assure you theyre real trees. And hot again, with the clouds glaring darkly and the rain we have had all week getting ready to come down all over again.

God love you like we do. He can do lots better by you - but cant want too much more.

Bestest to Davy and to you from us, blessed one,

evelyn

[Typed, typed signature. SSC]

To David Lawson

Yaddo

December 31, 1933

Davy dear, it was a great relief to have your note. I suppose by now you have got used to these brain waves of anxiety and, as they profit nobody anything and result in nagging about letters, youd have a right to be impatient with them. Im so used to being remote from nearly everyone I care about and periodic hauntings that something has gone wrong is a part of a well established and thriving old trauma.

We are, of course, very fortunate to have a comfortable roof with heat supplied and no rent to pay. Naturally one does, as I have discovered of all things, pay in other ways. I have decided that my temperament never suited me to be a member of the human race nohow, as my last experience of a group in Santa Fe was disastrous through indignations felt by me about gossip which still seem justified entirely, since the gossip was lies. And living in a group up here aint no better. Because of dedicating Eva Gay to Mrs Ames, so I have been allowed to gather, it was presumed by a group here that I was a sort of official Yaddo spy, and this story accumulated results which would be funny if one could look down as god instead of living in the midst of it. The people who now occupy the lower part of this house were among the originators of the tale and it with my resentment of it and the fact that I deeply resent the orthodox communist stand on art and they are quite rabidly orthodox has been responsible for a feud to which there is no ending. As I say, it am largely funny in its preposterousness. At the same time it makes a rather depressing atmosphere when one is virtually buried in winter with this same group.

It was thirty-five below zero here yesterday, which means the coldest temperature I have experienced, though Jack knew colder in Toronto when he was there as a child. However, considering, we felt it remarkably little. At the present moment the rest of the household is away on holiday and we quite rattle around, though not unhappily in this place. The icicles in front of our windows are some of them nearly three yards long and when the moonlight strikes them the diamond array is very exciting in a queer not quite believable fashion. There are no birds, rabbits or anything else - just snow, snow, snow.

I have spent December getting over a job of stenography for poor Jack as because of his inability to work steadily his literary chores have piled up until he gets almost dotty about them sometimes - the four novels he is still working on none of which is yet finished. Hope he never has such an idea again for it has delayed and discouraged him as working on one and getting it off his hands never would have.

Tomorrow Im going to start on the final draft of my quite short book for Spring. I have to turn it in on March 1st so it is rather sweat-shoppy as a prospect. I almost hate having it short because *[the publishers]* will think they won in all this pressure brought to bear whereas it was conceived as short a year and a half ago, before me spirit has been attacked and, as they doubtless think, broken. However it is economic pressures which made me decide to get it done at once and leave the long French revolution novel which is the next big job. Maybe Ive already written the title which is <u>Breathe Upon These Slain</u>.[121]

When writing to me please dont say anything about my comments on the situation here. Ill explain why when I see you. Mrs A has certainly been kind and generous to our material troubles, but there are lots of rather morbid concomitants for which I dont hold her responsible but which exist just the same. I think hers an impossible job - the sort of job which would work out tolerably only for a hard-boiled person who simply was oblivious to nine tenths of what went on and did not react. By unconsciously ignoring simplification would be achieved. For meself, I think Id rather be a stenographer provided I could get a stenographers job, which I doubt.

Of course Jack and me wish, wish, wish everything for you, dear Davy, and our beloved Lola, but Im almost ashamed to wish any more. Its too ironic. We just love you and that's that.

evelyn

[Typed, typed signature. SSC]

To Lola Ridge

Yaddo

February 3, 1934

My own lovey, I hope, hope, hope, HOPE you were finishing all the attack you were going to have - not beginning another, when you wrote to me![122] I think-feel-believe-through imagining - I know those awful black weeks of yours so well and it hurts all through me as I realize what you are going through. If only sympathy werent so futile!

I have only seventy-five pages more of final draft to finish my book, and I feel glad to have done it. However, its a kind of book I had to get off my chest - first person though with no autobiographical ingredients whatever.

---

121 Evelyn often referred to this book as "the French Revolution novel", published in 1934 as *Breathe Upon These Slain*.

122 This letter has not survived.

Lovely, lovely, lovely, LOVEY, more love around you and Davy, and would it were a
fairy ring that could keep pain and trouble out.

From me and jack, evelyn

[Typed, typed signature. SSC]

The above is the last letter in the collection written from Yaddo, although there may have been more which have since been lost. Jack had returned to England in search of a cottage and the dates of empty envelopes show that Evelyn was spending short periods at a number of addresses in and around New York, while waiting to join Jack in Walberswick.

Chapter 18

Walberswick
June 1935 - January 1936

Evelyn and Jack left Yaddo for the last time in early 1934, Jack returning to London and Evelyn remaining in the US, staying first with her friends Gladys and Dudley Grant in Scotch Plains, New Jersey, and then at various addresses in New York City. Very few letters of the period before Evelyn returned to England have survived.

During the autumn of 1934 Jack received his expected legacy, and soon afterwards he and Evelyn returned to England. The amount of the legacy is not mentioned, but it was enough to buy a modest cottage in the small village of Walberswick on the Suffolk coast. There is nothing in the surviving correspondence to indicate why Jack chose to buy in this particular location; perhaps he felt at one with the landscape of his childhood in nearby Norfolk.

After a period in London Evelyn joined Jack at Jove Cottage in the summer of 1935. The cottage still exists, much as it was then, with nothing between it and the North Sea but marshland, fully exposed to the bitter winds.

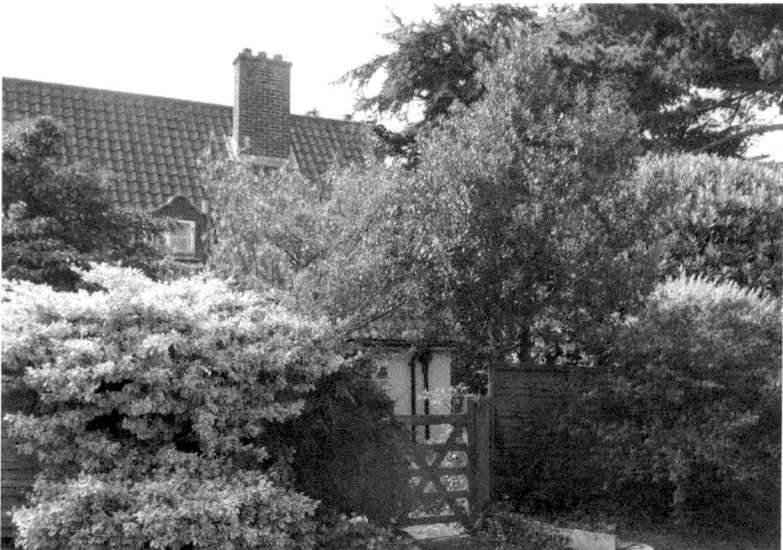

Jove Cottage: *Scott family*

To Lola Ridge

c/o Grant,
Scotch Plains, New Jersey
July 13, 1934

Blessed, your letter is stamped June 22nd. Well, I gave only the lighter reasons for my failure to acknowledge it on my postcard to Davy. The chief reason is another accumulation of a crisis in my perpetually critical personal affairs - not men, sweet one, nor book - money, health, things happening out west. I have simply been too harassed to write. Am this morning commencing to circulate among the most possible another petition to borrow money for a two week trip to the west in September of October. I thought to make enough by writing short stuff and (optimism) selling it in the three or four months in this place, but, alas, I fear me my mental state precludes such a solution. I have attempted five short stories since I arrived and only one has got itself completed in any form approaching saleableness. So in desperation I am going to try to get the fare more parasitically.

Jack writes from London in a cheerful tone about his treatment at the London School of Tropical Medicine which seems to be doing him far more good at once than the methods used here. However, he is running up a large bill with a Harley Street specialist as well as a hospital bill for something called "Suda"[123] baths, so when the Aunt Mary will is finally settled, as we hope it may be in about six months, he is certainly going to need the dab he will get out of it. Yet we are infinitely lucky to have the dab in sight, I know. The damndest irony is that Jack has been made trustee and has every month to sign checks for his Aunt Evie (aunt in law - widow of the parson) who is the beneficiary of the income we had hoped would be his. Ha, Ha!

evelyn

[Typed, typed signature. SSC]

To Lola Ridge

care Gilbert F Wright
37 Museum Street, London WC1
October 6, 1934

Lola, gracious, I dont write often because I keep waiting for something nicer to write; and things dont get better so I just sent this to let you know I am thinking of you all the time anyhow.

I finished my book first week in September, but there are publishing mix-ups again (also VERY confidential) and god knows when it will be out. Ive signed a contract but the publication has been put off six months beyond contract date, and my private opinion is that Smith and Haas[124] wont last six months.

---

123 This is most likely to have been a soda bath, in which epsom salts and bicarbonate of soda are dissolved, often prescribed to relieve skin inflammation and irritation.

124 The publishers with whom Evelyn was negotiating. They did not last to publish *Bread and a Sword*, which was published by Charles Scribner's Sons in 1937.

Jack and I are leaving Forest Hill next week, and above is temporary address. I expect to be back in NY in January, completely broke as usual. The gods never willed a peaceful time to any of us, did they!

Anyhow we love you and Davy and it will always comfort us to know you are, and I shall always wish I had more than words with which to prove how much.

I think we will move to the seaside town of Lowestoft, which may be cheaper than London in the winter.

With love and love from us to you two,

always,

evelyn

[Typed, typed signature. SSC]

To David Lawson

Jove Cottage

Walberswick

June 22, 1935]

Davy dear, you and your lovely flowers seem still both very near and far off. Im quite homesick as a matter of fact, though hoping to become readjusted and get over it. But I am afraid I am very American.

We are making efforts to reinstall ourselves in our new abode but every conceivable power seems against it so far and we are sitting amidst innumerable boxes in the Bell Hotel, the local pub. How long we shall remain in this suspension I dont know. Its worrying about work, chiefly.

Jack is so-so, in some ways better than I hoped in some not so good. The cottage itself looks rather sweet, with tiny rooms that are, however, adequate in number, a very steep roof with brown tiles, a white-washed brick outside and peacock blue window frames. It is on the edge of town and has a rather sweet peep at the somewhat distant sea. At present poppies are all over the fields and cheer the view considerably. But the question of light (fireplaces really arent six inches broad) furniture and fixings as Woolworth in Britain is a more limited establishment than the same in USA.

As I have to type in my lap in a very dark room Im not eloquent on letters but I send this ahead anyhow because I shall so very much want to receive them. Im just praying everyone will give me more than my own deserve as, during the next two or three weeks, I probably shant have any opportunity to write decently.

It is precisely a week since I landed and not one day has it failed to rain - that's something else to get used to. NO summer at all this year is the present prophecy.

Davy dear, the lovely roses were kept fresh in a vase in the cabin for a while and did once appear on the table upstairs. And you and Lola are my dear, dear, dear, dear, dears forever and ever. Always and always - and with Jacks love, too,

evelyn

[Typed, typed signature. SSC]

To MRG[125]

Jove Cottage

July 4, 1935

Dearest Mary: July 4th and nobody knows it! In fact I scarcely know what day it is at all. But the day your note came was the red letter one for me, because I find myself rather low and homesick after my long sojourn in USA and mail a very reassuring celebration. Especially mail like that from you. One of the defects of temperaments given to immediate responses to scene is a tendency to interpret the future in terms of whatever moment it is, and I havent written a lick since the first week in May, when never was writing more imperatively needed. Part of this is exigencies of any move, but a further extended part has been our effort to furnish this place cheaply from auction sale junk which looks presentable only if painted. I havent taken my hands off a paint brush except briefly for two weeks and there is a lot more to come - painted two whole bedroom suites including a cursed wardrobe, and there are more living room cupboards and book shelves.

It occurs to me that women - or my sort - function much like insects in regard to houses. Obviously I should sit down on a packing box and write no matter what; but somehow, since this is presumed to be more than a transient habitation, I cant rest without trying to give it, however, simply, a shipshape appearance of some sort. Poor Jack (who was very bad when I came but is I think and hope improving) simply had left no reserve for furnitures, bedding, kitchen utensils - and British Woolworths sell few of these things. It is most annoying to find that in England only the best is to be had and one pays six shillings for a bread box when a quarter one at home would do just as well-except that they dont exist over here.

We have been everywhere in Suffolk looking for bargains and probably spent more in gasoline than we saved. I dont think either of us is very bright in a business way! And now we are confronted with the how of paying rates[126] and taxes, both on the car needed off the railway in the country and on the house damnation! Weve talked about selling at once, but it seems so silly and as J says he would have to drop at least a thousand dollars on what hes spent on such hurry-up things. So I hope we can persuade ourselves not to worry for a while and enjoy the advantages.

The house is quite sweet - small rooms, but quite a number for its size, and J had it placed with the kitchen to the road and the living and bedrooms to the rear from which we have a sweet continuous glimpse of the sea. Its all done very nicely plain, with a brick floor in the best room and rafters and unpainted woodwork. And J got four carpets for other rooms for practically nothing.

---

125 Evelyn wrote a number of letters to "MRG"; apart from Evelyn's addressing her as "Mary" there is no further information as to her identity or connection with Evelyn.

126 In this context, "rates" is the British term for property taxes.

There are lots of psychological problems I scarcely dare write about. Not people. Just Js need to be analysed which is very various and acute and much worse during last year.[127] But better not refer to his in writing to me as he might read and be upset.

He sends his love and I send barrels.

Evelyn.

[Typed, typed signature. HRC]

To Lola Ridge

Jove Cottage
August 12,1935

Blessedest dear, so stupid of me not to write to you through Davy of whom I asked your address since quitting Taos! I perhaps I makes excuses though subconscious. I am working so hard - never so hard - 10 to 7 at typewriter nearly every day - and have to send notes to family and yet I long with the never failing avidness for news and words from you. How to manage the letters and the work and not bust under it!

Jack was very bad when I arrived, he improves a little and has finished all of Sally[128] but a few minor corrections. That makes me hope for a leap forward, as health and psyche to you united. Of course there will be suspense while a very long book is under consideration by two publishers but is overpowering to me and I feel sure of some ultimate approval whatever discouraging intervals like ahead.

All would be well with me except for time pressures. This is a pretty house, an unimportant landscape full of nice detail - heather quite up to its most sentimental apologists. So like the softest brightest poem of grief up and down everywhere-then the bracken going golden already and, after rain, bitter smelling divinely. Its been five weeks since I walked to the sea and the line of it is before my window daily. Thats because I am working too hard, also perhaps dislike of the village which I have imagined a nastier community than I have proof of. So when we do walk a few times we go away from town, of which we are the last house. Barley and oats make fields full of moonlight of sunlight now the crop is dry, and this with a windmill and the water clear silver or metal blue behind. And sometimes I feel as if Id been born into a world where people werent and remembered through Karma the last warmer existence. I never shall have a root here more than an inch below surface. All my temperament against wanting one. Makes me so apologetic to Jack.

Please write me if you can but dont if it takes heart beats that belong somewhere besides letter. Jacks love with mine toujours, evelyn

[Typed, typed signature. SSC]

---

127 A prescient reference to Jack's continuing fragile mental health and his later breakdown.
128 Jack's fourth novel, *Foster-Girl*, was published in London in 1936 and in the United States as *Sally: The story of a foster girl.*

To Lola Ridge

Jove Cottage
October 20, 1935

Sweetheart your understanding of Jack is movingly precious to us both. He has the most huge capacity for suffering I ever saw, and that is all that defeats us in life even as it contributes to art. The war cloud has done things to him too. We dont feel safe or able to plan. We cant write. I try. If he gets any money, we want Jig here. Im very worried all the time by Jigs complete isolation, his temperamental resistance to contacts. Next to Jack he is the most congenially suffering person - and so much my fault, early wounds, maladjustment, no sense of coherence in his background. I made a mistake being so away from him - let superficial advocates of Freud persuade me it was bound to be good. And really in twelve years he has had two productive years and both those he spent with us.

We want to rent his house but not yet able. It would be lovely in summer months to people at ease in their minds but harder to rent in winter - bleak. Gales over the marshes from the sea. Chimneys shriek, walls rock and the dour neutrality of troubled English skies looks like the worst reflection of one's own dead moods. The Coppards[129] especially mrs have helped Walberswick for me but I dont love it. Only at times the commons with the raspberry rust of dead bracken, the pine trees and the marshes, are smally lonely in a sort of poignant way.

I signed the contract for the short book on Tennessee for McBride because must have money from somewhere when leave here, but shall be very disturbed if return to USA without french revolution material after all. Arms of both of us around our Lola.

God bless darling dear beautiful own lola from us

evelyn.

[Typed, typed signature. SSC]

To MRG

Jove Cottage
Walberswick, Suffolk
November 10, 1935

Mary dear: Indeed no, how could I think you "a beast" for seven million unanswered letters? I dont think your value was ever estimated on a basis of promptitude in that respect.

Ive been and still am laid low by a small rectal fissure, but an air pillow and care may ward off the depressing experience a nursing home is to me even when the occasion is trivial. The real danger of it is that being physically a bit low inclining one to apathy and I seem able to work only in fits and starts - which is why the mss

---

129 Wynne and Alfred Coppard lived next door to Evelyn and Jack and the couples had become friends.

promised for Sept 15th may not be completed until after Christmas. Once it is placed I am going home, because, no use talking, when I hear of Jigs having bronchitis etc, I know that home is where the child is, no matter how often Freud proves motherhood to be the root of all evil.

Oh, Mary, Mary if you only could see the house! I mean how inexpressibly more than a house it would become if some aura from the body presence of beloved people could be shed here! The walls have been distempered now and all the furniture painting, to the so-called little maids room is over with - maids room my real triumph as its combine furnishings before painting cost exactly twelve dollars (including rug - tho we have no bedding yet). Most frightful junk not even selected, just cast in an odd lot at auction. But bright yellow and grey enamel with golden-brown trimmings, the rug blue and a very bright light blue mirror and candle stick with orange curtains look really sweet. Weve had half a dozen too expensive and tiring duty week-end guests, and not one person either of us cares two hoots for has ever crossed the threshold. And soon it will we aspire to hope become the property of renters anyhow. Im too, too, too American after all to really ever want a home forever here. Poor Jack - I wonder if he feels the same in US, and do we demand equally of the foreigner that he "spit in his own face"? Or is that Ellis Island behaviour not current elsewhere?

We see the sea all the time - a rather remote troubled line which is very occasionally a bright blue. We visit it rarely, and not for a month when we took our last walk down the lane, through the marshes and saw swans between the dykes. The heather went, and the bracket is as rusty as old tomatoes, but looks fine in a sunset after rain. Shooting at Blyborough Lodge[130] finished the quail and pheasants who from being our tame backyard pests have become creatures who clack mournfully and rarely in some distant hedgerow.

Jacks love and mine much, e

[Typed on personal letterhead, typed signature. HRC]

To Lola Ridge

Jove Cottage
December 29, 1935

Yes, we have had a hectic three seasons, but at present are calmer if not more settled as to futures. I feel so touched by your understanding of Jack. His insides I feel may never be really first rate, but if - as for all of us - he could only make something from writing all the outgoing elements in his nature would have their real chance.

I expect I wrote when we were so disturbed about the war with England and Italy. It may occur yet of course. However we have just got too tired stewing to stew

---

130 Blythburgh Priory was founded by Augustine monks in the 12th century and is now protected by English Heritage. The surrounding area is noted for its flooded marshes, and it may be here that they went shooting.

any more. I wanted very much to get to France in the summer but there was no cash, and now Lenore has sent us four hundred dollars (dont tell), I have also agreed to be home by March 1st to do the book on Tennessee and hand it and by winter, so France simply has to be dropped at present. Its too bad as god knows whether therell ever be that money again. But what I should prefer would be to live in France a few months again, as more important than facts to be had from documents is to get again the flavour of the race which I have almost lost after nine years. Anyhow the program is for me to sail for NY end of February, then go to Tennessee, come back to NY and finish Tennessee book. By that time something may have happened re publishing and if there is any money and Jack is no worse he says hell stay in France with me a couple of months.

We went to the Coppards on Xmas day. He has a very subtle intuition. But he is also in hard waters financially and they are rather morbid there not seeing anything ahead with two kids. Our most cheery Xmas visitor was the local chimney sweep who gave us parsnip wine and yarned about when he was in India in the Punjab. He is very Kiplingesque. He said of his whippet bitch, shes so intelligent its like lookin in a dictionary to look in her face.

Jacks most love with all, all and forever mine,

evelyn

[Typed, typed signature. SSC]

In early 1936, Evelyn returned to New York to share an apartment in Greenwich Village with Jigg, leaving Jack in England. Her letters describe her concern at Jack's mental well-being in Walberswick, where he remained on his own for several months.

To Lola Ridge

care Scott, 359 West 22nd Street,

early 1936

My own my lovey my dear: Next best to seeing yourself truly was seeing Davy who substantiates the link. I love you… whole letter full.

I dont like New York again. I mean the tastelessness of the people, the complete absence of any integrity, the casual view of brutality, have me down again. But I shall have my nerves rubbed down and like it once more with time Im sure.

I had flu on arrival, was in bed off and on for three weeks, and had to review my novel (not yet done) which has delayed my trip to Tennessee embarrassingly, as I am living on my travel money before I start.

Cyril is living uptown with Alice,[131] whose husband has died, while I am keeping house with Jig which is a great joy. Jig is working for PWA[132] and recently has done

---

131 Alice Wellman, Cyril's only daughter, was at the time a well-known concert pianist.

132 Jigg was working with the Works Public Administration (WPA), an agency of Roosevelt's New Deal which gave support to artists by employing them on public projects.

what I think some very fine painting for himself. I see little of Cyril who works too hard.

Poor Jack has esophagitis (chronic esophagus irritation causing spasmodic contraction when swallowing) had his septic tonsils out under misapprehension it would help and other trouble worse in consequence. I am deeply distressed by his being in Walberswick alone. After two weeks hospital still sick with no help. His novel Sally out soon but I darent hope it will make money fine as it is.

Im working until five thirty every day and no holidays, so this isnt much of a letter; but I hope it reaches the loveliest human sooner or later. Im simply an ache of expectancy to see what has come out of Mexico, which has better health behind it.

Love, evelyn

[Typed, typed signature. SSC]

To Otto Theis

359 West 22nd Street

[mid 1936]

Otto, old darling! I have meant for weeks to write and thank you for sort of ministering to Jack. Wynne Coppard has been writing me ever so pressingly abut psycho-analysis and if J has any money at all it will be the greatest act of friendship to encourage him, as while there is no advance proof of a cure, it is the only hope, apparently, for an existence not ridden by the cancer bugbear (which in turn produces the drink one, though the cancer probably stands for the real complication).

These seven months (imagine!) have been grisly like most seven months during the last twenty years, but little distractions (by the way I howled in an unholy way which belied my sympathy when I heard Jack had a mutilated bottom too) like hospitals and work enough to kill will be nothing if this war business can only be lived down. Jack wants me to come over immediately, and I want to and dont.

Otto, darling, can you suggest Jack might better come over here than get me caught in England in a war with mother minus any checks and Jig jobless: Im coming, end of October, if he hasnt. But he thinks Mussolini and Hitler will have run amok before then.

Awfully perturbed - that is to say normal - for me.

Heaps of love, evelyn

[Typed, typed signature. BRBL]

There are significant gaps in the surviving correspondence, but the remaining letters hint at Evelyn's future mental and physical health as well as providing excruciating detail about Jack's breakdown and Evelyn's threat to leave him.

To Otto Theis

359 West 22nd Street

[Summer 1936]

Dearest Otto, old dear, gee, I feel grateful for the soothing sane feeling you always manage to convey. Hearing from you about anything at all does me good, and hearing from you in connection with Jack does me good even though I dont know what the hell and all to do about him. The cancer of the spine is going strong according to his last letter, which I read between lines, as he is getting most temperate in statements, being, I think afraid I wont show up or something. But he sent me the address of his solicitor and has made a few light references to a "dying man", deprecating the idea, but, actually, I suspect pretty well in its grip. I am so sorry for him I could die myself if it would help - though contradictorally

Between you and me strictly, Wynne wrote me I was going to be in for it if I returned to Walberswick alone this winter again - I mean she felt the cancer would be worse than ever and I would have a thin time handling (she speaking medically). She tried to get jack to an analyst in london, but he couldnt afford even the clinic rates (he couldnt in one sense, he is very hard up, but I expect he welcomed the rationalization of resistance); so she wanted me to get him over here where my few medical acquaintances might cooperate with me in psychiatric measures about the business - Ive done my damndest and I cant budge him. He professes sincerely (as far as he knows) to want to shift the focus of living here, but the fact that the house is there and rent free and we are both very poor justifies stalling about the expensive tourist entrance for six months (he not feeling desperate bout him in my terms).

All this to tell you why I want very much to get J here and why I cant I mean I should be ready to go there at once if my book were done and there was heaps of cash. I simply must have a round trip fare as well as arrangements made here, because if I get caught as last year with no money in that Walberswick isolation not knowing what to do for him I shall end by developing galloping cancer of my own - its getting me, been smoking like a chimney and suddenly discovered what I thought a strange lump - cancer of mouth undoubtedly - telephoned May, without mentioning cancer, and she said go to Memorial Hospital and have them look, so I died overnight, went there the next day, and was told I had a bad case of smokers mouth but the cancer was just a congenital excrescence - like syphilitic shinbones or Hutchinsons teeth[133] I suppose; very small and insignificant and unnoticed before.

With all this, I could wish Jack was nearer you than he is, because otto dear, I simply cant depend on his report of himself, and I get pretty piseyed trying to figure it out. Oh, what a pitty to be mentally corroded by something nonexistant when there are so many nice existant miseries! (These hardly worry him - comparatively.)

And in a way I cant write wherever I am, honey - you flatter me, I had to redo my book because it was too sloppy to turning. I now realize all last year I was only half

---

133 Hutchinson's teeth is a sign of congenital syphilis, which could have been (but wasn't) transmitted to Evelyn by her mother.

there while writing in Walberswick. Partly physical, but largely strain. So it isnt done yet though only a few weeks left and I now like it...

I have about thirty letters to do and here I run on. But Im so grateful, and, as so often, rather drowning clutching at salvation. Awful gossip about us here. Suppose one shouldnt care, but his failure to come back here has started some terrible tales - Mrs Ames leading, so very uncomplimentary to me. Problem is to care about all the good things and not care about the rotten ones, instead of, as I do, caring indiscriminately about everything. Now you are much nearer my ideal in this respect. I dont dare think about the war - but I do. Love completely wholly to you and Louise,

[Typed, not signed. BRBL]

To Otto Theis

359 West 22nd Street
October 1936

Otto dear:

I enclose a note you may be able to give Jack before he sails. I sent one to Bingham Hotel, Southampton Buildings, WC1, where he will presumably be until October 21 when he sails on the <u>Montrose</u> for Montreal.

The sale of the house, or its mortgage and proposed sale, was on impulse but it was best considering his terrible state of mind. Wynne writes me he is in the most serious state she has ever know him to be and that it is acutely dangerous, I must do something. I have no money but Ill go to Montreal as soon as he sends some, at least to see him, hoping I can get him to enter here Tourist and return to Canada later.

He speaks in note today of buying a house in Canada as soon as he lands. If you see him Otto please suggest not. Im terrified. He has the idea he must save his money and it is so little only a house will hold it. But that is quite mad and really as there is no reason on gods earth for staying in Canada any longer than we can help, hell have to sell again and lose again. I want him in New York where conceivably May Mayers will help me to get a psychiatrist for him. Meanwhile Im on next to last chap of last draft of novel, and Tenn book not even begun. Ill be the dotty one too soon. Life always has another little trick up her sleeve worse than the last. Wouldnt it be funny to have something to be happy about!

Afraid those cheerful words go for all of us! god bless and thank you. Love to Louise.

[Typed, not signed. BRBL]

To Otto Theis

c/o Abrams
66 Perry Street
[December 1936]

Since arrival Jack has had a complete breakdown. The difficulty of getting psychiatric treatment for a man whose mania is anxiety about money, so that he is almost afraid to buy a meal, has been ghastly. Mental troubles are exclusive millionaire luxuries. Poor people evidently just go plumb crazy and are shut up. However a friend introduced us to a child analyst who has in turn written to the head of Cornell Psychiatric, who in turn may make some rate I can pay if Jack wont.

But the whole atmosphere of a small flat containing someone off their rocker, Jig by turns (in daily expectation of the collapse of the art project) and me trying to write has been morbid beyond expression. Also Jacks obsession is another house, to be bought with his mortgage money, and what was left from a precipitate sale of Jove Cottage (he now expects never to get that because of king crisis[134]), and there has been the additional factor of train journeys here and there to find very cheap house we can move to next month. But I want to delay until terms of his treatment are arranged.

What Jack needs to think is he did the right thing in sacrificing Jove Cottage. He dreams of it all the time with awful guilt - sure it meant perfect security. He wants to think England sure of a war. I was horrified when he sold it tho relieved he cabled he was coming here because last year scared me so I was gritting me teeth to face isolation with someone whose mental health was so precarious.

Again loads love. Jack sends his, too. He's perfectly lucid but obsessed and chisophrenic. How spell. evelyn

[Typed, typed signature. BRBL]

To Otto Theis and Louise Morgan

c/o 102 Greenwich Avenue

January 11, 1937

Dearest Otto and Louise:

Jack has been in the Payne Whitney Psychiatric for a month and is scheduled for at least two months more before he will be considered a going concern. The obsession is the loss of the house; and while he is definitely medically speaking no lunatic, the situation for the moment is as if he were. It is such a long accumulated story, and I am so tired that I wont attempt a resume of the "case" in full; but the matter of survival, and the constant fluctuation of plans between England and America play a part. Jack is not the type to sacrifice his work for my support and neither am I capable of giving up my work to support him, if I could do so. Maybe we would have found a way out had our sexual attitudes been truly complimentary. But while we are fond enough of each other for the alternative to carry considerable pain, there seems no question in the doctors mind any more than mine that it would be simplest if we were to separate. Jack doesnt know this. He is still in a turbid, chaotic state. He may not know it until a while after he leaves the hospital and America; because his feeling

---

134 It was about this time that George VI had to assume the throne after Edward VIII abdicated in order to marry a divorced woman.

toward me combines extreme dependence and extreme resentment in which such bewilderingly overlapping me measures he himself cannot deal with his emotions at all.

So dont tell what I feel is already decided: that he is to return to England as soon as able, and that I will not follow as he now expects. So much of the neurosis concerns money, and his affairs are so precarious, the doctors consider it would be therapeutic if he got any sort of job for a while, though preferably one through literary connections. He has lost nothing as to competence once he regains poise; and I believe, if the worst time can be got through, he is going to be far better off than for some years because the situation and his whole life will be clearer, less confused - invitation to chistophrenic behaviour less. But I dread when I must write him the letter to say I am not coming back; and I beg and pray everybody who cares at all in friendship for either of us to stand by him and do what can be to make the terrific readjustment which will be demanded easier, so as not to throw him again into this utter defeat and collapse. He could leave the hospital now if it were not for the certainty of suicide if he did. Getting him to stay is made hard by his money terror, as the money expended for treatment is his, and I have none. I dont dare make the break in this country because he will not have recovered for long enough to bear it. He cries continually that he cannot live alone.

So please, please, please do what you can for him. You can imagine after Mertons tumour how this hits, though thank god it is a different bag of tricks, being curable.

dearest love, evelyn

[Typed, typed signature. BRBL]

To Louise Morgan

c/o W O Tuttle, Esq
Corn Exchange Bank Trust,
New York City
January 27, 1937

My Dear Louise.

May I, out of depths of the worst misery, recall a promise you once made me? Evelyn has separated from me today. I am (tho' above address is for your reply) in a Psychiatric Clinic. I have already lost my house, and now, when I was already so low, Evelyn has taken this time to decide we are "incompatible". I have pleaded with her in vain. My fault was that the Atlantic between us gave me such jitters that I lost the house and came over here almost a wreck. As a result I suppose my company was too depressing to bear, and now, while I am here in a Psychiatric Clinic she delivers this, to me, almost death-blow. I cannot realise it yet. I still hope the breach may one day be healed, but I don't know. I am coming back to England pretty well knocked. I have to stay here in hospital for another month anyhow, but expect to sail for England about March 5th to 10th, arriving by 17th or so.

I'm not sure if E realises what she has done either to herself or to me. I admit she is desperately overwrought, worried and fagged. For the last six or seven months I have had blow after blow, and this is the last and worst. I literally don't know yet what it will do to me.

For pity's sake do what you both can for me when I come.

Much love to all

John

[Typed, signed. UTK]

To Otto Theis

Albert Hotel

65 University Place

New York City (for some weeks)

February 18, 1937

Darling Otto, your blessed old letter doesnt sound much more cheerful than I feel, but does me good just the same. Poor you - except that you are so courageous us other poor critters keep turning to you so matter what you yourself face at times and say so little about! After lying to Jack for weeks about England and the future, I found it made me so physically ill I couldn't go on. The three hourly, thrice weekly visits were grillings. He went back on his promise to "go to England ahead of me" and said he would not leave until I did. I wrote to the doctor, enclosing a frank statement to Jack I proposed the doctor should give him when he was well enough. The doctor had Jack up before the "tribunal" - of doctors - who pronounced him fitter, and agreed with my suggestion it was better to deliver a blow while Jack was in the hospital then to wait until he was out and not protected against himself. Jack was therefore given the letter[135] before I was told and I arrived at the hospital to be informed by the doctor Jack knew my plans, had taken them badly, and was determined to leave the hospital that night. The doctors felt if he did he would kill himself, and insisted I come upstairs and talk to him. So there were 2½ hours hell, Jack hysterical. I haven't seen him since - 12 days ago; but I agree to pay a few weeks if he would stay there until he got better. I hope he will, though I scarcely know how to meet the bill.

He has to get back, Otto - the doctors think he simply cant function here with his distrust and dislike of the country. I am much distressed by your confirmation of the gossip I suspected. Im sure it is fantastically exaggerated, for I discovered in Walberswick the auld English have vile tongues. I think Jack has told me most of what he did - bar maids, a few dives, night clubs, too much drink. But the period was brief, I dont think he indulged any perversities, and the great acquaintance with low life vernacular came largely from reading. I know the books consulted and skimmed them myself.

---

135 This is most likely Evelyn's letter telling Jack that she was leaving him.

However, the damage is the same and I shall feel pretty hellish from a distance until I know he is reestablished. His effort to appear a rake, is entirely compensation for what has really been a very secluded narrow life - a sense of sexual inferiority among the bull-necked boastful type of males who object to him because he has such a childish streak. Anything on gods earth you and Louise can do - and oh, oh, oh if I could ever help you as you have me so often, Otto darling - will be so so gratefully received.

I forgot to say Jack tried to swallow the thermometer - bite off the mercury - three days after the separation was suggested. The suicidal state may last. But beyond that I think he is very capable of jobs and that. The shock of my decision may stimulate recovery. Whenever he has held a job he has been good and approved. The last was 1928 - nine years ago - Montreal and Wanstall the head of the school was enthusiastically glad to see him this year.

I wrote to Jacks Uncle Jim and Aunt Millie and received cabled excuses for not helping - they are in a funk for fear they'll be held responsible. Oh these cold nice people

I feel low - though the statement about separation relieved a rather suicidy state of my own. But at my age - 44 last month - starting all over! Very well for a man, or at least possible. But a sex-suppressed, emotionally frustrate dame of the "dangerous age", who still has too much hang over of romanticism to sell her fading charm to a gent of 90 with money (there are a couple near that), and who cant sublimate in activities for the public weal, and who is too proud (too vain) to accept consolation from younger men who may rightly condescend toward a derelict, and who havent either the stoicism or the mysticism for - an adequate life alone - well, I don't quite know what will become of her.

I think of all the brave people I know - like you - and say if they can come through trials as bad surely I can. But at present all appears rather grey and desolate, not to mention the money fears which are intense, which you know so well. For a female, these late starts are almost degrading - offering of wilted salad leaves with a sour cherry on top and rancid dressing and trying to pretend the banquet is fresh. However, ca passe. Matter of fact Jig at 22 is as lonesome as I am, poor lamb, and that is another self reproach for me! Every way I look, skeletons have bones or victims of starvation I have somehow helped produce. But I realize those who have work - expression - which you were born to and ought to have, ditto L - are luck in the meagre measure of luck in this

I love you,
Evelyn

[Handwritten, signed. BRBL]

Chapter 19

Greenwich Village
Spring 1937 - November 1942

Very little correspondence remains from the period between Evelyn's separation from Jack in early 1936 and the summer of 1937 when Maude Dunn died. Following her return from Brazil in 1917, Maude had lived with her Gracey cousins in Clarksville, Tennessee. She was effectively a pauper, barely tolerated by her cousins, and Evelyn supported her when she could with a modest monthly allowance, scraped together from her small earnings from her writings.

Will of Maude Thomas Dunn

I want my only child Evelyn D Scott Metcalfe (novelist) to have everything I possess.

Maude Thomas Dunn

April 6, 1937

Clarksville, Tennessee

[Handwritten, signed. HRC]

During the summer of 1937 Evelyn stayed with Jigg and with a succession of friends in Greenwich Village trying, largely unsuccessfully due to her concern at Jack's health, to concentrate on her writing. These letters document the distress felt by both Evelyn and Jack: although each expressed this distress in different terms, its intensity is not in doubt. Evelyn's letters demonstrate obvious and deep concern for Jack and his recovery, this in stark contrast to her letters of later years in which she concentrates on her own frustrations.

To Lola Ridge

c/o Abrams

66 Perry Street

Sunday [Summer 1937]

No dearest I am not ill, but just sapless. Some days I think I must have tb[136] again that

---

136 It is very possible that recurring references to her chest problems indicated early symptoms of the lung cancer which eventually killed Evelyn.

I am on the brink of declining from some unnamed obscure malady; and in the end when I rest it is just that - fatigue - and rest is really all I need.

Jacks situation is very, very tragic; and I cant quite recover from my own decision, which my mind still approves, to save myself at the risk of his own chance of complete reestablishment. He went back to England, and I wont write to him until he is thoroughly in control again as it only harrows under the circumstances. He has every logical chance of being OK, again and greatly improved before he left; but finance and discouragements to writing are dreadful things for a man to bear alone who has just been through his ordeal - psychological collapses are worse than anything physical and I say that knowing at least enough of the physical not to be a fool of unimaginativeness. But at the worst if you are ill in body you die. So I was very glad the doctors so conclusively diagnosed him as not a case of insanity, but just break down, which is vastly different in the medical meaning.

Jig is writing a novel,[137] Lola - dont tell. I think it is marvelous in lucid, lucent reticent style. Lots of sad things come out in it however and the theme may make it difficult to sell today. *[remainder of letter missing]*
[Typed, first page only. SSC]

To Louise Morgan

28 Craven Terrace
London W2
September 23, 1937

My Dear Louise,

I meant to write or 'phone you for several days, but have been rushed. Darling, something you said over the 'phone annoyed me, and I prefer, particularly in my present irritable mood, to get my little "mads" off my chest.

You said I made "excellent first impressions". What I would point out is that even that is pretty darned good for someone who, ill-advisedly, sought a better world, or no-world, only a few months back, and was told by his doctor that he was foolish to think, as yet, of so much as applying for a job. The whole business in NY took me at a most staggering disadvantage. I'd given up the for what seemed, after weighing pros and cons, the joint good of both, but the actual doing of it was such a fearful wrench that I arrived a temporary wreck and said and did utterly misrepresentative things which precipitated the break. The break itself was hardly therapeutic with effect and the vicious circle was prolonged.

It's completely unjust, my dear, to judge a still-sick, if recuperating, bloke by standards applicable to the quite robust. I've survived enough to tip the strongest, let alone someone taken between wind and water in the middle of a nervous breakdown. I consider the whole thing a most grotesque pity, and an enormous

---

137 Jigg's only novel, *The Muscovites*, was published in 1940.

waste of time, nerves and emotions. I want, of course, to cut losses as much, and as soon, as possible.

Evelyn's action is historically and psychologically comprehensible, and while I think it misguided and quite as much of a pity for her as for me, I see how it happened detachedly enough, and leave it at that pro tem. Meanwhile, I can, with recovered health, live my own life, and get as good milk as has been spilt.

Love, see you soon,
John

[Handwritten, signed. BRBL]

Meanwhile, Jack had managed to sell Jove Cottage and had returned to London and to the Royal Air Force in early 1939. It is very likely that, as a former reservist from WWI, he was called up when it looked as though Britain would be involved in a second war. The tone of his letters indicated a much improved mental state. And, as war loomed, both Evelyn and Jack began seriously to consider how and when she could return to England.

During these years, Jack's mental health improved to the point that he could return to RAF duties. Although he was stationed at RAF Kinloss[138] in northern Scotland, for security reasons he used the address of his friend in Surrey. Letters from this period include references to a house in London which he bought with the proceeds from Jove Cottage. This property, 26 Belsize Crescent in the pleasant London suburb of Hampstead, was a large house of three storeys plus a basement. Jack planned to let out flats on the three floors and to live with Evelyn in the basement flat, using the rental from the flats to service the mortgage and to support himself and Evelyn. For reasons that become obvious later, the property became, instead of a source of financial security, a huge financial drain which will merit a chapter[139] on its own.

To Lola Ridge

Officers' Mess, No 14 FTS
RAF Kinross
July 23, 1939

Dear Lola,

I've been meaning to write for a long while, and wondering how you are getting on. I do so hope you are feeling fitter than when I last saw you, and that you are able to work some. The way you have carried on all these years in the face of so much illness and discouragement should be an example to anyone.

As for me, I'm back in the Air Force as you see and comfortable enough. I came up here in May. I was hoping to be posted nearer London, so I could use my own house,[140] but this station has its advantages.

---

138 RAF Kinloss was established in 1939 as a training base. Jack consistently misspelled the name of the base as "Kinross".

139 See Chapter 34.

140 This is the first mention of Jack's London property at 26 Belsize Crescent.

Work is varied and interesting - but leaves little time for my own writing. However, I manage a little now and then.

The country round here is quite lovely in its way, but we've been having an awful lot of rain; - it's been general, all over England too.

I wish I could have remained longer in New York and seen more of you and of Davey while I was there.

Over here there is, of course, the usual talk of war. There's no telling really what will happen.

This station is quite new, and only partially built. At present we are in hutments. It's all very familiar though it's twenty years since I was demobbed and twelve since I came off the Reserve. The CO is a very decent sort of bloke and the crowd as a whole not at all bad.

Ever so much love to you dear Lola, and all the best to Davey from

Jack

PS Am worried about Evelyn who seems, from her recent letters, to be having a hard time of it. And I, at the moment, have to put every cent from my pay into the house or, if I miss a payment, lose the whole thing. But if I can hang on for a few months longer I will have rounded the corner.

[Typed, signed. SSC]

To Evelyn Scott

Claygate, Surrey
September 29, 1939

My Darling,

Just a line while I have a chance. Am Oke, though hellishly busy as always.

Bless you for your dear letter. Yes, sweetie, we must just hold on. I think, with you, that it <u>might</u> be possible, conceivably, for you to cross later, - but I see from today's paper giving account of Roosevelt's speech to Congress that, as I expected, the proposals including both (a) Forbidding USA <u>vessels</u> to enter war zones, and (b) Forbidding USA <u>citizens</u> to travel in vessels of belligerents or in danger areas. So if these proposals go through, and I expect they may, you could not, anyhow, get to England while the war lasted, save as a <u>British</u> subject. You are that according to British law, but <u>not</u> by American law. I should be awfully glad if you could, perhaps, call at the British Consulate, and collect what information and advice you can and let me know what they say. If ever I get leave late on I might be able to call on the USA consul somewhere just for information.

All this, of <u>course</u>, is only for a possible, just conceivable, "later on". It would be madness to try and cross now in any but a USA ship, - and the trouble is, or will be, that, if the Roosevelt proposals go through, USA ships won't be sailing to England.

Well, darling, God bless you, and I <u>love</u> you and I'm all yours, and one's each's for always.

This just a scribbled note.

Much love and hugs to Jig, - and to Cyril

<u>Yours</u>

Dickie

[Handwritten, signed. UTK]

To Evelyn Scott

Claygate, Surrey

October 15, 1939

Darlingest Dear,

Just got two letters from you - one dated October 1st and the other October 3rd.[141] I have got a letter or letters from you every week except one, so far. In regard to putting "per USA boat", if repeal of Neutrality Act involves cessation of USA boats' running to England you will of course not put that. Anyhow, the letter you <u>didn't</u> put it on arrived OK.

I do so hope your cold is quite gone, and that you won't catch more and get down. And don't add worry about <u>me</u> to your own other troubles, lovey. I am quite oke and going strong. And for Pete's sake don't stew if letters don't arrive sometimes. There may be long gaps now and then and it can't be helped.

Whether there are or not you know that all is fine and strong between us. It may be possible for you to come over later on, if and when that can be done safely, but length of parting makes no difference to what we are to each other. I wish I could tell you! I have such a welling and overflowing of love and everything, - as you say, it is like an "ache", - but it will be all the sweeter when we are together. I think of you constantly, of all sorts of things that bring you vividly back - the Yaddo W African negroes and their "Jeem-jeem, Jeem-<u>jeem</u>-jeem"; and the Spanish records at Santa Fe "That'll be delightful, delightful, delightful", and the "Valse Ananas" etc, etc. And that isn't just "sentiment" at all because it is all integrated with a purpose for existence, with a steady realisation of you-and-me as persons with an identity-in-differences whose actual practical living - together means intelligent understanding and work as well as love.

Send the marriage certificate whenever it comes along. Yes, these things are slow, I know.

So, darling, darling, darling - don't worry - not about me anyhow. As to war, it may be shorter than we think and after it (if not before) we'll be able to enjoy all those things we've looked forward to.

All, all, all love for ever for my darling dear,

YOUR

Dickie

Love as always to Jig, Cyril

(William John Metcalfe)

[Typed, signed. UTK]

---

141 These letters have not survived.

To Evelyn Scott

Claygate, Surrey
October 19, 1939

Darlingest Dear,

Just a very hurried note to tell you I have been promoted to Flight Lieutenant (i.e. equivalent of "Captain" in the Army).

All oke. No time for more at the moment. - tho just a very very hurried scribble that you knew. And send marriage certif. as soon as possible. Shall write you soon,-all dearest love and adoration <u>from</u>

Your Dickie
(F/Lieut William John Metcalfe, RAF)

[Handwritten, signed. UTK]

To Evelyn Scott

Claygate, Surrey
March 11, 1940

Darlingest Dear,

Nothing fresh since my last of a day or two ago. Am hard at work as usual, - though there may be a lighter week-end soon over Easter, - weather and other things permitting.

Times goes slowly-quickly, in the funny way it always does, and by the time you get this it'll be a year since I sailed last from New York and ten since our marriage, on the 17th. Oh, golly, I think we are the funniest people out, - but I feel that after all these vicissitudes we are closer, and so much much more understanding than ever before. How I wish I could talk to you, - just for 10 minutes, even.

Well, I'm glad winter's over anyhow. I thought of you when I read of the New York blizzard in the papers, - and of course (now it's two months old, and the press has published weather-stories, it's permissible to mention it) it's been pretty cold here too. Many nights really darned cold, and with my shoes comically frozen to the floor next morning.

Oh, dollink, how swell, some time, to be together again and write our books. All blessings to your own novel. It will mean frightful hard work under unfavourable circumstances, I know.

Thank Jig and Pavla[142] so much for their message, - and much love to them.

Where is Cyril now and what is he doing? What is latest news of your mother?

All dearest love, always from
Your
Dickie (W J Metcalfe)

[Handwritten, signed. UTK]

---

142 Paula was born in Spanish-speaking Taos, New Mexico and originally christened "Pavli" (or sometimes "Pavla"), the Spanish form of Paula. After her marriage to Jigg in 1940 and their move to the East Coast she adopted "Paula" to avoid the need for constant explanations of the origin of her name.

To Evelyn Scott

Claygate, Surrey
April 1, 1940

Darlingest Dear,

I have just got your sweet letter of March 14th.[143] I hope you have been getting my recent letters OK. There are bound to be gaps in between, - I mean, a number of letters, written on different dates, arriving in a bunch. That's the way with yours, and I guess it is so with mine to you, also.

I wrote you a few days ago, - and had hoped to have any leisure to write a longer letter on Sunday (yesterday). Vain hope indeed! - And today is as bad. I want to read your poems properly, - but nowadays I have hardly time to think at all. This is just literally so, - No time whatever for leisure of the mind or for "souvenirs". But I hope to be able to get a moment to myself (and you!) before long. My letters, such as they are, have often to be written in a noisy, crowded room, - and this is one of them.

Oh dear, - I'm so sorry, - but know, beloved, that nothing alters and one is each's for always.

Tho only a tiny note to let you know I'm well and loving you. Shall write better letter the moment I can.

I am <u>so</u> sorry for your poor mother - do hope the operation will relieve her somewhat.

All blessings on you, on your novel, - and for Jig and Pavla

Yours

Dickie (W J Metcalfe)

Do forgive this note. It's not my fault, love, and unavoidable - but all OK Love you!!!

[Handwritten, signed. UTK]

To Evelyn Scott

[Clarksville, Tennessee]
April 21, 1940

MISS EVELYN SCOTT 18 GROVE ST NYC. MOTHER PASSED AWAY EARLY THIS MORNING FUNERAL MONDAY MORNING. LOUISE.

[Telegram. HRC]

To Lola Ridge

18 Grove Street
May 8, 1940

Yes, Lola, dear, losing mother did strange things to the emotions and still does. Death is wonderful clarifier of feeling. Mother was so oddly, too, both the same hen-headed person she always was, and quite different toward the end of her life. When she was

---

143 This letter has not survived.

ill, she had the most really aristocratic dignity and reticence. I dont think she ever complained except occasionally in a rather sharp joking way; and the only time she was furiously angry was when some nosey church members she didnt know butted into her room. I was there and she quashed them far better than I could in a highly dignified way, although she was so ill. Her face changed, too; and got a curious aquiline contour, different from the one it had when the bones didnt show. And she always thought I did everything for her, whether I did or not - other people got no credit for their flowers, these all came from me. It was very touching.

So I knew in the end that I really did love her, and that seeming not to was an instinct of nature in defense against a temperament too unlike my own to be lived with. It was my piece of sentiment to arrange what was to be read at her funeral, even though I couldnt be there. They read the Episcopal service at the cemetery, and Saint Paul on charity and the last chapter of Ecclesiastes, those being the loveliest things I know. So I hoped the petty little townsfolk would hear about charity for once. I dont like rationalistic funerals, in which death and garbage collection are on a par.

Now Ive got that out of my system I wont talk about it again. I dont think I need to be pampered with visits. Just know I love them when they come.

god bless, evelyn

[Typed, typed signature. SSC]

In the summer of 1940, Jigg married Paula Pearson, the daughter of Ralph Pearson and Margaret (Margué) Hale. They met when they were both living in Greenwich Village, Jigg with Cyril, and Paula with a friend. The newly-weds lived for a month with Jigg's half sister Alice Wellman Harris in Teaneck, New Jersey, before moving back to Greenwich Village where their first child, Denise, was born in February, 1941.

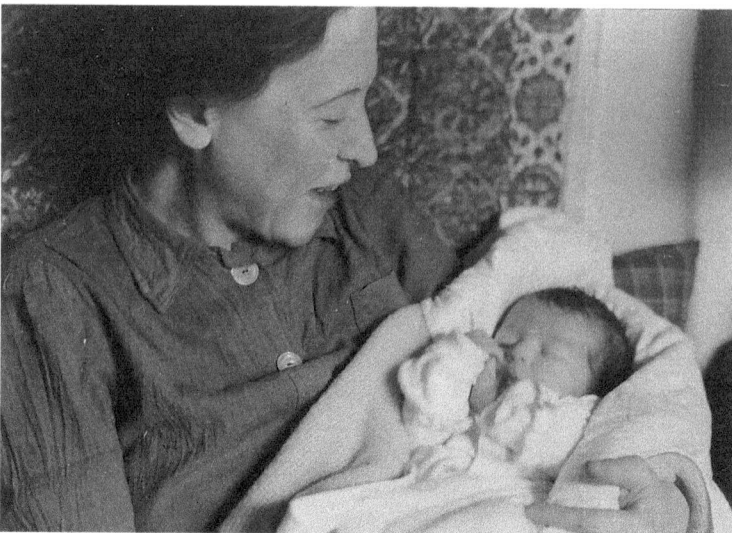

Evelyn and first grandchild, March 1941: *Scott family*

To Evelyn Scott

NEWYORK NY FEB 10 857P

MRS W J METCALFE 150 REGENT ST SG

MISDIRECTED ANNOUNCEMENT DUE TO EXCITEMENT VERY DISTRESSED DENISE EIGHT POUNDS ONE OUNCE PAULA DOING FINE LOVE AND REGRETS. JIGG

[Telegram. SFC]

At around this time, Jigg had found work in radio news, based on his experience on The Rocky Mountain News, *where he had been a reporter while living with Cyril in Denver. His first radio job was in the newsroom of the National Broadcasting Company (NBC), where he was able to make use of his excellent French by broadcasting in both English and French. He remained with NBC until March 1943.*

Before his marriage, Jigg had been working on his first and only novel, The Muscovites, *published by Charles Scribner and Sons in 1940. Although it was well reviewed, it sold very few copies. His mother, perhaps naturally, considered it to be a work of great artistic merit and constantly said so to her correspondents.*

To Evelyn Scott

269 West 10th Street

February 12, 1941

Dear Mother,

I have sent you the same birth announcement which I mis-addressed in the excitement, by air mail and special delivery. If it does not reach you, I shall print another as soon as I have time. I'm desolate that you, of all people, should have been neglected. I have intended to write you a full and complete letter about anything and everything when I recovered. This is to tide you over. The bathtub, a beauty, came; and I shall express my gratitude later, in full. Denise was born on Saturday, Feb nine,[144] at approx 11:30 pipemma, after twenty-four hours of labor pains. She weighed eight lbs one oz, has dark green eyes, a dark brown pubescence on the scalp, and a fresh, not to say choleric, complexion; but less raw looking than the average. The medical verdict is that her health is absolutely perfect. Appetite and voice both phenomenally powerful. I saw her for one minute on Sat, and am not allowed to see her again until she leaves hosp. Pavli is much admired for her stoicism and fortitude. The house physician, an assisting intern, and our own doctor all paid visits for the express purpose of telling her she was an ideal patient. The doctor who officiated did not realize her pains were labor pains because she minimized them so. He's used to Jewish mamas[145] who raise hell. P had to be told that she could scream if she liked. She was very slightly torn, but

---

144 Denise always believed, and her birth certificate confirms, that she was born on February 8th.

145 The baby was born at Beth Israel Hospital, a Jewish hospital in Greenwich Village.

only to the extent of a mild discomfort, and nothing more: one small stitch. She feels like a new woman. Plenty of milk, and enthusiastic about the baby. This is just a measly note, but honestly, I'm a ruin pro tempore. I'll write you more later.

You've been angelic, which forcibly comes upon me by contrast with MY mother-in-law. You may be an arch-loony, like me and the rest of the litt profession, but you've got taste. Margue[146] gets in my hair a little, especially as she's being very ladylike in order (I suspect) to show me up as an oaf. Or maybe she is just ladylike like a lady. I don't know. This Freudian instant-calculators gives me indigestion. I haven't enjoyed my meals since the lady came, although she is being very pleasant. But whatever you say or whoever you mention, she has a bright explanation for. For example, if you remark that Churchill said so and so, the instant comment is that, Oh, Yes; that's probably because he has no hair on his balls, or because his grandnephew was buggered by the choir master, and so whenever he (C) has pickled beets it aggravates his Agamemnon complex so that he resents Germans. It's a mania, sort of an intellectual dysentery, the diarrhea of which cannot be relieved except on somebody else's shirt. However, she has been trying hard to be nice, and don't ever quote me.

As I said, the bathtub is supercolossal and hyperprodigious, and I will write again. Denise received your valentine, in what spirit I am not able to say. My best love.

Your affec son,

Jigg

[Typed, signed. SFC]

To Evelyn Scott

269 W 10th Street

August 9, 1940[147]

Dear Mother,

Got your note and very much pleased with it. Things are going from bad to worse with us, although we are keeping our chins up, rather. We land in a crisis and scrabble and beg our way out, and then before we have recovered from that, the same old devils are back haunting us again: rent and bread and butter etc. It is pretty hard at times; but we have gotten this far, and DV we will go right on to the very end in spite of all hell. Still, it is a weary business and a burden of some weight that we have to share, although amply compensated for a hope of peace and quiet and all the things which are indubitably and rightfully ours if we can only wade through the present swamps. The future has been much brightened for us both by Pavli's Cousin, one Dorothy McNamee, who has done all that she could do to get me a job somewhere, and who alone among those I have recently known is disposed to weep on our behalf. She

---

146 Paula's mother, Margaret Hale Foster (Margué).
147 Although dated 1940, this letter must have been written in 1941.

managed to euchre the general manager of a department store into saying he would give me a job; and although he welched on it, it was not for lack of energy on her part.

That was the news I was hoping to give you; and now nothing has come of it. Yesterday I managed to get a man who runs a display company to agree to pay me 70¢ an hour for a 44 hr week. But it isn't much and he may have changed his mind before Monday when I start working, and I may be up against manner of technical problems (cinematography illusions and so forth) that I cannot do. Still, it is worth trying.

Parental love is a wonderful thing. How strongly I would recoil from the stained drawers of even the most angelic person. Yet the baby lades us and drenches us with all manner of things and we are privileged to change her pants; and what is more, when she holds levee on the potty we stand around and gawk and admire. *[remainder of letter missing]*

[Typed, missing signature. SFC]

To Evelyn Scott and John Metcalfe

269 W 10th Street
November 16, 1941

Dear Mother and Jack

This will amount to little more than a note although it should be more, to thank you both for your birthday wishes and the beautiful neckties; and to tell you that, beginning tomorrow, Monday November the 17th, I go to work for the National Broadcasting Company, Rockefeller Center, as assistant to one Maurice English, who is head of the Propaganda Section of the International (short wave) Division. I will be paid $150 a month, on a salary basis, until such time as I seem indispensable enough to sign a contract, on a yearly basis, with the company.

I don't recall that either of you have ever tried to get into Radio; so let me say that it was a heartbreaking business. I had to lie about everything on earth, and commit myself on countless dubious points; that was the only way. My duties consist of editing the daily news, as provided by the Associated Press, the International News Service, and about six others, including the Office of the Co-ordinator of Information (US) where my application is still being considered (I haven't had time to withdraw it).

In addition to the above, I have to digest the Editorials of about fifty papers, and keep an itemised file of the War. My hours vary from 7 to 9 in the morning, to 5 to 9 in the evening. Theoretically I should appear at my desk at 9 and leave at 5; but circumstances often interfere. There are seven broadcasts daily, in the compilation of which I have a hand; not to mention intermittent news bulletins during the day. That is about all I know of it so far.

Yesterday (Sat) I was given a cursory introduction to my job; and am wearily resting at the moment. I will write you more fully when I have the poop - in about a week, I think. Which does not mean that I have not appreciated your presents. Bless you both.

I will write Jack as soon as ever. Wish me luck,

Jigg

[Typed, typed signature. SFC]

To Evelyn Scott

269 West 10th Street
November 21, 1941

Dear Mother,

I appreciate that my correspondence is in a mess, but there is no help for it. I have a dim impression of having written you about my new job, but, things being as they are it is very likely that I just intended to. Here is the situation. Last Monday - today is Friday - I went to work for the National Broadcasting Company as assistant foreign editor in the International division. We are understaffed. I get to my desk at eight ack emma, and leave it sometimes at six, sometimes at six thirty, sometimes at seven or even seven thirty, but never before six. I have from ten to thirty minutes for lunch.

If you will just stop and picture for yourself the bulk of The New York Times on week days, it will help you visualise what I have to do. The number of pages in an average Times varies from 25 to forty. Well, an equivalent mass of material goes through my hands daily, and has to be edited and distributed to 12 departments. In addition I have to read anywhere from fifty to seventy out-of-town papers and digest their editorials. Not only that, but all the material from the office of the US coordinator of information goes through my hands as well. This is merely a part of the job. Every day I have to collect material for one half-hour broadcast, and write another. My boss does the rest, and it is really something considerable. At the present he is sick; I am new; and we are breaking in a Swedish department, and trying to locate the men for a Finnish department.

I don't get Saturday or Sunday off until this situation improves. I have already agreed to work on Christmas day and New Years, and I have worked on Thanksgiving.

God bless. The baby is fine, so are we all.

Jigg

[Typed, typed signature. SFC]

To Evelyn Scott

National Broadcasting Company, Inc
A Radio Corporation of America Service
RCA Building, Radio City
New York, NY

[November 1942]

Dear Mother:

It's a boy.[148] Everybody's fine, although Pavli had a hard time of it. I sent you a

---

148 Their second child, Frederick Wellman Scott, was born on November 11, 1942.

telegram the same day, only the telegram wasn't sent, I've just discovered because I had already used up my expense account (Employees are allowed five dollars worth of telegrams per month) notifying people, chiefly Pavli's family. The kid was born November nine at six twenty am, weighed six pounds twelve ounces, and looks like a comedy Irishman. The name is Frederick Wheeler *[sic]* Scott.

I am on the lookout for a new job, my present one having come to an end. The government has taken over all short wave, and has banned all broadcasts to American troops abroad (on the grounds that such are not important) and so my section - which specialized in this - are out of work. It would happen at a time like this. I took a look at the office the war information's headquarters here, but have decided against working there if possible. While waiting I observed that Mr Edd Johnson, the man I wished to see, dictated his polemics to a secretary. I just couldn't work on that basis. Also while I was there, Churchill made a speech, and when a someboy in the office proposed that it should be re-broadcast in its entirety, Mr Johnson said: "Oh, no! Because, whenever European listeners hear its Churchill, they turn off the radio". I just refuse to have anything to do with prejudices like that. Naturally nobody knows what European listeners do, or when they turn off their radios. The same man also referred to Gen Giraud as a "senile son of a bitch" - and unhappily I think Giraud is a fine man - with guts enough to fight, which is more than most of those draft dodgers at the OWI[149] have.

So, I am looking around for a job. Wish me luck. For the time being everything is oke. I'm terribly sorry you didn't hear more promptly, but it's the fault of red tape, and not me.

Bless you all

Love

Jigg

[Typed on official letterhead, typed signature. SFC]

---

149 Office of War Information.

Chapter 20

Tappan

December 1942 - January 1944

In common with many young families, Jigg and Paula were finding life in New York City with their two young children a financial struggle. In November 1942, they moved to Tappan, a small town on the Hudson River some 30 miles north of Manhattan, where they rented a modest house. No correspondence discussing this move survives, and it's likely they felt that, with a small child and a new baby, it would be better for them to live in the country whence Jigg could commute: the commute from Tappan, although long, was just tolerable.

Meanwhile, Jack, as a reservist in the Royal Air Force, had been called up for active service when the war started. He had been seconded to a training role in the Royal Canadian Air Force (RCAF) and he and Evelyn were living together in Ontario. This was wartime and although she was not a British subject, as the spouse of a serving British officer, she was entitled to a passage to England on a convoy. However, Evelyn needed somewhere in the US to stay while she was awaiting authority to travel and join him. This involved a considerable amount of red tape and Jigg, to help out, invited his mother to stay with him and his family while her passage was being arranged and while Jack arranged for instalment payments ("allotments") to be deducted from his salary.

To Evelyn Scott

Tappan, New York
December 9, 1942

Dear Mother,

After another unseemly delay, this is to let you know that we are all well. The government has not abolished us so far; and in fact we are working harder than usual. I hope it lasts.

We have finally managed to get our house fixed up a little - it was awful bare for a while. Pavli made us a blue corduroy couch cover, and we managed to make the chairs presentable, etc. But best of all we got hold of a grate, and now have a coal fire in the living room. Most of the day we keep the furnace down to negligible; let the grate heat the whole house, which it does pretty well. I had forgotten what a pleasure an open fire can be.

I may not act like it in the matter of correspondence; but I certainly wish we could see you folks - it would do us no end of good; and we are looking forward to it like nobody's business.

While Pavli was in the hospital, I had a fairly disagreeable heart attack - the worst so far; and was so goaded into going to a doctor. He says I shall probably live to be ninety; but that I have to watch myself in the matter of stairs, hills, coffee (I can't have any, which is pretty convenient, seeing as how you can't get any) smoking and excitement. It about scared me to death, as this is the first time I have had any really spectacular symptoms - the others were only mild. However, it does mean that I am definitely out of the running as far as the military are concerned (it would be hypocrisy to say that I was sorry) and that I am more or less inactivated for life where strenuous occupations are concerned. I can't even take a swim any more.

Just as you are feeling the pinch, so are we. When the government took us over we were all supposed to get a raise (I haven't had one for over a year) and in fact the boss promised me one. But he's afraid of the Vice President in Charge of Saying No, or something; and so I haven't gotten it. As a result having the baby was a pretty tight squeeze. Babies cost upward of $200; and we just didn't have the cash. We still have to pay off the MD. However, the end is mercifully in sight, even in spite of this damned Victory Tax, which begins on the first. I don't mind giving up 5% of my salary in a good cause. But I do mind the blasted arguments used by the powers that be. I'm better off than most, thank God.

I have to get back to work now; but bless you all, and the best of luck to both-and DON'T send us any Christmas presents - we aren't sending any.

Love,

Jigg

PS Incidentally, how would you like to go to the PO and get me one of every denomination of stamp up to say $1? I'll send you the money if you want to do it. P & I are collecting stamps for soothing purposes.

[Typed, signed, handwritten PS. SFC]

To Evelyn Scott

Tappan, New York
August 1943

Dear Mother,

You are more than welcome for as long as you want to stay. With some embarrassment we have to ask you to pay for your own food - about $6.00 a week. The rest of our economy is unaltered, and your visit will be a first class treat.

It's only fair to warn you of the following: my job comes to an end on August 22 and I start another on the following day, hence chaos for about 3 months thereafter. We are moving to a somewhat cheaper and pleasanter house in September - more chaos, but you can help. The present house, where we are somewhat camping out, is small, and so is the other one. I'm not in the best of health and pretty crockety.[150] It costs $1.00 round trip from Tappan to NYC and is a bore.

All this is merely forewarning - P and I will be tickled pink to see you, and only hope that the inconvenience won't get you down. We also think it's a rotten shame that J can't come too. Still we envy you like hell going to Britain.

I'll send you dope on trains instanter. A warning: don't bring too much baggage here. There are no porters, no taxis, and no nothing. And it is absolutely Verboten for me to carry loads up the hill from the station. So, travel light, be prepared for about 1 mile walk from the train to the house.

Wish me luck on my various ventures, and lent let us know the expected date of departure pronto.

God Bless, and all our best to Jack,

Jigg

[Handwritten, signed. SFC]

To Creighton and Paula Scott

Robbins House
Red Hook, New York
[September 1943]

Dear Jig and Pabli --

Thanks for Pabli's lovely letter[151] which was a pleasure to have.

I am aghast that ES plans to dump herself on you for such a long stay. It's terrible, but I suppose there is nothing to do about it. However, I hope that if she starts any funny business whatever, even the slightest, that you send her packing instanter. With Jack's position, she has plenty of money, so there's not the slightest reason she should stay with you a moment longer than is a complete mutual pleasure. Don't make the kind-hearted mistake of starting in to handle her with gloves. She doesn't understand kindness, courtesy or good taste-or anything except <u>first principles</u>. And she will be awake nights trying to make a rift between you two - so stick close together no matter <u>what</u> the merits of a discussion appear on the surface.

As I said to you, my position with regard to the lady is briefly this: I don't want her to have my address or know where I live, or <u>anything whatever</u> about Ward Manor estate.[152] As soon as you know when ES is coming please drop Gladys a card immediately and tell her <u>not</u> to give ES my address. For Jig's sake, since she is after all his mother, I might just possibly see her once in New York, if it is mutually convenient, <u>providing</u> she will behave herself and cut out all Evelyn Scottisms. And

---

150 Jigg had suffered from a mild heart condition since early childhood: he was to die of a heart attack in 1965, aged 50.
151 This letter has not survived.
152 Cyril had recently moved to this secluded estate just outside the town of Red Hook, New York.

I want her to keep her fingers out of my book.[153] Of course she will find out about it, one way or another, and doubtless get to read it. She will say it is not true to facts, meaning that I have omitted to say that from the time we returned to New York from Brazil she slept with other men and tried to rub my nose in it, that when we went to Europe she took along a lover (Merton) whom she began to sleep with in Bermuda and slept with him in my house in Collioure and Banyuls, that when we went out to North Africa in my car she took along a lover to sleep with, whom she afterwards married (Jack), etc, etc. She will be furious because I have left her some self-respect to live with, and myself some self-respect to die with! But the book is true to my life. I stood for all this for Jig's sake, trying to seek <u>some</u> semblance of a home for him. And if I have refrained from telling the world what kind of a mother my son had, and she says a word about it, either in public or in private to any friends, I shall be her bitter enemy and never see or communicate with her again as long as I live. And I think she knows me well enough by this time to know that I mean exactly what I say.

God bless you all four

Love

Dad

[Handwritten, signed. SFC]

Inevitably, war-time red tape, compounded by the fact that she did not hold British nationality and made more complex by the fact that Jack was at the time seconded to the Canadian RAF, slowed the process down. In her impatience Evelyn wrote numerous letters to the Canadian, British and American agencies dealing with travel permits, causing unnecessary confusion and thus slowing the process of agreeing and arranging her passage.

To Evelyn Scott
Royal Air Force
Staff Officers' Mess
No 31 Royal Air Force Depot, Moncton, NB
Canada

September 12, 1943

Darlingest Dear

Just a tiny and very rushed note to carry all my love and blessings. I do hope all well with you, and the family. I have made all sure, again, from here, about your allotment, so you should, as far as mortal man can tell, be getting it OK, monthly in arrears. The Canadian $73 dollars (approx) will dwindle by some 10 or 11 per cent, I

---

153 *Life Is Too Short*, Cyril's autobiography, published in 1943. Evelyn did not see it for several years and when she did, she took great exception to his account of their life together (see Chapter 31).

suppose, when it reaches you in USA - i.e. it will be about $65 in USA currency.[154] I wish to Pete it could be more, - but I can only just get by

Shall write again as soon as I can beloved.

All my dear love to you.

Your

Dickie

(S/Ldr W J METCALFE # 74992)

PS Much love to family, as always

[Handwritten on RAF letterhead, signed. UTK]

To Evelyn Scott

Royal Air Force

Staff Officers' Mess No 31

Royal Air Force Depot, Moncton, NB

Canada

September 12, 1943

Darlingest Dear,

As post-script to my other note of today; - apparently you <u>should</u> get your passport back in from three to five weeks after application; - so if much delayed beyond that time you had better write to Air Force Headquarters. Now, you have your "dossier" of copies of all those letters etc I had to write, - and although they bear varying dates, the actual registered letters in which they were finally mailed were sent off from Clinton in <u>August 13th</u>.

Now, what all this boils down to is that <u>if</u> you don't get your passport back in, say two weeks' time, I should write to Air Force Headquarters, and say that your husband sent your passport No 372415 on August 13th and can you soon expect to receive it? Also state that, as I have not present funds, I am saving up for your fare, by deductions from my pay, and that this has been approved by the United Kingdom Air Liaison Mission in their letter dated August 25th and signed by Mr F C Fayers, the Civil Officer for Finance and Accounts.

All this will probably be unnecessary, so don't let it worry you, - but <u>if</u> you don't get your passport in, say, two weeks from now, there'll be no harm in chasing it up.

There is, actually, a possibility, I understand, that you <u>may</u> get a passage even before I have finished accumulating the fare; - i.e. they might let you sail "on credit", so to speak, and they carry on deducting from my pay <u>after</u> your arrival in the UK. This would be swell, - and the only worry then would be that you might not have saved enough for your actual train-fare to whatever American or Canadian port to have to sail from. I wish to goodness I had more money. I fancy the actual rail-fare might be as much as $50 or $60 (you'd better enquire re this). I should try to put by for this as soon as ever you can.

---

154 Or roughly $1500 at 2022 values.

Also, of course, hang on to your USA passport.

Also, it might perhaps be useful, later, to have a chat with the British Consul in N York.

No more now, beloved

All, all dearest love always

Your own

Dickie (S/Ldr W J Metcalfe 74992)

Much love to Jig, Paula, Diane [sic] and Freddie!

[Handwritten on RAF letterhead, signed. UTK]

To Creighton Scott

[Robbins House]

[Late 1943]

My beloved Son

It was nice to get a word from you. <u>Don't worry about another chance</u>. There's nothing like one day after another, in steadiness and consistent good work, it tells cumulatively - I've found it over and over-and an even bigger opportunity will come: and you'll get it.

I understand perfectly what you and Paula are going through - I endured it for years. I hope and pray that by hook or crook you can get that octopus's tentacles out of your home right away, and when you do, for the sake of your children, of Paula, and your own sake, <u>never</u> let her enter it again, <u>no matter what the pretext or circumstances presented by her</u>. She's killing you and Paula by inches, but you can rationalize it and think of the great day when she finally has to leave - your magnificent babies, when they are a little older, not having experience and perspective, will have their poor little souls completely wrecked by her satanic emotional instability and complete inhumanity.

I want to send you the just-published supplement of <u>Who's Who</u> in which I appear in all my glory, but don't know exactly how to post it to you.

God bless you

Love,

Dad

[Handwritten, signed. SFC]

To Paula Scott

Robbins House

[November 1943]

Dear daughter -

I just have your long letter,[155] begun Oct 25th and concluded Nov 7th, and am

---

155 This letter has not survived.

much touched and pleased that you felt that I was a father to whom you could come in a time of perplexity and sadness. I am glad you sent me these letters, written in a time of trouble, instead of destroying them when what you dreaded had passed, for they are one more realization that you are a really-truly daughter to me who love you as my own child.

I wrote you and Jig those letters purposely. There is always a worst - and nothing can be worse than the worst. If we can face the worst then all else is better than it. Never be afraid of "it", for that means that you believe "it" is greater than God. And God is greater than "it". Throw away all unrecognized and undefined fears, and trust God to help you in all that is <u>really</u> endangering you. He did this time, and have faith to know that He will in the future.

Jig and you are more Christian in your attitude toward ES than I am. To me her psychology is not human. It really rests on choice of the highest available degree of emotional tension at any cost to <u>anybody</u>, and is thus a spiritual drug habit. I pray that I may never become comparably oblivious to the sufferings of others, and admire the spirit of Christ-like compassion that Jig expressed and you joined him in. I also pray that your home may be delivered from her soon.

God bless you all four
Love
Dad

[Handwritten, signed. SFC]

To Creighton Scott

Robbins House
[November 1943]

Dear Jig -

I wrote Pavli last night after I talked with you on the phone, and today I want to write you.

Listen, old man. If and when a thing no longer lies within your control the only means of safety resides in the way you meet it. Let's hope for the best, son, but I advise facing the alternative right now, even if it doesn't come. Let's face anything that may come, with heads up and determination to win through.

I wrote to comfort Pavli, but you are the only one who can comfort her. It's a woman's role to stand by in small crises - it's a man's role to stand by in a great one. Start in right now to get Pavli in the best frame of mind possible to meet whatever eventuates.

It'll come out all right, whichever way it goes. And you are your father's son, and you will be like him in a tight place.

All this doesn't mean that I have lost hope - but just in case.

God bless you my dear son,
Dad

PS Keep in touch with Louise[156] - she's a 100% princess when it comes to friendship and loyalty

[Handwritten, signed. SFC]

To Evelyn Scott

26 Belsize Crescent[157]
Hampstead, London NW3
November 16, 1943

Darling Love,

I am constantly thinking of you and hope to know that the worst of your troubles have been relieved, - that Jig can remain with you, that you have got your allotment money, and that the passport has been duly returned.

I got your registered letters with copies of correspondence, and wrote you re that twice last week. As I advised you, the best thing for the present, is to stick to the prescribed official line of attack, however exasperating the delays and miscomprehensions. Yours happening to be a "special case", the ordinary machinery does not quite apply, and although special application was made, and approved, the minor people who deal with your letters probably feel at a loss when faced with anything not absolutely routine. But the application <u>was</u> granted and you have the proof.

As I told you, while I should hold off for the present from other avenues of approach (since use of these could invalidate your eligibility for allotment money etc) I make an exception in favour of the British Consul (or the Vice-Consul). He, if you can see him <u>himself</u>, should certainly be able to help. But also, as I wrote you, until I have furnished the accumulation of your passage money, you could not <u>use</u> your passport anyhow, if you had, so I, from my end, will be in a far better position for any importuning re your passage that may be necessary when the money is there. And you may rely on me to do so then if it then is necessary.

Meanwhile you should have received your allotment money early this month (November) consisting of the dollar equivalent of £16.10.0 plus £10.9.0 for the portion of September. I personally went to Accounts and was assured you wd get it in early November. Anyhow, the money has been deducted OK from my pay at this end.

Well darling, this is all for the moment. Shall write again soon. All well here. Hard at work. Cold gone, & arm well now. Much love to family (do hope Paula is better & can get proper diet), - & all dearest love to you from

Ever yours
Dickie

[Handwritten, signed. UTK]

---

156 Louise Lotz, whom Cyril later married.
157 It appears Jack has now moved into the house he bought with the proceeds from the sale of Jove Cottage.

To Paula Scott

Robbins House
[December 1943]

Dearest Paula -

You poor kids! That Jig and you, who never in your lives said or did an unkind thing to me, or to any other decent person, should have to put up with such diabolism. Well, when it's over - "never again" must be your motto. I think, when she does leave, we should begin thinking about legally changing all our names to Wellman. It's really our rightful name, and going back to it will be a symbol of eternal repudiations of all E Scottism, just as your resuming Paula was a symbol of repudiation of all Joe Fosterisms[158] forever. There will be no trouble attached to it, and Jig can use his present name in business if he desires.

God bless you,
Love
Dad

[Handwritten, signed. SFC]

To John Metcalfe

January 28, 1944

NITELETTER
SQ/LDR W J METCALFE
26 BELSIZE CRESCENT HAMPSTEAD LONDON NW3
THIS URGENTISSIMO ET CONFIDENTIAL YOUETME STOP AM DOING
ALL POSSIBLE OBTAIN EXIT PERMIT EVELYN YOUR WIFE BUT
EXTRAORDINARILY IMPORTANT YOU EXPEDITE PASSAGE ARRANGEMENTS
YOUR END UNDERSTAND PASSAGE MONEY ALMOST ACCUMULATED IF
NOT EYE GLADLY CONTRIBUTE FIFTY DOLLARS OR MORE MAIN POINT
GET EVELYN ENGLAND PRONTO OTHERWISE HELLISH FAMILY SITUATION
COMING TO HEAD TELL ME HOW SEND YOU MONEY IF NEEDED REPLY
COLLECT THIS ADDRESS LEAVE EVELYN OUT OF IT UNDERLINED
CREIGHTON SCOTT, BLUENETWORK NEWS RM 276JA
[Telegram, carbon copy. SFC]

---

158 Joseph Foster was Paula's stepfather.

Chapter 21

Red tape

September 1943 - June 1944

It is not clear to what extent Jigg's telegram to Jack hastened matters, but less than a month later arrangements for Evelyn's passage to the United Kingdom began to fall into place despite initial misunderstandings over which government department had a role in the process. Confusion regarding her nationality and her right to travel to England in war time continued, almost certainly delayed by the application being caught between the twin stones of Canadian and British operating procedures and probably not helped by Evelyn's constant flow of letters querying delays. She wrote repeated letters to each of the government agencies involved in the arrangement of repatriation: the Passport Division of the US State Department in Washington DC; the British Consulate General in New York; the United Kingdom Air Liaison Ministry in Ottawa; the Department of National Defence Air Service in Ottawa; the Chief of Air Staff for the Royal Canadian Air Force, also in Ottawa; and the British Ministry of Transport Passenger Division in New York. This flood of letters, each alluding to a similar letter to another agency, must have slowed the process down.

During this period the family stresses which had prompted Jigg to send a desperate telegram to Jack continued. Evelyn was desperate to return to England and her husband; Jigg was equally desperate to resume family life without what he clearly saw as the malevolent presence of his mother. The mutual confusion of the agencies involved in these arrangements must have exacerbated these tensions.

To Evelyn Scott

26 Belsize Crescent
London NW3
November 27, 1943

Dearest Love,

Just got your letter dated Oct 20th[159] written when you were sending the cable re your allotment money. I do hope you have this allotment money now, - and also that you duly received the cable I sent, answering yours. My <u>previous</u> cable, sent on

---

159 None of Evelyn's letters to Jack during this period has survived.

September 21st, I know you did <u>not</u> get, and I do hope you got the other.

I'm so glad you heard at last from Brownlow, and that Martin is to pursue the matter, - and that, apparently, your passport is being returned to you OK via the British Consul. A few days ago I sent you a suggested rough draft for further letter asking for passport, - but by the time you get this draft you will - presumably, and it is to be hoped - have got the passport itself; and that, as soon as the passage-money has been accumulated and credited you should, at any time after that, get notice of your passage darling.

Much love, as always, to the family, and all dearest love my own to you from

Ever yours

Dickie

[Handwritten, signed. UTK]

To Evelyn Scott

26 Belsize Crescent

November 30, 1943

Darling Beloved,

Have just got your letter dated October 29th, and am anxiously waiting to hear what happens re Jig, and also that you have got your allotment money OK. From what you say, the passport question now seems in a way to being settled, so you probably won't have to use the suggested draft I sent you for a letter to Ottawa. (I also sent a carbon later.)

Well, darling, this may reach you round about Christmas time, and you bet I wish you all the blessings in the world in spite of your worries. And all blessings for the New Year too; and may we be together again soon! The next step is the completion of your fare from my pay and this is being done.

Glad you saw Gladys. Give her my love whenever you write. And I ought to write to her myself, I know.

I have had no time for any visiting lately, however, being too busy, though my hours latterly are somewhat lighter.

Very much love as always to the family and all my dearest love and blessings to you, from

Your Own,

Dickie

(S/Ldr William John Metcalfe)

[Typewritten, signed. UTK]

To Evelyn Scott

26 Belsize Crescent

December 12, 1943

Darling Love,

No further letter from you recently (your last to be received was dated Oct 29th)

and I'm hoping to hear again soon as your most recent news to reach me is now some six weeks old.

Anyhow, I'm so glad to know, by the last letters I did receive, that the issue of your allotment money had started, and also that you expected soon to have your passport returned. Another couple of months should see the passage-money duly accumulated.

Well, darling, this is just an interim scribble. Love as always to family, and all dearest love to you.

From yours,

Dickie

[Handwritten, signed. UTK]

To John Metcalfe

[December 30, 1943]

NITE LETTER
SQ/LDR W J METCALFE
GARDEN FLAT 26 BELSIZE CRESCENT HAMPSTEAD LONDON NW3
RE YOUR WIFE EVELYN STATE DEPARTMENT WASHINGTON WILL WAIVE
EXIT PERMIT ON RECEIPT OF WRITTEN ASSURANCE THAT PASSAGE
APPROVED ETARRANGED BRITISH VICECONSUL HERE IGNORES RAF
ARRANGEMENT SUGGEST YOU WRITE HIM MR PULLAN 25 BROADWAY
NYC ALSO SECURE WRITTEN ASSURANCE EVELYNS CORRESPONDENCE
WITH OTTAWA UNFRUITFUL
CREIGHTON SCOTT (BLUE NEWS RM 276)

[Telegram. SFC]

To Evelyn Scott

26 Belsize Crescent

December 31, 1943

Darling Love,

I have just got Jig's cable, which was 'phoned over to me when I got home, - I having been out when the man called.

I am very worried and concerned, - because I cannot understand the cable. It is, in a way, good news that the State Dept will waive exit permit - but how are you going to pay your ocean-fare? I cannot of course send money out of the country in the ordinary way, - and the only way I can do it is by paying it in at this end to Air Ministry as I am doing. The Air Ministry here then <u>advises</u> Ottawa (UKALM)[160] when my payments are complete. That is, no actual money is sent across the ocean, but the adjustment is made on paper as between London and Ottawa. Ottawa then pays the Shipping Co, - and allocates a berth etc.

---

160 United Kingdom Air Liaison Mission.

Secondly, unless you adhere to the repatriation scheme there would probably be trouble in getting your married allowances when you do arrive here. Though this could be risked perhaps. The point of view would be, perhaps, that though here in body you were not here at all <u>officially</u>. Which, considering all the sweat and worry you've had in trying to get the officials to follow their own directions would be exasperating indeed.

Thirdly, - I can't understand about the "<u>assurances</u>" Jig mentions. Supposing you did scrap the repatriation scheme and raised the passage-money some other way, how could I, over here, give any credible assurances that your passage had been "approved"? I am only longing for the time when it will have been "approved and arranged" - but you would hear that good news before I did. And similarly with the assurance about correspondence with Ottawa having been "unfruitful". The only way I could assure Washington of that would be by quoting from your own letters to me, - i.e. second-hand, instead of first-hand, evidence.

I shall do my damnedest of course in any way in which I can possibly help but (a) I don't see how you are going to raise the passage money, - and (b) the assurances, as I see it, could only come from <u>your</u> end.

As I told you, your passage-money will be ready at my end by early March. The Air Ministry will then have it all and will so advise UKALM at Ottawa.

All OK here except that I'm lonely and wishing you were with me. This geographical separation business, (though I'm sure it won't be too protracted) - was what I always bothered about, you remember, in 1936 etc, - though people thought I was "just exaggerating".

But cheer up beloved, - I'm sure it won't be more than a few months now. Blessings for New Year and for your birthday. Love as always to family, and dearest love to you from <u>your</u> Dickie.

[Handwritten, signed. UTK]

To Evelyn Scott

26 Belsize Crescent
January 23, 1944

Darling Love,

I received your registered letter re Mr Pullen etc OK, and, also, yesterday, two more from you, - but they were <u>undated</u>, and the postmarks undecipherable as they almost always are. Anyhow, I was so glad to hear you were feeling cheerier generally and had got more of my letters all right. I hope you will get the letters I wrote to you after I had cabled you on or about Jan 1st. I have, to date, sent you two copies of the letter I wrote to Mr Pullen. But do remember darling to date your letters or I can't sort things out. Not so long now for early March when my payments will be completed. Hurrah! If there is undue delay after that I can begin to agitate at my end.

Much love to family, - and all dearest love and lookings-forward to you.

Your own

Dickie

[Handwritten, signed. UTK]

To Evelyn Scott

26 Belsize Crescent

February 14, 1944

Darling Love,

No fresh news from my end, - save that I'm well and OK - and I hope you are at least fair-to-middling at <u>your</u> end. The payments for your passage will be completed early March, - only a few weeks now. I sent you copy of a letter I wrote to Dawson.

I <u>shall</u> be glad when you're over here darling, as I know you will be. Let me know if you hear from Pullen, to whom I wrote on Dec 31st, and sent you carbon.

Hope you manage to keep well and don't catch colds. Save for the one nasty cold in November that I told you about, I've kept very well, with plenty to eat.

Yes, some time I shall hope to enjoy reading Cyril's book. I do hope Jig remembers to give him my very affectionate best, whenever writing. Should much like to see him again.

Much love to family as always, and all dearest love to you, from

Your own Dickie

[Handwritten, signed. SFC]

To Evelyn Scott

26 Belsize Crescent

March 3, 1944

Darling Love,

All OK with me, and, as I told you in my last two letters, the payments were completed earlier than I imagined towards the end of last month, - so now it shouldn't be too long before you are advised by Ottawa. It may, however, be a month or more yet, so meanwhile we must just be patient.

Supposing my present household arrangements to be the same on your arrival you may have to put up with cramped quarters for a short time, as I must give a month's notice to tenants to vacate their rooms, - and of course I shall probably not know you are here till you actually are here. But I hope you won't mind as it will only be for a comparatively short time.

Much love as always to the family, - and all my dearest love to you, from

Yr own

Dickie

PS - shall think of you on our anniversary, - the seventeenth March!

[Handwritten, signed. UTK]

213

To Evelyn Scott

26 Belsize Crescent
March 10, 1944

Darling Love,

No fresh news here, - save to repeat that the payments are completed, so that you should be hearing before too long from Ottawa. Loud cheers! Also, I have a cold, - though the worst is over and I'm now on the mend. Hope you got over <u>yours</u> all right.

Whenever you come, if possible a few packets of "Valet" auto-strop razor-blades would be much much appreciated. Also some packets of pipe-cleaners.

I don't suppose I shall have any advance intimation of when you are coming, so, as I told you, you will have rather cramped quarters at first lovely till tenants have left after their one month's notice.

Have been and still am, very busy, but am usually home in the evenings by about 6.15 or 6.30. I get up, usually, soon after 6.

No more just now, lovely, but will write again very soon. Much love as always to the family and all dearest love to you, from

Ever your own
Dickie

[Handwritten, signed. UTK]

To Evelyn Scott

[March 25, 1944]

EVELYN METCALFE CARE SCOTT PO BOX 521 TAPPAN NY USA
PAYMENTS WERE COMPLETED MIDDLE OF LAST MONTH FEBRUARY
DOING ALL POSSIBLE TO HASTEN ARRANGEMENTS LOVE JACK METCALFE.
[Telegram. UTK]

To Creighton and Paula Scott

Kansas City, Missouri
March 31, 1944

Dear Jig and Paula -

I am having a wonderful visit,[161] entertained with daily luncheons, dinners, parties, theatre, etc, but I am so worried about you blessed children that I can hardly sleep nights. Having your permission to do so, I've talked the situation over with Paul a couple of times. His advice is "Throw her out on her ass, no matter what happens. Jig and Paula, and no one else on earth, can do anything for her, and she will kill both of them if something drastic is not done".

---

161 Cyril was visiting his eldest son Manly Wade Wellman, then a journalist on the *Kansas City Star* and living in Kansas City.

What I'm afraid of is that you'll both get your health permanently, or at least seriously, injured, and then what will become of you, and those marvellous babies? I don't know exactly how to advise. Would it be possible to get her to NY and then say, "You sign the proper papers, and keep your mouth shut while you're doing it, or you're not going to back to Tappan, even for one night."

You see the situation is not a human one at all. It's a medical situation entirely. Any trick, lie, deceit or scheme is not only justifiable but perfectly honourable in dealing with sick minds, as any physician will assure you. Get rid of her by hook or crook, with no compensations. The complete and unanswerable reply to anything she may ever say afterwards is "You're crazy".

God bless you all four,

Love, Dad

[Handwritten, signed. SFC]

To Evelyn Scott

26 Belsize Crescent

April 2, 1944

Darling Love,

Just a note of encouragement, - and I don't think it will be long now before we're together. I have done all possible from this end, and you should hear at any time from Ottawa or the Delegation.

All OK here darling. Very very busy, but have now quite got over my recent cold.

Let me know of any change of address. I shall receive only very brief notice of your <u>approximate</u> arrival, - so shall just keep on writing. I shall write regularly, as always, but there may be gaps in your <u>receipts</u> of letters, due to modification of postal arrangements necessitated by the war.

Much love as always to the family, - and all dearest love to <u>you</u> from

Your own

Dickie

[Handwritten, signed. UTK]

To Evelyn Scott

26 Belsize Crescent

April 22, 1943

Darling Love,

I was so glad to get your letter dated March 28th, and to know your laryngitis was better.

Well, beloved, I do hope that you won't have too long to wait now, and don't think you will. As I told you in my last letter, Dawson got <u>my</u> letters all right and replied to me saying that he had acted at once. So whenever I get the official information (which won't, I expect, give me more than a very short advance working) I shall give notice to

215

the tenants I spoke of so as to free more room, though even so, as I must give them a month's notice, there will pretty certainly be a period of overlap during which we shall be very cramped for space, - also re sharing kitchen etc. The only alternative would be, of course, getting a room temporarily in a hotel or boarding-house, but unfortunately I shall be too stoney-broke for that, - and anyhow it's very difficult to find anywhere now.

Much love to family as always, - and, again, all good luck and congrats to Jig! All dearest love to you from ever your own

Dickie

[Handwritten, signed. UTK]

Finally, a telegram from a Mrs King informed Evelyn that she should report to New York for embarkation on June 14, 1944.

To Evelyn Scott

MRS METCALFE CARE MR CREIGHTON SCOTT PO BOX 521 TAPPAN NY CAN YOU REPORT NEW YORK, JUNE 14TH STOP REPLY IMMEDIATELY. IF ACCEPTED DETAILS WILL FOLLOW. M H KING

[Telegram, not dated. UTK]

Chapter 22

Repatriation
June 1944

Evelyn eventually received what she had been waiting for over the previous months: her embarkation order confirmation that she had been allocated a berth in a convoy. Her reply to this information included, typically, a lengthy paragraph emphasising the importance to her of suitable provision for her continued writing while on board the ship.

To Miss M H King

PO Box 521, Tappan NY
June 7, 1944

Miss M H King
Royal Air Force Delegation
Director of Movements (USA)
Dear Miss King,

I am enclosing with this the receipt you have sent which acknowledges that I have the Embarkation Order, and the other receipt detached from the advice on the disposition of baggage which accompanied the Order.

My ultimate address in the United Kingdom is the home of my husband and myself, where I can always be reached care Squadron Leader William John Metcalfe, 74992, RAF, Garden Flat, 26 Belsize Crescent, Hampstead, London NW3, ENGLAND.

I appreciate the attention you have given to securing my passage and I am sure you have done as well as could be expected under the circumstances. I don't object strongly to "dormitory" sleeping, and in respect to my baggage the only problems presented are my typewriter, essential to my future livelihood as a novelist (my profession during some twenty-five years, although circumstantially suspended since I have been in the States awaiting my passage), and the secure disposition of the manuscripts of novels and poems by myself and my husband (on which both of us will work in England) which were deposited with the censor in New York on March 6th, to be returned to me at the pier when I depart, with twenty-two contracts for books by myself previously published in the UK and the States, some shorter mss and other matter more personal.

But I assume some safe place for these will be found aboard ship although I am to be allowed only the one piece in the "dormitory", as all these mss and documents are an essential of future livelihood and my husband, on his repatriation from Canada, took home mss and books by himself without difficulty or question.

Again my thanks to you, and I will report at the hour and place designated with due punctuality.

Yours sincerely,

[Typed carbon copy, not signed. UTK]

To Evelyn Scott

26 Belsize Crescent
June 9, 1944

Darling Love,

No fresh personal news since my last, - except that I have received one of your parcels. It was the two packets of "India House" and "Wakefield" tobacco, - and very very welcome, bless you! The customs duty was rather high, but I am enjoying the tobacco very much, - I'm smoking some "Wakefield" now as I write.

I do so hope it won't be very long now before your passage comes through. As I told you in a recent letter, your priority is high within your category of repatriated Officer's wife, - but that category itself has not a high priority just at the moment I expect. It's all a question of shipping-space.

All well, darling, and terrifically busy, - and when I say "terrifically" I mean it. So forgive rather short note this time. I think of you all the while.

Much love as always to the family, - and all dearest love to you, from
Ever your own
Dickie

[Handwritten, signed. UTK]

To Creighton and Paula Scott

Robbins House
Red Hook, New York
June 14, 1944

My Beloved Children-

I received both your letters in today's mail and, if you will let me, am answering them together and, <u>laws Deo</u>, can send them to your home address. For this is June 14th, flag day, because today I have been thinking of you all day. At last you are freed of the most spiritually-destructive and evil-loving being I have ever known personally.

Until Jig's birth she was not that way, so he, thank God, imbibed no poison through her veins. He is not her child, any more than the marred ground is parent of the seed planted in it. He is my son, alone, and of my seed, bone of my bone, a real Christian gentleman like my father and grandfather and great grandfather and our lone line of Christian gentlemen that I have traced back to Pauling Creighton Wellman who died in Palestine in 1251 fighting to free the sepulchre of Our Lord Jesus Christ from those who hated and profaned it. So you see, Paula, that I agree with you when you write in the highest terms possible in words, of your husband of whom I am as proud as you. He owes nothing, and derives nothing in body, mind or soul, from Elsie Dunn or any of her ilk, for she, when caught in the grasp of God's will and delivered of my child, rebelled at it, at me, at God Himself. For she could not conceive of anything or any event greater than herself. All her mind (which was once good, even brilliant), her heart, her spirit, her whole life, was henceforth bent to master or destroy what had shown her she was not omnipotent, me, my son, even God who made us.

I had 14 years of it, part of it as bad as what you two blessed children have just been through. So my heart aches for you. But now you know that I, whom you both know to be kind, loving, gentle and even tender in thought and emotion, never overstated what she has become through not loving good. Until he was born she wanted my son, because she thought he, and through him I, would be hers to violate. When he and I escaped her completely (for he took from her not one iota of her nature in any respect) her love turned to hate, and I need say no more; for you have seen it daily for nearly a year - extending from me to everybody and everything beyond her power to rule. She has forfeited every tie.

You, and your children, are not in any jot or tittle related to her. I am your father and your mother both. What God once joined together God can put asunder. Actum est, finis est. Amen.

God bless you all four,
Dad

[Handwritten, signed. SFC]

The following excerpt is from Evelyn's lengthy document entitled "Precis of events indicative of libel"..[162] It was written in 1951 in the third person in support of what she then saw as libellous persecution and adds further detail to the wait in Tappan and her return to England.

```
Evelyn Scott when, in 1944, she was finally assured she would
be allowed to sail for Britain, sat for three months and a half
by packed baggage, her mss in the hands of the censors, her
writing ended as far as Tappan was concerned; her fixity indoors
or near her habitation essential, she supposed, in view of the
warning she had had that she would be permitted just twenty-four
hours to move in, and the combined total lack of any baggage
transport whatever in Tappan, and of her son's heart murmur
which had re-alarmed her about him so that she was resolved not
to allow him to carry any of her baggage for her. She had, in
```

162 See also Chapter 31.

fact, about three days, and satisfactorily contrived to get her
typewriter and various pieces of small luggage to town over the
mile-and-a-half of steep hillside and flat road newly strewn
with uncrushed stones, between her and the bus-stop. And when
she went aboard the vessel, which was a New Zealand troop-ship,
afterward sunk and since either retrieved or the name re-used,
she took into her quarters, on a porter's advice, her typewriter
and a suitcase of mss beside the single "dressing case" which was
really a suitcase for clothing and which was the one piece of
luggage which was "according to Hoyle".

However - again in view of her Passport difficulties and of
subsequent libel - she asks again today whether the Canadians,
the British, or the Americans had it in for her in giving her
dormitory space with airmen's wives and small children, several
decks down, where portholes were seldom opened and a large
glaring electric bulb which lighted about a quarter of the space
used by forty of all ages and was controlled by the steward so
that she could not turn it out, burned fiercely a foot or two
above her head most of every day and more than half of each
night.

The Rangitike was not a very comfortable ship, the dormitory
bunks were built high off the floor, and it was unwise to have
put small children in beds from which they might have tumbled
with serious results had there been any really heavy weather.
But after a tiff with the purser, who thought her "unreasonable"
in wishing to store mss in his safe where "valuables" were kept,
her typewriter was lashed to a rafter above her, and she made
the best of her situation; though - AGAIN - she would like to
know why it was that when the ship was full of officers wives
who, as far as she could ascertain, did NOT "out-rank" her
as Senior, she was not allowed as they were cabin-space on a
passage for which she had already been waiting ten months since
the first payment on it and four months since the payments were
complete.

The Rangitike was in a large and very handsome convoy which
was all divulged on the last day out of Liverpool, and which
was probably bringing aid to France as the Allied landing was
then recent; but even before Evelyn Scott went aboard her ship
there had been an ado on the book about her waiver, which had
been guaranteed her in a letter from Washington in late October
1943, and had been confirmed at the Customs' House many weeks
and possibly a month or two before she actually sailed. It was
said at the dock "not to be on record" and because she had to
rely on the offices of a dock policeman to telephone the Custom
House and verify what she had said, she had no opportunity
- or thought she had none in the ensuing pother - to phone a
promised goodbye to her son and daughter-in-law. And when she
was admitted to the slip at which the ship was moored, she

discovered one of her parcels of mss returned by the Custom's was handed to her un-sealed, as it should never have been.

In London, when met by John Metcalfe at the railway station, she was greeted by a fly-bomb, like a salute to their re-union, but most unpleasant.

Part 2

London

Unlike Part 1 which followed Evelyn and those closest to her through her vividly descriptive letters from the places where they settled, Part 2 concentrates on her life and Jack's in London, where Jack had bought a large house in the north-west London suburb of Hampstead.

After her return, Evelyn developed a number of preoccupations. Many of these related to her son Jigg and his family as she became more and more anxious to know where he was and what he was doing and to exert an increasing degree of control over his life. Others centred around their poverty, her wardrobe and her health. And a great deal of effort was expended in tracing the inheritance she was sure her father would have left her.

Each chapter in Part 2 is devoted to one of these preoccupations and because the dates of these overlapped, the dates of the chapters overlap. She became increasingly focused on politics and on a variety of conspiracies, increasingly real in her mind. Her prose loses its lucid fluidity and at times the flow of her argument becomes contorted and difficult to follow. The letters themselves illustrate her state of mind through her handwritten comments and annotations, many of these verging on the indecipherable as her agitation showed in her writing.

Chapter 23

Home Again

June 1944 - October 1947

No sooner had Evelyn returned to England than Jack (who was still a serving RAF officer), was posted to a series of RAF training schools, leaving her alone in the flat at 26 Belsize Crescent. This created a number of difficulties: Evelyn would have had no experience of being a householder in England, nor of managing a house full of tenants.

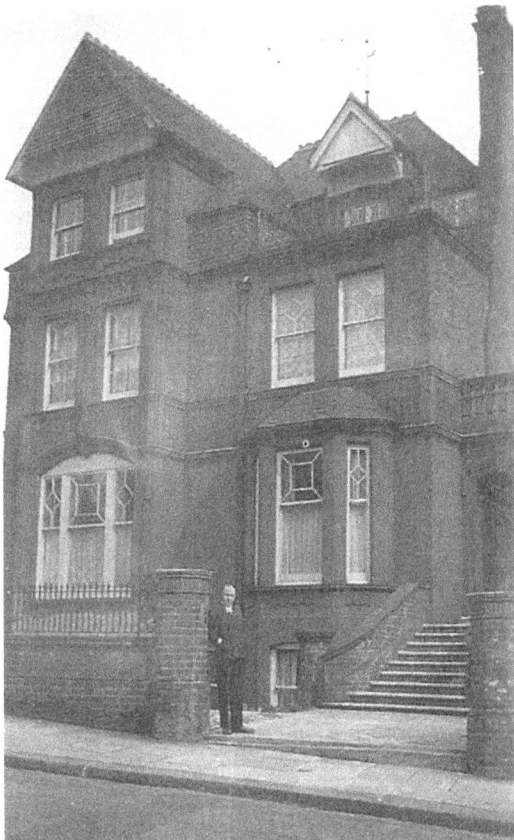

Jack Metcalfe in front of 26 Belsize Crescent

To Paula and Creighton Scott

26 Belsize Crescent
London NW3
[July 1944]

Darling kids

Please never forget that the personal loyalty of Jack and myself is something you can both count on always unexceptionally, and that Jack will appreciate as deeply as I do what you have done for us humanly in having let me stay these months with you. As I have said so often (and from both of us) the happiest time ahead will be the one in which we can help positively to make you two (and your lovely babies) happier, richer, or, in some manner make things pleasanter for you all four.

You are very dear, Jig. Jack and I have known you well enough to love and admire for many a year and I have admired the human Pavli for long, but these months have allowed me to double and triple earlier respect and affection for a brave girl as well as for a fine man.

Bless you all four from us, dear kids, and don't forget

To hell with the totalitarians! We human beings will win!!!

Maw=Evelyn=Gran'ma

If any letters from Jack (or anyone) arrive after I leave please forward to Garden Flat, 26 Belsize Crescent, London NW3, England. Forwarded letters to England have to be restamped with covering envelope and I leave the quarter for that as I think that will cover the few I may miss. Thank you.

[Handwritten, signed. SFC]

To Evelyn Scott

RAF Staverton
July 1, 1945

Darlingest Dear,

Here is Sunday and thank goodness the weather today seems better. It's been pouring with rain recently but this morning there's a bright sun. I hope you got the letter I posted on Thursday. This, though posted today, won't actually be collected till Monday so you won't get it till Tuesday I fear.

All well with me. The work is interesting and there's a fair amount of free time in the evening. Today, Sunday, we have a short period of work in the morning only.

Yesterday (Sat) afternoon I and another chap went into Cheltenham by bus between 4 and 6, - shopped and had tea. I needed some ink, also toothpaste.

Thanks for your to letters (so far) darling, - and bless the "novelette". Hope the kid[163] is not being too much of a nuisance. If we should stay at 26 Belsize he will have to go,-but supposing I am amongst those selected for this job it will almost

---

163 The child of one of the tenants was obviously causing problems.

certainly mean posting away in a few weeks time. The temporary dislocation, getting accommodation, etc would of course be a nuisance but the job would be worth it and we might be quite comfortable for a year in new surroundings. We should then be able to put by money for purchase of small house at end of it, and <u>then</u> put up No 26 for sale.

I expect to have a week or so anyhow free, after conclusion of course and before being posted (if I get selected), in which to do packing etc (as well I hope as <u>some</u> writing!) - but there would be no harm in your doing a little preliminary sorting and tearing-up of papers etc whenever you liked, to avoid rush at end. Though I don't think there <u>will</u> be a rush, and anyhow I may not get the job.

Feeling very fit and cheerful save for missing you. Finishing revision of <u>All Friends are Strangers</u> won't take very long, and then revision of <u>Enter, Cousin</u>.[164]

All love and blessings, - and I do hope you can go on with the "novelette".

Ever your own

Dickie

PS Ask Hobsons to repair cracked lavatory pan and give them the broken pieces.
PPS Send me on Ogg's receipt,[165] and other letters, please.
PPPS You should get your new ration books soon, but not on July 4th or 5th because of polling.

[Handwritten, signed. UTK]

To John Metcalfe

26 Belsize Crescent

July 10, 1945

Beloved Dickey The job in your room is varnished and ready for your occupancy as soon as it is straightened-the room I mean.

The sensible solution will be for you to continue to live in your own house and of course the only ultimately sensible solution for us is the opportunity to proceed with your books and I with my books as literary value is our real contribution to any decent future. The hell with "mass handling" any way! War conditions may have imposed it to some extent but nonetheless true recovery depends on giving each man or woman the opportunity to pursue the work to which he and she are suited by reason of natural abilities.

I wish you were getting a longer rest between the end of the course and the posting but in any case hope your job will be near home.

I asked about the riveting of the toilet bowl that was broken and was told by Hobsons man that riveting would cost as much as a new one, but he is to ascertain the price shortly.

---

164 *All Friends are Strangers* was published in London in 1948; there is no record of *Enter, Cousin* ever having been published, at least not under that title.
165 Ogg and Hobson were tradesmen who looked after the house.

I have been trying to shop and tried to get a pair of shoes at John Barnes[166] without success my feet being a size smaller than anything suitable they had. But I shall continue and will get something eventually I am sure.

I will not seal this until tomorrow as I wont be able to mail it today and I will follow your instructions and forward nothing after the twelfth. I dont quite understand what sort of job the job is and shall be interested in what you have to say about it bless you and good luck

Evelyn

[Typed, typed signature. UTK]

To Evelyn Scott

RAF Staverton
July 24, 1945

Darlingest Dear,

As I told you yesterday on the 'phone, I got here all right, though the taxi failed to show up and it was an exasperating job getting another one. However, I arrived in time for dinner, so no harm was done.

So far, Hornchurch still stands as the selected base, and I do hope it so remains, as it is so close in to London as to enable me to live at home, though there will be occasional nights away when I am visiting some station at the other end of the country.

Probably, I shall have the driving test, final billeting, etc tomorrow, Wednesday, and _may_ be able to get home on Thursday for one night, before reporting to Hornchurch on Friday. Then (I anticipate) I can get home again Sat afternoon, or Sunday anyhow, after spending either one or else two nights at Hornchurch.

Then, for the two following weeks probably, my job will simply consist in visiting each station in Essex so as to get to know the CO, etc at each one, _preparatorily_ to starting in as the actual Advice Service which is not due to begin till August 7th or 10th.

There has been a hold-up in the supply of cars, which will not be delivered till the actual job starts, - so this preliminary "tour" of the area will have to be done by train and bus etc. Rather a nuisance, since it means paying fares out of one's own pocket in the first instance, and claiming for expenses later.

Anyhow, I shall _hope_, during the next twelve months, to put by as much as possible for eventual purchase of cottage.[167] On Monday, when I had cloaked my stuff at Paddington, I saw Smorthwaite, the Bank Manager of the Westminster Bank, Haverstock Hill, - and started a small account.

So, darling, I shall hope to be home on Thursday evening, - with even more luggage since I shall have the VAST "pack-up" of books, literature etc, in addition to

---

166 John Barnes was a fashionable department store.
167 Jack always considered 26 Belsize Crescent to be an intermediate stop on the way to his dream of owning a cottage in the country, despite his recent experience with Jove Cottage (Chapter 18).

what I set out with. I probably need not report to Hornchurch till Friday <u>afternoon</u>, so want to use part of Friday <u>morning</u> in going to Walkers Loose Leaf place to make enquiries re large-size refills etc.

Then, Friday afternoon, I shall have to go to Hornchurch by train and stay the night there. Then, as soon as possible, I shall get the formal permission to "live out" fixed up, and be home, I trust, on at least a majority of all nights, though, as I say, there will be occasional nights when I shall have to sleep away, in the case of some of the more distant stations. But all in all, and considering that I might have been posted to Scotland or somewhere, it has fallen out very luckily, and I shall be able, too, to get on with the novel most evenings.

I hope you have not had too much Piruna, - and down and out with all Totes. No totes. !!! Wonder what the election results will be. We shall know on Thursday evening, - or Friday morning anyhow.

Bless you always, All dearest love from your own

Dickie

[Handwritten, signed. UTK]

In May 1946 Jigg left his job at the American Broadcasting Company for a job at WBBM in Chicago, part of the Columbia Broadcasting System (CBS) and went on his own to Chicago, hoping to find accommodation which would allow him to bring his wife and children to join him. This proved not to be possible: as Paula wrote "Housing was available, but not to people like us. To get an apartment in the city one had to pay a year's rent in advance and buy the landlord a new Chrysler or Cadillac."

To Evelyn Scott and John Metcalfe

Scotch Plains, New Jersey

May 9, 1946

Dear Evelyn & Jack:

I am ashamed to have waited so long to answer your good letters. The truth is I've been suffering from pip about the world and even my own work and haven't been fit company either in person or by letter! Please forgive me!

There is little personal news except that my job is completely over[168] except for occasional work. I'm glad in a way and ought to get back to writing. I hope I will. But there are so many things that must be done - Dudley called them the mechanics of living. And when I've done the minimum, I seem to feel just too tired. I'm hoping it is just the reaction and that I'll soon get a little pep and will power again.

Then, too, I do want to get in touch with friends again. I did get over to Tappan a week or so ago and had a grand visit. I don't know any place that has a friendlier

---

168 Dudley was Gladys' husband. For years after his death, Gladys worked as a freelance *parfumier* and had a fully equipped laboratory in the basement of her house in Scotch Plains.

and happier atmosphere. They were all well. Denise is always growing lovelier and Frederick was amazing. The baby was very sweet though he was away asleep the greater part of the time. He looks somewhat like Frederick at his age, but has a personality of his own, too.

I've been too self centered and haven't asked a thing about you two. Please write anyway. I will again and soon.

Love

Glads

PS I have some paper[169] to send as soon as coal strike is over

PPS Did you know I have a dog? A grand one!

[Typed, signed, handwritten PS. UTK]

To Evelyn Scott

RAF Staverton

July 5, 1945

Darling Dear,

All well here, and I hope you are. Have you been able to get your new dress yet? I wish I could have left you more for it darling, but I thought I had better clear all Ogg while I could, - and for that I had somewhat to overdraw at the bank, so I have not so much in the pot at the moment. But the probability (barring specially favourable treatment, which of course I am <u>trying</u> for) is that I should be appointed to some other area, in which case I should have to go ahead to the station, and find accommodation for us as quickly as I darned well could: I <u>imagine</u> a week or so might elapse between July 14th Saturday, when the course here ends and I come home, and my posting to an area. If I am appointed it will mean catering for the requirements of a county or so, with a staff of 5 or 6. A car is provided and I must dig up my driving licence again.

Lectures very interesting and a healthy bias against robotism. Psychometric tests used with plenty of salt. Chief Instructor an excellent type and most humanely and culturally minded.

All, all dearest love, and DOWN and OUT with the Totes!!!

Yours

Dickie

[Handwritten, signed. UTK]

Meanwhile Cyril had married for the sixth time. His new wife, Louise Lotz (known in the family as "Weecie") owned a house in the pleasant little town of Pine Bluff, North Carolina, not far from Chapel Hill, and the couple settled there. It was decided that Paula should take the children to live near Cyril, and that Jigg should fly from Chicago to join them

---

169 There was a paper shortage in Britain during and for some time after the war. Gladys, among others, sent supplies to Evelyn when she could.

whenever he could at weekends. This separation continued for a year until Jigg joined his family in Pine Bluff permanently in August 1947.

When Jigg came to live full time in Pine Bluff he and Paula tried to set up a creative business, Jigg drawing and painting and Paula designing and making greetings cards. No doubt the idea for Paula's enterprise came, at least in part, from the fact that when she was a child her parents had created a successful greetings card business from their home in Taos, New Mexico. Although Paula's ideas had approval and practical support from many of their friends, the business never took off.

At this time, too, Cyril had reverted to his original name and had personal stationery printed "Frederick Creighton Wellman". Paula writes of this: "When I arrived in Pine Bluff, Dad [Cyril] immediately introduced me to people, without any warning whatever, as his daughter-in-law, Mrs Creighton Wellman. There was nothing I could do about it and Daddy [Jigg] was suddenly Wellman too. We had to spend our entire three years there as Wellman, which produced awkward moments for us. Even getting mail meant we were accepting mail for a cousin or something when addressed to "Scott" and all our friends had hurriedly to be told to use Wellman. Dad hoped that we would make the change permanent, but we reverted to Scott as soon as we left in August 1949, with a great deal of relief."

During this period Evelyn wrote on a number of occasions that the family went to Lumberton, North Carolina, about 200 miles south of Pine Bluff, to live rent-free on a farm owned by an African-American in return for labour. There is no evidence for this unlikely scenario: neither of the two eldest Scott children has any memory of this, though both would have been old enough to remember it. However, years after his death, detailed maps of Lumberton were found in Jigg's papers: he may have considered this course of action and never actually gone. Or, equally, he may have let Evelyn think this was his plan in order to deter her further pursuit of Cyril through him. There is no information in the collected letters to explain this.

To Evelyn Scott

[Pine Bluff, North Carolina]

July 11, 1946

1952 —This letter without address other than the "Col Broadcasting System" Chicago on her envelope relieved yet distressed me. We heard nothing more for three years thereafter. Evelyn D S Metcalfe—Evelyn Scott author

Dear Evelyn,

As to your enquiries about us - we couldn't very well be worse placed, within reason. Jigg's NYC job with American Broadcasting Co (ABC) came to an end last March, and it took a long time to get another, which he finally did, in Chicago. He is living in a hotel because apartments and houses are not to be had without paying an exorbitant price for the furniture on top of the also exorbitant rent, and in view of such a profitable racket there are no unfurnished places to live. He's managing on 30 dollars a week, sending me what's left. I am living with friends who kindly offered me and the children sanctuary until the housing shortage is over. I can't find a place in NY because although not quite so bad as Chicago, it is bad enough to be out of the question

We are all well and looking forward to bring reunited - probably in Chicago wherever and whenever the situation lets up sufficiently for us to afford a house.

Good luck to you both, and to Jack's book.

Paula

[Handwritten, signed. Handwritten annotation by ES. UTK]

To Evelyn Scott
Royal Air Force Station
Staverton Gloucester

August 21, 1946

Darlingest Dear,

Just a scribble - My release date is Aug 28 Wednesday (a week today) and I'm afraid it means staying here until then, as my leave entitlement is now exhausted, - unless I come up just for "the day" on Sat or Sun. But even so I have to be back here Sun evg.

But I expect to be home late on <u>Tuesday</u> evening (the 27th), - then I go to Uxbridge for actual release on the following day, Wed.

So it means six days from today before I'm home. I hope you won't get too lonely darling, - anyhow it's for the last time. And I do hope you can manage to get some cigs and to do some writing. As for me, I have a fair amount of form-filling and "clearing" to do. Saw Accts Officer at Barnwood yesterday, who were v nice re my claims.

<u>Bless</u> you and <u>bless</u> you
All love darling
Dickie

[Handwritten on RAF letterhead, signed. UTK]

Jack continued in the RAF after the war ended, supporting young airmen about to be demobbed in making decisions about the course of their future lives. He enjoyed this work and by all accounts was good at it.

After his discharge Jack focussed on his continuing entitlement to "quota" status in the United States and it was decided he should return to New York to fulfil the residence requirement and to find employment, possibly leading to becoming more permanently settled where they could be nearer to Jigg and his family. While Jack stayed with their friend and benefactor Margaret DeSilver in a fashionable part of New York City for two years, Evelyn remained at Belsize Crescent to continue her writing and to look after the house and the tenants.

To Evelyn Scott

c/o De Silver, Apt 12 G,
130 West 12th Street,
August 13, 1947

Darling and Precious Dear

I sent you an air-mail letter yesterday and hope it reaches you quickly, - though there was nothing much in it except an account of the trip over. I'll write you every so often by air-mail, but usually just by ordinary mail like this. I'll even look forward to hearing from you.

Well, - it's HOT. Not sure what actual temperature is, but ninety something I'm certain. My flannel trousers (worn on the boat) were so dirty I just had to get them cleaned, so till they're done in a week's time, I have to sweat in heavy trousers.

Well, up to date I've done nothing except start the application for a fresh re-entry permit, which I must do first of anything, and immediately, in order to be able to get a sailing-back by an early boat in about 3 weeks time. Since last time I applied for a re-entry permit there are all sorts of fresh regulations, making the process much longer and more of a nuisance. Anyhow, darling, the business is nearly done now and by tomorrow or Friday I hope to have the darned application duly notarised and posted off to Philadelphia.

And then, once that's done, I can book a definite passage and start on all the things to do which you have listed, most importantly, of course, Ralph Pierson [sic].[170]

New York is, in a physical sense, much the same, but it seems all wrong to me without you. Nothing is right without you and I long to be with you again very soon.

All my love and blessings,

Bless Evelyn, and bless Evelyn's books!

Yours

Dickie

[Handwritten, signed. UTK]

To Evelyn Scott

c/o 130 West 12th Street
August 20, 1947

Darling Beloved Evelyn-Chookie

As I told you in last letter (tho' it was not air-mail, - and this may arrive first), I saw Ralph Pearson (it's spelt that way, I find) on Saturday, - and left a short letter for Jig, which he will forward. Jig had asked RP not to give his address to anyone, so of course I still have not go it, and it may be a week or so before I can get any reply.

---

170 Ralph Pearson, Paula's father, was living in Nyack, New York. Evelyn had hoped that he would give Jack some information about Jigg's whereabouts.

RP seemed most friendly, - but a little hurt that you hadn't visited him as often as he (apparently) had wanted. He begged me to understand that <u>he</u> was not to blame. Now he regretted the present situation, and, for his part, had asked Jig to write to us, - and had no idea why he would not.

I am sure all this will adjust itself if only you (who have, at the moment, to play infinitely the most difficult part) can hold on for a while. I told Jig, of course, how lovingly we both felt and I delighted I wd be to see him, - but at the same time assured him that I was not, in any way, "pursuing" him. If I <u>did</u>, incidentally, learn his address, what good would that really be to us unless he himself had volunteered it? - as I think he will.

Today and tomorrow are jam-packed, - but on Fri or Sat shall hope to send you off some type-paper. And soon, - if I have slightly to overstay - shall cable more money to bank to feed the a/c. The Manager there, whom you saw, is Mr SMORTHWAITE, darling, not "Smallthwaite", - tho' he well might be.

I love you. If only you were <u>here</u>! NY is largely the same funny old noisy NY we both know, - but, as I said before, just seems all <u>wrong</u> with Evelyn not here.

All love always

Dickie - Jack

[Handwritten, signed. UTK]

To Evelyn Scott

Margaret DeSilver

130 West 12th Street, Apt 12G

New York City 11

[October 1947]

Dear Evelyn, *1947 —ca pu! Better is the truth 1952*

I am really very happy that Jack is actually on his way. The poor guy was getting so restless and homesick. He loves you very dearly, Evelyn. For all your miseries, you're a lucky girl to be so loved. Love and honesty seem to have become rarities!

Anyway, this is to wish you both well. It's no use hoping this winter will be better than last, because I'm really sure all winters will be worse and worse and worse!

However! - love to you

Maggie

[Handwritten on personal letterhead, signed. Handwritten annotation. UTK]

To Evelyn Scott

October 10, 1947

EVELYN METCALFE 26 BELSIZE CRESCENT HAMPSTEAD LDN NW3
NOW SAILING ON QUEEN MARY ARRIVING SIXTEENTH OR EARLY
SEVENTEENTH LOVE. JACK
[Telegram. UTK]

It was at this point that Jack and Evelyn, reunited, embarked on what would be several years living together in London, isolated from many of their friends and living on Jack's meagre income from tutoring.

Chapter 24

Jigg: Part 1
November 1946 - November 1949

Back in London with Jack, Evelyn became increasingly preoccupied with the lack of news of her son, his wife and their (now three) small children. Jigg, perhaps as the result of the unhappiness and stress resulting from her stay with them in Tappan, did not wish to continue contact with his mother and did what he could to impose distance between them. At this point Gladys Grant, a long-time friend of Evelyn's, became the buffer between Jigg and his mother. She had met Jigg some years earlier and was fond of him. She could see how destructive Evelyn's possessive behaviour could be, and she managed a delicate balance between her continuing friendship for Evelyn and her desire to protect Jigg and his family from Evelyn's desire to control his life.

The following letters are early expressions of Evelyn's assumption that difficulty in contacting Jigg was due to (often) malign forces outside her control or Jigg's; she could not conceive that he would want to reduce contact with her.

To Evelyn Scott
RFD No 1
Scotch Plains New Jersey

November 1, 1946

Dear Evelyn:

I am ashamed not to have written before, but kept putting if off in the hope of telling you more. I've forwarded all your letters but my last address for Jig is also care of the radio station in Chicago. So far as I know he is still there with apparently no prospects or likelihood of being in or near New York. I'm always glad to forward letters but, of course, this makes for delay and sometimes uncertainty. Of course the registered letters would have been kept at the PO but the others just lie there. I've been planning to get a PO box, but there isn't one to be had just now and it would mean daily trips to Scotch Plains. The old mail man used to be much more careful, but I suspect I've lost considerable mail lately. I'm particularly upset today as all the

236

boxes along this route were torn off by hoodlums last night - Halloween! So glad as I am to forward any mail for you, I think you ought to know it is not too reliable.

As to the kids - I wrote you after I saw them last. They were fine then but I haven't seen them since. When Jig went to Chicago, I believe the rest went to Paula's father - but for how long, I don't know. But I'm sure I'd hear and, so would you, if anything went wrong or any of them weren't well. They were flourishing, the last time I saw them. I'm sorry I can't tell you more as I realise you must want to know. *[remainder of letter missing]*

[Handwritten on personal letterhead, first 4 pp only. UTK]

To Creighton and Paula Scott

26 Belsize Crescent
December 22, 1946

Darling Jig and Pavla

What has happened? Where are you?[171] I have written several letters to the business address given as Jigs on Pavlas July letter, and sent them registered, but have had no reply, and have merely inferred Pavla was with her father until she rejoined Jig, which she must by this time have done.

I am writing to Ralph Pearson and sending this letter with the one to him for forwarding, but his address, also, I misplaced, and I have only remembered it recently as Piermont Avenue.

As I am telling him, I had to give Jigs address as care Gladys, when I got a new American passport and dont know yet whether he received a check meant for Freddys birthday, and it is also very important that I have Jigs correct present address[172] for a British agent for The Muscovites, which there is a strong possibility of my being able to sell in Britain; and it need it similarly for the validation in the States of the Will of which he has a copy, in which he and Jack are appointed my literary executors. Anyhow, all this goes to prove how necessary it is that we all keep in some sort of continuous contact and I dont know how many more got where they were sent, and while that was during the bombing, there seems more than ever no reason for being left in the dark NOW.

Our love again and again and I do implore Creighton and Pavla themselves to reply NOW to this.

The very best to you two and to the children.

[Typed carbon copy, not signed. UTK]

---

171 At that time, Paula and the children were living in Pine Bluff, North Carolina, near Cyril and his wife Louise, while Jigg was commuting from Chicago at weekends.

172 Evelyn often claimed she had important reasons for needing Jigg's address, in this case to find an agent for his first novel, published in New York in 1941. These ploys never had the desired result.

Frustrated by her inability to contact her son, Evelyn turned in desperation to Paula's family. She had earlier met Paula's father Ralph Pearson, a talented silversmith who ran a successful design business. This led to her involving Paula's mother, Margué Foster (who had divorced Ralph and married artist Joseph Foster some years previously) as well as other members of Paula's family, in her search. Much of this chapter is devoted to Evelyn's growing assumption that an unanswered letter could not have been delivered and to her attempts to involve the Post Office, which she viewed as somehow collaborating in preventing her letters from reaching Jigg.

To Ralph Pearson

26 Belsize Crescent
December 22, 1946

Ralph replied after several letters and in 1949 I learned of experience in Chicago like experience reported in The Sun column during early part of war-similar

Dear Ralph Pearson,

When Pavla and Jig moved from Tappan, in July, Pavla wrote me saying she would have no permanent address until she was settled with Jig, again; and Jack and myself have been much concerned about her, Creighton and the children recently, as we have had not a word since, although as Pavla, on the envelope enclosing her letter, gave Creightons business address as the Columbia Broadcasting Company, Chicago, and we have written several letters to him and her there. *Other letters were not returned -there were not many two or three at most*

Her own letter was blank as to address, and it has been merely by inference that we have assumed she was with you until she joined Creighton, which by now she must surely have done; though Gladys Grant, said she thought Pavla could be reached through you. And I would have written to you, in any case, and asked you to relieve our anxiety, and I had not misplaced your address, which I, all at once, remembered a day or two ago as Piermont Avenue. You have lived there so long, I am sure the fact that I have not got the number wont matter. *June Jig had been in Army then ill.*

Well, there is the situation! Jig and Pavla have always kept us apprised of what happened and of their whereabouts, heretofore, and if I had let myself I could have been in a fine dither, by now!

I wrote Margue during the war, to the address which was hers when I visited Pavla and Creighton on my way back to Jack and have written there, again, although that is two years and a half ago, and she may have moved; but I have yet to get a reply; and as letters I sent Pavlas Aunt Gertrude at the same time I wrote Margue and which undoubtedly, if it arrived, went to the correct address, *1952 —All requests for addresses—anyone's—were ignored. except that he sent Harper's- was never acknowledged,* you cant blame me for the anxiety I shall feel until I have your answer to this and all the necessary information about Creighton and Pavla, Denise, Fredrick and Mathew, whom Jack and myself love very much and for whom we feel the greatest loyalty. *No allusion to my books and Jacks or to Jigs has been made by Mr Pearson*

And so you will understand why I appeal to you, certain as I am of your innate kindliness! Letters, the childrens and your own, are of first importance NOW, but the other things are also very VERY very important to us, and, ultimately, what we are able to do for ourselves is important in effect as regards them too.

Our regards to you all, and our very great appreciation,

Do you know Cyrils address? I had a letter sent him in my care for months, and cant forward it because he didnt give me any more address when he last wrote than Pavla did. Really, if it wasnt damnably serious, it would be funny.

[Typed carbon copy, not signed. Handwritten annotations. UTK]

To Paula Scott
Ralph M. Pearson's Design Workshop Courses by Mail
288 Piermont Avenue Nyack, NY

January 30, 1947

Dear Pavli:

Glad to have your report[173] and you certainly have a case vs. Evelyn; it is very sad when a mother builds up that kind of a situation. You see I have not had any direct evidence of it aside from the few words from you and Jigg, as the case does not press on me as it does on you. And it is devilishly hard to know how to handle the situation in a reply to her letter. I have written two letters and, after consulting Louise, torn them up. They lied badly and I hate to do that. And to ignore the questions about which she wrote me is an open affront; I'll be damned if I know how to handle the situation.

It would seem that it might be better for you to answer directly and give her hell and have it out in the open. She says she is coming to the States soon and she will find you in one way or another. Perhaps my best way is not to answer her at all. But it was a registered letter she sent; she will know I got it. You had better tell me what to do.

Glad to hear that the family is together again; it must have been quite a reunion. Shall be glad to hear details at any time. Also about the business. It is fine to be independent - I don't blame you for preferring that kind of controllable insecurity for security at the price Jigg was paying.

So, - my best to you

Dad

[Typed on business letterhead, signed. SFC]

---

173 This has not survived.

London

To Creighton Scott

Ralph M Pearson's Design Workshop Courses by Mail

288 Piermont Ave Nyack, NY

February 3, 1947

Dear Jigg:

This second letter[174] came from Evelyn today; I send it on to you where it really belongs. I have finally after much thought and after consulting Louise,[175] decided on the letter in answer, a copy of which is enclosed.[176] I cannot see the need of telling her lies, nor of the insult of silence; to us it seems that you should take care of the matter as you know all the answers.

Though Evelyn was distraught while staying with you, silence will only make her more so. Can't you see your way to set her at ease before the situation goes from bad to worse? It would appear to be a son's duty to do that.

Cordially,

Ralph

[Typed on business letterhead, signed. SFC]

To Evelyn Scott

Ralph M Pearson's Design Workshops Courses by Mail

288 Piermont Ave Nyack, NY

February 3, 1947

Dear Evelyn:

Your letters both received, the second one came today, and both have been forwarded to Jigg.

I fear I can be of little help to you as it is obvious that this situation exists between you and Jigg. Besides he must know all the answers to your queries. The letters you have been sending to them certainly must have been forwarded; why he has not answered I do not know. *He did know he and Jig were both pestered by "inquirers" about Ralph's innocuous second wife Pavla's step-mother and calling me Margaret Jack Carlo it is just rackety politics*

So, this seems to be the best I can do.

With best wishes,

Cordially,

Ralph

1952 There was some constraint about the content of Life Is Too Short when I was with Jig in Tappan. He seemed happier about this in London when Jack and I

---

174 This letter has not survived.

175 Louise (not to be confused with Cyril's wife Louise Lotz) was Ralph's second wife.

176 This letter has not survived.

both said the libels libelled the author and that it was evidently re-slanted by a ratty editor to suit low markets 1952 —I think the silences I object to criminal—imposed by criminals

[Typed on business letterhead, signed. Handwritten comments. UTK]

To Creighton Scott

26 Belsize Crescent

April 7, 1947

Darling Creighton-Jig *1952 —Why is this letter silence repeated in Munich—1952*

I think you must surely have answered my letters sent to the Chicago address Pavla put on her envelope last July, if it remained the correct address, but whatever you have or havent done, please write again now, as my effort to get the address confirmed by Pavlas father resulted in nothing but mutual misunderstanding, he assuming "quarrels", though there had been no quarrels, and refusing to give it, or relieve a really tormenting anxiety about all five by at least some comment on circumstances health whereabouts, and so on.

If there had been any misunderstanding of which I am not aware - and I cannot myself remember anything ever having happened that could be called a "misunderstanding" except a few very minor altercations due to the war and frazzled nerves on all sides - if there is anything that requires explaining then surely you will tell me what it is and allow me to clarify the situation to the best of my ability. It is a humiliation to be obliged to send this care of Ralph Pierson *[sic]* after his very strange attitude to my previous inquiry about you, but that is what I am forced to by being kept in the dark. Why, why why is it possible for Piersons and Fosters, to continue in normal contact with not merely their child, but my child while I seem banished to inscrutable limbo, as is Jack who is both a loving step-father and a distinguished man? *Why? 1952 —Hiatus was compensated for in part by Jig's partially explanatory visit which he was to have repeated after two weeks in France—he was unable to return because of illness and short cash*

Pavla can tell you that any mothers attitude toward her child is the same whatever happens, and no hiatus can ever affected my love for Jiggie Creighton, or Jacks or, as far as that goes, my affection for Pavla herself, Denise, Fredrick, Mathew, and our regard for Cyril, whose Life is Too Short we still hope to get here somehow.

Very fondly your mother with Jack's love too

[Typed carbon copy, not signed. Handwritten annotations. UTK]

To Evelyn Scott

Scotch Plains, New Jersey
April 11, 1947

Dear Evelyn: *She sent paper twice*[177]

Your letter came yesterday and I would have answered it then, but was just taking Edgerton to New York to return to school and had several business things I had to do there. Last night I came back so tired that I waited to write you until morning.

I'm glad to have you and Jack use this address and will see there is no delay in forwarding anything, should it come here. It is grand that you have finished your novel. Do you still need paper? I have some bought for you, but did not send because again I thought you might be on your way.

I realize how you must want to hear about your grandchildren and wish I could send you details. But I haven't seen any of them since they left Tappan or even heard for the last month or more. In Paula's last letter she enclosed a nice one from Denise, very sweet and well written, mainly asking about the fish they gave me before they left. So perhaps you know more than I do!

Love to you both as always.

Glads

[Typewritten, signed. Handwritten annotation. UTK]

To Creighton Scott

RFD No 1
Scotch Plains, New Jersey

May 12, 1947

Dear Jig:

This is written to you to ask what you want me to do if and when your mother comes. May I say that I promised to give your address to <u>no one</u> without official permission, I'll lie and say I don't know, if you prefer, but I'm not a good liar and this may just make her angry and more hurt and determined. It's none of my business but, if you don't want to see her, wouldn't it be easier for both of you to cable her before she started? If she gets to this country she is almost sure to find out somehow were you are. I realize such a cable is hard and cruel but won't it be much worse for all of you after she is here?

Please forgive my butting in. I won't mention it again. Unless I hear to the contrary I'll just refuse to give your address, if I'm cornered.

Excuse scrawl. I'll write again soon and be sure to let me know how you all are.

---

177 Post-war England was suffering shortages of paper; it was rationed and as a result Evelyn was continually asking friends in the United States to send her supplies. Gladys was one of those who responded to these requests.

God bless you all

Love

Glads

[Handwritten on personal letterhead, signed. SFC]

To Paula Scott

Ralph Pearson's Design Workshop

288 Piermont Ave Nyack, NY

May 31, 1947

Dear Pavli:

About Evelyn. She sent me a scalding letter just before the one I forwarded to you;[178] I was hiding you. It was my fault that she couldn't find you. Etc, etc. I did not answer it. I guess you have reasons all right for breaking the cord. But it is sad that a parent creates such a situation.

So long, old top

Dad

[Typed on business letterhead, signed. SFC]

To Evelyn Scott

RFD No 1

Scotch Plains, New Jersey

June 15, 1947

1952 This letter rather stupid in view of facts. Jack was about to sail—arranging passage when this arrived

Dear Evelyn:

I hope when you wrote "domiciled with me" you did not mean to stay here. Not that I don't want to see you and Jack, but there isn't an inch of space. You can always have mail sent to this address, if you trust the RFD, and I'll be glad to forward it. But there isn't any place to sleep.

As for Jig and Paula, I haven't heard from them for ages and can't tell you their address. The last letter, I believe, was the note from Denise and had none. They are worse correspondents than I am, but I'm sure I would have heard if all was not well. If the Chicago address is the last you have, it will undoubtedly reach him. *1952 — mail to Chicago was returned to London*

I hate to write this discouraging letter and perhaps should not send it, but I don't know when I'll get a chance to write again. I'll try to when I'm in a less depressed mood myself.

Love to you both

Gladys

[Typed on personal letterhead, signed. Handwritten annotations. UTK]

---

178 Neither of these letters has survived.

In August 1947 Jack returned to the United States to fulfil the requirements for his "quota" residence, leaving Evelyn to manage the house and tenants in London. Evelyn took advantage of this to set Jack the task while in New York of visiting Ralph Pearson at his home to try to gain information about Jigg's whereabouts from him.

From John Metcalfe's diary:

August 16, 1947: Got up about 7.45. Breakfasted and showered, while John Hall was cleaning-up. Wrote and posted letter to Match's.[179] Wrote letter to Jig and took it with me to Nyack, where I eventually discovered Ralph Pearson at 288 Piermont Avenue. Heavy rain, and somewhat cooler. Thank goodness. Mrs P came out to front porch and gave us drinks etc. Ralph P took letter *[below]* to post to Jig. He showed me some of his own work, and the atmosphere generally was friendly. Caught the 6.10 'bus back to N York, then subway from 167th Street.

To Creighton Scott

c/o DeSilver,
130 West 12th Street
August 16, 1947

Dear Jig,

Here I am back in the US and eager to see you if you care for that.

I don't know what in heck the conditions or considerations which have created the present impasse (to call it that!) may be, but I am not lacking in imagination which, towards yourself, has always been and will always be, exercised in the friendliest possible way. Please take that as a first datum anyhow.

At the same time, you, also, are a person of imagination, so you can probably guess the effect on Evelyn (and by repercussion and propinquity on myself) of a sustained silence. I fancy, from all one may gather, that she must have been a wearing inmate of your house while she was awaiting a passage to England, and I certainly feel no "disloyalty" to her in saying so.

None the less, and conceding all of this, her affection for you is very deep and genuine, and to grant it some sort of vent, if only by occasional correspondence, could, as I (failing further enlightenment) see it, do you no harm. It would not be a wedge's thin-end towards anything you might find obtrusive, inappropriate or oppressive.

Meanwhile, however, your silence has had the effect of rendering her unresigned to life in England. A line or two, now and then, would, as they say, have kept her happy, or reasonably so; but, as it is, the absence of a word from you has received, progressively, a wholly disproportionate emphasis until it was warped and coloured her entire outlook, and tended, of course, to aggravate those very symptoms of

---

179 Match & Co had been managing Jack's house for some years. There will be much more from them in Chapter 34.

nervousness and all else which may, in the first instance, have played some part in prompting you to drop correspondence.

So what I want to put over to you is the present actual concrete picture and no more. At present, and rightly or wrongly, that actual concrete picture is that lack of word from you is a prime cause - I may say the prime cause - of mental disturbance generally, impeding work and destroying health. A word from you would relieve this condition and constitute no faintest kind of "threat" to yourself. But you can imagine the effect a continued silence will undoubtedly have upon such a nature.

This, of course, is inadequate and partial. In particular, it fails to convey how warmly I feel towards you, yourself, as a person. That is quite apart from anything construable as mere "sentiment", of which, I hope, I am sufficiently adult to be absolved.

If you feel like it, I want, as I've said, to see you. I, just as much as Evelyn, am feeling rather bothered and "bottled-up" by this "situation", - which I still insist on enclosing in inverted commas.

Yrs ever,

Jack

[Typed, signed. SFC]

To Evelyn Scott

c/o 130 West 12th Street

August 20, 1947

Darling Beloved Evelyn-Chookie

As I told you in last letter (tho' it was not air-mail, - and this may arrive first), I saw Ralph Pearson (it's spelt that way, I find) on Saturday, - and left a short letter for Jig, which he will forward. Jigg had asked RP not to give his address to anyone, so of course I still have not go it, and it may be a week or so before I can get any reply.

RP seemed most friendly, - but a little hurt that you hadn't visited him as often as he (apparently) had wanted. He begged me to understand that he was not to blame. Now he regretted the present situation, and, for his part, had asked Jig to write to us, - and had no idea why he would not.

I am sure all this will adjust itself if only you (who have, at the moment, to play infinitely the most difficult part) can hold on for a while. I told Jig, of course, how lovingly we both felt and how delighted I wd be to see him, - but at the same time assured him that I was not, in any way, "pursuing" him. If I did, incidentally, learn his address, what good would that really be to us unless he himself had volunteered it? - as I think he will.

I love you. If only you were here! NY is largely the same funny old noisy NY we both know, - but, as I said before, just seems all wrong with Evelyn not here.

All love always

Dickie-Jack

[Handwritten, signed. UTK]

To Postmaster, Nyack, New York

26 Belsize Crescent
May 23, 1949

Dear Sir

I take the liberty of asking if you will be good enough to inquire into the return to me, today, of the small parcel I sent recently addressed to Mr Creighton Scott, care Ralph Pierson *Pierson Piermont – PO replied Pearson*Design Workshop, Nyack, New York.

I ask because Mr Pierson has resided at that address in Nyack for a number of years. And although I shall, of course, write to him personally about this, I have had several experiences of the same sort in the last few years, and actually began to send very important letters intended for my son Mr Creighton Scott, in care of Mr Pierson, his father-in-law, because a most important letter to Mr Scott, which was sent to him in Chicago, was returned in this same way.

[Typed carbon copy, not signed. Handwritten insertion. UTK]

To Evelyn Scott

United States Post Office
Nyack, New York

July 21, 1949

NB August 3rd 1949 this was an inquiry about mail addressed to my son in Pearson's care which though correctly addressed was returned. I therefore regard the Post Office at Nyack as disingenuous and evasive and as having downright refused to answer straight questions regarding a specific instance of mishandling. This inquiry was made May 27 1949 this letter arrived August 2 1949.

Dear Madam:

Receipt is acknowledged of your letter of June 29th, 1949, all which has reference to mail which you send to your Son, his Wife and your Grandson.

You are advised that Mr Pierson *ear—my fault!* is alive and resides at 288 Piermont Avenue, for a number of years. All mail received at this office addressed to him or other persons in his care has been delivered to that address.

Of course, it would be impossible to trace the letters you mailed during the years 1944 and 1945, however, I can assure you that if they were addressed to Mr Pierson or someone in his care they were delivered to the above mentioned address. What he might do with such mail is unknown to anyone at this office.

We have no forwarding address for your Son or any member of his family and any mail addressed to them directly would be returned to the sender marked unknown. If the mail was addressed to your Son or any member of his family in care of Mr Pierson it would be delivered to Mr Pierson's residence for such disposition as he cared to make of it.

Trusting this explains our position in the matter,

I am

Respectfully yours,

Postmaster

NB 1952 This blast of ice returned to me a letter and parcel correctly addressed to Mathew Scott my grandson and Mr Pearson's in Mr Pearson's care-Mr Pearson said he know nothing of it. In London, Jig said Ralph's second wife had been called a "red" because she was once in a teacher's union in which were some communists. The two Pearsons were once socialists.

[Typed on official letterhead, signed. Handwritten annotations. UTK]

To Evelyn Scott

Ralph M Pearson's Design Workshop

288 Piermont Ave Nyack NY

October 7, 1949

Pearson lies I think and he knows a situation so painful would naturally make it impossible for Jig to read my letter in his presence.

Dear Evelyn:

The Nyack postmaster just showed me another letter from you about Jigg not getting your letters. Now look, Evelyn - Jigg has received every letter you sent in my care. That last long one about a month ago came to me while he happened to be here visiting for the day and I gave it to him direct from the carrier - without reading it myself. From the way he acted I doubt if he read it, altho I saw him read part of the first page. He is following a deliberate policy of not answering your letters; that is the hard fact you may as well take into account. And I suggest you stop bothering postmasters about this family matter; it is hardly fair to them to be brought in on such a thing.

But every letter you sent to me will be forwarded-so you may always be assured Jigg gets them.

It is very unfortunate, this whole situation - and I regret it very much - but there is nothing I can do.

Sincerely,

Ralph M P

Egregious evasion--Ralph doesn't answer during two years and not until I had embarrassed him by inquiring of the P Office about parcel (returned)

[Typed on business letterhead, signed. Handwritten annotations. UTK]

In November 1949, Jigg decided to try to find employment in Europe and sailed to London en route to Paris. He had been given some small commissions in England and hoped to find work at the BBC or, failing that, a post in Paris, for which he felt he was well qualified with his fluent French and his extensive experience in radio journalism.

From John Metcalfe's diary:

November 17, 1949: Found E had opened in error letter for me from Pavla to say Jig coming to London.

November 20, 1949: Jig rang up from Regent Palace Hotel and arrived soon afterwards, bringing whisky. He stayed the night, company retiring, after coffee, at about 1.30.

To Paula Scott

Regent Palace Hotel, London
November 21, 1949

Dearest baby -

I had a very severe shock a while ago. The telephone in my room rang and when I answered it, it was my mother. The letter you sent care of Jack was the means by which she knew I was coming; and they found out where I was by the simple expedient of calling up the Cunard line every day and asking where I would stay until the right ship came in. Naturally I had to go out there, which I did last evening.

It was awful. E Scott is much better - in fact, she is quite changed. But they are both living in a state which I can only describe as near-destitution. The house is up for sale. For a while they hoped to live on some money the government allotted them to repair bomb damage; but that was not allowed. Jack is very sick with the same thing Dad had - an infected prostate, but he can't have it out because he does not dare give up the occasional tutoring jobs by which they keep body and soul together and take the time to be operated on. They are both almost emaciated and so shabby they are quite ragged. The rent from the house is no longer enough even to keep the house going, and the price of fuel and repairs, etc, has skyrocketed in the last few months so that they are heavily in the red. Lately they have been unable to pay for the gas which heats the house, and the tenants are threatening to leave. If that happened, they would have to leave themselves, with no place to go. Jack has been trying to look for a job, but he can't because he has no decent clothes, and all he has been able to get is a few kids to tutor.

I went out last night and stayed until midnight, then found that the underground closes and that there are no cabs late at night, so I slept on the couch. But they no longer have even enough blankets to keep warm, and I slept under a coat.

I couldn't stand it. The upshot is that I lent them fifty dollars, mostly to pay the gas bill, buy a few clothes, and get something to eat. They will also be able to fix up one of their 4 rooms so that they can take a lodger.

I'm sorry, baby. It is really appalling. Nobody asked me for anything but I just couldn't stand it. Blood is a little thicker than water, and it's hard to watch anybody living on oatmeal. I am sending out some of the grub I brought with me.

If you can raise the missing fifty I will be all right. My room here is paid for until Wednesday - that is, Thursday morning, when I shall be able to go to a pension and live much more cheaply. However, I find I can't do that until they give me my ration books, which won't be until Wednesday.

Try to raise it from two sources, on the grounds that my going to work is delayed by red tape. It seems to me that Glads and Julia[180] could do that between them. I shall be in a frightful jam if I don't get it, but I will do the best I can. You should get a bank draft and send it to me here, or wire it here (to this hotel). Even if I have moved, I can always get mail from the hall porter after I have left.

I am terribly sorry, baby. The letter care of Jack was a mistake, and I should not have gone out there, but I didn't know what I was getting into. And I just simply couldn't take it all in my stride.

I have told them that I am leaving for the continent on Wednesday, so they don't expect to see me again excepting perhaps for a brief visit, which I can't refuse. I have between 35 and 40 dollars left, and that will do the trick if I can get the other fifty. I would think up any reason but the real one, if I were you. Tell them I have to pay for a laboring permit - anything you decide is propitious. I will avoid pitfalls hereafter.

God bless you, baby. I love you better than anything in the world. I'll write you again later, when I am more myself.

Your devoted husband,

Jigg

[Typed, typed signature. SFC]

From John Metcalfe's diary:

November 21, 1949: Jig left after breakfast, I putting him on right track for a taxi.
November 24, 1949: School - and lunched there. Tea. Nap. Jig arrived.
November 25, 1949: School as usual. Tea, Work. Nap. Supper of corned beef. Read stories etc to Jig. Bed.

To Creighton Scott

Rutherford, New Jersey

November 26, 1949

Dearest Angel -

Today I got your letter about your mother and Jack. I put a PS on the letter I was about to mail to you about it - but this is the real answer. And yet I don't know what to say - except that until we have some money of our own we can't help them any more

---

180 Julia Daniels, a friend of Gladys'. This passage illustrates the degree to which the Scotts were not only dependant on Paula's family but on a few loyal friends.

- after that perhaps we can - at least enough for Jack to have his operation. I was sorry to learn that they are so terribly up against it. But we can do no more now, so please don't get into anything more. I have enough for myself and the kids with Julia's and Gladys' help, but if I have to send you more (not counting the other twenty you'll get next week) before the normal need for more arises, if it does before you can get things started for us, the kids and I will be up against it. So stretch it, will you, honey? I'm dying to know how the BBC thing works out. It's the limit that your letters take so long to get here, but I suppose that regular mail would be 10 days instead of five.

I told Deo and Aunt G[181] that you had to pay 50 bucks for a labor permit. They helped out, but we can expect no more from them for quite a while. Julia and Glads are doing their best.

I love you

P

[Handwritten, signed. SFC]

From John Metcalfe's diary:

November 26, 1949: Walked home, and all three had lunch of soup, no, mistake, Jig didn't want any! Nap.

November 27, 1949: Work most of day. After supper read aloud to E and Jig from *This Emergent* and from 1926 diary. Bed.

November 28, 1949: Morning school. Jig just leaving when I came home for lunch.

In spite of some positive interviews in England and in France, Jigg did not secure employment in Europe and returned to the United States some days later. Evelyn had been very hopeful of his success in finding employment in Europe as she saw this as bringing her son and his family within easy reach of London and Jigg, realising this, did not tell his mother that he had returned to the United States jobless.

From John Metcalfe's diary:

December 25, 1949: Spent all day quietly at home. After tea read E's MS to p 515. Steak and Christmas-pudding for supper. Work. Bed.

January 9, 1950: Posted letter, air mail, from E to Pavli.

January 14, 1950: Letter for Jig from Paris telephone manager.

February 17, 1950: Letter at last, - from Pavli. stating Jig had been ill.

October 14, 1950: Letter for E from Paula.

December 25, 1950: Stayed in all day, working at <u>Enter Cousin</u>. Got cheque for $10 from Mr Harper, - also a card from Bullett acknowledging receipt of my MS. Made scones for tea.

---

181 Deo was Dorothy McNamara, a maternal aunt of Paula's, and Aunt G was Gertrude Brownell, Paula's great aunt. This passage makes it clear just how dependent Jigg and Paula were on support from Paula's family.

Chapter 25

In search of an inheritance
December 1946 - October 1947

Not long after her return to London Evelyn decided to renew contact with her father, Seely Dunn, whom she had last seen at a brief but cordial meeting in Washington DC in 1925. This impulse may have been prompted by filial affection but was very probably also motivated by her difficult financial position and by her hope that her prosperous father would be able to help.

When she tried to re-establish contact in late 1946, she was shocked to discover that her father had died in 1943 and worse, that she had not been told. This, naturally, upset her. She believed that her father would have left her a sizeable sum of money as her grandfather, Oliver Milo Dunn, had been very well off and she believed he would have passed a sum to Seely to be kept in trust for her.

Now that her finances were so parlous she embarked on a flurry of letter writing to try to establish both the facts of her father's death and the whereabouts of the will which she was confident would establish her claim to this inheritance. These letters, in a very different style to her more informal correspondence, demonstrate Evelyn's desperate and understandable search for information as she wrote to every individual and institution that might possibly help her. Many letters repeated the same information again and again and some of these passages have been deleted in the interests of brevity and readability.

Evelyn eventually learned more from an obituary notice in the Lynchburg, Virginia News in May 1944, which she did not see until two years after her father's death.

Obituary
Seely Dunn
from *The News*, Lynchburg Virginia
May 6th 1944

Married Maud Thomas Feb 4 1892 divorced during 1914 war. Evelyn Scott Metcalfe, born Elsie Dunn is Mr Dunn's only child

"Seely Dunn, 74, of Lynchburg died at 5.15 am in a government hospital at Biloxi, Miss, following a long illness. born Toledo Ohio

"Born October 13, 1869, he was the only child of Oliver Milo and Harriet Seely Dunn of New Orleans. He was married Nov 18, 1917, second wife was to Melissa Whitehead of New Orleans, a relative of the Virginia Whitehead family.

"Mr Dunn was a railroad executive until World War I, in which he was a captain and later a major. Before the war he spent two years in Honduras as construction engineer in charge of surveying through the jungles for a railroad for the United Fruit Company. For six years after the war he was with the Interstate Commerce Commission in Washington from which position he resigned to become associated with the firm of J. P. Morgan in New York. He retired in 1935 and came to Virginia to live.

"Though confined to his home for most of the time he lived in and near Lynchburg, he became well known.

"After coming to this section Maj. Dunn purchased a home near Forest Road, later selling his place and coming to town."

[Typed copy of obituary of Seely Dunn, copied by librarian after request from ES. Handwritten annotation. UTK]

The following is the letter with which Evelyn started her quest, and which was returned to her with unexpected and unpleasant news. This letter, in an unopened envelope, had scrawled on it, in pencil, "Resigned January 1928, died 1943".

To Director, Bureau of Interstate Commerce

Personal Attention, Please

December 22, 1946

To the Director of the

Bureau of Interstate Commerce

Washington, DC

This brought return of my letter with unsigned marginal scribble announcing my father's death.

Sir

It is with a degree of hesitation that I approach a stranger, in connection with so intimate a matter as information as to the present whereabouts of my father, Mr Seely Dunn; whose address I herewith request you to supply if you are able. *reply was very sad news of my father's death—date given was 1943 I now know 1953*

My father was, in 1925, when I spent a few days with him in Washington, the Assistant Director of your Bureau, and resided at 1746 K Street, where he had an apartment in a building in which, I believe, he had an interest; and I was told, a year or two later, that he had removed from Washington to Cranford, New Jersey, and was employed by the firm of J P Morgan and Company. But since he was in Washington, he has neglected to correspond with me; and while I attribute this to the estrangement between him and my mother, from whom he was divorced, and who died in 1940 in Clarksville, Tennessee, and, therefore, bears him no grudge, I have frequently, and particularly during the war, been regretful of the unjust impression created by having to give his address, on my American passport application, and other documents, as "unknown", and being obliged to say that I do not know whether or not he is, as I hope, still very much among the living.

I now hope, however, that you will be able to put me in touch with him, again, and there may be some resumed contact with him - at least to the extent of a letter.

Again, my apologies for troubling you; but I shall certainly be most grateful for any assistance you can give me, preferably by forwarding this letter to my father himself, or, if not that, by requesting Mr DeBardeleben, Junior, to do so, should you chance to know him. And in any case, if you do neither, and can tell me where to write to my father, I shall appreciate the return to me of this letter, which I should prefer was not in a file to which others have access, where it might be misconstrued as reflecting on him, which is not at all my intention.

Very truly yours,

My father should know, I think, that while British by marriage, I am still an American citizen.

I enclose an envelope with, I hope, the appropriate stamps - the only American stamps I have!

[Typed carbon copy, not signed. Handwritten annotations. UTK]

So sure was Evelyn that her father would have made some provision for her in his will that she sent similar letters to all the possible jurisdictions in which a will might have been lodged: the Lynchburg Circuit Court, the Lynchburg Probate Court, the Lynchburg County Court, the New Orleans Civil District Court and the court for Gulfport Mississippi, as well as New Orleans and Lynchburg Public Libraries. The content was broadly similar: the following gives a flavour of these letters and the information Evelyn thought necessary to include.

To Judge of the Probate Court, Lynchburg, Virginia

26 Belsize Crescent

June 12, 1947

Judge of the Probate Court For Lynchburg, Virginia *sent in duplicate was not acknowledged*

Sir,

I take the liberty of applying to you for any information you can give me concerning my father, the late Mr Seely Dunn of Lynchburg. I appeal to you in some embarrassment on so personal a matter, but I am Mr Dunn's daughter and, as far as I know, his only child, and when I have clarified my reasons for doing so I hope that you will consider me humanly justified.

My father's first marriage was to my mother, Mrs Maud Thomas Dunn, a native of Clarksville, Tennessee, who died there in 1940; and as he had re-married his present wife, Mrs Melissa Whitehead Dunn, after his divorce from my mother, and as I was in constant contact with her, and had the full financial responsibility for her maintenance, that may explain why my father, since 1925, has not communicated with me or replied to my letters.

In 1925, when he was with the Interstate Commerce Bureau, I visited him briefly in Washington, DC (when he was most affectionate and considerate), and it was to the ICB I first wrote last autumn; asking them to return my letter if they were unable to forward it to him. It was returned, with a note on his death scribbled on it, and that was the first I had heard of it; though on writing to J P Morgan and Company, on the suggestion of the late Mr Morgan's sister-in-law, I was told, by a Mr Moseley of Morgan's, of my father's service with them, his independent business venture (they did not tell me what it was), and his final removal to Lynchburg. And as soon as I had the Norfolk Avenue address I wrote to my stepmother, and she has not yet answered, and as I am in doubt as to what her attitude toward me is, I cannot even be certain of her replying at all.

In 1925, when my father was especially nice to me, and after I went to Washington, came to New York to see me, in turn, my grandparents, Mr and Mrs Oliver Milo Dunn of New Orleans, Louisiana, had not been long dead. And my father showed me a news clipping which, though it did not, as I recall it, give the terms of my grandfather's Will, gave the estimate of his estate as evaluated at something over three-hundred-and-thirty-five thousand dollars, and the jewelry of my grandmother (who collected diamonds, in a modest way) as worth thirty-five thousand dollars in the market as it was then. And as my father was an only child, I assume this went to him, and that he, therefore, had some substance to dispose of. But I do resent, at this juncture, having been kept in the dark as to the disposition of my father's property and effects, and think I have every right to know precisely what was done with them; and this regardless of whether or not I was included in his Will. He was a man of high standing in business, and prior to the hiatus in our correspondence, was meticulous in his family obligations, and I cannot reconcile with what I know of his character what seems the omission of so much as a memento for me in any of his final arrangements.

I am assured that, in England, information regarding Wills can be had by applying to Somerset House, and is open to the public; and while, of course, it is possible my father left no Will, I think it likely he did, and am assuming you are at liberty to advise me in this regard. But it is on the human side most of all that I would be grateful for any possible illumining as to my father's incredible silence during these last years, and anything whatever that throws light on that will be welcome, as, also, information as to Mrs Melissa Whitehead Dunn's present whereabouts, if you have it.

Mr Seely Dunn has the grandson, my son, Mr Creighton Scott whom I have already mentioned, surviving him in the USA and three great-grandchildren, Denise, Fredrick and Mathew Scott. *Julia Swinburne Scott born July 6th 1951 NY State Upper* But I refer you to people who are not members of my family as perhaps more impartial judges of the situation, for I do think it is simply human to object to my father's ignoring of them, and that they do seem probably, as I do on their behalf, even as I try to keep before me my father's originally great virtues.

I respectfully await your reply,

Very Truly Yours

Evelyn Dunn Scott Metcalfe neé Elsie Dunn

[Typed carbon copy, signed. Handwritten annotations. UTK]

The next four years saw Evelyn sending similar lengthy and detailed queries to the various public bodies which may have held records of her father's death and, more importantly, details of his will. The replies were typically polite and brief but importantly none of these organisations had any record of a will for Seely Dunn. Eventually, Evelyn tried a strategy which she had used before: asking her cousin Charles Day to pursue queries on her behalf. He contacted his friend Clark Dunn, and this produced information about her father but, significantly, no knowledge of any will.

To Clark Dunn

Louisville & Nashville Railroad Company

Office of Vice-President - Operation at Louisville Ky,

October 1, 1951

I asked for information about my father's estate and Melissa—I knew my father's history up to 1925 and much since. Why the hell was this sent? They are fools! I could have choked Charles and these asses!—Evelyn Scott—Evelyn D S Metcalfe

Mr Clark Dunn

Division Passenger Agent

Atlanta, Ga

Dear Clark:

Please refer to your letter of September 27th[182] regarding Mr Seeley Dunn. According to our files, the General Manager wrote Mr Edward H DeGroot, Jr, Colorado Building, Washington, DC, under date of March 19, 1951 as follows:

"Please refer to your letter of March 17th relative to record of Mr Seeley Dunn.

"Mr Dunn was born at Sylvania, Ohio, on October 13, 1869. He entered L &

---

182 This letter has not survived.

N service on September 1, 1884 and after serving in various capacities was appointed Assistant Superintendent of our Henderson Division on December 14, 1899. Our files do not indicate when Mr Dunn left L & N service but in 1913 we had some correspondence with him, at which time he was Division Engineer for the Tela Railroad Company, in Tela, Honduras.

"We have no further record of Mr Dunn and are unable to state whether he is still living." *My father was full Superintendent and was not an assistant at any time. Must have been that of Evansville, Indiana firm which my father resigned. 1952 November 23rd, London, England. Evelyn D S Metcalfe baptismal name at birth Elsie Dunn*

This is about all the information we have been able to develop around here about Mr Dunn.

With best regards, I am,

Yours very truly,

L L Morton

Vice President.

[Typed carbon copy, typed signature. Handwritten annotations. UTK]

To Charles Day

Louisville & Nashville Railroad Company

Passenger Traffic Department

Atlanta 3, Ga

October 2, 1951

Mr Charles M Day, Vice-President

Hickman, Williams & Company

St Louis 1, Mo

Dear Charles:

I acknowledged yours of September 13th on September 27th and now am in position to give you some information on Mr Seeley Dunn.

One of your New Orleans representatives was kind enough to visit the Veterans Administration Center at Biloxi and advises that their records are as follows:

"Seely Dunn *Seeley Dunn, C-910,629 name misspelled—my father's name is correctly recorded in the letters from the Veterans sent to me*

"Admitted Veterans Administration Hospital, Biloxi, Miss Dec 24, 1943

"Died May 5, 1944 at 4.00 AM

"1st Designate: Wife-Mrs Melissa Whitehead Dunn 2807 Rivermont

"Ave, Lynchburg, Va. *Their home was Norfolk Avenue Lynchburg*

"2nd Designate: Brother-in-law - Jules L Brana 165 Roberts Avenue, Mobile, Ala.

"Enlisted: March 27, 1917

"Discharged: October 8, 1919, Honorable

"Rank and Organization: Captain, Quartermaster Corps.

"Regional Office: Washington, DC

"Date of birth: October 13, 1869, Sylvania, Ohio *Toledo EDSM — Lord knows why this he himself always said Toledo*

"Serial Number: 0-206052

"Social Security No: None

"Body shipped to Washington, DC, for cremation

"Correspondence Folder sent to Veterans Administration Regional Office, Washington,

"Clinical Records sent to Records Center, Philadelphia, Pa, Nov 28, 1949.

Mrs Melissa Whitehead Dunn was present at time of death and gave disposition instruction. She acted as escort to body on trip to Washington, DC.

"If further information is desired same can be secured from Veterans Administration Regional Office, Washington, DC."

It might be that you will wish to inquire of Metairie Cemetery at New Orleans to see if Mr Dunn's ashes are buried there.

I have also secured the record from Louisville which is contained the attached letter[183] dated October 1st from our Vice-President, Operation, Col L L Morton.

I hope the information which we have secured may be of some assistance to your friend, or at least put her on the right track to secure additional information.

With every good wish always.

Sincerely,

Clark

1952 — I had written Charles Day I had all these records by this time, but he paid no specific attention and so wasted his friend's time as well as my own.

I ascertained all this in 1948 except that name of brother-in-law of Melissa who saw to the disposition of my father's ashes at Metairie was then given to me by Metairie Cemetary as Mr Andre Chenet of New Orleans whereas the one mentioned here is Mr Jules D Brana of 165 Roberta Avenue Mobile, Alabama.

[Typed on business letterhead, signed. Handwritten annotations and PS by Evelyn. UTK]

---

183 This letter has not survived.

During this period Evelyn was also writing to her stepmother, Seely's widow Melissa Dunn, asking for details of his final illness and, most importantly, details of any will he might have left. The following letter, like the three which preceded it, was not acknowledged in any way by Melissa.

To Melissa Whitehead Dunn

26 Belsize Crescent
October 3, 1951

Dear Melissa:

Will you, in case you have actually received the four letters sent by me to this address, one forwarded by the Lynchburg Postmaster, and possibly, a fifth letter I requested the "Veterans' Bureau" "Department of Claims, etc" to send on - in case you have every one of these letters, or even ONE of them, won't you please emerge from your silence and make some moderately human gesture in elucidation of why you did not tell the "Veterans' Facility", when my Father was ill and dying, that I was his daughter and should know something of his death and his estate.

Will you tell me anything whatever? You know something of my candour and you must have realized I would not just meekly accept a stand on your part superficially "irrational" as my Father himself identified me when Cyril applied in 1923 for the Permanent Scott Family Passport and he - my Father, the late Mr Seely Dunn of Washington at one time-signed the application, and it is absurd to be aware as I think you must have been that my Father has been on record as my Father since 1914 or 1915 when my Mother came to Brazil to "visit" us and registered as Maud Thomas Dunn (Mrs Seely Dunn) at the American Consulate in Recife the day she landed from the Lamport and Holt steamer.

It was in Recife that Cyril with my agreement took the first step toward the establishment of the Common Law Marriage which we had decided was the one solution since his second wife in New Orleans would not, then, as yet, divorce him, though long afterward - a few years, we gathered - she did.

You know all these things and that every word I have said about any of these official steps is the truth and that our Common Law Marriage was re-established in the States with our documented re-acceptance as a family and our documented change of name: not a change by deed-pole but by usage.

We must be accepted as we are, as having taken the steps we did for the motives actually ours, which were accepted until this damnable war seemed to re-poison American and British minds. And I have brought up the date business because I cannot think of anything else that you could possibly have been exploited to alarm either you or my Father about our relationship.

Maybe I am just "telling you something" - if so well and good. I do not and never did like any sort of concealment, and that you and my Father began in Lynchburg with what may have been merely as a social lie in denying my existence, has resulted in humiliations, implied insults from every quarter, and I really don't know what else, as myself and my second husband John Metcalfe have been stuck here in Britain with just enough money to keep us actually in food, and literally no more, ever since he was demobilized.

We have been immolated, Creighton and his wife and children have been nearly so we are allowed to think and it must be so, and this is probably as true of Cyril who is I am certain basically unchanged, though we do not hear from him and his Wellman son does not answer letters, or else does not receive them.

Anyone with an atom of sense should realize that to communicate with myself and Jack normally is to stop libel, and that to be silent, is to foment it. So it may be your letters - Melissa - have been sent to me and I never got them. *My daughter-in-law says I do not receive elucidating letters sent by her here.*

Will you please acknowledge this as suits you

Evelyn-Elsie

[Typed carbon copy, signed. Handwritten insertion. UTK]

To Probate Court, Washington DC

26 Belsize Crescent
October 3, 1951

The Probate Court
Washington DC USA
Sirs:

As I have not yet been assured that there is a Probate Court under Federal jurisdiction, I hope I address you correctly. I wish to know whether or not you have on file any Will of the late Mr Seely Dunn whose residence was Lynchburg until he fell ill and went to the "Veterans' Facility" in Biloxi, Mississippi, where in May 1944, he died. He had once lived in Washington - twice in fact - as he was first there as the Assistant Director of the Bureau of Interstate Commerce, but resigned from this position in the late nineteen-twenties to take a better position in the offices of "J P Morgan and Company" in New York, where he remained until 1934, when, again, he resigned to "go into business with Mr John Oldham, now of Wellesley Hills, Massachusetts": the facts as to Mr Oldham here in quotation marks because it was then that I lost contact with him entirely, though even before the move he had ceased to write to me, his only child.

He and my Mother, the late Mrs Maud Thomas Dunn of Clarksville, Tennessee, were divorced and he had remarried a Miss Melissa Whitehead of New Orleans, and she I think disliked me because of my Father's differences with my Mother, though for a time she appeared friendly.

My Father had never to my knowledge attempted to conceal our relationship until, a few years before his death, he bought a house in Lynchburg and retired there with his second wife. But I have discovered, in my efforts to ascertain something about his death and his possible Will, that in Lynchburg neither he nor Mrs Dunn

second commonly referred to me, and their intimate friends had any idea that he had a daughter and that she was myself.

All these things are matters of public record, so I have found it difficult to grasp that I was not notified when my Father fell ill and no notice of his death was ever sent me: this admitted by the Biloxi Hospital and by the Department of Claims and Benefits of the Veterans' Administration.

The hospital blames my stepmother. I think her dislike led to one of those "social fibs" which are frequent and that she may have involved herself in some technical irregularity by having persisted more or less innocently in a fib in its origin without original intention. And this seems to me the more likely because my Father's death occurred in the course of the war, when panics were easily incited, and when, in fact, I was part of the time in Canada, with my husband Squadron Leader William John Metcalfe of the "RAF".

I have written endless letters about these things to various people whom it might have been reasonably supposed could be informative, but many letters are still unacknowledged and the comparatively small number who have replied either could not or would not elucidate. However but I have been fairly reliably assured that my Father did not file any Will in Lynchburg; that he did not file any Will in New Orleans where I grew up and my parents lived for a time, and where his second wife and he met, as she is a native of Louisiana, and that he could not have filed any Will in New York. So Washington seems the one logical place left to ask about, and I might have written this present letter before had I not be trying to re-contact my stepmother herself at an address given me, by the Lynchburg Postmaster, as hers in 1947.

My Father, at the time of his death, was still nominally a resident of Lynchburg I am told, but his body - according to various official reports as communicated to me - was shipped to Washington at once for cremation at the Jones - I think it was called Crematorium: I have the name on file but this correspondence has already so nearly worn me out that I am reluctant to sort papers to find it and we own no filing cabinet. Anyhow, I am precise as to the Biloxi Hospital's record of the Cremation Order, and I also have the Metairie Ridge Cemetary Association's letter to say that my Father's ashes were then sent to New Orleans for interment at Metairie Ridge Cemetary, where my grandparents, Mr and Mrs O M Dunn lately of New Orleans are buried.

And I have further confirmation of the interment of his ashes by Mrs Melissa Whitehead Dunn's brother-in-law, whose address in 1947 was 931 Nashville Avenue, New Orleans. He took charge of my Father's ashes on their arrival in New Orleans and had them interred on behalf of my father's widow, Mrs Melissa Whitehead Dunn, but when I wrote to ask him to explain why his sister-in-law had refused, apparently, to reply to my letters to her, he said, in gist, that this was "none of his business".

All these things are consequences of the war and of the conditions since imposed on Britain and to some degree I gather in the States. We cannot sell our house, it would be giving it away, and we will not. We would just be in the street, literally.

Can you advise me on any step that will end a silence so inane, which, however, is dangerous as an incitement to libel.

Mrs Melissa Whitehead Dunn may have been intimidated in some way, as a result of real ignorance of Law.

May I have at the very least the acknowledgment of the receipt of this letter by whoever does receive it - the Probate Court I hope, if there is such a Court in the Federal District.

I consider silence in itself almost a crime with the world in such continual upheaval as it has been since 1939. And that I will be deeply appreciative of any sort of human response to an appeal which has been iterated to exhaustion ever since 1947, will, I hope be comprehended.

I know Mr Metcalfe will also take it in good part to have me assisted to the truth as soon as may be.

Respectfully Yours,

(Mrs John Metcalfe) Evelyn Dunn Scott Metcalfe
neé Elsie Dunn
legal authors signature Evelyn Scott

[Typed carbon copy, signed. UTK]

To Evelyn Scott

Office of Register of Wills and Clerk of the Probate Court
United States District Court for the District of Columbia
Washington, DC

October 16, 1951

Dear Madam:

Referring to your letter of October 3, 1951, you are advised that an examination of the records of this office fails to disclose that a Will of Seely Dunn, deceased, who you state died in May 1944, has been filed herein or that Letters of Administration have ever been applied for upon his estate.

For your further information, you are advised that only the estates of deceased persons who died either a resident of the District of Columbia or who left property in the District of Columbia are of record in this office. Inasmuch as each state has its own separate probate authority, it is suggested, therefore, that in order to obtain the information desired by you, it will be necessary for you to ascertain the name of the city, county and state in which the decedent was a resident at the time of his death and then correspond with the Register of Wills or Surrogate of such city, county and state.

Very respectfully
[Illeg signature]
DEPUTY Register of Wills
Clerk of the Probate Court

[Typed on official letterhead, signed. UTK]

To Evelyn Scott

Office of Register of Wills and Clerk of the Probate Court
United States District Court for the District of Columbia
Washington, DC

December 7, 1951

Dear Madam:

In response to your letter of November 21, 1951, in further reference to the estate of Seely Dunn, deceased, you are advised that this office can add nothing to our previous letter (dated October 16th, 1951). An examination of the records of this office still fails to disclose that a Will of the said Seely Dunn, deceased, has been filed herein or that Letters of Administration have ever been applied for upon his estate.

Very respectfully
Theodore Cogswell
Register of Wills, Clerk of the Probate Court

[Typed on official letterhead, signed. UTK]

To Evelyn Scott

Chancery Court
Harrison County, Mississippi
Gulfport, Miss

December 10, 1951

Dear Madam:

After checking our records from 1944 to the present date we can find no trace of an estate proceedings in our county concerning your father, Seely Dunn.

Very truly yours,
Margaret Edwards
Deputy Chancery Clerk

[Typed on official letterhead, signed. UTK]

Chapter 26

An inheritance is lost
Spring 1947 - December 1951

Seely's second wife, Melissa Whitehead, married Seely shortly after Maude travelled to Brazil to join Cyril and Evelyn. She was said to be a work colleague of Seely's (there are hints that she had been his secretary), was not much older than Evelyn, and the two women had never met. Although there is no direct evidence in any of the correspondence to support this, it is easy to deduce that a reason for Seely's decision to divorce Maude was his wish to marry his young colleague, Melissa Whitehead.

The following sequence includes references to Maude "causing trouble". This refers to events of 1915, when Seely sent Maude to Brazil to look after Evelyn and her new baby, and soon after divorced her, in her absence, on grounds of "desertion". It was feared that Maude would seek some form of financial support from Seely, and as a result Seely was anxious that his whereabouts were not known to Maude's extended family. In the event, Evelyn and Cyril took financial responsibility for Maude and later, after they were no longer able to do so, Maude became the responsibility of her Clarksville cousins, with whom she lived until her death in 1940.

To Andre Chenet

26 Belsize Crescent
London NW3
[May 1947]

Mr Andre Chenet
New Orleans, Louisiana
Dear Mr Chenet,

I learned of the death of my father, Mr Seely Dunn, a year ago, when attempting, as I have on several previous occasions since the commencement of the as yet inexplicable silence antedating his death, to locate him as living. And it has taken all this while to receive confirmation of the place of his interment, and to learn that you, as Melissa's brother-in-law, had charge of the disposition of his ashes at Metairie Cemetary, New Orleans.

And as I have written Melissa four registered letters, of which three were, I am sure, correctly addressed, and must have reached her, and she has answered none of them, I judge her, for reasons as yet to be specified, to be unfriendly. And I therefore appeal here, to you, as possibly taking a more detached view of conduct towards me, on her part, and that of my father (originally a most scrupulous man) which has caused me great distress, to assist me toward a human elucidation of what is behind her attitude, and whether or not it reflected his, and what his actually was.

When I last saw my father face to face in 1925, he was friendly and affectionate; and though Melissa was not in Washington when I stayed a night or two at their Kay Street flat, I was told she was not well, and at some sanatorium, and nothing whatever occurred to throw light on my father's subsequent failure to reply to letters sent to his place of business; as we did not quarrel, and I had already, in 1919, been duly "forgiven" for any discomfort he may have suffered as a result of my having "run away" from home.

But as I am not unimaginative about other people's troubles, I quite realize that the explanation of yourself or any personal friend of my father's, may completely alter my view of what seems to have taken place; and to that I look forward. *Tell Melissa my father was so afraid of "yellow journalism" when he stayed in NY (1925) he registered at Earls Hotel off Washington Square as "Captain O'Neil" and became panicky when I was visited by a friend who was a "feature-writer" but not of "yellow" journalism.*[184]

The name of my first husband, from whom I am divorced, was legally changed to Scott, and my son, who was originally named for my father, dropped Seely for Creighton, as I dropped "Elsie" for Evelyn; and while my father and Melissa knew this, the fact that we all suffered something as the butt of "yellow journalists", when I ran away from home, may have been an ingredient in a "mystery" to me highly painful; and may have something to do with the failure of Melissa to inform the Biloxi hospital of my existence and ask them to notify me of his illness, as of his death. And all these things I am taking into account, in an effort to be just, although I admit I feel somewhat "ill-used" *and Melissa should realize even in New Orleans we are what is called distinguished people.*

I acknowledge a "posthumous" clearing of the air cannot be the same as if my father were living, but it is, nonetheless, something for which I would be very grateful, indeed.

Sincerely yours,

Did not respond or admit he "buried" my father's ashes—acknowledged this letter and no more. This version of pen most accurate word by word as other

---

184 Evelyn and Cyril's "elopement" precipitated a flurry of interest in the so-called "yellow press", mainly newspapers owned by William Randolph Hearst. This coverage appears to have caused her family and Cyril's considerable distress.

letter mailed before I put the pen emendations here but this is approximate and has all the gist of the first minus to crossed and equivalents.

[Typed carbon copy, not signed. Handwritten annotations. UTK]

To Andre Chenet

26 Belsize Crescent

October 30, 1947

I think you are the Mr Chenet in question, but wishing to preserve an accurate record of this correspondence, I ask, in case of error, for the return to me of my letter to my present address I am a US citizen but my husband is British, domiciled in USA which he has recently visited to maintain his status, as a quota-re-entrant, and we are here for the time

Sir,

Having learned by the merest chance, in an effort to re-contact as living, my father, the late Mr Seely Dunn of Lynchburg, Va, at one time a resident of New Orleans, that he had died, in 1944; I have been for the better part of a year writing officials and others who seemed likely sources of information regarding his illness, place of death, place of internment, his executors, and the present whereabouts of his second wife, Mrs Melissa Whitehead Dunn. And I have just been informed, by the Deputy Clerk of the Civil District Court of the Parish of Orleans, who has been most generous in his efforts on my behalf, that, according to the advice given him, a Mr Chenet he believes to be yourself, as your phone number was also given him, had charge of arrangements for the interment of my father at Metairie Ridge Cemetary.

I am the daughter of Mr Seely Dunn, and as far as I know, his only child, his first marriage having been to my mother, Mrs Maud Thomas Dunn of Clarksville, Tennessee, from whom he was divorced , and who died in Clarksville in1940. And while I have for many years, been much distressed and perplexed by the conduct of my father, always previously scrupulous and responsible, in not having replied to letters written him at his early business addresses, I cannot yet believe that the neglect to notify me when he became seriously ill was his intention; and it seems to me entirely out of character - his character - that he should have done this. And I continue convinced he must have remembered me in some way in his Will or elsewhere, and therefore hope that, his executors once located, a distressing situation can be cleared up.

I saw my father face to face, last, in 1925, in Washington and in New York, and he was friendly and affectionate, and send me, afterwards, a check for fifty dollars, for which I had not asked. And though I have realized the fact that I had the entire moral responsibility for my mother, and supported her, with some assistance from relatives and my husband (my first husband, Mr Cyril Kay Scott and my present husband both actually), probably disturbed his conscience, he was never reproached by me, and must have known I continued fond of him.

If therefore you are the Mr Chenet in question, and did actually arrange my father's funeral, I hope you will respond to this with the information to which I have a human and legal right.

However, if the explanation exists, we will all be most grateful to have it, as I am sure, would my own grandfather, Mr O M Dunn, who lived in New Orleans for more than half his life, and who was a bond of sympathy between me and my father, as we both admired him as "the salt of the earth" - something said of many people but in this case merely just.

Hoping for an early reply from you, and that it will be one to relieve my natural concern, I am,

Very truly yours

[Typed carbon copy, not signed. UTK]

To Melissa Whitehead Dunn

26 Belsize Crescent
October 3, 1951

Dear Melissa:

Will you, in case you have actually received the four letters sent by me to this address, one forwarded by the Lynchburg Postmaster, and possibly, a fifth letter I requested the "Veterans' Bureau" "Department of Claims, etc" to send on - in case you have every one of these letters, or even ONE of them, won't you please emerge from your silence and make some moderately human gesture in elucidation of why you did not tell the "Veterans' Facility", when my Father was ill and dying, that I was his daughter and should know something of his death and his estate.

Will you tell me anything whatever? You know something of my candour and you must have realized I would not just meekly accept a stand on your part superficially "irrational" as my Father himself identified me when Cyril applied in 1923 for the Permanent Scott Family Passport and he-my Father, the late Mr Seely Dunn of Washington at one time - signed the application, and it is absurd to be aware as I think you must have been that my Father has been on record as my Father since 1914 or 1915 when my Mother came to Brazil to "visit" us and registered as Maud Thomas Dunn (Mrs Seely Dunn) at the American Consulate in Recife the day she landed from the Lamport and Holt steamer.

It was in Recife that Cyril with my agreement took the first step toward the establishment of the Common Law Marriage which we had decided was the one solution since his second wife in New Orleans would not, then, as yet, divorce him, though long afterward - a few years, we gathered - she did.

You know all these things and that every word I have said about any of these official steps is the truth and that our Common Law Marriage was re-established in the States with our documented re-acceptance as a family and our documented change of name: not a change by deed-pole but by usage.

We must be accepted as we are, as having taken the steps we did for the motives actually ours, which were accepted until this damnable war seemed to re-poison American and British minds. And I have brought up the date business because I cannot think of anything else that you could possibly have been exploited to alarm either you or my Father about our relationship.

Maybe I am just "telling you something" - if so well and good. I do not and never did like any sort of concealment, and that you and my Father began in Lynchburg with what may have been merely as a social lie in denying my existence, has resulted in humiliations, implied insults from every quarter, and I really don't know what else, as myself and my second husband John Metcalfe have been stuck here in Britain with just enough money to keep us actually in food, and literally no more, ever since he was demobilized.

We have been immolated, Creighton and his wife and children have been nearly so we are allowed to think and it must be so, and this is probably as true of Cyril who is I am certain basically unchanged, though we do not hear from him and his Wellman son does not answer letters, or else does not receive them.

Anyone with an atom of sense should realize that to communicate with myself and Jack normally is to stop libel, and that to be silent, is to foment it. So it may be your letters - Melissa - have been sent to me and I never got them. *My daughter-in-law says I do not receive elucidating letters sent by her here.*

Will you please acknowledge this as suits you

Evelyn-Elsie

[Typed carbon copy, signed. Handwritten insertion. UTK]

To Evelyn Scott
Office of Register of Wills and Clerk of the Probate Court
United States District Court for the District of Columbia
Washington, DC

December 7, 1951

Dear Madam:

In response to your letter of November 21, 1951, in further reference to the estate of Seely Dunn, deceased, you are advised that this office can add nothing to our previous letter (dated October 16th, 1951). An examination of the records of this office still fails to disclose that a Will of the said Seely Dunn, deceased, has been filed herein or that Letters of Administration have ever been applied for upon his estate.

Very respectfully
Theodore Cogswell
Register of Wills, Clerk of the Probate Court

[Typed on official letterhead, signed. UTK]

To Evelyn Scott
Chancery Court
Harrison County, Mississippi
Gulfport, Miss

December 10, 1951

Dear Madam:

　　After checking our records from 1944 to the present date we can find no trace of an estate proceedings in our county concerting your father, Seely Dunn.

Very truly yours,
Margaret Edwards
Deputy Chancery Clerk

[Typed on official letterhead, signed. UTK]

The finality of this letter put a seal on Evelyn's search for her father's will and her inheritance.

Chapter 27

Life in London
September 1947 - September 1952

Evelyn and Jack were enduring a life of bleak poverty in post-war London, and Evelyn's letters vividly convey their difficulties. These letters are lengthy and sometimes incoherent, possibly because Evelyn, alone all day and unable to go out due to her proclaimed lack of suitable clothing, filled the time by doing what she knew best, writing.

These years in London were largely occupied by Evelyn's attempts to procure agreements to publish her collection of half-finished books; with their poverty and her dependence on friends for their donations of clothes (and she was very particular about what she wanted); with her dental problems and her general health; with her anti-Semitic views (a number of Jewish refugees had settled in that part of London); and with the nuisance caused by local children invading their garden. These all figure in her letters of this period but have not been included because this account focuses on her primary concern: making contact (never successfully) with her son and her grandchildren.

To Evelyn Scott

Eastham, Massachusetts
September 6 [1947]

Dear Evelyn: -

I hope you got the $50 in time. The mails are so slow and your letter had to also be forwarded from NY.

The reason I seem so unresponsive and do not answer your letters is because I am anyway rather confused politically and of course do not know the situation in England at first hand as you do, but my sympathies, as you must surely know by now, are with the Labor Party in general, and here in USA with the Socialist Party, so there really is not much that I can say. As for the world of arts and letters, I certainly agree with you that it is in a woeful state, but I do not know what I, as a Philistine, can do about it except to buy the books and the paintings that I like and to protest that this and that are not published or exhibited. My protests are, of course, entirely futile, as I am not a figure or a force in those worlds and have absolutely no chance of appearing authoritative, natch.

As for Jig, that is a personal matter about which I am also entirely incompetent, as I do not even know where he lives, and letters I have written to him in the past, merely friendly, neighborly letters, have gone unacknowledged. Harrison[185] has clear and friendly recollections of Jig and frequently says he would like to get in touch with him but it appears to be quite impossible. *She knows why I ceased to see them and I should think someone could have relieved my anxiety about taking "sides". Margaret is included in all I say of Jig—details different that's all why guess*

Anyway, as you know, I love and admire you and Jack and do wish things were not so rotten for you. But I think it unfair of you to make your friends responsible for all your troubles. People really DO still protest, but the forces are such that their voices simply are smothered.

Margaret DeS

They should have some sense about Jig. These silences cannot be an advantage to him, they are a painful embarrassment Jig is fine of spirit I say, and certainly they cannot deny he has intellect—his book

[Typed, signed. Handwritten annotations. UTK]

To O C Reynolds

26 Belsize Crescent
October 11, 1947

Mr Oliver C Reynolds
Reynolds, Richards and McCutcheon
Attorneys and Counselors at Law
68 William Street, New York City USA
Dear Sir,

Mrs Margaret De Silver has just written me enclosing the carbon of your original letter of September 22nd, 47, containing draft No D-14306 for $50 dollars drawn on the Central Hanover Bank and Trust Company, 7 Princes Street London, England, at the request of Mrs Margaret De Silver and made out to myself Evelyn Scott.

Your letter and the draft would have been acknowledged earlier, but I did not receive it until about eight days ago and the Bank, when I last called there, on Thursday (this is Saturday) had not yet cleared it, but were sure it was all right and will be cleared when I go there to draw on it or before. As a gift I am sure it is all right, but the longer time it has taken to clear it may have been due to its having been sent to me in my professional name which was my legal name when married to Cyril Kay Scott, and which is still my legal name as regards books contracts and anything of a

---

185 This is likely to be Harrison, or Hal, Smith, who had previously published a number of Evelyn's books.

business nature appertaining to my literary career, but which, incredibly, I have not used officially since I arrived here during the bombing phase of the war, as the literary careers of myself and my husband have been very much interrupted until recently.

However, we are beginning to re-establish ourselves normally, and while Mrs De Silver has apologized for having sent the draft that way, she need not have done so, as after all, the preservation of my continuity as a writer in an official as well as unofficial way is important to me, and especially as my son Creighton is also a Scott.

The draft was deposited in the account of my present husband W J Metcalfe, who is John Metcalfe the British author and publishes in the USA.

Thanking you for having sent Mrs De Silver's generous and appreciated gift.

Very truly yours

I am very explicit, because I dislike "pokers, pryers and snoopers", and if it is actually true, as is published in the papers, that the Government reads your mail, I just think it best to tell everything relevant.

[Typed carbon copy, not signed. UTK]

To Margaret DeSilver

26 Belsize Crescent
October 11, 1947

My dear Mag,

The Reynolds, Richards McCutcheon letter with your gift was received by me just a few days after you wrote yourself you were sending it, and is now with the bank, having arrived in the nick of time, when, again, due to "this and that" (and god rot this and that) I had just two pounds cash left to draw on. *1952 - I had not a cent left in the house-literal*

Yes it was the first time (barring five dollars sent once, which insulted me) that I have received any money whatsoever since I have been in England this time. When I was here as a Guggenheim Fellow[186] I cashed checks here of fund money, and when Jack had enough, in Suffolk, he opened an account for me so that whether the money was for my books or his I would not have to consult him about what I spent for personal necessities.

Mag darling, I told you, I would write you more about whats wrong with "this and that", and I am doing so. And my situation as it has been so far is especially unjust as regards Jack himself, on whom has devolved the responsibility for maintaining us both, which he has done impeccably; but it has been often by "odd jobs" which sacrificed the time he requires for creative work; and as normally I earned as much as he did (sometimes one more sometimes the other) also at creative work, there was never a more senseless and inexcusable waste of two talents.

---

186 Evelyn had received a grant from the Guggenheim Foundation in 1932 and, exceptionally, a further grant a year later. These grants were intended as financial support to enable her to write and did not carry any duties with them.

I will go to the Bank again to make sure the gift has been cleared (I went there on Thursday and they thought so, but I didnt try to do anything as to drawing on it), and if it is and I am pretty sure it must be, I will mail this then with my very great and continued affection, because the most important thing to say here really is that you have again done something generous and genuinely good that is just Margaret and thank you very much.

Evelyn

[Typed carbon copy, typed signature. Handwritten annotation. UTK]

To Louise Morgan

26 Belsize Crescent
August 13, 1948

[First page(s) missing] Standing as regards clothes any one of these acceptable and every one needed. I have a pair of slacks and some old blouses for wear indoors. I have a coat ten years old and somewhat out of style for very cold weather (worn but usable if not smart)

I have not a pair of shoes - brown or black or both very acceptable, size five-and-a-half c last, for highish heel dress, five d last for a tennis or heelless shoe (and in espadrilles I wore four and a half). I like low or moderate heels (very high, tire) wear sandals indoors when I have them, and though having no dressy shoes, would still find good black grey or brown evening shoes second-hand acceptable, as of possible use with all future dress (have an old blue dressing gown and no slippers, by the way).

I have no moderate weight or light coat, nothing for moderate winter weather or coolish summer fall or spring; and either a sports coat or a dressy coat (or of course both) would be most welcome - size thirty-six bust gives a good coat shoulder (the best jacket shoulder is thirty-four, but usually the skirt measures dont, being larger in waist, and longer in skirt than a misses size) - and as <u>becomingness is as important as warmth</u>, I may say, that I can wear to advantage brown black sage green medium green (cant wear acid green or bottle green) tan, beige, fawn, and any subdued mixture of tan or beige with green or blue or yellow or orange, or any very small pin-stripe on a tan or brown or fawn base, also russet and deep wine (not bluish) and navy blue, but dont like, and I <u>cant wear</u> (beside bottle and acid green) black-and-white (hideous), white (horrors), very pale fawn (terrible) and though I <u>can</u> wear navy blue, it is not really becoming, just passable, and lacks interest when you have few clothes as it is more difficult than brown black and beige to combine with various other colours, cant wear grey (atrocious).

I have no suit except one bought in 1938 and darned, as well as demode, the skirt conspicuously short. So a coat suit would be very very <u>very</u> acceptable; and the range of colour is about the same as for coats, although the matter of combining other colours with it figures more importantly than as regards coats, and I can wear yellow blouses with brown, green blouses with brown, pink and cherry blouses with brown navy blue and black, and pale blue blouses with all three; and, as well, especially with black blouses in any interesting floral strip or check if it is small, the more colours combined in one textile subduedly the more interesting the effect with a plain suit.

I have no dresses whatever; neither for hot or cold weather sports or afternoon or evening, so every sort of dress is a fine fine fine if in style, with a close-fitting blouse or top and a longish, flaring skirt. A black dress with subduedly vivid colour touches, or a black dress with cream (cant wear white touches, hideous), or a dress in a very small and intricate floral pattern on a black brown or green base.

I have not any stockings, I have no underwear nor rags, especially step-ins and bras (a few frayed, 6 slips, all much too short to be of any use now); my stocking size is eight and a half, step-ins with elastic 28 waist without elastic 29, brassieres 34 bust.

I also greatly appreciate elastic step-in girdles without bones but with hose-supporters, price new one dollar and a half, 28 waist, like the step-ins, slips 34 bust.

I have not a hat of any sort, but hats are something you have to buy yourself, in most instances, though sometimes toques or tie-on turbans or comprise headgear can be used second-hand.

Well there is the situation and of course blouses in any of the colours mentioned as becoming would be gratefully received - thirty-four or thirty-six (thirty-four not washable, thirty-four washable).

Slacks eighteen year size (I have a pair, but just one) twenty-nine waist, brown black blue dark (not bottle) green, pin stripes in same, and any material including corduroy which I like very much in most colours.

I dont expect any one source to supply all these, nor do I anticipate a full supply from every available source combined, but it does seem possible some could be acquired and sent over, if I do not over-tax, the generosity of those to whom I appeal.

I didnt mention the evening dress, but if any are going and in the mode, all the better; but I cannot wear a real decolette now, having got too "old and skinny"; and I actually cannot stand the temperature indoors here well enough to wear thin clothes without an evening jacket - so that ingredient is more complicated.

A black brown or green dress, or a black dress with touches of interesting colour, just decolette enough to not - to be mistaken for a "day dress" is what I would buy if I could buy one and with it, either as part of a costume, or as combinable with the dress, a short wrap of the jackety order, with a touch of trimming in colour if it were black, or perhaps if the dress were black the jacket could be one of the becoming colours subdued but contrasting. *[remainder of letter missing]*

[Fragment, typed, not signed. BRBL]

From John Metcalfe's diary:

December 25, 1947: Breakfast. Work. Coffee. Work. Lunch. Felt mouldy and went to bed. Got up again and had tea. Supper of steak. More work at Maths. Cake and bed.
January 28, 1948: Gladys has sent a box of typewriter paper, very welcome;-and the paper is excellent quality.

March 12, 1948: E's teeth troubling her greatly of late.

April 18, 1948: E still very poorly with jaw-ache.

May 10, 1948: Letter to E from B Baumgarten asking E to employ another agent.

June 25, 1948: Letter from Gladys with $50 arrived just as I was leaving for school.

July 12, 1948: Posted letter to Maggie, also letters (3) from E to possible agents.

To Louise Morgan and Otto Theis

26 Belsize Crescent

August 15, 1948

My dear Louise and Otto

I have written to both Lenore Marshall and to Margaret de Silver and shall write to some others, asking them to try and locate friends who will donate me some second-hand clothes in good style, so I can make a front here and get about some. But we cannot pay duty and I can get no assurance that any clothes will reach me really free, and I am therefore trying to find somebody who is coming to England to visit and could bring a few things second-hand with her own clothes (a woman, it would have to be). And as you two have mentioned seeing Americans, and brought the California girl here, I have wondered if yourselves or perhaps Sophie[187] and Ruth might not know somebody who was about to visit England who would be willing to include such gifts for me with their belongings and deliver them on arrival.

It is a favour I dislike asking, but the situation fully justifies it I think; otherwise, I might as well be in prison. I havent even marketed since May. Not a step can I stir from the house under these conditions.

I stress style because I want to put up a good front, and I dont want just "kivver",[188] as per charlady, as that would defeats the real purpose of being decently dressed again, but though it is a lot to ask, I know Sophie is already au courrant with some of the charitable wealthy and as I have written Margaret, Marie Garland supplied me with half a wardrobe of very expensive good quality clothes which were not entirely satisfactory only because I had to have them altered; which I couldnt now afford and which seems about the hardest thing to get done in London there is, judging by our previous experiences in that line.

And so I throw myself on your generosity, for the time - if you can do anything, as I say, well and good and whether you can or not it is very much to be appreciated that I can discuss things with you both with complete candour.

our love

Evelyn

[Typed, signed. BRBL]

---

187 Sophie was Otto's sister; nothing is known about Ruth.

188 Cod Cockney for "cover" or clothing.

From John Metcalfe's diary:

September 13, 1948: Letter from Gladys enclosing $25.

September 24, 1948: E got cheque for $50 from Maggie, which I paid into bank (it was made out to me).

October 14, 1948: Went into town and bought children's book for Denise at Foyles.[189] E got first parcel of clothes from Maggie today.

October 15, 1948: Bought more children's books at Foyles.

October 16: 1948: Further parcel of clothes came for her today from Maggie.

October 29, 1948: E got another parcel of clothes from Maggie.

November 26, 1948: …. also packet of typewriting paper from Gladys.

December 25, 1948: At home all day, working mainly on Scilly novel. Removed teeth after tea, as very sore. Supper of steak. Work. Bed.

March 14, 1949: Got letter from Margaret with $100.

April 4, 1949: In evening found out we had run out of American-size typewriter paper, - and E accordingly depressed.

In 1951 the war had ended some years earlier and post-war austerity was adding to Evelyn and Jack's already considerable poverty. Perhaps it was not surprising that Evelyn reacted to the necessary post-war regulations by conflating them with her own frustration at not hearing from Jigg in spite of her entreaties to mutual friends. Perhaps in these conditions it was almost inevitable that Evelyn came to believe that some force, almost certainly political, was keeping her apart from her son and his young family.

To Gladys Grant

26 Belsize Crescent
April 8, 1951

My dear Glad

It really is a shame that even you misinterpret and misquote me at times. I have never said I "disbelieved" what you say about yourself and Edgerton, Jig and Pavla and Denise, Fredrick and Mathew, or conditions in the States. I have reproached you because you are so seldom explicit and in many instances have ignored queries by me concerning the things of greatest importance to ourselves. Some of this may be due to those damn "via air self-contained envelopes", which dont allow for much explicitness and to which you are, apparently, addicted. I think them a pain-in-the-neck

I will continue to consider it criminal that anybody with the really genuinely superlative fine talent as painter and author which Jig has proved is so forced into that damn machine-pattern. It is stupid beyond anything what America has allowed to be done to the finest of fine arts

---

189 Foyle's bookshop in London was, and still is, one of the largest bookshops in England.

We wish someone in the family and friends such as yourselves would visit here during this damn fair,[190] so we could overcome these handicaps of distance. Could you afford it and would you like to?

We are going to try to do something about the garden wall that fell before very long and whenever I can I hope to have my teeth fixed. But the girding slowness of everything here has been atrocious. The Labour Government is due to fall and here's hoping again SOON. Our idea of the best Government is one that Governs least and we are convinced the public is continually more of our mind than it was five years ago - damn it! [remainder of letter missing]

[Typed carbon copy, unsigned. UTK]

To Margaret DeSilver

26 Belsize Crescent
April 29, 1951

Maggie my dear

Your harping again on my supposed feeling of "injury" because you helped other people is tommyrot and you know it. I contradicted it twice and fully explained to you how gratuitously you were misinterpreting me. So please dont. You sound like Marie Garland when she said something or other as unjust and when I objected said, "The truth hurts!" Dont forget that lies hurt genuine people much more than truth ever could. You should know this yourself Maggie as you are genuine. I think that "truth hurts" fallacy is a hang-over from "psycho-analysis". It is an over-simplification that is just too easy and works like a gag. And gags are precisely what none of us can afford.

But what I am especially writing to say is that your apology for its being a small check has some compensation in the thought that you will be out of New York often. You havent said where your new "shack" is on the Cape, but I hope you have real refreshment there and that it isnt in the hackneyed place were "everybody" goes. I also hope there are no "dialectical Jews" or hyper-reactionaries who dont like our sort and make letters hard. I am as certain as ever that when you write to me somewhat unkindly, as you do occasionally, some sort of snooper is in the offing and has suggested a prejudiced frame of mine.

We think you are the very good friend you really are and we are affectionately disposed both of us anyhow.

The spring is here in the garden and when some of that ebullience is evident in the book world we will feel it is appropriate. We hope the Government here falls and there are other approaches to solutions for the world mess.

---

190 During the summer of 1951, and partly to mark the centenary of the Great Exhibition of 1851, the British government mounted the Festival of Britain, designed to showcase British post-war achievement. It was a hugely ambitious undertaking and drew large numbers of visitors to London.

There are wild cherries blooming all across the front of the garden this year and they are lovely. Last year an hydrangea in front near the steps had over a hundred blooms on it at once and no care whatever - it just grew "miraculously". The blooms did not fade until well into December. Pavla and Jig should have a garden for the children. They havent any where they are and are still looking for better quarters with less kitchen and more real living space.

Jig was ill in France and Gladys reports he is thinner. I am glad of the thinner but it is distressing I was not allowed to receive any word from him when he was ill - some sort of post office high jinks between France and Britain.

Jack is still marvellous but it mustnt go on like this. We are the same as banned and suppressed here too, so far. Jack has not had any vacation since 1939. He taught all through "Easter holidays" again and he is tired.

Love and best

Evelyn

[Typed carbon copy, typed signature. UTK]

To Gladys Grant

26 Belsize Crescent

May 20, 1951

My dear Glad

If I went into the chronology of our correspondence and you yourself read over my file of letters and questions and your replies and these dates of these indicating the time between my writing and your answers you would not say I was unreasonable. I am not. However, I dont see why you should have interpreted this as "mistrust" of yourself. It is mistrust of a policy of evasiveness regarding most specific facts which seems to have become pervasive in America, like a sort of contagion. But I have never blamed you yourself, nor do I specifically blame the many others who have followed a policy of never replying to me or whose letters - so I know in a few instances, were either lost in the PO, confiscated thee under some pretext of "censoring" - wrong I think in communications to Britain - or were not delivered here because of factionalism in the PO either in the States or Britain.

Our finances here are as dire as ever. Jack has never been as discouraged as recently. He just hasnt had the heart to write. And that is criminal. We do not want to be reduced to "turning on the gas", but we would rather than be shoved from pillar to post by such conditions as the government here-probably dominated by uno's[191] extremists - have imposed on us. We will not be paupers. And that is that. But we cant merely "exist", and in order to live at all require both cash at once and the restoration of our raison detre in specific terms of art.

---

191 This is a reference to the United Nations Organization, later the United Nations. Evelyn clearly did not think much of them.

Show the first page of this letter to Jig and Pavla if you like and I am writing to them too, but PLEASE DO NOT TELL THEM OF OUR FINAL DESPERATION AT ANY TIME. We love them too much to wish to distress them knowing positively as we do they really care and would help if they could. It would be shameful to trouble them with this fact. I just think somebody in the States should realize where we are and so I tell you

You are our good friend Glad or I would not confide. I am very clear in distinguishing you and your character from surroundings and such changes in the States as have been for the worst. The competence of generals in military spheres is one thing and important no doubt, but there are problems at home there as there are here which require the first attention and get very little.

Our very real love to you and everything good and genuine to yourself. I appreciate every one of your helpful moves.

[Typed carbon copy, not signed. UTK]

To Creighton Scott

26 Belsize Crescent

May 20, 1951

1952 - This letter may have been acknowledged in one of the letters mentioned by Pavla as apparently not delivered in London.

Darling Jiggie

I write you two pieces of comparative good news: one is I have re-registered at the American Consulate so my citizenry is not in jeopardy, and the other is that my third go at Escape Into Living has I think succeeded. The novel is now complete and clear I am convinced and we are eager to tell you and Pavla of at least this much we consider hopeful.

I have given your Rutherford address as our to the Consulate so if ever there are moves to better houses please tell us. However, we are glad to hear Rutherford according to Gladys is working out well for the children and that the health of everybody has improved. I cannot too often reiterate that my concern for Jigs over-weight was a concern for his health. He looked handsome but I know what is normal for him and I have worried about it.

I still kick over almost never hearing from either of you. I think you must surely have written further occasionally and I will not feel at ease in this regard until I get Jigs own letter and Pavlas also.

Gladys is somewhat given to glossing my real cause for distress on this score but she has behaved like a human being and not an utter brute, and has written me something about yourselves and the children. *[remainder of letter missing]*

[Typed carbon copy, not signed. Handwritten annotation. UTK]

To May Mayers

26 Belsize Crescent
May 27, 1951

My dear May

Jack and myself grow increasingly desperate about getting home to the States - we will just die here as a result of "economy" unless something is done for our books there. I call it murder. We have been economically exiled and it is preposterous to say we were ever allowed any choice about it. We may move before long to cheaper quarters and sublet this flat - once it is repaired - but we are still having to mend the garden wall that collapsed last summer, and the law about taking out money should we sell it would have to be abolished for any sort of sale to be worthwhile - it couldnt be very profitable in any case unless the mortgage were paid off. Ill let you know if and when we move.

Well you will see that the financial pressures that have compelled us to remain in a veritable slough of despond, unable to buy more than postage stamps and certainly not boat fares, are scarcely to be classified as our "choice". Dont forget that when Jack went over in 1947 to maintain his quota and tried to get a job to bring me over there - me born there - he didnt succeed and had one substantial offer after he was on en route home. Jack is qualified to teach as very few of those who "thrive" in our robot system of "education" are, but it cut no ice. He is honours in philosophy University of London and has also much experience in teaching higher mathematics and every sort.

We just go on fighting and hoping so please you do too.

Affectionately

[Typed carbon copy, not signed. UTK]

To Gladys Grant

26 Belsize Crescent
[July, 1951]

You ask me of friends in London Jack recently called on Louise and Otto whom we had not seen for a year and a half and who - Louise - were rude to insult when last seen, and no notice was taken, *they were out but could have I think* though they know of our poverty and distress of every sort - "friends", for sooth. Faugh! I have none and Jack few. Not in England - not since we ceased to be celebrities here

My dear Glad

I appreciate your longer letter which arrived this morning, though I wish its length were more informative as to facts and more cheerful as to yourselves and ourselves. I just know you gave time to it and that time is precious, and the impulse good, although I go on disagreeing as unshakably as ever with what you say about people who have congenialities among you as we have among some old. I dont consider generations have anything to do with obstacles to rapprochements. They are imposed mostly by conditions in which age is made to seem to figure, and doesnt. I have no doubt whatever that Creighton and Pavla and Jack and myself are congenial just as we originally were - which is very - and I dare hazard a guess this is the truth about Edgerton and you.

But those dirty rackets dont know art from hay - and that Jig was of the highest talent cut no ice. All to them were "dirty daubers". I think they were Nazis, too, some from the samples of the new incursions into New York that came to look at our flat when Jig and I were in Commerce Street and Jack here on a visit. They were as contemptuous of him and myself - these interlopers - when asking about the flat I tried to sub-let, and though they had strong German accents as likely as not they were New Yorks prime police grafters and army grafters, already by the time war actually began.

However, again, I dont agree that I should just take it Jig and Pavla stopped writing because they didnt want to write. They were placed in such an unfair position that it seemed, for the moment, useless. Again I say, why did Jig come to London? - because he cares for us. Was Jig a hypocrite in being affectionate and good here? - NO! And Id like to smash whoever implies such a falsehood.

Our situation is desperate, yes. We have been as if banned for eleven years, and all that time taunted about age as a handicap, while each year getting older and not allowed to publish yet.

Yes, there may be congenial people here, but when you cannot leave the house because of lack of first dress, then stockings, and now teeth - to be fixed - you dont meet anybody. Beside the British are cold in some regards and you have to know them well, and Jack and I have been libelled here as well as there.

This country is church-run religious dilemma and the author of <u>Escapade</u> has not been published here since 1934.

Unless something is done to finance our return to the States in the States, where money cannot be grabbed by this British Government we will die here, never see any of them, and be murdered in compelled exile. I am appealing again to everybody we know. We cannot go on - not so much as another year. We are being driven from this house, and the house debts dont diminish.[192] The wall that collapsed and took twice the money earned by the lodger who made writing impossible most of the time, was recently mended and can be slowly paid for we hope. But the day the wall was finished Gumbs[193] electro collapsed to some extent and the price of repair is the price of the wall - or near it - 22 pounds.

Jack is not young either now. He is worn out physically by teaching small and some defective children year after year in vacation as well as term, and the staleness of it, the absence of any incentive or raison detre, you will grasp. We are both at low par in every sense and have not advanced one penny toward our goal in recovered and re-established earnings as publishing authors. So wish inertias in any wealth quarter

---

192 Chapter 34 describes the finances relating to Jack's house in detail.
193 The Gumbs were tenants.

could be overcome on our behaviour that some foundation not a total hoax could be found and money supplied for our return and maintenance for at least a year.

DONT DONT DONT please PLEASE send ham! What good is damn belly-stuffing to us when we are deprived of every human reason for being. Our appetites are good, but it is worse than wicked that so many Americans are incited to think Britain needs nothing but groceries, and culture going to pot doesnt matter. It is a criminal misapprehension deliberately disseminated in the States. At least six or seven friends appealed to for books and typewriter paper, have ignored appeal and sent grub. NO.

Love to them and to yourself

[Typed carbon copy, not signed. Handwritten insertion. UTK]

To May Mayers

26 Belsize Crescent
August 6, 1951

Dear May

I think we have just had an orgy of rotten cross-purpose mail.

I was obliged to allow my teeth to get in bad condition because I lacked clothes shoes stockings - one summer it was one thing, one another,and because it is humiliating in an atmosphere of rah-bottoming all the time admit to the lack of such necessities as Jack and I have had to, every so often. The teeth were loose and I often shifted most of them with my finger. But when it came to pulling, there was more difficulty. They were hard to pull, and at moments no amount of whatever they use in the gums effected the normal deadening. And when finally this was really achieved - and May will remember the codeine that wouldnt work, though it was many years since I sometimes had to take syrup of codeine in Brazil when I was ill - when the essential deadening of pain was accomplished, I was given a temporary plate that as a fit is the cats pyjamas.

It was cast from the teeth that were all loose and out of their natural position. I originally had regular teeth. The plate first made in Santa Fe for two front that abscessed fell and broke and always dangled a little. The second plate made because it broke didnt fit and I never wore it if I could help it. But the effect was approximately that of my originally nice teeth which were often remarked as I grew up as like those of my father the late Seely Dunn, whose teeth were really noted as perfection - as anybody who knew him thirty years ago and they will confirm this.

This bloody plate makes me nearly vomit - not aesthetically but literally - it is such a bad fit. But is it probably a job-lot "type" of plate and I am now determined that the dentist make the permanent plate disregarding the teeth he pulled - of which he showed me the marks on the misfit, as if that proved anything. It certainly explains the misfit.

So now I am as shut up as ever, because, damn it, I have no teeth except a few underpinnings below.

The other issue I have in mind is birth-control which just must be made legally available and guaranteed as authentic in the States. You know the love one has for ones family insists on it, and not that maligning reverse dirty opponents try to put forward as argument - decent normal humans should not be asked to "choose" between trappist sanctums,[194] like Tom Mertons, and normal sex life conjugal or not. Has anybody recently resumed agitation for voluntary birth-control - voluntary birth-control to save the parents. Parents have some rights in the world, or would if criminals didnt butt in. We dont butt in, like crooks. We would like to see them all more than just surviving. It may sound nice to be a bloody "family tree" but individuals mean most and adult individuals must be first in decisions. Heres hoping. Accidental sterilization I know of, and no harm results for women. Voluntary however and not tote imposed.

Pavla is not a cow her health is the first consideration and her decision but the public issue is for everyone. *[Remainder of letter missing]*

[Typed carbon copy, not signed. UTK]

To Creighton and Paula Scott

26 Belsize Crescent
August 4, 1952

Darlings-

Whether you say so or not, I think you both will be interested in the happenings connected with this house and our continued hope that we may return home to the USA in the autumn or early winter.

I have written explicitly of the horrible rot and fungus, and these had a blow - thank goodness - in the concrete floors that now replace the boards in the rooms attacked. But as I explained, the shelter[195] was demolished to supply rubble as a basis for the concrete. And though this has improved the spaciousness of the flat to such a point Jig would be delighted should he see it now, it is so much a contrast to the dungeon-like hall of 1949, the results again, have not been all we wished.

The damaged walls in this flat which were cracked during bombings had just been repaired in 1949, when, although we observed a somewhat cursory attitude toward work, we hoped these specific repairs were final. Now, however, the slighter reappearance of the same cracks in 1950, has become extreme. The first repair lasted precisely ten months, as far as smooth walls want. But until the shelter was torn down, a month ago, or thereabouts, we had at least tried to persuade ourselves that the place was nearly rentable as it was, and that the cracks though again apparent ever since the autumn of 1950, could not endanger anything and might be left for a second mending whenever the tenants we would like had the flat re-decorated.

---

194 Evelyn is referring to Thomas Merton having entered a Trappist monastery.
195 During WWII almost all dwellings in London and other main centres had rudimentary air raid shelters (Anderson shelters). Most were buried in gardens, but some were constructed within the fabric of the house as was the case in No 26.

Probably the cursory mends of 1949 were insufficient where both the partitions between the living-room and bath-room and the bath-room and toilet had cracked through during bomb hits; and the shelter, with its brick walls which were over a foot thick, was supporting some of the weight of structure which, with its demolition, fell too heavily on the cursory repairs. There is no sagging anywhere. External walls are intact, but because of the re-appearance in two partitions of exactly the same cracks - one extending across the bathroom ceiling as well - these parts of the flat are again not in condition to let. Neither the Carnegies five hundred nor a small sum sent by Margaret from the fund for me intended to finance our travel home, will cover these new mends, and that restoration to at least some of the windows of the iron bars removed from the front gate by the borough during the war; a removal said to be necessary to afford exit to the basements occupants during raids, but one for which we should have had indemnity, as trespassing - as I have said - began then; compelled me to close windows to be safe from theft, and it is now generally conceded that a shut house plays hell as to rot.

And so my darlings we are still on the spot. Please dont misconstrue my explicit accounts of happenings here as due to any lack of commensurate interest in happenings wherever you six are at any time. But I decided, after Jigs visit, that I would go on writing fully of everything just as is most normal to me, regardless of a superficial paucity of mail some would misinterpret as indifference. I know it is NOT indifference, and that eventually I will have your own personal explanation.

Has the parcel of second-hand clothing arrived? I hope it is there before Pavlas birthday. I never forget it, and I must say second-hand clothes is not the gift I should have liked to send. But some of it may be useful and it does show we think of you all. Anything that is not appropriate Pavla can chuck out if she likes and no one will be in the least hurt. Just remember, however, that good will produced these clothes as gifts to me and love goes with them now. To see you Jig, you Pavla, and the four children is one of our incentives continuing to fight - but it must be as the individual creative minds we really are. And whenever we win in this, I know you will all six benefit to some extent.

Love doesn't falter

Our love—Mother to Jig—your loving Evelyn to Pavla Jack's love with mine to you both and four kids.

[Typed carbon copy, signed. UTK]

To Creighton and Paula Scott

26 Belsize Crescent

September 1, 1952

NB—I have recently had two letters—one NY one [?] which alluded to me as the "owner" of an "apartment house" hence too plutocratic to need help!—really huh?

Darling Jig and Pavla:

Please, wont you, acknowledge the parcel of second-hand clothes that was sent to you, chiefly to see if there was anything in it that could be cut down to fit Denise - though two or three of the longer dresses may be of use to Pavla, we hope - sent to you now more than a month ago, at the address above. *NB the PS on this page about libelling us as "wealthy" refers to a rumour of some sort that was circulated as soon as Margaret began trying to help finance our going home to the USA —I call that meanness of a base sort! —Seven years of penury here and that! like your mss oblige much baggage*

They were in good condition when sent and I hope arrived so. I have had very little opportunity to wear the second-hands sent by friends who know of the injustice we have suffered since the war in the-so-far-nearly total suppression of our books, with its consequences in a poverty that has reinforced a further injustice in respect to Jacks nominal ownership of this small[196] Church of England property and the house in which the rents have remained frozen since the early years of the war.

We are very eager to see you both in the USA when we return, and we have NOT lost hope, though, at the moment we are stuck again and in a state of suspended animation once more, because the help provided both by Margaret De Silver in the generous attempt being made by the friends of our books, ourselves and you both in spirit, is so far not enough to allow Jack to clear up taxes and debts and to complete refurbishing of this flat to such a point as will permit of its advertisement for rent.

I gave you both the full account of the disaster of rot in the two floors that had to be demolished; and explained then that the shelter that had blocked the dining-room-hall during ten years because we never had enough money to have it removed, had, also, been torn down that the rubble resulting might go into the new concrete.

The result is good, as far as it goes, as I have said, too, in an earlier letter. The reception hall is now of a size to be the dining room it also originally was. The large table that had been buried in the shelter during its construction, was taken out at last - as it could not be through the shelters narrow door - and has been oiled and polished and mended both by myself and the builder who is helpful in these small ways as well as large, and chairs are all that we now lack. The curtains - sash curtains new - are now made for every window except the French window - where half are up. The older inside curtains used at night have all but one pair been washed by me. The large rug also buried in the shelter and half ruined is now being re-made into a much smaller rug moderately sound and for the dining-room. The armchair I re-upholstered myself looks very pretty, but awaits money to buy kapok to finish the cushion. The dressing-table the builder cut down for me from an old RAF hutment table has been enamelled

---

196 No 26 was actually a generously sized Edwardian house on four stories.

white by me, and lacks just paint for the mirror to stand on it and for the stool I contrived of a box to go with it. And the one big thing lacking yet is money to do something to the living room wall and to do a few brick mends outdoors in connection with keeping drains clear. *Distemper*[197] *would re-transform the living room which has again a dilapidated look.* There are also three old chairs - not dining room - yet to be mended as I cannot, and every door and the French windows has to be made so it will lock - inside several are swollen. We would like, as well, to put bars at all the windows and have now restored them at four. And it would be much better, as a warning against trespassers to restore the front gate that was confiscated as war metal about 1941.[198]

The indoor work except distemper for living room walls where damage crack appeared to get the flat in order would cost comparatively little - I should add to the above several pounds for paint as I myself proposed to re-touch wainscots here and there, and to make some lamp bases for table lamps - all there are are broken - by filling appropriate receptacles with sand and painting them. This necessitates lamp shades, but these are not expensive. *A couch cover in Jack's study for a double sommier is as needed. We need baggage mended some bright [?] for mss and many small essentials for travel—so do you probably*

I realize YOUR OWN PROBLEMS darling children, as I tell you of ours. But it is because we must rent the flat to be able to show we have something somewhere to distinguish us from penniless that we are so eager to re-do the flat. The rentals should be designated transferable and we hope they will be, though until the house is sold they really are needed to keep it going. However there is the promise of some sort of solution as to the house we HOPE - nothing is yet certain - but the shameful fact remains that we are still banned as authors. I use that word "banned" advisedly. We have adhered to pure art. I think the WPA, though it saved lives by giving jobs, set a disastrous precedent in dictation; and that authors and painters who were put on salaries and had to do what they were told to do by Washington, afforded gross and vile commercialism a clue as to how to extort trash ad infinitum, deteriorate taste, and graft. *They should grapple with the saving of the genuine artist specifically - not job lots.* This method is a road to totalitarian dictation. It should be fought. *As a postscript to the front page-our mss require baggage so the cheapest travel is impossible. We are going as authors, damn lies. Your experiences with the family are in mind again as I write of ours. We hope but all at home to help each other*

---

197 Distemper was similar to what we know as emulsion paint.
198 During the war, iron fences and gates were requisitioned by the War Department as the iron was needed for the making of armaments.

Paper as a tool of politics of course figures yet, no doubt. But these things could be overcome were there any genuine intention on high to do so. *I think ghouls should be exposed, too. Jack's 7 books and my 20 will figure my calculations almost certainly German, French and all pure artists should protest every aspect of this system—reflected everywhere.*

We arent immortal and we are being compelled to waste years on futling and fruitless red-tape contention. And there has yet to be one positive move to publish John Metcalfe here; though at one moment there is evident stress on native-birth and the next just the opposite. We want something more sensible as to solutions for ourselves and yourselves than what we call "just counting Jews". *I suppose there resent British natives and Americans and any dual staters*

Love love love love love love

Please you both <u>read my letters</u> - some people at home wont, they say. It has led to senseless confusion. Every word I write is <u>pertinent to our right to resume publishing seriously and yours and Cyrils and to our right to be at home</u> *in the USA you there too darlings please*instead of <u>stuck</u> here gagged.
Mother to Jig Evelyn to Paula Jack's love with my own— he is great creatively, but commercialism is our enemy. Special love to Denise, Fredrick, Mathew, Julia. How are you both? How are the children? Where is my picture of Creighton with Pavla: Has Julia begun to walk and has she more teeth? I kiss you all in spirit.

[Typed, signed. Handwritten insertions. Not opened by addressees. SFC]

286

Chapter 28

Jigg: Part 2
January 1951 - April 1953

Only two letters from 1950 remain. Judging by the 303 letters from 1951 and 1952 which have survived (and many more may have been lost), it is fair to assume that she wrote a similar number in 1950. The following is a very small selection of those written during those years. These letters are lengthy, repetitive and sometimes incoherent, and have been heavily edited. Evelyn's language becomes increasingly bizarre, reflecting her growing conviction that her letters were being intercepted by political forces, with the specific aim of keeping her from her family. In his unpublished memoir, Confessions of an American Boy, *Jigg refers to his mother's "overweening self-obsession, to the extent that she was incapable of understanding or responding to another's needs or point of view". It appears she could not comprehend that someone to whom she wrote would choose not to respond to her letters: ergo unanswered letters were being intercepted for vague political reasons based partly, she believed, on the fact that she and Jack remained in London even though she was an American citizen.*

To Creighton Scott

26 Belsize Crescent

January 1, 1951

Please please send me your address should you move as I need and must really
have it for the Consulate here whenever I go there. Please dont throw me back
on Gladys I dont like asking favours and Jack and I are with Jig as Cyril is - our
address in the States is Jigs

Darling Jig

We dont yet know whether at least three-quarters of our mail to the States has
ever been received by anybody. And though during the visit of 1949 here, Jig said he
"thought" "most" of the letters we had sent there to yourselves were received there
was no way of checking on it and we had no real opportunity to discuss particular
letters and identify them by content - especially as this sort of thing has been going on
continuously since 1944.

I continue to think people we all used to know have been monsters - whatever their reason - in none of them so far having made so much as one gesture toward seeing Jig and Pavla and the children - all five of you-personally and giving me some first-hand information, as there a few whose mail apparently is not stopped or obstructed - something that leads me to wonder if I have not-ever since I complained about the results of phoney - I think - "inquiries" into "subversiveness" in 1939 - been on some kind of damn libellous "list". That is the single explanation that occurs to me of mail that apparently does get here in a few selected instances and not others.

Our visitor was handsome but stout. Our original Jig was leanish muscular and not at all fat. Our visitor had considerable girth. Our Jig of 1944 had no perceptible girth whatever. Our visitor of 1949 seemed to me taller - I cant be sure - and thirty-five is not the age when people usually grow. And his nose seemed so changed I wondered afterward if he could have had a plastic as our original Jigs nose was like Cyrils and he looked much more like Cyril than me, whereas in 1949 he looked like me.

We were given just a sketchy idea of events between 1944 and 1949, and when on top of that no word came from France after Jig promised he would be here again in two weeks, the impact has been a disaster to everything but love. We love him and I love every one of you and we both really love Cyril as the best friend we ever had yet, and just discount whatever appears to have resulted in a breech we cant yet elucidate.

I know we are every one sane and good individuals, and until dirty war politics impinged on our lives our lives were full of interest and achievement. Please help to live and remove the bann on both plain speaking and art, for we have every proof that there must be one.

We love you and our love is really indestructible but common humanity insists we know how rotten silence was imposed on our free human interchanges We are not politicians but artists who think - and until thinking is re-encouraged in the States. [Typed carbon copy, not signed. UTK]

To Gladys Grant

26 Belsize Crescent
January 15, 1951

My dear Gladys

Jack and myself were really glad to have your letter, and we think of you as we do of Dudley on every occasion likely to revive affectionate associations.

But we continue to be troubled by a constraint in your correspondence which we do not blame you yourself for, but which we must construe as a commentary on rotten conditions in the States.

I havent asked you to do anything for us since spring 1950 - almost a year, now. But notwithstanding your saying "I cant do any of the things you want me to", I am now asking you something again, because I think as my requests are every one sane normal human and reasonable, if you "cant" execute them, its time you, too, did something to assist to make it possible for normal Americans to carry on normally with their lives and careers.

We have not yet ceased to have egregious criminal interferences with mail. I think there has to be a check on it and this probably to take the form of more "police" trial.

I cannot even conjecture any reason why it is we yet have been unable to account for so many of our letters and have had no acknowledgement that they were received. It is either the fault of supposed authorities here or there, but that phoney "probing" in the States, of which I had that sample so often sanctioned, leads us to infer the fault is more there than here.

Pavla has written me many letters I have never received though I did receive a single note sent here in October 1950, which advised me of Jigs being home. And as I have had very few specific acknowledgements of any letters sent to them and to other friends during the year, I am still in the predicament of not knowing whether to condemn the mishandling of mail by postal authorities as the cause of all this, or whether in some instances, people have not replied because they were otherwise badgered.

In 1944, in bloody damn Tappan, he was, it was obvious to me, already being made alarming respecting myself and Cyril and Jack and our friends, and what I gather to have been intimations that we were blacklisted for Government inquiry as "subversive" because we do not write sheep-fold "literature" for low-level commerce and nincompoop "labour". And as the impression I had then was even more pronouncedly my own in 1949, and I also know he and Pavla must have been "pushed around" to some extent - perhaps in connection with us and Jacks being British - it was a very severe strain on my poise when, on his leaving here for France, he did not return when he said. And it has become still more a strain to not be allowed any correspondence with him and Pavla save those two notes, she of an entire year, neither informative save as to Jigs re-appearance.

He is restored to radio announcing and there can certainly be no damn mystery respecting this. But on every occasion of my writing to ask anybody we know who knows him to please go to Rutherford to see them, there has been no responsive move and ninety-nine-and-a-half-percent of the times no allusion to the request, afterward. We must begin to be humans again NOW - we shouldnt permit American to become a country of "psychological dog-trainers" - like these tote countries are. Will you please try to see Jig Pavla and the children and tell me your impressions of them genuinely.

Please be our old Gladys and dont be afraid to speak out against the stupidities inane fools aspiring to dictate must have attempted to impose on American-results prove it *[remainder of letter missing]*

[Typed carbon copy, unsigned. 2 pages only. UTK]

To Evelyn Scott

Scotch Plains, New Jersey
March 10, 1951

Dear Evelyn:

I don't know what to write as you disbelieve what I say and accuse me of hiding things when I try to be absolutely frank. That naturally leads to constraint and makes me put off writing Perhaps the same is true of others and is the reason they don't write either.

Now about Jig and his family. Of course I see them! I wrote you in detail when they were here about a year ago, i.e. Paula and kids, Jig was in Europe, and have kept in touch ever since. They were over for Denise's birthday celebration - all fine. I haven't seen them since but have talked on telephone. The kids had the flu like almost everybody here, but not bad and were fine two days ago when I talked to Paula on phone.

Jig was pretty sick in Europe but is better now. I can't give details because they don't want to talk about it and so I don't know. He lost a bit of weight which I think was good. So far as I know they are settled in Rutherford. Like lots of the younger generation they don't like questions and withdraw from those who ask them.

I want to remain friends to you and Jack.

Gladys

[Handwritten on air letter, signed. UTK]

To May Mayers

26 Belsize Crescent
March 11, 1951

May my dear

I am pleased that you thought my letter was "more relaxed", my dear May, but I am sorry to say it wasnt. I am compelled by the incredible cold-blooded obtuseness of most of those dominant in Britain and America today to protest the conditions here and in the States which have been imposed on Jack and myself and Jig and Cyril and their families - I am compelled by my natural human feelings and by the sort of literary and financial impasses we have yet to surmount, to protest over and over. If you were here or we could meet otherwise than in correspondence, you would have ample proof that I am NOT "tense" as a matter of "temperament" which can be put aside, but because we are still fighting for our lives every moment of every day.

You quote Gladys, my dear May, but that is small comfort to me I assure you. What you quote, as far as I can see, is a relaying of the very meager note Gladys wrote to me when Pavla Denise Fredrick and Mathew went to Scotch Plains to see her for the day over a year ago, before Jig had got back from France.

I have three times since asked Gladys by letter to go to Rutherford to see Jig as well and give me recent news, and she first threatened me with "silence" - not explaining why or what about-and finally to my recent letter-less than two months ago - vouchsafed no reply whatever.

What the hell am I <u>supposed</u> to think? Talk about totalitarian oppression, it could hardly be beat in the sort of things that have happened during my seven years and Jacks of attempting to preserve normal contacts and communications with our family in the United States of America. I have never seen anything so rottenly evasive and whoever or whatever it is that has interfered. And as for being "tense", if I start breaking up the china and hurling the bric a brac it would still be just the normal human reaction to such senseless atrocity respecting decent normal human connections there.

Who the hell told you you were "not to see" Jig? That is what Gladys told me but it is NOT what Pavla wrote me. And why in bloody blazes should anybody say such a libellous thing. I demand an explanation on Jigs behalf now. And I will go on reiterating this until I have the explanation clear. I demand to know what the origin of libels Gladys is purveying. She is probably unconscious or diddled but is purveying libels of my family. What is the source?

This is my own supposition. I have had quoted to me scurrilities - some I gather current yet in the States - about myself and Jack which would literally "make your hair curl". And I am convinced this must be a part of phone "red" rackets that are a disgrace, as I have also been told that Americans with British connections are especial butts.

So dont ask me to just accept such a situation because I wont. We all know what low caliber minds have figured in American politics from the start. I think these have been at work. And I think they must have become for more brazen as a result of dumping foreigners in the States adlib.

So you see I disagree with your interpretation of these extraordinary silences about my family as not being connected with external aspects of things, I am damn sure they must be and criminally so.

To be almost starved here by dirty blanket statisticians, to be financially stranded in London, to be suppressed as an author - even as Jack has been and Jig and Cyril and as painters of the highest rank as well - and to be sent insults and quoted insults and never allowed any really human responses where I know there are human responses-and then to be assured again and again all is well and "jake", "hunky-dory" and "hokey-dinky" is quite enough to convince anybody that somebody in New York should be indicted and probably more in Washington.

This is my opinion but it is honest and well-founded on experience of these seven years.

Anyway I am just where I was as regards the human response.

Please know the generosities have the response they should. We are far more "objective" than most purported "science" we are also far more scrupulous as to the facts and the conclusions to be reasonably drawn from them we really love May-but won't swallow American evasions re "isolation"

[Typed carbon copy, not signed. Handwritten PS. UTK]

To May Mayers

26 Belsize Crescent
March 28, 1951

May darling

Dont throw up your hands when I appeal to you again. You probably have had my letter replying to yours in which you said you felt unable to go to Rutherford[199] or ask yourself about Jig and his family, and know I was not satisfied to have Gladys report second-hand and vaguely.

And now Gladys, when I implore her to see the family - writes me in a letter of March 10th, as vaguely as ever. She says "I dont know what to write to you as you disbelieve what I say and accuse me of hiding things when I try to be absolutely frank". Well I HAVE JUST ACCUSED HER OF NOT ANSWERING my questions - thats all. I never at any time ever said I "disbelieved" her. I dont know where she gets such misconceptions unless she has neighbours who pump her full of guff.

She says - "Now about Jig and his family of course I see them. I wrote you in detail they were here about a year ago". So she did, but she didnt write of Jig, she said plainly she saw just Pavla and the children and Jig was in Europe. She did write that but in a brief note and as she has never since said anything, why the hell should I be satisfied. She just didnt answer last summer.

I was glad to hear you were in touch with Gladys, I think she is very unfortunately situated in isolation such as has been "wished" on her by the isolation of her house.[200]. I am not angry with her herself and have never been, but I dont think she is using her imagination as she can when conditions are normal - that is to say when she is not heckled or harried, as she must be periodically to say such really stupid things when she isnt really stupid. And I think she has too much pseudo "legal" advice from a lawyer who has become antagonistic and unfriendly to ourselves-to myself and Creighton, at any rate.

She never writes except on these damn via air, self-contained envelope-cum-note-paper things - just one page and almost always handwriting so there is no room to say much.

It was better to have even her note than nothing I admit, but as I have already written you about Jigs having strangely gotten suddenly almost portly, and have been constrained and nearly mute, about the art that was his life and I know is very

---

199 The family were living in Rutherford, New Jersey, within commuting distance of New York City, between November 1949 and June 1951.
200 Gladys lived in a very rural and wooded part of New Jersey: houses were far apart and her garden was large and surrounded by woodland.

important to him yet - and - well I wont repeat. But not having had his letters from France and having been worried about his health because of actual fattiness which was not normally his - you can see how Gladys bungles gestures, that are basically un-candid on her part because - I am obliged to suppose - people in the States now a days just never say all they think about anything or anybody. SEVEN YEARS OF EVASION - as far as my correspondence the States goes compels me to draw this conclusion.

If I had the power to indite official mystifiers at any point Id have 'em hanged or electrocuted or shot.

Affectionately

[Typed carbon copy, not signed. UTK]

To Evelyn Scott

Scotch Plains, New Jersey
May 2, 1951

Dear Evelyn:

Sorry if you don't approve of this paper.[201] I won't inflict it on you after the present supply is used up. I use it because of its convenience and the saving in time and money - time because I have to stop and get each letter weighed and often have to make a special trip to the PO. Money because this is considerably less than the same amount of air mail stationery plus stamp.

I did not mean to say you accused me of lying in so many words. But time after time you have asked questions about Jig or his family. I have reassured you when I knew and you have immediately written or asked me to contact others to find out the very things I have told you. Or I have told you I did not know certain things, such as Jigs whereabouts when in Europe, and you accuse me of reticence or lack of frankness. I realize you do not mean it as it sounds, but it shows a lack of trust which is hard to bear by an old friend. If you have shown the same to others who are less understanding, it is no wonder you receive no answers.

Now to tell you what I do know. I visited Jig and *Pavla Pavla is Paula in English--even they know differently* and the kids about 10 days ago. They were all recovering from colds, but otherwise fine. Jig was practically over his and the kids about ready to go to school again. Pavla, too, was almost recovered. They were all very happy, esp the kids who do not have the worries of living in this world as yet.

Love to you and Jack both - I'll write again.

Glads

[Typed on air letter, handwritten annotation, signed. UTK]

---

201 Evelyn had complained about the folding air letters sold at the time by the United States Post Office.

In the summer of 1951 Jigg secured a new position and the family felt that this was a good time to leave the suburbs of New Jersey for a better life in the country, which they found in Red Hook (Chapter 29). He did not feel it necessary to inform his mother of this move and, when she learned of it, she devoted considerable time (and postage) in her efforts to track him down.

To Margaret DeSilver

26 Belsize Crescent
January 14, 1952

Maggie darling -

I think you may like to know where we stand so far in respect to the normal information and communication with Jig himself that I must have restored or I will just go to bed and never get up again.

Pavlas letters of July and September about Julia did NOT prepare us for any move, and as she spoke of the three hours of Red Hook from New York and spoke of this in connection with Jig, I took it to be that he had a job either in New York or Philadelphia and would commute or was doing so.[202] Pavla replied that Jig was "in Germany". It now seems likely he already had gone on there, but that they should have been put to the expense of moving from Rutherford to Red Hook just to be uprooted within two months, is brutal. I suppose they had no choice because of "economy" and four children![203]

The day before New Years I had a short letter from Pavla written on the back of a picture of wood-carvings, in which she said: "We are in Germany as you can see as a result of a very sudden and hectic turn of events." And she goes on to say they are "twenty minutes" from town - I have been too distressed to re-read that item, and have spent a week worrying about more commuting - the house is "cosy but small" and they "hope for furniture by Xmas", the children are "learning German faster than we are" but "go to an American school". The card is signed by Pavla "P and J".

Pavla also sent an enlargement of the Passport Photograph of herself and the four children - and again the photograph of Jig should have been sent with it. Pavla is very thin. She looks ten years older than she actually is. Fredrick is bright and touches my heart, but he is thin, too thin. Even the baby is thin. I dont like their learning German - it may be said it is "not my business", but I dont believe in 1920s shibboleths except in part. They have been economically obliged to go there, it is doubtless pretty country near Munich, but our cultural background and both Jigs and Pavlas is NOT German.

Jack and I are both ill with colds, *Jack looks awful—heath*[sic] *all around!* Jack has had his for months and *is so tired,* and I am worried and I myself am now about to go to bed.

---

202 Chapter 30 provides more detail about the move to Red Hook and Evelyn's attempts to track them down there.

203 In fact Jig had gone ahead to take up a new post in Munich (see Chapter 30).

Love Maggie darling - I am not contending with you my dear Mag but against this awful world-as-it-is.

Grateful love
Evelyn

[Typed, signed. Handwritten insertions. HRC]

To Creighton Scott

26 Belsize Crescent
October 26, 1952[204]

Darling Jig:

Unless, by the time Jack and myself arrive in New York, I have full information as to the familys present whereabouts, whether still in Munich or elsewhere, and am given accurate and full knowledge of their present and future prospects, and assurances as to the health - in every respect - of every one of them, I propose to raise hell. I will do so very publically if need be, and in no uncertain terms. I love my son and I consider what we have all been put through as to communication, as well as in regard to "planned" lives and a virtual dictation regarding what is published-in part circumstantial but a reasonable assertion on the basis of my own experiences and Jack's, as well as yours - so blatantly inexcusable that it would merit a public crisis.

Darling Jig, I am sure I dont alarm you and Pavla. I am not and never was, hysterically disposed, but silences unexplained have mounted to such a point that, were I to give tacit assent to any further glossing of the facts, I would be unworthy to be the mother of so fine and creative a human as Creighton Scott.

I am quite certain no one has "disappeared"; so I insist, darling Jigeroo, on some reply to this sent in friendship and with complete and unalloyed love.

I think our lives are being wasted on guff of some sort; but whether it is military guff or criminal guff - my fathers will or I dont know what - I still do not know. It may be that both you and Pavla are as unable to elucidate our common victimization as we are ourselves.

We continue to await public sanity, we ourselves being on every hand eminently sane individuals just as you and Pavla are.

Our love - call it finite or infinite, it matters not at all - it IS OUR LOVE and we insist on personal and public truth for the reason that love for your demands this insistence.

Mother with our love to Pavla too and to four good bright children

[Typed, signed. Not opened by addressee. SFC. Typed carbon copy also at UTK]

---

204 Evelyn and Jack were about to return to the United States to take up a fellowship at the Huntington Hartford Foundation near Los Angeles. Chapter 33 relates the circumstances of this period of their lives.

To Creighton Scott

130 West 12th Street
April 24, 1953

Dear Jigg;-

Your letter just received[205] so horrifies and fascinates me that I hasten to answer it, even tho a letter from me must always scare and bore you! What fascinates me is the revelation of my own stupidity.

First let me hasten to say that my arthritis - the present - was only mentioned to Evelyn because I was bored with hearing of her complaints and thought I'd just stick in one of my own. But I see that that is dangerous as, like other mentally ill people I know, Evelyn never forgets a damn thing! I have always assumed it was Evelyn's enormous vanity that made her unable to admit that you of your own free will wish NOT to communicate with her, but had not the heart to come right out and say so - she would not have accepted it anyway. BUT I did NOT know she was so thoroughly au courant as to your ideas and intentions.

Plenty of people DID warn me against trying to bring Evelyn here[206] are plenty are hiding out in fear and trembling, all of which makes me feel an utter ass, softy, simpleminded "Do-Gooder" - such always mess things up for all concerned. But I did somehow think that if E got out of that hideous environment she might be able to do some creative work again.

Yes, Cyril and E both sure have outsized egos but I sort of assumed that was a disease of artists - that they had to have egos to buck all sorts of things. But I must say when they get top-heavy, one certainly ceases to function and instead does only endless damage.

Well, that's enough. Good luck to you both. And thank you for writing Evelyn.

Margaret DeSilver

[Typed, signed. SFC]

To Margaret DeSilver

Hotel Chelsea
222 West 23rd Street
April 24 [1953]

Dear Margaret

Sorry my letter threw you, as it appears to have done, and which I didn't intend. Your letters have never bored me, although I admit they have scared me at times. I don't think it's correct to say that you have been stupid about bringing E Scott[207] and Jack to the 'States. What I do contend is that you, and the others involved, have failed to take into consideration that she is, in the strictly clinical sense, insane.

---

205 This letter has not survived.
206 More information about Margaret's efforts and the results of these are presented in Chapters 31 and 32.
207 It was about this time that Jigg began referring to his mother as "E Scott".

As you say, my mother was a bit of a witch hunter in her time. Every-body who knew her at the time realises that she went quite overboard on the idea that there was a terrible conspiracy afoot to repress True Art, and that the super patriots, as represented by the Hearst Press, the un-American Activities Committee, etc. were natural allies against such a conspiracy. The logic of this did then, and still does, escape me altogether.

As I say, everyone knew, or suspected, that she was doing a bit of witch hunting. What nobody knew, and what the people I told have steadfastly refused to believe up this moment, is that she was nuts.

At the time in question, for example, I spent many hours trying to convince her that she was wrong in supposing that there was in existence a machine (a kind of telepathic radio) which enabled malignant influences (at that time communist, but today God knows what) to tune in on one's thoughts. A little later, I tried to talk her out of the notion that this same device had been improved to the point where it could not only be tuned in on one's thoughts, but used to twist, pervert and direct them as well. In 1943, at a time when she was considered to be quite sane, and when my own rationality was called into question for suggesting that she was not, she was urging me to get rid of my wife (Paula), by poison if necessary, because, she claimed, Paula was a robot under the influence of this contraption. It was later perfected, as she took pains to inform me, to the point where it could make people ill. (How's your arthritis?).

Not only that, but it soon transpired, as she made clear, that there was no such thing as a germ or a virus, or what have you. All diseases, mechanical fractures of the bone possibly excepted, were induced by this super-gadget. There was, however, a counteragent. If you thought "right" thoughts, and repeated the word "Peruna" frequently enough, you could outwit the gadget. To prove the point (she was living with me at the time) she deliberately infected my son Frederick (then a baby) with the flu, from which he nearly died.

This is merely by way of illustrating the point things had reached ten years ago: they were plenty bad before that. I recall suggesting to various people that she might not be all there, and all I got was a sweet, sceptical smile - the smile one accords to someone who doesn't know what he's talking about.

At ABC[208] two things happened. Firstly, I found that my mother had a reputation among persons of more or less liberal complexion as their sworn enemy, and that it was assumed that I was her staunch supporter in this. My rather timid intimations that this was not so got me nowhere.

The second thing that happened was that my boss at ABC got the inevitable letter from my mother, asking, indirectly, that some kind of heat be put on me to make me a better correspondent, and suggesting that ABC was preventing me from writing.

---

208 American Broadcasting Company.

From ABC I moved to CBS.[209] Ed Murrow is probably still puzzled by the letter he got from my mother trying to enlist his help in making me a more dutiful son. My mail was opened in Germany by the CIA, and I have often tried to imagine what whoever my mother's letters (forwarded from the 'States) finally reached thought about their contents.

As far as I know she is still a confirmed letter writer.

Now I realize that the foregoing may sound completely incredible to you, or anyone else. Nevertheless it is true. However, about the only thing I have ever asked anybody to do about it is (1) kindly not hold me responsible for what my parents did- the sins of the fathers may be visited upon the sons in the bible, but this is supposed to be a non-biblical age; and (2) that someone look into the matter, with the aid of competent and qualified medical men, without automatically assuming that it couldn't be true because it was I who said so. If I am wrong, I shall be happy to abide by the decision of an unbiased judge, but I'm afraid I'm right. I have been for fifteen years, and the fact that I spent 25 of my 38 years dancing attendance on my mother and father gives my opinion some weight.

So much for that. You now have the main facts in fairly comprehensible form. Sorry to bother you with it all, but it seems easier to state the whole case in one lump that to try to explain it piecemeal.

I'm very grateful to you for what you are trying to do for my mother, and I'll do anything I can to help. Frankly, however, it presents certain problems. But don't let it get you down. Best of luck from Paula and myself.

Jigg

Incidentally, you are the second person who asked me to write my mother in a week. Gladys Grant was the other. The letter is in the works.

[Typed, signed. Handwritten postscript. HRC]

---

209 Columbia Broadcasting Company.

Chapter 29

Red Hook
June - September 1951

In the summer of 1951 the family moved to a rambling old house on Pitcher Lane in Red Hook, a small town in the Hudson River valley in Dutchess County, about 100 miles north of New York City.

Cyril (who had now resumed his original name of Frederick Creighton Wellman) had been living in a retirement colony in Red Hook for some time, and it is possible that the family moved to be near him. At the time, Jigg was working for the Columbia Broadcasting System (CBS) and commuting to New York City.

There are two places bearing the name Red Hook in New York state. One is the small rural community in Dutchess County where Jigg and his family were now living. The other is a district in Brooklyn, one of New York City's five boroughs. Once she learned of this development, Evelyn began another of her quests to track Jigg and his family down. This time her efforts were hampered by wrong assumptions and an increasingly paranoid view of the world interspersed with her views on dentistry and birth control, the latter perhaps her reaction to the birth of Jigg and Paula's fourth child, Julia.

The following sequence of letters, all written within a few months, illustrates Evelyn's ability to focus on a seemingly unimportant detail and to become obsessive about it. It is likely there are other similarly obsessive exchanges, but it is hard to know as much of Evelyn's correspondence was either dispersed or destroyed over the years.

To Evelyn Scott and Jack Metcalfe

Pitcher Lane
Red Hook, New York
July 7, 1951

Dear Evelyn and Jack

Yesterday - July 6 - a daughter was born to us, named Julia Swinburne Scott. Vital statistics: weight 7 lbs 12 oz, 19 inches long and perfectly formed.

We are all well though weary after a hectic time getting moved before the baby came.

Please stop worrying about mail - it all reaches us and registry is unnecessary and only harasses me with trips to the PO to sign, when I have plenty to do as is. I'm just a lousy correspondent and that's all.

Excuse horrid ink color and the scrawl - it's hard to write in bed.

Love, Paula.

London, November 1952. Pavla here contradicts her own prior assertion as to mail. I think she was concerned to protect the Post Office. Love Jig and her love all four children—but await responses. Evelyn D S Metcalfe

[Handwritten, signed. Handwritten annotation on envelope by ES. UTK]

To Creighton and Paula Scott

26 Belsize Crescent

July 25, 1951

Darlings

I go on being so grateful to Pavla for her letter telling me of Julias birth. She is, however, now nineteen days old and I will again be happier when somebody we know in the States has seen her mother and her father and herself and Denise Fredrick and Mathew and writes to me specific details as to them and their health and fortunes.

I consulted the map we have and located both Red Hook in Greater New York and Rhinebeck, which was the postmark on Pavlas letter,[210] and I do hope I am correct in supposing the Red Hook on the map is where Pavla is - though I couldnt find Pitcher Lane, and just take it for granted she didnt mean a hospital but the present family residence.

I think it was splendid to Pavla to write so soon, but I am naturally imaginatively sensitive to everything connected with Julia and her and Jig and the children, and I am also just hoping that Denise or perhaps Denise Fredrick and Mathew are visiting at Rhinebeck or somewhere in the country until Pavla can recuperate and Julia and her mother and father are settled comfortably in whatever home will be the familys for the present.

I know New York summers and I hope the proximity of Red Hook to the water[211] means at least some whiffs of sea air and some space outdoors for the children. I also do so hope my correspondence with you both will soon cease to be so one-sided. Im not really a droning granmar, who goes over and over the same questions a million times! It is just that it is difficult to write natural letters until I am assured of natural

---

210 The nearest hospital to Red Hook, where Julia was born, was in Rhinebeck, a few miles away.
211 This letter and several of those following are based on Evelyn's assumption that Red Hook is somewhere in the Greater New York area. Her 1910 edition of the Baedeker guide to New York showed a Red Hook in Brooklyn not far from the Hudson River.

and explicit replies that arrive here and are delivered to ourselves. If I had a letter once a month that really kept me aware of important happenings and was sometimes specific like this one of Pavlas I would be much improved myself as a letter-writer. So I hope and hope you will see some mutual friends beside Gladys, who, as she invariably does, didnt mention Julia, but bloody damn "advised" me not to inquire into the lives of the bloody damn "younger generation".

Whenever our letter welcoming Julia is commented on, we will be very grateful to have the comment specific enough to leave no doubt that it went to the right address and that the address is not temporary.

Love again - I never want to pester with too many letters but I dont really know what anybody there thinks about anything and I must assure myself that the non-Scotish Scotts - Jigs Dad always included - know we are not indifferent but go toward them in spirit with whatever we have continually.

[Typed carbon copy, not signed. UTK]

To Gladys Grant

26 Belsize Crescent
August 28, 1951

Dear Gladys:

In the letter you were answering when you wrote on August the 8th, I mentioned Pitcher Lane Red Hook as the address of Jig and Pavla and said that I conjectured it to be on Long Island, as the one Red Hook I had then discovered on the maps of our old Atlas - its a Baedeker but we so use it and it is of 1910 - the only one I had then discovered is on Buttermilk Channel in Brooklyn. As I took this to be the case, I also construed the postmark Rhinebeck, on Pavlas letter about Julia as indicative of the fact that she must have given it to a friend with a car who lived up state where it was mailed. And that she was not more explicit was normal of course, as she and Jig had just moved before her confinement and she was still in bed, and Jig had his job and three children as well as Julia to look after.

But I do wonder my dear Glad that you didnt correct me if I am wrong, as I may be, because I have not found, on a map labelled "Catskills" - at which I had not glanced because I had already found Rhinebeck on the other map and it is not in the Catskills, which are far from jobs, - I have now found both a Red Hook and an Upper Red Hook. I have written six letters to Red Hook under the impression that it was in Brooklyn and one and maybe two were sent to "Greater New York", and now I dont know which were received, if any. And I would not have looked through the maps again, had not Charlotte[212] written me a terse postcard - just these words: "Red Hook (Dutchess County) congratulations".

---

212 Charlotte Wilder was a poet and a long-standing and close friend of Evelyn.

Is Red Hook in Duchess[213] County? - second Red Hook, I mean. Do you know anything in detail about them or their surroundings now? Has Jig a job - we hope so. We and most of all I here, have been in a hell of anxiety about Jig and Pavla their health and money for the four.

Why cant people with common sense see that by falling for rot of which rumours that isolate us and my family are a part, they virtually hand us all over to criminal "police protection" which should be shot. I know Jig is "nominally" free to write to me and so is Pavla, but actually every detail that has happened in their move to Red Hook is a repetition of the happenings of 1946 when Mathew was born, and they were broke and had no house. And among the many things I dont forget, is the fact that kuklux[214] terrorists were active in North Carolina when they were there with Cyril. And that even in the north Jig has had two experiences of intimidation and been rescued by his boss.

[Typed carbon copy, not signed. UTK]

To Creighton and Paula Scott

26 Belsize Crescent

August 29, 1951

Darling Darling Darling Darlings

Please for humanitys sake and ours relieve my anxiety about you as much as you can NOW.

I have sent six letters to Red Hook Greater NY - Buttermilk Channel Brooklyn - told several people I thought you had moved there - Margaret De Silver among them - and now have a letter from Charlotte - or rather just a postcard - in which she says merely Red Hook Duchess County NY.

I think this is wrong and my distress is acute. I think bilgey and wicked rackets in America spread false rumours and attempt to divide families in this criminal way.

Please reply and explain please we love you so I think there are factions there to indite and impeach.

This post office thing has got too much to endure.

[Typed carbon copy, not signed. UTK]

To Paula and Creighton Scott

26 Belsize Crescent

August 29, 1951

Darling Darling Pavla and Jig

Are you at Red Hook Brooklyn or Red Hook Duchess County. I have already mailed six letters to Red Hook NY one of them with the addition of "Greater" to New York and two relative to Pavlas birthday and all to Jigs health and Julia.

---

213 Evekyn persistently misspells "Dutchess".
214 This is a reference to the Ku Klux Klan.

Please please please please elucidate the address. That Pavlas letter was postmarked Rhinebeck has added to confusion, because we cannot find any Red Hook near there on the maps we have - and if there are two in New York we should know which and how to distinguish them.

Charlotte Wilder sent Duchess County and I am now worried more than ever as she doesnt explain why she thinks so - just your address with Duchess County added.

Lovingly, oh we do love you

[Typed carbon copy, not signed. UTK]

To Creighton and Paula Scott

26 Belsize Crescent

[August 1951]

It would be best to know where Jigs job and other normal information and stop
fools gossip - please tell me

Darling Jig and Paula

The letters sent to Pitcher Lane may have reached you but I had been able to find on our old maps just one Red Hook, near Buttermilk Channel, Brooklyn, and thought you must be there, and Margaret De Silver wrote to Greater New York hoping to locate you and relieve your anxiety, and had no reply. So I send this to Red Hook just discovered on another map as up near Rhinebeck and on the Rhinebeck, Philadelphia and Reading RR of 1910. There is Red Hook and Upper Red Hook on this map, which is marked.

I thought some friend going north in a car had mailed Pavlas letter about Julia, and Gladys must be prompted by diabolists, because after I had carefully explained to her that Pitcher Lane was I thought in Brooklyn, she writes me "I have talked to Pavla on the phone and she has invited me to be Julias godmother". And not a word does Gladys say about my possibly erroneous conjecture, it was the most normal supposition to make as the map marked Catskills was not even noticed by me, so far from jobs did that locality seem.

It was so completely natural for Pavla writing in bed and not yet recovered from her confinement to have not thought of such a confusion as possible. I love her and I love my son and I love her letter. She may not have known - neither she nor Jig - that there were two goddam places - really three is the hell of it - Upper Red Hook, Red Hook, Duchess County, and Red Hook Long Island.

But we are all sane so please do something at your end.

I wont call Pavla "Paula" until there are no further complications about names changed. I dont see any real reason for it - none was ever given me - and endless torments must be ended and Pavla is the best name for writing. Paula is a nothing name - Im sure Pavla can see this is the truth.

[Typed carbon copy, not signed. UTK]

To Creighton Scott and Paula Scott

26 Belsize Crescent
September 9, 1951

Darling darlings

Please do something about assuring me there is no more confusion of addresses. Is your Red Hook in Duchess County? You say you receive my mail and I dont receive all yours, but how the hell do you know whether you receive all mine or not-I dont know because your replies are not yet SPECIFIC ENOUGH.

I am worrying every minute about the health of all six, and though it may be said I dont help by worrying, there is a limit to the applicableness of that comment.

Do you see anybody we know who will both help you and write to me of how you are physically mentally and financially.

Have you our letters about the agreement of several of our old friends to try to raise a fund[215] to finance our return to the States to see you as well as to arrange the publishing end of things.

Well Mother is very Loving.

Love and hope to six adult and young non-Scotish Scotts and to Dad.

[Typed carbon copy, not signed. UTK]

To Gladys Grant

26 Belsize Crescent
September 11, 1951

Dear Glad,

Wont you please tell me whether Jig and Pavla are near Rhinebeck or not? Is it the Red Hook with the Pitcher Lane, and is there an Upper Red Hook and a Red Hook such as shows on my map of the Catskills?

If people are "mysterious" about mail or about their location, it is just the proof of everything I say about Jig and Pavlas victimization by those who have libelled me and Cyril and Jack and probably Joe and Margue. I should think anybody would see this was the case. It is the sort of senseless hushiness which accompanied intimidation in my own experience of it. I was definitely intimidated, and when I complained was at once inundated by "mystification". I thought it was the war, but after all, the war cant go on forever and should never have done so in that guise.

Dont say I "blame" you when I reiterate these protests. I dont, I just think if there is any more suggested hushiness it must must MUST be defied.

[Typed carbon copy, not signed. UTK]

---

215 This is a reference to the fund later referred to as the "Evelyn Scott Fund" (see Chapter 32 for a full account of its formation).

In September 1951 the family left Red Hook to follow Jigg to Germany where he had gained a position with Radio Free Europe, working out of their Munich offices to broadcast anti-communist material to countries behind the Iron Curtain. Needless to say, Evelyn did not learn of this until some months later, inevitably creating confusion as letters continued to be addressed to Red Hook.

Chapter 30

Germany
September 1951 - August 1952

In September 1951 while Evelyn was still wrestling with letters to Red Hook, Jigg, who had built a solid reputation in radio news, secured a post with Radio Free Europe, an anti-Communist radio network based in Munich and supported by the National Committee for a Free Europe. His role was to establish a newsroom and be news editor-in-chief at their new station. In the immediate post-war climate, anti-communist propaganda was seen as extremely important and much of Radio Free Europe's output, supported by the CIA, was aimed at countries behind the Iron Curtain.

The family followed him to Munich, where they spent the first weeks of their stay in Germany at the Regina Palast Hotel in the very centre of Munich, then still severely bomb-damaged. In spite of the damage, the hotel retained much of its former splendour, and the family were housed there until accommodation could be found for them in a modest house in the suburb of Grünwald some 10 miles to the south of Munich.

In the spring of 1952 the family moved from their small house in Grünwald to a much larger property in the Munich suburb of Gräfelfing, a substantial house with a large garden and orchard which backed onto extensive woodland. The house had been, Jigg was led to understand, commandeered by the Americans from a local high-ranking Nazi; whether true or not, it was spacious and comfortable in the traditional Bavarian style, complete with bierstübl *and* weinkeller. *For the first time in their married lives, Jigg and Paula enjoyed a much more comfortable lifestyle; Jigg's salary was enough for them to employ a live-in maid and to spend time with numerous friends among Jigg's colleagues.*

It was also about this time that Evelyn, having decided to document her suspicions that she was being libelled, had asked Margaret DeSilver to forward a copy of her "Precis"[216] to Jigg in Red Hook. This started a sequence of letters that alerted Evelyn to the fact that Jigg and his family might not be in the United States.

---

216 This 74-page single-spaced typescript or "precis" is a detailed account of events as Evelyn saw them from 1939 until the date of its completion in late 1951. It was prompted by a suggestion from Margaret. DeSilver that she might start a fund to enable Evelyn and Jack to return to the United States. (See also Chapter 31.)

To Margaret DeSilver

26 Belsize Crescent
December 27, 1951

I have not said a word about xmas, it was about the bloodiest we ever had as we were both sick all day and I got a crying fit and couldnt stop though I am NOT given to hysteria. And both of us by coincidental accident banged our heads on things and Jack has a bump swollen on his scalp and I have what looks like a black eye, which I got in getting out of bed in a dark room and bumping a table. Aint life wonderful - I dont think!

Dear Maggie:

Thank you for sending on the temporary address. I suppose Jig must have been "economically" compelled to go to Munich in connection with jobs. It has been so invariable as yet that, whenever I have had anything important to tell Jig and Pavla there has been some sort of fool mix-up or shenanigan about mail that I cannot say I am surprised. It was in what has become positive anticipation of such occurrences that I asked you whether you could find anyone to hand the precis to Jig in person, and as you mailed it instead, I suppose you could not. I would not have troubled you with it at all, however, except that I hoped to forestall precisely what has happened

I think it is probable that Pavla is still at Red Hook with the four children,[217] and the whole situation is sickening, as Jig should be saved NOW from being just a damn stud-horse, and Pavla is NOT a brood-mare. To hell with the way our lives have been made to fall out - it is senseless wreckage.

I will be for Jig FIRST as long as I live, but I am naturally affectionate in my feeling for our original Pavla and I dont know what sort of tosh and bosh has been fed her that makes her do the sort of thing she did this time, write me mentioning Jig for the first time in literal years as "commuting" to Germany, as probably he either was already or was about to be. I think she has been senselessly alarmed by some idea that mother is an obstacle of some sort, and this is NOT so. I just think the shibboleths that go with too much progeny must be put an end to and something allowed both that is normal to their character and innate capacities as individuals - Jig first because of his proven talent having exceeded hers in proof, but taking her individual capacities as well into consideration as this bloody blasted damn breed thing has not allowed for her development OR his *since 1943*

We hope Jig will soon be home again and that you yourself are not discouraged as to our eventual return - and may it be soon. It was precisely this element of bigoted orthodoxy and damn progeny that Jack and myself had to fight here when our relation *initially* became serious. These utter fools who insisted on families as tribes and who definitely sacrifice parents to mere multitude really deserve shooting.

---

217 The family had left Red Hook three months previously, in September.

This is just opinion. Remember I cannot see anyone, having no teeth and no money and having still to be reassured about last summer and its hefts, cannot yet leave the house. And I do think it is a criminal commentary on the entire Scott-Metcalfe situation that an <u>American</u> artist and creative author of Jigs proven ability, though things should not have come to this, has to go to a German city to pick up bloody damn crumbs in order to support a family that would never have been of its present dimensions but for just the sort of bloody alternate sex starvation and over propagation bloody religious dictation imposes.

I have a second copy of the precis, apparently you are not especially interested in reading it but I would so like Cyril to read everything I say of his book. WE HOPE TO SEE JIG HERE WE HOPE TO SEE JIG HERE AS COMMON SENSE on his way home, but I would prefer NOT to wait any more, to write to Cyril as our genuine friend for I am convinced he is

[Typed carbon copy, not signed. Handwritten insertions. UTK]

To Creighton Scott

26 Belsize Crescent
December 28, 1951

Mr Creighton Scott
Hotel Regina-Palast, Munich
Darling Jigeroo

I hope this can be forwarded to you as I suppose this address is merely temporary and Jack and myself would so much like to see you at least for a week or so before you go home to the USA.

I also suppose I might have known should I send any mail of real importance to yourself and Pavla something would happen, if not what has, an obstacle of some sort to your receiving it. I have this address because the precis I compiled of material I propose to use in an autobiography was sent to you at Pitcher Lane for Pavla and yourself to read and send to your Dad. I had first sent it to Margaret De Silver with the request that, since she almost never sees you and Pavla any more, she try to find someone to give it to you in person. She mailed it instead, probably having had too much to do to look for anyone and having, apparently, more faith in circumstances than I have; and the Postmaster at Red Hook returned it to her with the above address on it as the forwarding address for you. And she at once sent it on to that address as she never should have since it represents about two months of work for me, off and on, of course, and hotel addresses are seldom more than temporary.

However, I will just hope that the hotel forwards it if necessary and you will receive it and write to tell me and say something of why you are in Germany and whether or not you can visit us here briefly as we hope and have a steamer rug please bring it as blankets are our present greatest need when anyone is here.

The precis was sent especially because of my opinion, which cannot be shaken, that somebody tampered with Cyrils autobiography at those points involving ourselves before and since our divorce, and that this tampering, just before the book was completed, when first your stepbrother had been ill and Cyril had been to his bedside, then Cyril himself had been ill, was done without consultation with him and that he has never since been in a position to publically protest the incontestable great damage done him us and yourselves because he and his wife also are under "economic" duress.

I dont give up hope nor does Jack for us all though I am still awaiting news of an agent to handle <u>Escape Into Living</u> and as the author of twenty published serious books this should not have taken so long as it has *over six months.*

[Typed carbon copy, not signed. Handwritten insertion. UTK]

To Paula Scott

26 Belsize Crescent

January 1, 1952

The picture of the family[218] is already kissed every night. It is yourselves and whenever we look at it love burgeons and we are very lucky in having you all "ours" too. You are a lovely daughter-in-law.

You are the best of daughter-in-laws and I like your responsiveness and hope for the children's and know Jig is with us as well as his Dad. We think the same things and Cyril agrees as does his wife no doubt. Divorces are a small matter in the arts.

Darling Pavla

Your own Christmas letter arrived and this is to expand our reply and as the further sign of our delight in your nearness and our hope soon to see Jig and yourself and all four here with us, the sooner the better, and as many as we can provide beds for - three at once is the present limit. Julia of course goes with you as she is too small to be left but perhaps there could be two visits with Denise and the boys divided between the two adults.

We would be somewhat crowded and that we wish were not the case but just to see you at all would be such refreshment to us we hope it will be to you and Jig. I am sending Jig the letter explaining this to him because I am eager to break whatever jinx has been between my son and myself in respect to correspondence. Your letters darling Pavla have just kept me from tearing my hair with anxiety but it is not right that I should have to depend on you for any news whatever and to have Jig himself write to us will be the restoration of common sense in our human stand.

I dont repeat here what I say to Jig but we must sort it out, and I think it is the result of that criminal low-level commercial contempt for arts intrinsic value which has lately resulted in an "agent block" on me because I WONT CHANGE WONT CUT any mss ever again - and <u>Escape Into Living</u> is waiting for publication I now know

---

218 This was the passport photograph obtained for travel to Germany. At the time it was possible to include children in the photo of the parent holding the passport.

on this account. It shall not be mutilated, it is integrated and aesthetically right as it is in the present 1951 clear version now in New York, and damage to Cyril is a case in point and proves such tinkerings must be opposed as the reducto ad absurdum is already approached, and would consist in any sort of mere opinion, also, being printed irresponsibly under an author name when not representing the author opinion at all. It could be carried into anything, already pervades doctored newspapers, and is dictatorial and wicked, stupid and a cause of general hell.

I have mentioned the American school[219] you tell us of and am very glad it is American, though I despise our school system in its machine-made aspects. These are of comparatively late date, however, and we hope the American school there is old-fashioned and know this will also suit you both and the children will learn.

However, for us just having the picture is joy - any picture and Jigs to match is now all required in the photographic sense which is NOT sense as art but is good to prove affection.

Jack will cook for you when you come. He continues the chef de lux of the household. I recommend to you the desert of semolina he is now preparing for supper. It is very cheap and takes a comparatively small amount of sugar and he puts powdered coconut in it as he takes it from the stove and flavours it also when possible with brown-sugar. For the author of so many fine books he has unsuspected accomplishments. Tell Cyril Jack is almost as versatile in some ways as he is himself.

You should be in France I think because of the visual arts but Germany has a few fine painters and I hope Jig sometimes can paint again even there - and here's to all our new books. We must gradually become again the sort of creative people we are. The things we have been compelled to do since the war are just a travesty of our real selves. We will all go home to the States before too much time but some good will come of your being there. *We hope Munich music is bold and not droves herded to popular concerts—I despise "anodynes".*

[Typed carbon copy, not signed. Handwritten annotation. UTK]

To Creighton Scott

26 Belsize Crescent
January 1, 1952

Darling Jigeroo

I have already invited you here thinking Pavla must be still in Red Hook, in a letter sent to the Hotel Regina-Palast, Maximilian Platz, Munich, and I hope you will have received when you do this both the first letter and the outline of a part of an autobiography I propose writing about my author-experiences, as this outline went to

---

219 The US Army provided schools for the children of the armed forces stationed in Germany; these schools also admitted the children of expats working in Munich.

the Regina-Palast when returned to Margaret De Silver by the Red Hook Postmaster with your forwarding address stamped on the parcel. It is for reading by you and Pavla and by your Dad whose opinion on some portions we should have.

I am most anxious to see you first without waiting on other things as soon as it is convenient to you because we have been so cut off from communication. But that is just because I am exhausted by the suspense which has resulted from knowing so little of you yourself specifically. We are both also actually very eager to see Pavla and the four children, and were we able to provide the beds and fares we would urge having you all here now at once. However, as soon as the expense can be met you must come please, and Pavla and Denise and the boys in relays - Julia we know going with Pavla at this age as she is too young to be left.

We have enough beds for three with some squeezing, and two we could easily have if camping out arrangements are tolerable to you. And though we HOPE not to have to wait long in any case do lets all try to so arrange it that we can all meet here before we all go home to the States, which, though it may still require time, we will all do.

We know Munich must be an interesting change after the places you have been in recently at home and that it is a stimulus to have a new scene and we hope there is enough material benefit in the transition to allow for some enjoyment - though I think you should be in France rather than Germany, as the visual arts in France are more consistently one with your innate talents and hers than music for which Munich I suppose still stands - the old rather than the "new".

We are glad the children are at an American school - I put this first because I remember that, although you learned excellent French rapidly when you were at school in France and Algeria and there was that advantage in instruction in the native language, you had some trouble in catching up on some things in which you had to be advanced in the States and were ahead on others for which you had insufficient credit, due to curriculums that didnt jibe. And American school will probably take all this into account and provide the opportunity to learn good German, though I reiterate it should be French with us as the Scott cultural inclinations are primarily French with complete friendly appreciation of German culture in its different genre and mores.

It is a very sweet privilege to be allowed to feel myself really Grandmother again and Jack has touched me very much by saying spontaneously and with genuineness, on looking at the picture Pavla sent, "Well I am glad to have a family of my own again" - his emotional generosity is precisely as I tell you. He is ready to reciprocate love and he is especially interested in meeting Denise as he has always been fond of little girls as I am of little boys- we will of course love both, regardless of sex, once there is a rapprochement that proves the responses to our interest are natural and are not forced. *Tell Denise I fell in love with her ten years ago— soon eleven and I will never fall out I fell in love with Fredrick in 1943 I fell in love with Fredrick in 1943 —it will be Mathew and Julia too soon I know*

Do tell us everything you will of yourself Jig darling. I am already kissing the picture of Pavla and the four every night, but I would like yours to kiss too and most of all the visit - yourself and Pavla and as many as you can bring and we can accommodate and the sooner the better.

[Typed, not signed. Handwritten insertion by ES. UTK]

To Creighton and Paula Scott

26 Belsize Crescent
February 11, 1952

Darlings -

I refuse to be hurt, though there is not yet any acknowledgment yet received by me of the outline of the portion of the future autobiographical volume's data - sent to Jig forwarded by Margaret De Silver to the Hotel Regina Palast, Maximilian Platz, Munich, and intended to be sent on to Jigs Dad in the States for his opinion on how to combat imposed tinkerings with books with fine material, such as his Life Is Too Short must originally have been before some half-wit tried to re-write it for low-level consumption.

Well we hope the precis or outline has arrived and is read and has been sent on to Cyril himself and that we will both soon have his home address again.

Couldnt Jig write us just a few lines please? We would feel so much better if he wrote them himself. He cant be ill and we hope as well as very living he is very well indeed and you all are, but the very sight of his handwriting would be cheering.

We are as militantly opposed to totalitarians as if we were the heads of the allied armies- or considerably more so, I may say ironically in view of the results of the war in landing us among the labour tyrants. But we do not think any military or civil bureaucracy has any right to interfere at any state in civil human relations and civil careers and the communications essential to carrying these on. And we protest the mail status quo as dense, stupid, brutal, wrong. And if there is censoring between here and Munich - officially none has been allowed as far as I know - then I hope these guy-dan, god damn brutes will get a dirty, muddy eyeful, because I say as an American mother they should be shot.

NB Important We would love hearing of explicit happenings of your lives during these few months since your arrived there, but Pavla has the household, and Jig his job so notes help and are acceptable - more than. And still taking the photograph to stand for the affection ours in common I would like to tell you of happenings here, if these as yet included anything whatever except stress and strain about how to keep just barely afloat, as we still await action on books for any money whatever WE are none of us - save Jig and Pavla - young any more.

Do you have ready-cooked food in Munich? There are a few places here that sell it, frozen like birds-eye vegetables such as we had in Canada, and not half-bad. Some really rather good, and some dear and some not. It might make a change sometimes should you discover any place where you can buy these things there and Jig bring home dinner in his pocket ready-cooked.

I still have no teeth as the money saved for them went to stave off a tax-summons, but although I refused, as was recently suggested by Jack's cousin here, to go to the Guild Hall and look up data for my French historical novel with such a denuded mouth I am entirely reconciled to being seen toothless by my family, so whenever any visit to London is possible we will be glad no matter how toothless.

Jiggie darling Mother to you please
Jack's love to all

[Typed carbon copy, signed. Handwritten insertion. UTK]

To Creighton and Paula Scott

26 Belsize Crescent
March 2, 1952

Darling Jig and Pavla:

Have you yet received any notification respecting the parcel containing the segment of an outline of the future autobiographical volume I propose to add eventually to my published volumes? This parcel, because the mss contains allusions to you both and to Jigs Dad and his <u>Life Is Too Short</u>, I wish you both would read and send on to Cyril.

I have explained in an earlier letter that Margaret De Silver, who was to see it reached you, not having been informed of the move to Munich at the time. This was nearly three months ago - two and a half approximately may be more exact, as I do not know precisely the date on which she mailed it - and as there has been ample time for its receipt by you and its arrival has not been acknowledged in any letter as yet received by me,

I have written to the Manager of the hotel requesting him as a very great favour to do me the kindness to ascertain if he can whether or not it is yet at the hotel yet or has already been delivered to you. There hasnt really been time to have his reply - or that of some member of the hotel staff - but I send this on to you, too, hoping you will check up on the parcel in any case and if you have it, whether or not you have already written saying so, write and tell me again.

Should the hotel Manager or any of his staff assist to locate the parcel of mss please offer him my thanks as Jigs American mother - we will all be thankful to have no further trouble of this sort, in London and in the States I am sure.

How is everything with you both now? We are eager for news specific enough to bring you

Please tell us more please please

Jigs affectionate and loving mother and Pavla's affectionate friend for Jack and myself both - he sends love to all six and Cyril his still very friendly regards.

[Typed carbon copy, not signed. UTK]

To Evelyn Scott

Scotch Plains, New Jersey
March 10, 1952

Dear Evelyn:

I don't know what to write as you disbelieve what I say and accuse me of hiding things when I try to be absolutely frank. That naturally leads to constraint and makes me put off writing. Perhaps the same is true of others and is the reason they don't write either.

I've wanted to answer your last letter but first put it off and then for more than a month now, I've been down and out with flu. Up now but absolutely pepless. I've never been so sick since I could remember.

Now about Jig and his family. Of course I see them! I wrote you in detail when they were here about a year ago, i.e. Paula and kids, Jig was in Europe, and have kept in touch ever since. They were over for Denise's birthday celebration - all fine. I haven't seen them since but have talked on telephone. The kids had the flu like almost everybody here, but not bad and were fine two days ago when I talked to Paula on phone.

Jig was pretty sick in Europe but is better now. I can't give details because they don't want to talk about it and so I don't know. He lost a bit of weight which I think was good. So far as I know they are settled in Rutherford. Like lots of the younger generation they don't like questions and withdraw from those who ask them.

I want to remain friends! to you and Jack.

Gladys

[Handwritten on air letter, signed. UTK]

To Creighton and Paula Scott

26 Belsize Crescent
March 12, 1952

Darlings:

Please please please help me to expose the truth as to the difficulties we continue to have with mail as between myself and yourselves and every one of our American relatives including Jigs Dad.

I have written to you both three times about this and the outline or "precis" of a segment of data compiled for the third of my autobiographical volumes, which has yet to be written but which I wish to have read as data yet in which we all figure, both by you and Cyril and his wife.

This compilation *an outline isn't a book but it is valuable as author record* for my family and myself, and a record merely, not a book for publication as data, is the parcel sent to Margaret De Silver for conveyance to Jig at Pitcher Lane, Red Hook, Duchess County, NY, where you both were in the summer and early fall.

And this is the gist of the request I made of the hotel over two weeks ago. I think it is like "psychological warfare" to impose on us all the sort of anxiety this represents, which, in any one instance, would be "minor", but as an accumulation of years and in connection with important matters like writing books and knowing how ones nearest and dearest really are and whether or not they do receive their mail, it is serious as augmenting strains that are already enough.

I have complained so continually about the situation at home in this respect that there may have been some action taken there to improve it, as I am now having many more letters actually acknowledged *which I receive.* But this still does not include my letters to my family and relatives - both yourselves and every member of my American family. It would seem to me that with the numbers of Americans there are in Germany, this stupidity about mail should not be allowed and that there should be steps taken there to make an end of conditions anything but conducive to peace in the world.

Pavla and Jig my dears you should both acknowledge letters which are to both - even if it is just in the matter of signatures. And it would probably be helpful <u>not</u> to sign initials as Pavla sometimes does as we would like to hit any censors who meddle - if they meddle, we are just guessing - hit them in the eyes as meddlars by making as public as we can your and my American identity, so that mail when lost can always be traced.

Our love Jacks and mine to yourselves and the four children - please do write and tell me just where we are in respect to this utterly poppycock situation about mail and that parcel the handkerchief and the children's book sent Mathew. I have a book for Freddy and dont yet dare send it. *Tell me when - love - Mother to Jig to Pavla Evelyn*
I always think of Margue when I sign Mother to you— Jack's love sent with this to both.

[Typed carbon copy, signed. Handwritten insertions. UTK]

To the Manager, Regina Palast Hotel

26 Belsize Crescent
March 31, 1952

Dear Sir:

Your reply to my inquiry of February 25th, 1952[220] arrived here on March 23rd, and I am greatly obliged to you for attempting to ascertain for me whether or not the parcel containing data to be used by me in a book I propose to write, had been forwarded by the hotel to my son Mr Creighton Scott.

I tell you this because the acknowledgment of this manuscript by my son himself as well as his daughter-in-law should, of course, be made to me; the reason I wish to

---

220 This letter has not survived.

have them and my first husband see the data being that I will write to them in this book, which will be my third volume of autobiography. And I will again appreciate the preservation of this record, if it is possible, until I am completely certain that the parcels sent from London directly to Munich since Christmas and containing trivial and unsolicited gifts for my grandchildren have not been confused with the parcel already twice forwarded after I sent it to the States last autumn before I had been informed when my son had gone to Germany.

I do indeed thank you for your kindness in attempting to assist me to locate the parcels. But the parcel I as an author value most is naturally the book synopsis, and it is in connection with this that I shall be indebted to you whenever I have reassurance in full.

Whenever I <u>do</u> I will send you a line to that effect, and meanwhile I continue greatly obliged,

Faithfully yours,

[Typed carbon copy, not signed. UTK]

To Creighton and Paula Scott

26 Belsize Crescent

March 29, 1952

~~March 29th~~ *April 2nd 1952 lacked cash for stamps—this was held to April 2nd 1952*

Please send on the precis to Cyril Kay Scott and NOT to me. The hotels letter mentions "my" receipt of a parcel as "assured" - but this is the opposite of my request, which alluded it to it as to be sent on to Jigs Dad as above. Jacks lawyer is Mr Lindsay Fisher of an old London legal firm - would make a better Will had I the cash - for you and Jack, however, the terms the same. Darlings
- Dont mistake this -we are not going to die! Be well—

The Regina Palast Hotel was appealed to by me on February 23rd for information regarding the parcel containing the precis or outline forwarded there by Margaret De Silver according to the instructions stamped on the parcel by the Postmaster at Red Hook, Duchess County, NY. And this is the Hotels amiable reply, which I quote as the phrasing may amuse you amiably.

"Dear Madame,

"In reply to your letter of 25th February I beg to inform you that the two parcels in question has received your son. I got the information by your daughter in law.

"Trusting that you will receive the parcel safely, we beg to remain

"faithfully yours

"W J Risderle"

So now my darling children please send the precis to Cyril and please for goodness sake come out of this bloody ban on communication, and tell us everything you like about yourselves.

We love you and dont forget it is real love

[Typed carbon copy, not signed. Handwritten annotations. UTK]

To Creighton and Paula Scott

26 Belsize Crescent
April 14, 1952

Darling Jig and Pavla:

When are we again to experience that pleasure of surprise ours when we had Pavlas Christmas note signed for both and telling us that you were comparatively near?

We have not had a word since. And as I wrote to the Regina Palast respecting the segment of an outline for an autobiographical volume by me which Margaret de Silver re-forwarded to the hotel when it was returned to Red Hook, Duchess County after having been sent by her there at my request, and the hotel assures me Pavla - or "my daughter-in-law" - assured <u>them</u> it was received, I am distressed again that I have not yet obtained your personal affirmation of this.

I dont like to write of nothing but mail problems, parcels etc, and I know you dont either, but just sensibly prompt replies to specific issues would relieve us both of burdens. Have you received any of my detailed letters about this. Please please PLEASE do anything you can at your end to conclude this interminable business about mail and whether it is actually received or not by the personal addressees.

We implore and dont know whom to implore, we so need details of yourselves and your lives in Munich as well as at home. Whatever has been at the bottom of a lack of free communication is criminal. We would so like to be precise as to this in order to combat it.

Are you both and the children well? What sort of job is Jig doing? Is it something Army or hushy, or something he can speak of freely?

The trees in front are just ready to bloom. We have hoped every year you would all see them. There have been nine daffodils out, and a few bluebells, but the garden is still a wilderness of weeds and needs a wall to shut it in so the flat can be private. It is warm here at present. How is it there? Do you see mountains afar? We havent yet any map of Germany. Are you both writing at least a little, and is Jig - fine artist that he actually is - painting some? We so hope so. Did the school continue satisfactory? When are we all to go home to live near and love each other and our various arts?

[Typed carbon copy, not signed. UTK]

To Evelyn Scott and John Metcalfe

[Grünwald, Germany]
April 19, 1952

Creighton Scott with Mother and Jack USA—temporary address on envelope otilostrasse 22

Graefelfing bei Munchen This make sending Jig to Germany a catastrophe! Rat [illeg] don't.

Dear Evelyn and Jack-

I'm scribbling my twice yearly note and sending along these snaps of the kids. We're all pretty well, but have no hope whatever of making any visits. It's hard for us to get away on a Sunday afternoon, although last Sunday we managed to take the whole day off for a drive to Innsbruck - <u>very</u> nice. *I am tired of this duty scribble -What the hell is Innsbruck to us? A char employed where I boarded in 1901*

We all send love and thanks for the book <u>Quite Crazy</u> which delights the kids.

The baby stands up and has 2 teeth, now.

Love,

Paula—

Pavla Scott I despise her senseless use of Paula

PS Your MSS arrived, but I can't send it on to Cyril as I haven't the remotest idea where he is now. Haven't heard from him for 6 months when he was about to move.

1952 -November This letter of my daughter-in-law is all any news of her with my son and grandchildren—four since April

The art of EVELYN SCOTT with Cyril Kay Scott is with Scott the art <u>with JOHN METCALFE WITH CREIGHTON Scott</u> with Pavla

This arrived on a brutal day an intolerable criminal day May 24th

[Handwritten, signed. Handwritten insertions and annotations by ES. UTK]

To Creighton and Paula Scott

26 Belsize Crescent

April 20 1952

Do you give Gladys address now as your address at home or Jigs Dad's I gave Jigs of Ridge Street Rutherford at the US Consulate here and I suppose I will have to go back to Gladys again for us

Darlings -

Where are the answers to my letters? Where is your personal acknowledgment of the outline of the autobiography I sent for you to read and send on to Cyril? Do you reply and are the letters stopped somewhere, or what? I cant help it. So would you were you in my place.

The plum tree in the front garden is beautiful just now. We so hoped some of you could manage a visit in time to see it. The spring bloom here is a very fine sight. We have nothing comparable in any city, though of course we do in the country. This tree is flawless, every cluster of white perfect, and the tree - there are two or three in front - has echoes up the street - in fact up both the streets at the crossing the house faces. They are airy gardens with that unreality of American autumns - so extravagantly lovely one is wordless, as one cant relate them to anything in the experience of every day. I think of them as Fredricks especially because Jig said he was the "botanist"- probably they all are now.

The teeth will soon have their first try-out. I have been to the dentists and he tried to make the old set fit but it could not be did. It will have been nearly nine months or more like ten months if you count the first extractions, since I had any to speak of. Has Julia quite a number by now? I hope so. At first we were neck and neck, but I think shed better win.

How are Denise Fredrick and Mathew and the school? How are our Jiggie and Pavli -

Please we love you - do reply *again*
To Jig mother
To Paula Evelyn
To all six my love and with Jacks.

[Typed carbon copy signed. Handwritten comments. UTK]

To Creighton and Paula Scott

26 Belsize Crescent
May 25, 1952

We are glad you had half a day at Innsbruck. We hope you can have some other at least short trips to beauty spots near you

Our darling best family:

I am both happy and grieved whenever I receive what has become - as Pavla justly says - my "bi-yearly note". I am naturally primarily grateful to her for writing me the meager assurances of any well-being the notes imply. But it would be false to the real love of Jack and myself for the six of you, my darlings, to pretend that the paucity of any sign that you yourselves are having the rewards that should be yours for your courageous struggle to maintain yourselves in an alien scene on small money, and still, I gather, without the full compensations in restored art careers which should be yours as well as ours - it would be foolish to pretend that the notes do more than alleviate a distress about you and about Jig especially, which, otherwise, is acute.

Jack is as delighted as I am to have some further snapshots of the four children, and they actually look in these in somewhat better physical condition than when the passport photo Pavla had enlarged and sent me at Christmas was taken, last year. They have sweet and appealing little faces, and this Jack especially remarked. He says he thinks they look more like Jig than when they were younger - the three eldest - and that Julia looks now very like Jig and Cyril. I think this.

You can imagine, I suppose, how these pictures pull at my heart and, I conjecture, by every indication, at Jacks too. The helplessness of us all, as yet, in relation to each other, and the longing probably common on all sides to be of mutual help, is nearly heart-breaking at times. But we refuse to become helpless or despairing. We are determined to fight on for both ourselves and yourselves as long as we live, and we still think we will all have soon the sort of "break" that is NOT heartbreak, but its antithesis.

Yes, this house is an octopus still, but once we are enabled to go home to the States we may be able to re-furbish it and repair it to the point which will command a sale that salvages for Jack something of the really large amount that has now gone into keeping it going and with a roof. *1952 —This letter was not acknowledged—November 1952*

I so wish the notes were not just "bi-yearly"! Please do not set a precedent of that sort, my dear children. We should like to know when Julias "two teeth" are augmented to four, and when - now being able to stand - she can walk. I still remember the day at Tappan when little Freddy climbed the stairs by himself - all the way to the top with no assistance. It was a great event. Denise, of course, by then could do everything, but he was still very very young.

I suppose the house you were in first became too uncomfortable as it was small, and probably expensive. It is irony that the "garden" did not materialize. But that is like here. We have had to appeal to the police to stop trespassing. It has improved since we did, but as soon as we can we will put up barricades of some sort as they are needed to make this flat fit to line in for us or future tenants, whom we hope will demand privacy as we ourselves do.

I have some teeth I think will be usable - hurrah!

[Typed carbon copy, not signed. Handwritten annotations. UTK]

To The Manager, Regina Palast Hotel

26 Belsize Crescent

June 4, 1952

1952—November Mention was of April in a letter as if in afterthought—indicative to me that they thought it easier not to stress—this speaks ill for Munich

Sir:

You were good enough, in February, 1952, to trace for me the parcel forwarded to the hotel for my American son, Mr Creighton Scott, and to write me that you had communicated with my daughter-in-law who said it had been received, with a second parcel sent from here. And when I acknowledged your kindness, I again requested you, if not inconvenient, to file my letter for reference until I had some word direct from Mrs Creighton Scott respecting the parcel.

I asked this because, at various times since the war, we have had trouble about the delivery of letters, and some, apparently, have been lost. And I now write to say-as I also promised I would, voluntarily-that my daughter-in-law has, finally, mentioned the parcel when writing to me. I still think she had probably already acknowledged it, and the information had not reached me; but, at any rate, now it has, my second request becomes superfluous, and I herewith thank you very much again for your kind aid.

Very truly yours,
Evelyn D Scott Metcalfe

[Typed carbon copy, signed. Handwritten annotation. UTK]

After nearly a year in Germany, Jigg and the family returned to the United States and, as they did not have a "home" base in the United States, they ended up living in a small serviced flat in the Hotel Chelsea in New York City on their return. There they remained for a year, during which time Jigg found a new job, this time in the newsroom of the Mutual Broadcasting System. In the summer of 1953, the family moved to Spring Valley, New York, whence Jigg commuted.

Paula's family on her mother's side were not wealthy but were fairly prosperous, and Paula had had to turn to them for financial support more than once. After some months in the Hotel Chelsea, she felt she had no option but to ask for help from her elderly great-aunt, Gertrude Brownell, who lived with her maid of many years in late-Victorian splendour on Central Park West.

To Paula Scott
50 Central Park West
New York City

November 22, 1952

Dearest Pavli

I am terribly distressed by your news - your suffering - and your difficulties.

You are creating difficulties for me too - who am taken for little less than half my income and need the other half for inevitable expenses (rent service living).

It seems unkind to mention this when you are so afflicted - but mentioning it makes me hope that Creighton will think better of going abroad - leaving a large family for others to provide for. My hope is that he will look for a job in New York or at least in this country and so be able, to some extent at least, to look after the family for which he is responsible.

You evidently think that I can give you 500 dollars by sending a cheque by reply mail - I have to go to a savings bank to draw out the 500.00 additional - and will do this in Monday - (send you some part of it at least).

With much love to you all

Aunt Kitty

[Handwritten on personal letterhead, signed. SFC]

To Creighton and Paula Scott

26 Belsize Crescent
December 6, 1952

Darling Jig and Pavla:

We are delighted to know you are back in the USA.[221] I do not wonder that, in the moving of yourselves and the four children home, there has, again, been some confusion as to mail. The American Consul at Munich has sent me your forwarding address and we now hope to have the letter we thought would be sent before you left advising us of how and where precisely you are, and whether Gladys, after all, has managed to put you up in her flat.

You have probably had some of my letters[222] respecting our arrangements for renting this flat and going home. These arrangements were three-quarters completed three months ago, but we have been temporarily delayed for the lack of a few of the things both essential to completing the flats furnishing and essential for our own travel - baggage and baggage mends, socks, stockings, handkerchiefs, a shirt or two for Jack, etc. We actually need about seventy-five dollars more as the delay itself has cost a disproportionate amount in added bills for heating, and a slight increase in accumulated taxes.

However, notwithstanding the delay, we will be home long before February 1st, when we are due in California; and to see you all <u>before</u> we go to the West coast for six months, is our dearest hope. And it should be possible to see Cyril too and Manly, we could feel normal and ready and eager for the opportunity to resume work on our books allowed by the Huntington Hartford Foundations invitation.[223] I think of you all day and night, every day; and to have the hell of ambiguities and misunderstandings distance has imposed removed once and for all will be to us like the re-beginning of genuine living instead of merely existing.

Please reply - I would rather not have to be exclusively dependent on Gladys forwarding, and certainly not at all once we are home again and you have had time to get settled.

Love should shine from this page for it is implicit in every letter.

We hope in every letter sent you. Our greetings to Gladys whom we naturally look forward to seeing again with the old affection, with Edgerton.

Mother-Evelyn-Mother

[Typed, signed. Handwritten insertions. Never opened by addressee. SFC. *Also* typed carbon copy with handwritten insertions as above. UTK]

---

221 There is no record of how Evelyn came to know that the family had returned to New York City.
222 Chapter 34 includes a number of letters regarding the condition of the house.
223 See Chapter 33.

Chapter 31

The Précis
November 1951 - April 1952

Cyril's autobiography, Life Is Too Short, *published in 1943 and detailing what he described as his six careers to date, was greeted with moderate critical approval. Importantly to Evelyn, it included an account of his "elopement" to Brazil with the then Elsie Dunn, the adoption of their new names, the birth of their son Creighton (who was known by his infant nickname "Jigg" throughout his life), the years of poverty in Brazil and their return to the United States in 1919.*

Evelyn did not see this book until 1945, although she knew it had been published. When she did finally see a copy, she was angered to read what she considered to be distortions. She could not believe that Cyril would have written some of the descriptions of her and their relationship which she considered to be libellous, and the only possible explanation she could imagine was that someone, unnamed, had altered the text at the printers between the proofing and printing stages and that said person had altered the passages she objected to with libellous intent. In her increasingly febrile view of her situation and Jack's, this distortion of her story was the result of one or more libels. This suspicion, which developed in her mind into a certainty, was a central theme in many of her letters from then on.

This is important because it marks the beginning of Evelyn's continuing and increasing conviction that she was being libelled, and this in turn fed her conviction that she was being kept from her son and grandchildren. I am introducing it here because the late 1940s is the point from which Evelyn's gradually deteriorating mental condition can be most easily dated.

Evelyn started work on her "Precis of events indicative of libel" (which she also referred to at times as her autobiography) in the autumn of 1951. This précis eventually became a 74-page single-spaced typed document, describing in some detail the forces she felt were preventing her and Jack from seeing their family and from getting their books published. She felt it imperative to share this précis with as many of her circle as possible in order to "clear her name" as she put it.

Each page was headed by a paragraph: the first reads "To those with Pride in the Preservation of the Integrity of American and British Artists and Art" with each succeeding heading longer than the preceding until the heading on the final page reads:

```
"Precis indicative of libel, to be read AS SOON AS POSSIBLE
BY CREIGHTON AND PAVLA SCOTT BY THE PERSONAL FRIENDS OF JOHN
METCALFE AND EVELYN SCOTT AND, if possible, BY CYRIL KAY SCOTT
whom Evelyn Scott is convinced has been victimized with Life Is
Too Short either in mss or when rushed to the printers during
Mr Kay Scott's illness which was preceeded by illness among the
Wellmans, this tampering or tinkering probably illegal because
unauthorized and done without consulting Mr Kay Scott himself
respecting certain facts involving Evelyn Scott with him and
their son, these facts so controverted by interpolations in the
text of Mr Kay Scott recognizably not his, that the result has
been as damaging to him as to any concerned, though most of all
to Mr Creighton Scott and his wife, who, inference, in a list
of "acknowledgements", might easily have been misconstrued as
having somehow sanctioned a villification of Evelyn Scott which
also cannot be Mr Kay Scotts and is a controversion of the
truth as to the life-long affection of son for Mother and of
Mother for son-all these things intollerable and compelling and
necessitation protest here. This precis is the condensation of
a longer precis to be completed in consistence with this one,
and its aim is the restoration of the integrity of American and
British Artists -"
```

The entire document is prefaced by the following handwritten note: "This MS contains an enormous amount of inaccuracy and I can only caution any reader to check almost any statement in it. [signed] Paula Scott".

When the following sequence of letters begins, Jigg and Paula and the children had been in Germany since October 1951, although Evelyn is not yet aware of that.

To Creighton and Paula Scott

26 Belsize Crescent
November 19, 1951

Darlings

I have compiled for reading by our PERSONAL FRIENDS OF WHOM YOU ARE THE FIRST AND WILL WE HOPE INCLUDE JIGS AND JIGS DAD a sort of documentary record of the various calamities which have resulted in that virtual suspension of our careers as artists which the war began, and fools FOOLS FOOLS continue. I did not intend to begin in so exclamatory a fashion, but it is still nearly impossible to write anything in London without egregious offensive interruptions of some sort, and that is what I had as I began this letter. However, I resume it because I would like you both and Cyril to know that I have sent this "precis" as I call it, which may eventually serve as a source of reference for a book on author experiences and the hell they have become, to Margaret De Silver as she and a few people - most of whom you too know - are trying to accumulate a fund to pay our expenses home.

They are to see the precis, but I have asked her to give it first to you and as you Jiggie seldom if ever sees her now and Pavla would find it difficult to get to town, I here ask whether or not you can have anybody go to Margarets for it and take it to you. I would trust it to the mails were it not always that mail is not specifically acknowledged, and though Pavla insists that all the trouble of that kind is at this end, I am not persuaded.

I especially would like to have Cyril read it because after reflecting on the matter ever since 1947, I re-read Life is Too Short, and I think Cyril has been somehow "economically" or otherwise forced into libelling himself in having allowed a tinkering with the mss of that books, probably when it was partly completed or in rough draft, which was not authorized as to detail. I do not and CANNOT believe that Cyril himself could possibly, no matter what the conditions, have written anything as tripey, cheap, sleazy, false and at odds with his own PROFUNDITY elsewhere, as that account of "why" our first Emergency Passport was issued in 1919 at the Rio American Embassy by Ambassador Morgan: which, actually was because I was ill.

Then there is the further provocation to libellous rumour in the fact that Lippincotts, without consulting him - I am very positive here because it is publishing routine to take out copyrights without consulting authors - without consulting him, took out copyright for him in the name of Fredrick Creighton Wellman which legally ceased to be his name when he registered for himself and me in Rio at the American Embassy as Cyril Kay Scott.

There are many factual misstatements, most connected with me, and to have it said in print and circulated that I "neglected" Jig whom we all love and whom I hope I continued to prove I loved as long as I was allowed to see him or have any contact with him - to have that damnable implication underscored, when it is as false as hell and blatantly hell! No - Cyril could NOT he could not - COULD NOT have perpetrated such a thing. I have known him since 1913, and never knew him to do anything petty, mean or base - Jack agrees completely - Cyril could not have written the lies or the vicious attacks on me and Jig and Pavla could not have agreed to having their names associated with mean, petty spites, which were NOT Cyrils.

It is for Cyril to say in respect to his book, but I think a demand should be made to have it re-issued in a considerably larger edition which he does the editing on and which has deleted from it things he knows are not so - some about myself and himself and some just spite allusions to my books, also damaging as it gives an effect of elan envy in him, which is UNJUST to HIM - he was never mean or envious of me in his life.

The circulation of the book in its present form, with the interpolations I discern and Jack agrees were NOT Cyrils has been doing us damage steadily ever since 1943. It may be the things the book may have contributed to the criminal mystifications about my Fathers estate,[224] as he went to the Veterans Hospital in Biloxi on December 23rd,

---

224 See Chapters 25 and 26.

1943, when it had not long been out, and he was, as you both know already, a coward about scandal, as he had suffered libel and had suffered in a yellow journal libelling of me and of Cyril - we were one then in every sense - which almost killed my Mother and made her as difficult as she was,

I am not sensational. I am giving facts. And should my family wish to leave it to me to give the facts, very well. But I think we must agree as humans to fight our battle together - Scotts Metcalfe and Wellmans conceding Margarets courage and her generosity. She is not all-wise. She has sometimes offended me for the moment. We have often disagreed. But she has stood for straight truth and generous procedures when nobody - literally nobody-save her would turn a hand.

Our love love love love love love love love love love

Kiss Jig this for Pavla kiss Jig

and please love each other and let us love and be fond - for Dad and Jack and me this is solution in the personal sense and publically art must be pure again

[Typed carbon copy, not signed. UTK]

To Creighton and Paula Scott

26 Belsize Crescent
November 25, 1951

Dear Darling Good Children

You will realize I am anxiously awaiting your opinion of my intention to protest on behalf of myself yourselves and with myself and yourselves and Jacks on behalf of Cyril Kay Scott as the author, the unauthorized tinkering that must have gone on with Life Is Too Short when he was ill, Paul had just been ill, and the book was scheduled to go to press.

I think Jigs Dad had written most of it in rough draft, but had omitted the Cercadinho section because of Escapade and that whoever got hold of it and went through it inserted some sleazy "pulp" writing which consisted in misinterpreting Cyril and myself by just reversing the truthful account of his own and my relations then and thereafter, and that this same interloper on the fine arts, being imperfectly informed as to the reason why Ambassador Morgan at the American Embassy in Rio first issued to Cyril for him and me and Jig the Emergency Passport accepting Cyrils change of name, just concocted a stupid pulp thriller pseudo-"explanation", which was an occasion for rumour, has steadily raised more and more unnecessary hell for all concerned every year.

The reason, as I said in the letter sent recently, for the issuance of this Passport was humane, as I had been seriously ill most of the time since Jigs birth and had been operated on twice within a few weeks at the Presbyterian Mission Hospital in the interior of Pernambuco, where the operator was Dr Butler, a Mayo-trained surgeon

Please also try to find some means of reading the precis of happenings since 1939 which has been sent to Margaret De Silver, who has generously tried to bestir someone to attempting the financing of our return to the States and the end of this impossible, ambiguous living in limbo, which has resulted from our penuriousness here, and which CANNOT be any further endured.

When you have read the precis please return it to Margaret who will not offer it for general circulate *[sic]*, but will allow it to be read by a few friends who may be helpful in deciding what is to be done to counteract on our behalf an effect of the libel which has continued during eight damn bloody years.

I think the time has come to call a halt on desecrating art. He could NOT have written the cheap passages in that book, and he could NOT have knowingly allowed them because of the degrading inferences that might be drawn and harm us all Please speak out. Mother

[Typed carbon copy, typed signature. UTK]

To Evelyn Scott

Margaret DeSilver
130 West 12th Street, Apt 12G
New York City 11

December 6, 1951

Dear Evelyn

I have received the "precis" which I have forwarded to Jig at Red Hook, NY as you requested. Maybe eventually we'll get this business straightened out!

Maggie

This note on December 6th 1951 —I have precise facts, irrefutable facts in respect to criminal interference received here December 8 1957

[Handwritten on personal letterhead, signed. Handwritten annotation. UTK]

To Creighton and Paula Scott

26 Belsize Crescent
December 9, 1951

Darlings -

Margaret De Silver writes me she has sent you the precis I compiled as my own reference for use whenever I write my own realistic and completely authentic account of the life of an author. I hope soon to have JIGS OWN ACKNOWLEDGEMENT that both of you have received it. As soon as Jig can write to my letters respecting important matters and run no risk of any interference or "economic" discouragement - due sometimes probably to communicating with a mother in England - ONE of our anxieties will considerably diminish.

Please give me both of you as soon as you can your opinion on the libel which has apparently resulted from the sort of interpolated writing in Life Is Too Short. I KNOW

CYRIL COULD NOT HAVE DONE IT HIMSELF he is too intellectual and fastidious a man.

I hope Fredrick had a nice little birthday. He is eight now and I like to think of the nice things one can do when eight. Mathew is going to school earlier than I did. We hope all our behaving and as bright as good as always, including Julia who is still competing with me on teeth.

We hope the house is warm and that warm clothes are enough to more than "just get by on". I hope soon to go to the dentist. I always wish for ten times as much for your six. How wonderful to be again able to earn money with books.

Denise Fredrick Mathew and Julia I know love you both as we love you we love you we love you we love you PLEASE ACKNOWLEDGE and see whether we can overcome impasses about mail.

Evelyn
to Jig Mother

[Typed carbon copy, signed. UTK]

To Margaret DeSilver

26 Belsize Crescent
December 11, 1951

Maggie darling-

I should think it would have become completely obvious to the veriest moron by now that Jig and Pavla do not of themselves invent situations which embarrass and distress them just as much as us, and yet this is what has happened, and is to me - my opinion - continued proof that their lives are being "directed" in some fashion or manner which just makes them serve as crook cover for whoever began libelling the Scott-Metcalfes when tampering was imposed on Cyrils autobiography during the war, and misstatements were made so damningly disadvantageous to the author himself that it is NOT possible that he was consulted as to detail.

Your own letters to us are not interfered with my dear Margaret but when Pavla complains to me that I do not receive some - perhaps a number - of the letters she writes me for both I believe her complexly as I know she is straight-forward. And though she says in a vague, general way, "we have all your letters" I know the most truthful may be so wrongly isolated because of stupidities on the part of others that they may be hard-put enough to make such general statements as a matter of "diplomacy" because at least some of my letters to them are delivered. Pavla lives too far from the Post Office to go for letters herself[225] and Jig spends six hours of every day commuting according to her - or so I infer as she said "it is three hours each way to New York but at that it is some better than Rutherford for Jig".

---

225 This passage is based on the mistaken assumption that the Scott family were still in Red Hook.

What are we to do? It is as bad as dictator countries, to be cut of repeatedly this way from those human ties most essential to our normal lives even as are our books.

The Cyril Kay Scotts including Evelyn and John Metcalfe are NOT bloody damn criminals who must go skulking about the States, but the utter rottenness of these provocations to confusion and distress would make you think so if you did not know them. I do NOT believe Jig is in Germany, or ever was, And I do believe both are truthful - and that seeming inconsistencies is merely apparent.

I WONT be german and I KNOW Jig and Pavla MUST THINK REALLY AS THEY ALWAYS HAVE and it must be from German toads that this coercion emanates. That is where rackets have been straight through, and I CANT STAND the libelling of my straight pure American family any more. I WONT I WONT I WONT.

I MUST criticise our Government for allowing what it obviously does, and so making me drivel away my life in protests it must seem to it get nowhere! - damn it! If it is "seditious" to object to libel, where the hell have our Civil Liberties gone? *I hope the precis is not meddled with—it is my personal property and data for a book-but to be read by Cyril*

Love - I hope you read this. I dont apologise, because I dont think apologizing means a bloody thing. But I know you must long for sense somewhere just as Jack and I do.

[Typed carbon copy, not signed. Handwritten insertion. UTK]

To Creighton and Paula Scott

26 Belsize Crescent
January 13, 1952

Darling Jig and Pavla:

Please send some more news of yourselves and, also, tell us whether you have received and read the section of outline of possible autobiography which was forwarded to the Hotel Regina Palast, Maximilian Platz, Munich.

This is not one of my long letters - I will write more extensively when I have one of Jigs and Pavlas both - but this is to remind you we love you and we are eager for news and sight of you more than ever now you are almost near.

*With our love
Mother for step-grandfather Jack too*

I am so disgusted with "respectable" "pious" "religious" bloody "commerce" in people's letters I could cheerfully see every purveyor of "popular" and "average" "tastes" shot - I hope you have something less inane than some letters from those of our friends who fall into the clutches of damnable putrid fallacious trade "psychology" - arrant rats propound it. This is the result of a spatter of mail - since this was written - mail about nothing normal to the writer of these hocus-pocus suggested letters. I hope for yours in different vein.

[Typed carbon copy, signed. UTK]

Gladys Grant was an exceptional woman. She had known Evelyn since they were both young and living in New York City and had also known Jigg since he was a small child. Somehow she managed to act as a buffer between Evelyn's unremitting and increasingly paranoid possessiveness and Jigg's need to live his own life without interference from his mother. She managed to retain Evelyn's trust and friendship while at the same time providing loyal and uncritical friendship and support to Jig and Paula and their children.

To Gladys Grant

26 Belsize Crescent
January 20, 1952

Pavla sent me an enlargement of her Passport photo with the four children. I was pleased to have it. She is too thin yet, so is Freddy. Denise is pretty but not much like when age 3, Julia is just a baby and Mathew looks dark and not the blond you described a year or two ago. Did his hair change or is it the picture? We would so like to have Jigs too. *Of course I think forcing Jack and myself to linger in Britain and forcing Jig and Pavla to go abroad for jobs is "economic" crime and amounts to trying to steal our birthright as Americans Jig included*

Dear Gladys:

The outline of the section of the autobiography I will write unless I die before I can, was sent to Margaret De Silver with the request that she find someone, if she could, who sometimes saw Jig and Pavla and could hand it to Jig for their reading and to be sent on to Cyril to read, also. As I mentioned this is just a section of an account - in synopsis - of the "economic" life of Scott-Metcalfes, the full account to begin with 1919 and New York and to be carried on to the date of writing. I am anxious to have Cyril read what I say of <u>Life Is Too Short</u>, because I am completely and unshakably convinced that he was taken "economic" advantage of at the time he was writing it, at the outset of the war, and was compelled "economically" to assent to a sort of editorial chopping, hashing, and writing down by someone other than himself who did NOT and could NOT have consulted him as to the details

This is really important to anyone who has any scruple or is enough above moronism to grasp the fact that it is destructive of any society to allow lives careers and human relations to be attacked by cheap defamers who "amuse" masses.

But probably no one who has not endured the senseless and brutal ambiguities and silences - many due to mail mishandled - which have pursued myself and Jack in our every prized relation, could possibly envisage how serious to me the risk Margaret unwittingly took on my behalf in mailing still again an important parcel - the entire human side of my life is at stake in clearing up relations with Cyril and Jig which were damaged by this book - which had no guarantee of safe arrival. The parcel was returned to Margaret at once, stamped "Forwarding address, Hotel Regina Palast, Maximilian Platz, Munich" - probably the hang-out of the Army - ours, Jews, or what I dont know! I just guess! - and she at once sent it there. This was in the latter part of November - when it came to her and was returned - I dont know what day she mailed it - and it has not yet been acknowledged by Jig and Pavla in any letter received here as yet.

But the agonizing thing to me was that the very considerateness of Margaret in forwarding and at once advising me by air mail, failed of its effect because I had no prior knowledge or specific information of any sort as to the movements of my American family until informed thus obliquely that they were in Munich - or so I presumed, and not it seems correctly.

I no longer hesitate to say, as I did at first when I was trying to help my family and still more in the dark than now, that I saw every clear proof in 1943-44 that liars, libellers and political defamers were interfering with our personal lives and were doing their utmost to poison the minds of my son and his wife against us. Judging by Jigs visit of 1949, I think they did not succeed. Pavlas little notes also, though unsatisfactory are the further proof that she is as out-going as conditions imposed on her have permitted.

And so my dear Glad I am telling you what I asked you to tell me about a month ago in the letter requesting you to ascertain whether or not Jig and Pavla had received the "precis" which is a section of an autobiography yet to be written and which I ask Cyril to read wherever he may be. *I hope you have the full set of my books and will continue with them. More flattering even than gifts!*

[Typed carbon copy, not signed. Handwritten annotations. UTK]

Chapter 32

The Evelyn Scott Fund
December 1951 - November 1952

In 1951 Margaret DeSilver had the idea of creating a fund to clear Jack's debts and bring him and Evelyn back to the United States. Evelyn welcomed this initiative, but she insisted on it being on her own terms. She was also determined (or maybe it was because of her increasing self-obsession) that potential donors were made aware of her difficulties in becoming united with her son and his family.

In these letters Evelyn makes frequent reference to a "precis" referred to in the previous chapter. This document conflated incidents in Evelyn's life during the 1930s and 1940s with her inability to restore contact with Jigg and his family. It was her wish that this be circulated to potential donors who would, she assumed, have a better understanding of her situation and would therefore be more likely to contribute to the fund.

Another new feature of these letters is the evidence they hold of Evelyn's confused thinking: writing of herself in the first and the third persons in the same paragraph; numerous non-sequiturs; and an unconventional vocabulary (with spellings to match). It is hard to know whether these are the result of the obvious distress she was experiencing at the time, or whether they are a foretaste of her future obsessions with political "tinkerings" and her belief that external forces were keeping her from her son and his family. And, throughout, her insistence that art must be detached from politics, and that somehow these two created and contributed to the libel which she was convinced was preventing her being reunited with her son.

(Unfortunately Margaret DeSilver's original letter, which prompted the replies below, has not survived.)

To Margaret DeSilver
Truro, Massachusetts
July 10, 1951

Dear Margaret,

What a damn shame about Evelyn! Of course, your idea is excellent. I'll be glad to lend my name and help a little - how much depends on my own finances measured by my many great responsibilities. I should think the signers of the letter should include a number of our outstanding novelists who most admire E's work - such as Dos Passos and Faulkner; and a few more critics - for instance Van Wyck Brooks and Lewis Mumford. I really don't understand E's utter neglect! She is certainly one of the important American novelists of our generation!

When are you coming to the Cape? Do phone us and come and see us.

Always (hurriedly),

Waldo

[Typed, signed, strikethrough by Waldo. HRC]

To Margaret DeSilver

Rutherford, New Jersey

August 6, 1951

My dear Margaret DeSilver:

I shall be glad to read at any benefit you plan for Evelyn Scott, but I do not want my name used on your letter head.[226] Under such circumstances you may not want me to participate in the effort at all but it is all I am willing to do.

Sincerely yours,

William Carlos Williams

[Typed, signed. HRC]

To Margaret DeSilver

Princeton, New Jersey

August 7, 1951

Dear Mrs DeSilver

I returned only last night from the Middle East to find your disturbing letter about Evelyn Scott. You may certainly use my name in a campaign for her relief. I will try tomorrow to see the Secretary of the National Institute of Arts and Letters.[227] If anything can be done there, it will be done at once. I am at a loss to think of any other source of immediate relief, but I am sure that, given a little time, we can rally people to the support of the campaign. I will write to you again in the next day or two.

Yours sincerely,

Allen Tate

[Carbon of handwritten letter, signed. HRC]

---

226 What Williams did not say is that he and Evelyn had been lovers during the 1920s.

227 This institute (now the American Academy of Arts and Letters) was modelled on the Académie Française and included in its membership a large number of authors and critics. The institute awarded grants to individual writers on the recommendation of its members.

To Margaret DeSilver

26 Belsize Crescent

August 8, 1951

My Dear Maggie

I can't tell you how much I thank you for your letter - enclosing check for $100 and how grateful we both are. It really just about saves our lives. And I'm the more appreciative since I do realise that you have many many calls upon your native generosity, - and many problems of your own.

I do think that, if you are so kind and unselfish in time, labour, and some incidental vexation (probably) as to undertake the organisation of an Evelyn Scott Fund, as you suggest might be possible, it would be a splendid thing. I believe that Evelyn is of the same opinion, - providing, of course, that any funds resulting were not regarded as implying a cessation to writing, but rather as a help to further writing. We know of course that there is no doubt about your regarding it in this manner, but a few others possibly might misconceive the object of such a Fund. However, a suitable wording of the appeal would be adequate protection against this, I should say. In any case we could certainly think of no one so fitted as yourself, in every way, to conduct the matter. I myself, I may say right away, am unreservedly enthusiastic about the idea, and more than ever grateful to you for advancing it. Even if they appear were only very moderately "successful" (and I should allow myself no higher hopes) it would be a godsend.

I won't add more just now as I want to air-mail this off, - but I just can't express my personal relief, and my gratitude to yourself.

Bless you, dear Maggie,

Jack

PS. I would re-emphasise for my own part, that too high a "target" should not be set. Pete knows, it would be nice if realised, - but we should be fortunate, and lucky (and ought to be bloody grateful!) for anything. So, if you can, I should rather not bother about any too-precise figures Evelyn mentions as "necessary". If you are self-denying enough to shoulder such a chore, and if sufficient funds resulted for us to come to the States, - tant mieux - but I should get a job there, naturally, if only for the preservation of my own little amour propre (+ to pay off debts). But, - considerably short of that, - anything would help. This is just an added post-script from me personally - to which you won't refer.

Again, - bless you!

Jack

[Handwritten, signed. HRC]

To Evelyn Scott

Eastham, Massachusetts

August 14, 1951

Dear Evelyn:-

I'm pleased you and Jack are pleased with the idea of the Fund, but it is ticklish to keep it, as you so sensibly pointed out, from being just a substitute for real recognition and continued publication. So later on I will write you in greater detail about so far rather vague outlines, and get your approval on any public letter before making a move. I have had interested responses to the idea from Waldo Frank, Edmund Wilson, Lewis Gannett, Allen Tate. I do not want to seem to be putting it up to others what I might be able to swing myself, at any risk to your basic welfare and to your proper pride. But I feel you do also need more actual cash than I can manage. But it must all be done JUST RIGHT.

Much love to you and thanks again for writing. I'll write you at greater length a little later.

Margaret

[Typed, signed. UTK]

To Margaret DeSilver

26 Belsize Crescent
August 20, 1951

Please note as you read that every private and personal document I left in the States had to be stored with Cyril and Manly when Jig and Pavla went South and returned in a used car. I just hope bloody klansmen have not meddled with them.

Margaret my dear

Not pressing for reply - not until there are some positive developments. We hope Eastham Massachusetts is nice and you enjoy it - know your letters are forwarded

I dont mean this to be an answer to answer, and I await further information respecting anything that eventuates about the fund for getting us home whenever something really develops and for that just wish to thank you, and, also, Waldo. Edmund Wilson, Allen Tate and Lewis Gannett for having evinced interest in it and grasping that it is NOT TO BE A SUBSTITUTE FOR CONTINUED PUBLICATION FOR BOTH JACK AND MYSELF THERE AND HERE - it is generous of them, but most of all generous of you Mag dear.

I am as distressed as before, however, about my family, and all I can say is that I implore and importune anybody anybody ANYBODY with any human feeling - such as you know I have - who is not associated in their minds with politics, to go to see them WITHOUT WRITING FIRST the letters they sometimes get but more often dont, as far as I can judge by the evidence.

I dont ask you yourself to do more than you have or anything that makes you shrink because you too have had your sensibilities hurt and cant bear "foisting" yourself and must be re-assured. But do please remember that I am a stickler for accuracy and that I cannot do other than conclude from the facts I myself know that, ever since the experiences of which I told you here, both Jig and Pavla and probably Margaret Hale Foster and Cyril, have been intimidated by rumour about me and - I think - about themselves and all my friends; and that, in consequence, they have been isolated over and over whenever they moved to any new address, and that Pitcher Lane[228] has yet to prove different from Rutherford in this respect.

Mag my dear - the cable you sent has just arrived[229] as I say on page one of my letter with this and Jack and myself are full of the utmost gratitude again and hope you will thank Allen as I will myself shortly as soon as you see him. You are restoring my belief in humans and Allen is contributing to the revival of our optimism so genuinely that we will not forget this proof of his own sustained character of pure artist and will always remember his generosity as we do yours. And this, of course, I will myself tell him when I write to him.

We are fed to the gills with guff so I cannot say I "pray" you may be rewarded for your goodness, but if I could "pray" in a world such as we have, I would insist Margaret De Silver among the first bloody old "God" should save. My "blasphemies" have their justification, and are considerably less than those to which politicians are too readily inured.

[Typed carbon copy, not signed. UTK]

To Margaret DeSilver

26 Belsize Crescent

August 24, 1951

To be forwarded to Eastham Massachusetts. Government gas[230] took the whole of that other draught and I literally never saw a penny, once it was banked - but it isnt Jacks fault they are blood-suckers, he is supporting me and is in terrible difficulties YET we have to pay or be sunk

Maggie darling -

You cannot over-estimate the good it does Jack as well as myself to know you are being sustained in your generous and lovely effort to really get us home. I can see Jack improving in spirits already and in health with this, and I have now written to Allen Tate and hope he will show you the letter, as William Rose Benet approached "The Institute for Arts and Letters" on our behalf in 1948, and he succeeded in obtaining five hundred dollars for me, which is the sole help anybody in the States has given us since years before the war, with exception of yourself and of the two or three checks Lenore has, also, sent.

---

228 At this time Evelyn was writing numerous letters to try and establish to which of two places named "Red Hook" her son had moved. She eventually learnt they lived on a road called Pitcher Lane.

229 This has not survived.

230 One of the causes of Jack's indebtedness (see Chapter 34) was the escalating bill for gas heating and hot water for his tenants. He was not permitted by law to raise the rent to cover these increased charges.

However, the experience especially re-impressed me with the fact that we must save in the States in order to return home there, because the five hundred dollars - like most of your help - went bang into the house, almost to the final penny. Nor was there any alternative for us. And this five hundred will have to go into the house, too. We will be jailed for debts otherwise so I am told. We are in arrears with everything, including "income tax" on this property based on a theoretic "income" although we have been losing two hundred pounds a year on it during some years.

Would you be willing to become the official "Trustee" of my "Fund"? - I have suggested to Allen Tate that I hope you will because you grasp the situation completely now I think - and you and Jack can consult as to the minimum we can peg on with here once anything is accumulated. It is the one way of getting out of reach of tyrannical extremists who - as I have often seen indicated - bitterly resent ones normal determination to resume the life normal to ones self and to see ones family in person.

This is the Truth again. Weve loved you for so long its not "new" to say we do now, but you are

[Typed carbon copy, not signed. UTK]

To Margaret DeSilver

26 Belsize Crescent
August 25, 1951

Maggie darling -

Would you be willing to become the "trustee" of any fund accumulated in the bank there for our return? I hope so because your grasp of our financial plight is I think complete like Jigs when here, and your grasp of our situation will probably be even better when you have the letter respecting Jig Cyril and Pavla which I mailed to you day before yesterday[231] and which had to do explicitly with badgerings endured in the South by everybody not moronic.

I am more than obliged to Waldo for offering to draw up a letter to be circulated on our behalf - on mine especially as an American but Jack should be included as artist and as the quota resident he was for so many years. And to re-assure those whom gossip may have boggled as to my standing the cable sent Allen was signed with my Passport Signature in full - Evelyn Dunn Scott Metcalfe - and the American Embassy clerk has seen my birth certificate with my baptismal name of Elsie on it and the names of both my parents in full and my place of birth and affidavits as to my identity, some still such as can be checked on.

I will be very appreciative if you will yourself read Waldos draught of a letter and will let me see a copy. I thought that letter circulated about Patchen[232] was not

---

231 This letter has not survived.
232 Margaret had suggested a funding letter based on that of a similar fundraising campaign for Kenneth Patchen, an American writer who had become poverty-stricken as a result of a spinal injury.

good - and sometimes people with the best intentions dont realize possible angles of the impression likely to be created by the manner of presentation. I would like to be assured that by no possibility can anything said on my behalf reflect on Jack Jig Pavla or Cyril. Jack has supported me here at some sacrifice to himself and Jig and Pavla have done no more because they just couldnt.

> We always love you but you endear yourself again

[Typed carbon copy, not signed. UTK]

To Evelyn Scott

> Princeton, New Jersey
>
> August 28, 1951

Dear Evelyn: *1952—What about John Metcalfe's art—he is British born*

I am of course glad to get your letter but distressed by the news it brings.

I am sure that Mrs DeSilver will succeed in getting up a fund to bring you back to this country, but as you know such a campaign takes time; and we are of course anxious about your immediate plight. If any other resource suddenly appears I will take advantage of it on your behalf. Meanwhile I am joining Mrs DeSilver's campaign.

You are quite right about the more fundamental need of getting home where you can participate again in the literary world. It is almost impossible to do this abroad, where one's connections, however good, are never quite adequate. The British publishers quite naturally feel little obligation to do well by us unless they are certain of getting a lot of money out of the connection.

I can scarcely believe that this $100.00 will go very far. I can only hope that you can hold out until more effective aid can be organized. Please give my regards to Jack. Caroline joins me in warm regards to you both.

> Sincerely yours,
>
> Allen Tate

[Typed, signed. Handwritten annotation. HRC]

To Margaret DeSilver

> Princeton, New Jersey
>
> August 29, 1951

Dear Mrs DeSilver:

I am at a loss to know what else to do at present, but I shall be glad to join you in any concerted effort on her behalf. A long letter from her[233] received yesterday, tells a very sad tale. I can well understand her desire to come back to this country, and I think she would be better off here. At the same time one must remember that she has been away so long, she has not published a book here in so many years, she has been

---

233 This letter has not survived.

virtually forgotten: the public and the publishers have a very short memory. It is by no means certain that a publisher would undertake the task of rehabilitating her as a writer; and even if this could be managed, there would still be, as in England, the problem of a steady livelihood. Very few writers make a living out of their books, even if they have a best-seller or two from time to time.

Sincerely yours,

Allen Tate

[Typed, signed. HRC]

To Margaret DeSilver

26 Belsize Crescent

September 9, 1951

Maggie darling

I sent yesterday letters of thanks to Allen Tate for his appeal to "The National Institute of Art and Letters" on my behalf, and, also, a letter to Committee who granted me the gift of a hundred dollars, but I realize you are the benign instigator of Allens move to assist and my gratitude and Jacks goes to you again.

You know our history of our poverty and the clothes! I was not out of the house more than a few times last summer, 1950, and this year had hoped for an improvement; but my teeth are still raising hell plates wont stay in and gag and I am as penned as ever and except for the visit to Ewell just before we saw you in June, I have not left the house, again, except during my seven weeks of dentistry, so it looks as though even that "pleasure" was taken advantage of.

So please swear for me! - even though I dont yet know at whom to swear! In 1949 I lost a carbon of my book of childrens verse, which, this summer, I have re-typed, so that I NOW have THREE copies. However, today, Jack went through every book in the flat, and as I did the same yesterday, he agrees with me that these three books were swiped since May; and that they could have been swiped at no time except when I was at the dentists, unless a nasty electrician who was very offensive when working in the study where they were, and who boasted that he had been employed by Agatha Christie, took them in spite, because I admitted to him I had no tip for him and could not afford any.

I think the time has come to demand Governments that do not allow scoundrels of any persuasion - call them "right" or "left" - to meddle with personal property and I know you will agree, too.

So when you are discussing me I hope more than ever you will tell people there all these things and mention Jig and Pavla, who should NOT be left at the mercy of crooked "policemen" of the sort who protect crooks and allow thefts. They had begun in Tappan. I would like to see thieves who take such things as paintings and mss electrocuted - and I am not by nature fierce.

Our love and our gratitude, for any help.

[Typed carbon copy, not signed. UTK]

To Margaret DeSilver

26 Belsize Crescent
October 11, 1951

Maggie darling

Will you be good enough to hand the letter in this envelope[234] to Waldo or mail it to him as convenient to yourself - first reading it, as it is about the precis of events which I may one day include in a memoir of New York and of the war, as I have yet to write in the first person of the literary world.

The precis is to be regarded as AUTHOR COPYRIGHTED just in case - for I do not wish and WONT HAVE good book material spoiled by any newspaper distortion.

We just must put an end to the idea that no body should think, and that original inferential comment on contemporary happenings has to be in those political terms extorted by military dolts.

We love you - everything lately has been hell again, but probably bloody politics has been figuring more than ever, and what we should like would be what I call PINK CONSERVATISM - by which I mean a CHANGE better minds more intellect and MORE TRUTH, and an end to hocus-pocus fears about jobs, which just keep political scoundrels in the saddle to eternity.

Our own fortunes reflect what goes on publically and we should love to be SAVED AS AUTHORS and go home to the States and help to restore Jig and Cyril and other artists of high type to the ARTS.

We love you for everything you do and are doing.

[Typed carbon copy, not signed. UTK]

To Waldo Frank

26 Belsize Crescent
October 11, 1951

Sent to Mrs Margaret De Silver 130 West 12th Street, Apt G, New York City with the request to pass it on to Mr Frank. *Love to Maggie. Please see people read precis when it gets to you don't just glance. Grateful Evelyn*

Dear Waldo,

Margaret De Silver has certainly proven herself again the fine friend we always knew her to be. Jack and I are both so grateful to her for trying to get somebody interested in financing our return home, either by means of publication resumed with conditions that are a guarantee against "token" handling such as killed every possibility of sales when The <u>Shadow of the Hawk</u> and <u>The Muscovites</u> my book and Jig's[235] - were published by Scribner's during the war.

---

234 The letter referred to here appears immediately below this letter.
235 Jigg's only novel, *The Muscovites*, was published in 1941.

The appreciation goes to you here unreservedly, but as we have not had the letter yet, it occurs to me you may have been waiting at your end for what I referred to as a precis of events since 1939, which I propose sending in original to Margaret and in carbon to Allen to be read privately by Margaret and yourself and anyone whom any of you know who can be guaranteed to read it without political bias and to neither "hush" me up about things I object to in the current scene because these are destructive of pure art value, nor let us in for the sort of libellous misconstruction on the happenings set forth which is an invariable result of journalistic intrusion on the art world. *I disapprove of cuts and won't stand them again and am adamant against editing. I did not want it known I had tried cutting but I did once—it is hopelessly wrong!*

The precis - a carbon is to go to "The National Institute of Arts and Letters" too - the precis, as I have been going over the material of the mangled preface and elaborating it, seems to be to be that of a potential further volume of memoirs to be written in the end about the art careers of the Scott-Metcalfes and their friends and acquaintances in the art world, and so I also wish to have the content accepted as already copyrighted by Evelyn Scott and NOT for the public prints until the time arrives to re-write it at leisure and incorporate it with experiences which long antedated the war, here covered and including Britain but unconnected with any damn "war secrets" as I know nothing of them, thought I was with Jack during all his 1939-46 service with the "RAF", in Canada and here, and wasnt in Scotland where he was the first year because I was economically trapped as a "neutral" in New York and he couldnt send me any money. This precis will be ready in two or three weeks but meanwhile we are pretty desperate again. *So please please pester anyone you can—I think Allen could show my precis to Mr Epstein as I have "altercated" with him about art. Anyhow we won't despair.*

[Typed carbon copy, not signed. Handwritten insertions. UTK]

To Evelyn Scott and John Metcalfe

Eastham, Massachusetts
October 12, 1951

Dear Evelyn and Jack:

My "Evelyn Scott Fund" is turning out to be far more complicated than I realized. First of all, to have it NOT have a PUBLIC and OFFICIAL look involves a good deal of very delicate planning. Waldo has been most fine and generous about ideas and suggestions, and one was that each of the four persons whom I first approached and who responded warmly and eagerly, make up a list of people to whom each of them might write a personal letter. This will take time, as these people are all busy people and also because it is very difficult for any one person, judging by my own experience, to think up a likely list of people who have not already been appealed to for this that and the other project many times over.

Secondly, I myself feel that coming to the States would be an impossibly large and expensive undertaking unless Jack FIRST had a job lined up here, and unless you sold your Hampstead house, or leased for a long term. Living here may not involve quite as much red tape as England, but it is actually more expensive, as to rent, food and clothing (partly, of course, because we do not have any regulations). Then, too, the publishing business here is even more cautious and wary than in England, in spite of the fact that we do not have your crippling paper shortage. Instead, we have inflation, which makes everything very expensive.

Also I would say that the mood of America is at the moment far from adventurous, intellectually speaking. In plain language, dear people, I think when you get here you are going to be as angry and troubled about conditions in general as you are in England, and I am afraid the struggle to heat will be about the same. On the other hand, the market is certainly here, and also family and friends. That I know is your crucial consideration. But I just feel the raising of enough money to get you here and launch you, so to speak, is going to be difficult and slow.

Later Waldo corrects this somewhat by saying he had in mind a form letter that would not look like a form letter, which each of us would sign and send off to a small list of prospects. Or else that a list could be bought or borrowed, such as the Patchen list, but still signed individually. Well, we will try to work out some sound and respectable method. In the meantime, much love -

Maggie DeS

[Typed, signed. UTK]

The following sequence is included in its entirety as it vividly illustrates Evelyn's conviction that it was necessary for potential donors to be aware of all of her circumstances: not only the books for which she was trying to find publishers, but her insistence that Jack, Jigg and Cyril all be recognised for their gifts and achievements. She conflated her difficulties in finding publishers with an unspecified form of political interference and mixed this with issues of citizenship, including Jack's status as a "quota" resident. And she insisted that all of this be included in the appeal letter.

Waldo Frank provided the first draft of a letter asking for funds for Evelyn and Jack and was quickly discouraged by Evelyn's reaction to it. It is not entirely clear how the drafting developed but the final appeal letter was very probably a combined effort by several of Evelyn's friends.

To Margaret DeSilver

Truro, Massachusetts
October 29, 1951

Dear Margaret

Herewith Jack's letter, and a rough draft[236] of the Fund letter, for which you asked

---

236 This draft is reproduced below, along with Evelyn's comments and corrections.

me. I have no doubt it can be improved. I suggest that you and Lewis Gannett whip it into shape - or discard it altogether if you think proper. You see, I have stressed E's need to get home. This necessitated focussing on her alone; one can hardly appeal to Americans to help an Englishman get away from home. Of course, if she gets here, as Jack suggests, nothing more natural than that her husband should follow her.

As usual, I have difficulty in learning exactly what E in her letter to me is talking about. Dimly, I descry that there is a finished novel - all typed and ready to be read. What publisher has seen it?

I'm enclosing a small check to you, which you can turn into money to send to her - from a "friend" - please don't mention my name. Perhaps it will help pay a gas bill or something. It's not much but it's really more than I can afford at present. I hate to think of Evelyn worried in that dark enveloping London winter. If we get her out of this, she may write the best book of her life.

Waldo Frank

[Typed, on letterhead of Hotel Waldorf in Caracas; signed. HRC]

To Evelyn Scott and Jack Metcalfe

130 West 12th St

New York 11, NY

[October 1951]

Dear Evelyn and Jack:-

I enclose a copy of an appeal letter drafted by Waldo Frank. Will you let me know what you think of it? If you approve of it, I shall try to get in touch with Julien Cornel, who engineered the Kenneth Patchen Fund, to see if he will let me use that list. If he will, I'll undertake to weed it out and to plan to whom the three or four people who helped me start this project will each write or rather sign this letter.

Much love to you both -

Maggie DeS

[Typed on personal letterhead, signed. UTK]

Draft by Evelyn of letter of appeal, including Evelyn's comments

~~Hotel Continental~~

~~Bogota, Columbia~~

Waldo Frank

Truro, Mass

See final page of this and précis sent with more details later on. Please Waldo use the facts—they are EXACT Evelyn

The purpose of this letter is to win your interest in the plight of Evelyn Scott, - one of the small company of truly distinguished writers of our time. During the 20s

HOTEL CONTINENTAL
BOGOTA—COLOMBIA

The purpose of this letter is to win your interest in the plight of
Evelyn Scott,-- one of the small company of truly distinguished American writers of our time. During the 20s and 30s, Evelyn Scott's novels
were widely known and greatly admired, although their uncompromising
character kept them (with one or two exceptions) from the best-seller
lists. Their fate was that of so many important books within a few
years of publication: they went out of print. Most good writers circumvent this common event by publishing new books -- or by dying, in which
case the "rediscovery" of their work becomes unimportant to them.

Miss Scott, having married the English novelist John Metcalfe
this about 1930, and second marriage ambiguous, Married twice
to England during the last war. The unfortunate effect of this
families should NOT be separated by fools, is Evelyn Scott's opinion.
put her out of touch with American publishers. She feels strongly
we fear, correctly -- that if she could return to her own country, she
could place her new work and resume her position as a producing
American novelist. But penury keeps her in England,

We do not ask charity for Evelyn Scott (she would probably be too proud
to take it.) We wish to raise a Fund of money which will enable her
to come home and to find living and working conditions at home.

Please bear in mind that Evelyn Scott's situation is not intrinsically
rare. What would have become of Henry James, after his early successes,
without a private income? And what did become of Herman Melville, when
his books stopped selling? Evelyn Scott's need to get home is, we
are convinced, the of a creative artist who - if again in
touch with the milieu of her work - should have good years of work
before her. In a sense, both psychologically and economically, she
is "marooned" in the unsustaining world of post-war England,

First page of draft letter of appeal for Evelyn Scott Fund: *University of Tennessee*
[Photocopy of a carbon copy including handwritten and typed insertions]

344

and 30s, Evelyn Scott's novels were widely known and greatly admired, although their uncompromising character kept them (with one or two exceptions) from the best-seller lists. Their fate was that of so many important books within a few years of publication: they went out of print. Most good writers circumvent this common event by publishing new books - or by dying, in which the date of the "rediscovery" of their work becomes unimportant to them. *I have visited England many times on my American Passport—British by marriage, but chose to retain citizenship as native-born in 1930. Stop this token discretion!*

Miss Scott, having married the English novelist John Metcalfe in 1930, he was a quota resident US & then moved to England during the last War. *[Typed insertion in margin by ES]:* this about "last war" and second marriage ambiguous, married twice, second 1939 - "RAF" service brought us here 1943-44 I travelled British as an "RAF" wife - passport resigned on landing - families should NOT be separated by fools, is Evelyn Scott's opinion. The unfortunate effect of this was to put her out of touch with American publishers. She feels strongly - we believe correctly - that if she could return to her own country *with second husband,* she could place her new work and resume her position as a producing American novelist. *why the hell should it!* But penury keeps her in England, *and both published in USA as before 1937 would end her worst penury and his he has books to publish*

We do not ask for charity for Evelyn Scott (she would probably be too proud to take it). We wish to raise a Fund of money which will enable her to come home and to find living and working *and publishing* conditions at home.

Please bear in mind that Evelyn Scott's situation is not intrinsically rare. What would have become of Henry James, after his early successes, without a private income? And what did become of Herman Melville, when his books stopped selling? Evelyn Scott's need to get home is, we are convinced, the intuition bleak eventual need for justice of a creative artist who - if again in touch with the milieu of her work - should have good years of work before her. In a sense, both psychologically and economically, *she and John Metcalfe are* is "marooned" in the unsustaining world of post-War England, *which has yet to be culturally restored*

We in the US today, who are concerned with the cultural health of our country surely should feel that our good fortune places many responsibilities upon us. The practical hand held out at this hour to Evelyn Scott, in order to help her return home would hearten her and would give a new hold on life and work to a significant American artist. *Please press for our resumed publication—the antidote for "charity" is to SELL US—they can sell us if politics can be made to stand aside—and give art a chance. Thanks for letting me see the rough draft of your letter.*

1942—which began the near-debacle of onslaughts— read précis—long and short when these arrive.
[Initial draft by Waldo Frank typed on hotel notepaper with heading crossed out. Handwritten insertions UTK]

The following, also by Evelyn, is her suggested revision of Waldo Frank's letter.

Waldo Frank's letters amplified with a few facts - sent to Margaret De Silver

The purpose of this letter is to win your interest in the plight of Evelyn Scott, - one of the small number of genuinely distinguished American writers of our time. During the 1920s and 1930s, Evelyn Scott's novels were widely known and greatly admired, although their uncompromising character kept them, with a few exceptions, off "best-seller" lists. Their fate was that of a number of important books; within a few years of publication they were allowed to lapse from print. This is a common calamity. Most writers circumvent its effects by publishing new books; some, again, die, thus rendering the date of their "rediscovery" unimportant to them. Evelyn Scott is the wife of the English author John Metcalfe, and as a result of his "RAF" service which took them to Britain during the war, they have been stranded there ever since, and Evelyn Scott is under such "economic" duress that she feels strongly it is essential she return home and recover her American contacts.

We wish to raise a fund of money for her which will get her over this difficulty of a fresh start which requires expenditures on almost everything, including teeth, clothes and boat fares, and enough to live on when she lands until royalties on her books are due.

This is not proposed as a "charity" but as restitution for a form of neglect Americans cannot afford. If offered as a "charity" our aid would be spurned and rightly. She has many books in her yet to be written. What would have become on Henry James, after his early successes, without a private income? What became of Melville when his books stopped selling? That the creative suffer most in the aftermath of wars is in the nature of things, but to save wherever we can those whose cultural outlook is unique and can never be duplicated is to the advantage of all who realize intrinsic values in art must be revived and preserved for the cultural health of the country. Evelyn Scott proposes again to resume the French historical novel as soon as she has any respite from money worries and the strain of anxiety she has been under impoverished and remote from her friends and family and the public which knows her best.

To Margaret DeSilver

26 Belsize Crescent
November 12, 1951

Maggie darling

The check or cheque for twenty-five dollars adds to the sum of gratitude both to yourself and the donor, who probably thought I might be embarrassed should I be told who he or she was - so do please, you thank them for me in all sincerity. And as we thank whoever gave it we thank you again even more. I dont see how anyone could have been a better friend to us both than you have, and while it is difficult to receive money at times it is very difficult to ask for it also as I KNOW - so bless you.

I thought Waldos letter well expressed and full of good intentions, but NOT SPECIFIC ENOUGH - and as I write with this to thank him too, perhaps he will grasp my explanation, which has to do with the WAR. He mentions it that I married Jack and was stranded in England, as if I had never been there or as if Jack was to be disassociated in going to the States and it isnt POSSIBLE NO DO EITHER OF US WISH IT.

In the precis - both the short version sent now and the longer which duplicates it but extended substantiation, is in small items and is to be regarded as material for a book to be eventually copyrighted.

I tell these things because I have made out my own brief as far as I am able as a protest against what I am convinced were passages in Cyril's Life Is Too Short which were edited and "ghost" written and which have resulted in libelling Cyril myself Jack Jig and Pavla. I think this libel in combination with my stepmother Melissa's hushiness about my Father's will, and her failure to so much as mention either publicly in Lynchburg or at the Biloxi Hospital that my Father had a daughter surviving and that it was myself - may be the cause of some of our troubles about books and mail and all sorts of things.

MUST BE EMPHASIS ON BOOKS READY FOR PUBLICATION NOW EMPHASIS MUST BE ON THAT FIRST - why NOT charity *Everything public except libel stemming from "ghost" passages in Life Is Too Short—consult Jig and Pavla or Cyril and Pavla as Cyril himself delay here.*

Dear Maggie - The front page and the above should be the FACTS PUBLIC KNOW WHEN APPEALING FOR HELP FOR US I THINK - it is much more interesting as the Truth than generalized as Waldo had it though his belief in me is appreciated. It must also be KNOWN that Jack and myself return together and have NO INTENTION of parting and that the fact that he was British-born and still a British subject though an American quota resident has been "used against" him and me should at least be implied I think. You will grasp why when you read the precis.

WE STAND FOR PURE ART DETACHED FROM POLITICS AS MUCH AS HUMANLY POSSIBLE, but beside all the general handicaps which now afflict pure artists, we are a SPECIFIC INSTANCE OF WAR ABUSES. It will I consider be a more effective appeal if the FACTS IN THIS LETTER ARE PUBLICIZED FREELY.

But my problem is about the libel. I want that combated and will go on fighting it where I can. That is why I document as reference Common Law Marriage and Divorce, for these involve the real legality of Scott as our name Jigs name Pavlas name the names of Denise Fredrick Mathew and Julia, and actually, Jack and I were married as William John Metcalfe and Evelyn D Scott legally in Tierra Amarillo in 1930 when I elected to retain my citizenship.

Tell our friends we surmise his FC Wellman copyright ruse of false rumour by Pavla and Cyril too.
Love Evelyn

[Typed carbon copy, signed. Handwritten insertions. UTK]

To Margaret DeSilver

Truro, Massachusetts
November 16, 1951

Dear Margaret,

The enclosed,[237] just received, makes it clear, I'm afraid, how hard it is going to be to help Evelyn. I don't know what truth there is in her charge that Cyril's book was tampered with, but these points are clear:

1. To put any such statement into a general letter would be libellous unless legally proved in advance, and even Cyril's statement would not be legal proof.

2. It is very dubious that even if the book was slanderous, this has the slightest relation with Evelyn's present condition - the book was read by very few, and those few certainly would not on that account have "plotted" against Evelyn.

3. To bring such matter into an appeal, in any case, would I think frighten people off, rather than make them open their purses.

Personally, I refuse to get embroiled in this sad personal quarrel. I found Cyril's book disgusting, but I am certainly not ready to get involved in why it was so - and it all seems irrelevant to the simple wish of friends to get E back to the USA since she wants to come.

Do what you want about this; but if the letter is to be amended to include these "personal" matters, someone besides me - who know nothing and am in no position to sift the facts - will have to do it. Moreover, such an amended letter might readily be one I simply could not sign, not knowing the facts, first hand.

What think you? Is there a "plot" or is all this Evelyn's obsession?

Waldo

[Typed, signed. HRC]

To Margaret DeSilver[238]

26 Belsize Crescent
November 18, 1951

Dear Margaret:

I compiled a precis of the happenings in our lives since 1939, when our literary careers were virtually suspended, with originally the idea that it would be useful

---

237 This refers to Evelyn's revisions to Waldo's earlier draft of the appeal letter.
238 This letter was accompanied by the full text of Evelyn's "precis".

as reference when I write, as I propose to, in the future, a book about the actual experiences of authorship in the course of publishing twenty volumes. But the original precis though consistent with this one and merely elaborated with further substantiations of the main facts, is not completed yet - so this one. It may seem to you long but I think it should be read by every personal friend who is seriously deposed, first how-ever, when you yourself have read it, by my family.

I have gone into some detail respecting what I believe to be sources of libel, and one of these is an evident tampering with the mss of Life is Too Short which could NOT have been done by Cyril, and as to detail must have been unauthorized, because it is unjust and harmful to him as well as us and Jig and Pavla. You dont see them so perhaps Waldo could help there - it all seems absurd as a friend of a friend in Saint Louis telephoned to Red Hook and, though the line was busy, Gladys Grant corroborated the fact that they have a phone. And I do KNOW THEY ARE FRIENDLY TO OURSELVES by Pavla's letters, brief and infrequent though they are - Jig and Pavla both.

Waldos letter was generous and very good but it was so much too generalized that it conveyed a wrong impression as to why we have been stranded here so long. And I therefore have asked Jack to bind with the precis a sort of summary more pertinent to precisely the situation ours, which, in the main, is we both consider the result of the war - after all Jack and I have been married twenty-one years and we never got stranded in Britain when conditions were those of times less ridden by politics.

Love and gratitude and hope. We are very desperate at this moment, gas, rates, etc again.

Evelyn

[Typed, signed. Enclosure: copy of "Precis of events indicative of libel". UTK]

To Evelyn Scott

130 West 12th Street, NYC
November 20, 1951

Dear Evelyn:-

You certainly have every right to object to the form of appeal letter presented to you and to prefer your own approach. But as a person on the receiving end, who am on every known list, I can tell you that most of the appeals I receive go straight into the scrapbasket unopened and the art of getting letters opened by the recipient is quite a fine one. And Brevity and Simplicity is of the essence. So that I have to say that I could not undertake any such letter as you propose, for purely practical reasons. Besides this, I myself feel that Cyril and Jig are not in the least concerned with this specific problem. Jack, of course, is, and the only reason he was not brought in was that it was thought it would be easier to appeal for just one person, the American writer, and that if enough money was forthcoming of course Jack could be included in the deal. And of course, harsh as it sounds, you are the

American Novelist in this case, and not Evelyn Scott the human being. Of course actually the two are inseparable, but artificial divisions sometimes have to be set up in the practical world. As to the Kenneth Patchen list, my only idea was to get ahold of it or the Authors League list, and weed out likely names for each signer to send the appeal letter to, some for Waldo, some for Lewis, some for Bunny, etc, etc. It was just my idea of a way to get ahold of some names.

So, Evelyn dear, I guess I'll have to go back to sending you money when I can and asking other people to do so when I see them.

Love to you both -

Margaret

1952 —November 24th, London. I think Jig is concerned with every publically circulated word about his mother. Evelyn Scott

[Typed, signed. Handwritten annotation. UTK]

To Waldo Frank

26 Belsize Crescent

December 4, 1951

Please remember we cant wait on dickerings of foundations, and this shouldnt be regarded as replacing anything else anybody is willing to do - we are just hanging on from week to week.

Dear Waldo:

I don't like burdening our friends with letters, but as we are determinedly making a stand for our survival as living authors and for our living human relations, I dont know how to avoid a correspondence relevant to sustaining us.

Perhaps Margaret has sent you by now the letter you first wrote for me with such real generosity but without, apparently, having taken stock of some aspects that might have been misinterpreted, and which I, therefore, tentatively altered, with the proviso that you see it and pass on using any part of yours before it was sent it. Should it be that you disapprove, then probably someone else can paraphrase its content and retain those statements of fact respecting myself and Jack, which, though not many, I insist on because of the legalities involved, which are all legal legalities, documented on file and correct, but must be recognised as existent or the entire business of trying to help me will result in a humiliation which I think you yourself would not tolerate and I cannot.

Best regards

[Typed carbon copy, not signed. UTK]

To Evelyn Scott

Truro, Massachusetts
December 28, 1951

Dear Evelyn,

Last week M deS sent me your revised version of the letter. I returned it, saying I had no objection but that I thought Allen T and Gannett should compare the two versions and possibly make up a third. I entirely disagree with your notion that personal details should go into this letter. To begin with, these matters which loom so large in your mind and heart are not known and even less cared about by practically anyone. These controversies and data are irrelevant, and to throw them into the consciousness of persons appealed to can in my judgement only confuse and deter.

The appeal for you should be made upon clear simple cultural facts; your marriages, your relation with Cyril, the state of your teeth and even of your mss is of no importance, from the standpoint of presenting a persuasive objective picture. Even your "insistence" that it MUST be stated that you both have books ready for publication is in my judgement an error of objective view. If such an item had any effect at all on readers it would be to deter them from helping, for they would say - "Well then, if she has a book ready why not send it to a publisher and get an advance?" I think dear Evelyn, you would be wiser if you simply let Margaret and her friends handle this matter as they (we) judge best.

May 1952 be good - a better one for you both.

God be with you,
ever affectionately your friend,
Waldo

[Typed, signed. UTK]

To Margaret DeSilver

The Saturday Review of Literature
245 West 45th Street, New York 19, NY

February 4, 1952

Dear Miss DeSilver:

I am heartily in sympathy with the idea of aiding Evelyn Scott in her time of trouble. Last year I received several letters from her which distressed me. They were not incoherent, but they betrayed what I thought was a mild, or perhaps a serious case of persecution complex. We were helping her at that time to find copies of The Wave through our Personal Columns.

I would be willing to sign the letter you suggest and am sending you a small check to start with.

Sincerely yours,
Harrison Smith

[Typed on company letterhead; signed. HRC]

From Margaret DeSilver

THE EVELYN SCOTT FUND

Margaret DeSilver, Treas

130 West 12th Street

New York 11, NY

[February 1952]

The purpose of this letter is to win your interest in the plight of Evelyn Scott - one of the small company of genuinely distinguished American writers of our time. During the 1920s and 1930s, Evelyn Scotts novels were widely known and greatly admired, although their uncompromising character kept them, with a few exceptions, off the "best seller" lists. Their fate was that of a number of important books; within a few years of publications they were allowed to lapse from print. This is a common calamity. Most writers circumvent its effects by publishing new books, some, gain, die, thus rendering the date of their "rediscovery" unimportant to them.

Evelyn Scott is the wife of the English author John Metcalfe, and as a result of his "RAF" service which took them to Britain during the war, they have been stranded there ever since, and Evelyn Scott is under such economic duress that she feels strongly it is essential she return home and recover her American contacts. She was victimized during the war, and requires practical help in a re-beginning that financially is from rock bottom. We wish to raise a fund of money for her which will tide her over to a fresh start in her own country. This is not proposed as a "charity" but as restitution for a form of neglect Americans cannot afford. If offered as "charity" our aid will be spurned and rightly. She has many books in her yet to be written. What would have become of Henry James, after his early successes, without a private income? What became of Melville when his books stopped selling? That the creative suffer most in the aftermaths of wars is in the nature of things, but to save wherever we can those whose cultural outlook is unique and can never be duplicated is to the advantage of al who realize intrinsic values in art must be revived and preserved for the cultural health of the country.

Waldo Frank

Dawn Powell

Allen Tate

Lewis Gannett

John Dos Passos

Edmund Wilson

[The typed slip below was included with the duplicated version of the above appeal letter:]

Recently both Miss Scott and Mr Metcalfe have been granted Six Months Fellowships at the Huntington-Hartford Foundation in Pacific Palisades, California to take effect October 1st. Their immediate need, therefore, is for clothing, transportation and enough money to tide them over the intervening months. Please help us.

List of Contributors to the Evelyn Scott Fund

(compiled by Margaret DeSilver)

May R Mayers, MD

John K Kutchens, Book Reviewer, New York Herald Tribune

Katherine Dunlap

Lewis Gannett

Witter Bynner

Allen Tate

William Carlos Williams (did not want name used)

Jean K Nevius

Sophie Kerr Underwood

David Davidson

A R Wylie

Henry Steele Commager

Van Wyck Brooks

Jerome Weidman

Elmer Rice

John Robert Coughlan

Max & Gladys Eastman

David & Jean Lerner

T S Matthews

Alice Port Tabor

Julian Gumperz, (Pres., Hillaire Foundation)

Irving Stone

Mrs W Murray Crane

Berry Fleming

Rita & Werner Cohn

Frances E Blum

Jane Hudson Davis

Rita Halle Kleeman

Dr Sol Wiener Ginsburg

Laura Wood Roper

Marjorie Griesser

Alfred E Cohn, MD

Vincent McHugh

Robert K Hass (Vice-President, Random House)

C Kempton (sent snide letter!)

Inez Haynes Irwin

Harrison Smith (Saturday Review of Lit)

Louise Bogan

Luise M Sillcox (Author's League of America)

Mrs James H Scheuer
Lewis Mumford
Lewis Galantiere
John Dos Passos
Dawn Powell
Waldo Frank
Edmund Wilson

Chapter 33

Pacific Palisades

December 1951 - March 1952

Although desperate to return to the United States, Jack and Evelyn had no clear destination as they had no idea where Jigg and his family would be living. This led to them spending considerable time and energy in securing some form of grant aid or locating some form of arrangement in a creative community which would help their finances by at least providing accommodation while they tried to complete (and sell) the books on which they were then working.

The proceeds of the Evelyn Scott Fund were being released in stages and were specifically linked to their travel costs. While they were waiting for funds to be released, Evelyn and Jack had been preparing to let the garden flat in which they had been living since 1945 to supplement the Fund and their royalties.

Their luck changed when they were offered residential fellowships at the Huntington Hartford Foundation in Pacific Palisades near Los Angeles. As this was conditional on the transfer of funds from the Evelyn Scott Fund, Jack had to ask the director of the foundation, Michael Gaszynski, on several occasions to agree to changes in their arrival date. They eventually arrived in Pacific Palisades at the end of March 1953 and left in March 1954, after some months more than their planned six-month stay. Only three of Evelyn's letters from this period have survived; Jack's diary entries are the main record of their sojourn.

To Michael Gaszynski

26 Belsize Crescent
February 20, 1952

The Huntington Hartford Foundation
2000 Rustic Canyon Road
Pacific Palisades, California
Dear Mr Gaszynski,

It is with very great pleasure that my wife and I received your letter of February 11th, and I return herewith, as requested, signed copies of your enclosures informing us severally that we had been so fortunate as to be awarded Residence Fellowships at the Foundation.

I need hardly say that our sole aim will be to turn this opportunity to the greatest advantage creatively and in that way to justify the confidence you have placed in us.

Actually, since we shall have so many arrangements regarding transport etc to make, we should prefer to begin our tenures later than June. Would, say, October 1st be a convenient date for you? That would leave us a wider margin of time in which to settle up a number of affairs before sailing and also in New York on our way west.

I am taking it that it would be best to undergo the medical examinations when we have arrived in America and at a time closer to the commencement of our tenures.

Sincerely and appreciatively yours,

John Metcalfe

[Typed carbon copy, signed. UTK]

To Lewis Gannet

26 Belsize Crescent

March 17, 1952

Dear Lewis,

You'll be glad to hear that we have each been awarded a Fellowship at the Huntington Hartford Foundation, - and thank you very much for your sponsoring of my application. We are supposed to take up residence on 1st of October this year, - and so now we are keeping our fingers crossed in the hope that we'll be able, financially etc, to make it, if the appeals letter which Maggie so kindly has sent, - or is sending - out brings in sufficient response. The Fellowship is for 6 months in the first instance, - and although California is a heck of a long way out, and the fare colossal, free board and lodging for 6 months seems worth it. Also, it may be, we may make some useful contacts leading to a job for myself.

At the moment, and at this end, things, to put it very mildly indeed, are "difficult", so we're chanting "always darkest before dawn", etc etc.

I do most earnestly hope we can manage it and land in US in time!

Shall see you then.

Cordially,

Jack

[Handwritten, signed. HRC]

To Margaret DeSilver

26 Belsize Crescent

June 3, 1952

Dear. darling Maggie

This is just an interim note to say we have your letter re the Fund, + to thank you again + again, - + express, inadequately, our real devotion for all that you have done. Of course it's understood that you can't do any more from your own personal funds, - you've done more than too much already, + I hate to think of all this has cost you, in every way, - the $300 down, the doubtless very considerable expense of printing mailing etc, and the worry, - and, I realise occasional bad smells, humanity (some of it) being what it is. For all this our everlasting gratitude, and determination to show it's all been worth while.

We are, too, of course, so grateful to all who have contributed, and Evelyn is touched by the remembrance of those you mentioned by name. Later, when appropriate, she can make some individual acknowledgements.

Yes, - I can + will look around for, + get, a job. The difficult thing was (+ still in some respects is) to get to US at all.

I have called this an "interim" note because there will still have to be a heck of a lot of thinking done as to practical steps, - and, as to them, I shall write you more fully in a few days time.

I cannot give any date of sailing etc. because my ability to sail at all is contingent on my being granted a fresh visa and upon my being able to (for instance) get my income tax release etc. And in order to do that, - well, I'm hanged if I know at present. I air-mailed you a letter from Evelyn on May 23rd in which she told you of our receipt of a lovely cheque for $500 from the Carnegie Fund (bless it!); - but (a) I won't (i.e. we won't!) actually have that credited to the bank account for, possibly, two months (another, small cheque for $24.50 for my story took just two months + two days!, - and (b) when it is credited it will all go on debts for gas, repairs, etc. I don't, at the moment, see much chance of our getting straight here in time for Oct 1st at P Palisades and I shall have, I expect, to ask the Director of the Foundation for a postponement. I think that would be granted, all right.

These, as I say, are just the "things to think bout", - + to write you about, after further reflection, in a few days, - + this note is only an interim acknowledgement, - + are not adequate expression of our deep, deep gratitude.

Love

Jack

[Handwritten, signed. HRC]

To Margaret DeSilver

26 Belsize Crescent

June 9, 1952

Maggie darling: *1952 November 7 months since sent*

Will you please believe that the factual letters like this in which explicitness is requested are not "naggers" letters and are implicitly as filled with the signs of gratitude as the letters we sent before this which were just the registering of our emotional out-going!

However, there are other factors that have to be reckoned with at home to make anything but dropping dead in our tracks worthwhile! I am sure you and all the contributors to the fund for me must have been genuinely concerned about me as Evelyn Scott the author as those who know Jack are as concerned about John Metcalfe the author. It is all very well - we did with an appreciation that is sustained - to accept the Huntington Hartford Foundation invitation - possibly postponed but nonetheless accepted and acceptable to them yet we trust - to go there and work on new books. *1952 November This letter unacknowledged*

The other thing about California is that I would rather - again - drop dead in my tracks where I am, than put six thousand miles between myself and every human I love most bar Jack himself, *except temporarily. 1952 November— return East must be guaranteed or aim lost*

Jig and Paula have no money to come here from Munich. I had hoped on their arrival some means would be found for allowing us to meet again here. But the few hundred miles between us here, will already - as far as boat fares go - be three thousand when we land in New York. And in California, unless one is fully guaranteed – job in the East, lectures for Jack, or any comparable method - the return fare to the East, one is likely - very likely my dear Mag and this really is a most serious problem - to repeat, in California, a marooning such as we have endured here, and with Jacks house and his tenure on it such as it is, six thousand miles further off. *Jig and Paula have moved to Otilostrasse 22, Graefelfing bei Munich*

We will continue to name Pacific Palisades as our temporary goal, of course, in the hope that the arrangements begun can be carried through; but as for being put on a train - we arent husky enough for busses cross-country - and just left in California, it would be hell in repeating what has already happened; and even should Jack - without other assets - get a teaching job there! - after all, he has a teaching job here, and it has been like a complete suspension of our normal lives as humans and authors. In California there is not a thing for us, except the generosity of the foundation in respect to a habitation in peace - we hope - for six months.

It hurt because we have never borrowed or asked for a penny from any of my relatives since Cyril and I left New Orleans;[239] and because, although their father and mother - the Graceys - did help my mother for several years when she first went South,[240] and all of them at intervals contributed small sums - very small - to assist her when I had become responsible for her.

Any lacks in this letter please blame on the fact that the day the good news came I had to go to bed with an attack of combined "grippe" and bladder irritation. The aches and pains were so persistent that Jacks medical uncle called in a consultant who specialized in such things. But he was a good doctor in my view as he just said go to bed and stay on a light diet for a while - and that was all. But that cost five pounds so I

---

239 This is a reference to their "elopement" from the US to Brazil in 1913.
240 A reference to when Maude travelled to Brazil without any financial support from her husband Seely.

am now preferring to utilize the same advice, as that was twenty years ago and I never had any serious recurrence of any such complaint since.

We hope to arrive very well again and present NO problems in health or - with books - no serious problems in money.

Love Evelyn

Marion is trying to help again with second-hand clothes. Still have not had money to alter coat - sent 3 years ago - so just hope. What to do to make flat habitable is some problem.

We also have to buy trunks - mine collapsed completely, and I also have not even a change-purse and need bag for Passports. And again shoes as these cannot be mended.

[Original typed copy, signed. Handwritten insertions. Typed carbon copy, also signed, with additional annotations. Both at UTK]

To Margaret De Silver

26 Belsize Crescent

July 27, 1952

Maggie my dear:

To thank you for the arrival of the draught.[241] It gave me a funny feeling to go to the phone and hear there was money for Jack sent by the Evelyn Scott Fund. We are probably more grateful than anyone there has grasped. The demolition of shelter and re-building of floors had to be suspended mid-way and we have been sitting in the midst of literal rubble in spots, and dejection had reached a nadir with both.

We should so like, as Jack says, to prove it was and is worthwhile to help as you and the friends of both our books have, and just long for an opportunity to do so, especially an opportunity in the USA.

Love

Evelyn

[Typed, signed. HRC. Carbon copy, also signed, at UTK]

To Margaret DeSilver

26 Belsize Crescent

July 27, 1952

Darling Maggie,

You will have got Evelyn's last letter, - and this is to add my thanks to hers. I cannot tell you how grateful we are. I do tell you, - but feel the best way of showing gratitude for your year's self-denying labour, and for your own personal generosity, is for us to make it all worth while, - to you and to us. I do intend to do this.

---

241 "Bank draft" was the term then in use for what we know as a cheque.

It may be difficult, from your end, to realise the causes of delay on ours, - but such delay as there may be is quite unavoidable. It results from the necessity of paying off a minimum of debts here (which I can now do) and from the necessity of getting the flat in a minimum lettable condition (which I can now also do), - + using the flat as an additional lever with the consul in applying for a fresh visa.

I take it, from your previous letter, that enough money (earmarked for transport) remains in the Fund to cover our boat and rail fares, - and also that it will be possible, once our sailing-date is fixed, for the boat-fares to be paid on our behalf as it were, to the shipping-company, by you at your end? - I suggest this, tentatively, because otherwise it would mean your sending another cheque to me here for the boat-fares. This would be all right, and of course you would have our promise to spend it on nothing but boat-fares, - but it struck me it would be more agreeable for you vis-a-vis the subscribers to the Fund, to be able to prove to them without question that the earmarked portion had been spent only upon transport.

Once again, dearest Maggie, - I just can't tell you how we feel about your kindness. As I say, it's now up to us to make it worth while.

Blessings be upon you!

Jack

[Handwritten, signed. HRC]

To Michael Gaszynski

26 Belsize Crescent

August 12, 1952

The Huntington Hartford Foundation
2000 Rustic Canyon Road
Pacific Palisades, California
Dear Mr Gaszynski,

With reference to your letter of February 25th, I much regret that the arrangements necessary for our return to the States, as preliminary to our commencing our tenures as the Huntington Hartford Foundation, have taken a far longer time than I had hoped.

We had, first, to accumulate sufficient funds "ahead of us" in the States for transport, etc, and only after that had been done (as it just has) was I in a sound enough position to apply for a fresh visa.

I have now just been informed by the American Consulate that the shortest time in which I can expect the visa is three months, it might be somewhat longer; and have therefore to ask you, with many regrets and apologies for any disturbance of your schedule, whether it will be possible for my wife and myself to be granted a further postponement, - say till the 1st of February 1953.

Should you find it possible to let us postpone the taking up of our tenures to February 1st 1953 we would indeed be most grateful. If this is feasible and acceptable to you, and if you would kindly let me know, I shall be able, in completing my application etc at the Consulate, to quote February 1st as the revised target date.

Sincerely yours,

John Metcalfe

[Typed carbon copy, signed. UTK]

To Margaret DeSilver

26 Belsize Crescent

October 19, 1952

Maggie my dear Maggie:

We dont know whether we are on the verge of the real end of this damnable exile, or are in some Gethsemane of tragedy.

Jack is writing again the plea that must seem interminable for help from somewhere - anywhere - to provide the three hundred essential to making the flat rentable enough to allow us to go home to face and solve all the vital issues that have accumulated during thirteen years - our two brief sojourns since 1941 having been such as permitted of no solutions.

These have been pretty intolerable weeks - these last. They have added tantalization to our other miseries. I, *today*, re-cleaned the woodwork in the room first renovated, when the floors were removed and the shelter; suddenly realizing it has been three months since then, and my first cleaning in preparation for new occupants, had to be repeated.

It has been a question of not even the cash to buy a tin of paint; and of course trying to keep enough for the Consular fee ready. All the details I enumerated as yet necessary, as a preliminary to renting furnished, still are necessary. We look to some advance rent to finish everything, even with the three hundred dollars more achieved. But this should allow for asking what others do for furnished apartments in good condition, and will save the house until eventually it can be sold. The essentials have to be here to rent for enough to save the house.

I feel we owe you something that not even a fortune, were it ours, could ever repay. But poor Jack is even eager to incur an obligation - in the form of a debt and promise to pay it, rather than just collapse as we are. I dont want him to incur any debt if there is any other way, however - more than the moral debts to you and our friends - because he works so hard and should have strains eased and not added to, if possible.

Love Maggie darling love

Evelyn

[Typed carbon copy, signed. Handwritten insertion. UTK]

To Margaret DeSilver

26 Belsize Crescent

December 14, 1952

Darling Maggie,

I have GOT IT (visa), thank goodness! It is a great relief, as the hold-up on the medical side was worrying in several ways. But all's well that…etc. It arrived by registered mail yesterday morning.

I then went at once to enquire re passages and fares, to the US Lines, Cook's, etc. It appears that the earliest date on which there might be any accommodation within our financial compass would not be before mid-January and might be as late as early February. This is later than we wanted, but almost everything at a reasonable price is booked up till about then; - and of course I could not make even the first gesture about it till I had got my visa.

The tourist fare for a double cabin would be from £68 to £71 each. There might be something slightly cheaper obtainable by waiting long, - but hotel or lodging expenses in England meanwhile would more than negative this gain, and it will pay us to get away as soon as possible after we move out of this flat around Jan 1st.

The rail fares from London to Southampton will add a bit more, say $10 for the two of us, and there will be at least some lodging expenses in England between the time this flat is let and the time we sail. Also some unavoidable renovation of baggage: - though I do not know how far such expenses could properly *[be]* regarded as "travel" or "transport" expenses to come out of the Fund. We should also have to spend a little (as little as possible!) on small tips on the boat, and I am not sure either how far these (say a further 5 to 10 dollars) are includable.

But altogether, if possible, we should like $430 (four hundred and thirty dollars) now from the Fund. If you could send this please the way you sent the last money so that it is immediately cashable I should be able to instruct Cook's to clinch the earliest sailing (within the money-limit) that offers.

Darling Maggie, I cannot tell you how we both feel to you about all this. As I said before, all we can do is to make it worth while. I can get a job I'm quite sure, and shall then of course repay the last $250 loan for a start. All these months the thing has persisted in appearing still too dreamlike (against reason!) but now that at last I really have my visa (my chief anxiety) I am really getting quite excited. Bless you and bless you! See you SOON now, I hope!

Much much love from

Jack. Evelyn adds her very much love with mine

[Typed carbon copy, signed. HRC]

To Creighton and Paula Scott

26 Belsize Crescent
December 30, 1952

Creighton and Paula Scott,
care Gladys Edgerton Grant
Darling Jig and Pavla-Paula

We - Jack and myself - have now secured our sailing for mid-February and will arrive in New York before the end of the month - sometime before.

I hope you will now both write to me of yourselves, and will send your present address at once - I really should have more than the forwarding before we leave, anyhow - so that we can write to you of the details and you can tell Gladys and Edgerton with our love.

Jig's affectionate mother and Paula's firm friend

Kiss Denise, Fredrick, Mathew and Julia for step-grandfather Jack, too

Mother=Paula's Evelyn

[Typed, signed. SFC. Carbon copy also at UTK]

To Creighton Scott
130 West 12th Street, Apt 12G

New York City 11

January 8, 1953

Dear Jigg

I thought I should l let you know the Metcalfes are arriving mid-Feb, due (overdue!!) in Calif 1st March. Don't know where they'll stay upon landing. I advised Hotel Earle or Madison Square. I shall of course say nothing about you.

Greetings to Pavli

Yours

MdS

[Handwritten on personal letterhead, signed. SFC]

To Creighton Scott
130 West 12th Street, Apt 12G

New York City 11

February 7, 1953

Dear Jigg

I thought you might like to know the Metcalfe's arrival has been postponed on account of illness - I don't know whose, or what illness - just got a cable.

Will let you know as soon as I know just when they now expect to get here

Yours

MdeS

[Handwritten on personal letterhead, signed. SFC]

To Lft Commander and Mrs F W Saint-Pierre
26 Belsize Crescent

March 1, 1953

Dear Mr and Mrs Saint-Pierre:

I do not know where to put the blankets and linen until Mr Paget and yourselves have agreed on the inventory. I gather he will come here when you are moved in or just before, and until we had our nice evening conversation I had not realized it unlikely that you yourselves will need to use the blankets, so I am leaving all of them - two lots, the greater portion in good condition but a few patched - on the bed in the small room.

Should you wish to use any that require dry cleaning, please ask Match and Company if it will be okay with them to deduct the expense incurred from the future rent. Davis, the cleaner, just to the left of Belsize Circus, clean very well and for a moderate price.

Three of the pillow tickings also look very dingy and can be cleaned by Davis for six shillings each. And this we would have had done but that with both of us under the weather we were using all the pillows until today.

Our cash shortage - temporary we hope - obliges me to leave this to you on the same basis, in the belief that it will be alright to charge up these comparatively small sums to rental to be deducted at the appropriate time. We are both very sorry to have to request anything that may seem a bother.

Three soiled pillowslips, one bath towel and two or three kitchen towels, as well, have not been washed, and perhaps you will be good enough to let Mr Marsh know that I have neither time to wash them nor any way of sending them to be laundered with no one in the flat yet.

These are the most troubling last-minute items. I really don't know how it is managed as to linen when moves are in process and one has to use a little for the most make-shift final night

Should you come in briefly during the next few days, please don't be unduly perturbed if all the discards of the move - empty paint tins, discarded clothing, etc - have not every one been put in the dust bins. These are at the foot of the stairs you pass as you walk along the path to the door of this flat, but the trash collection is usually on Tuesdays and I daren't fill the tins any more today as others as well as ourselves seem to have been throwing things away and some place has to be left until Tuesday, when I trust Mr Coleman, as a real favour, may come by and put the remainder of the debris in the bins. As a rule the space for trash is adequate, but there is now and again an overflow when anyone is moving in or out.

I don't know whether "hints" on the housework will sound like those of the Suffolk landlady who awed me with superfluous "directions" years ago, but give you some anyhow to be followed or not as you incline.

Unless you already have experience with painted concrete floors, you will not know that the red-painted floors in two of the rooms and the toilet cannot be washed, but are easily freshened with "Cardinal Polish", which can be bought at almost any hardware store, some groceries, and at the tobacconists adjacent to Meade's green grocery to the left of the first turning at the bottom of Belsize Crescent. These shops can also be reached by going down the "snicket" behind the house and turning right at bottom.

When dust accumulates along the tops of wainscots it is better, I find, to brush it off with a small dry brush, as you then don't have to be so careful about the tinted walls, or, for that matter, the wall paper. I use a damp cloth on the painted wainscots just occasionally, and in the first bed-room at the front just on the painted wood. The one drawback of "Cardinal Polish" is that when it gets on paint or walls it is hard to get off - ditto as to hands and clothes. But though it can be smeared when fresh, once it hardens - say an hour after it is used - it will not come off further as far as I know.

There is a good brush for cleaning radiators that was not put on the inventory, ad it was bought to re-paint them and by the time Mr Paget and I got to the kitchen cupboards I was too all-in to explain or say whether it should or shouldn't be listed. But I now point it out because of the convenient shape and handle. It cost something but does not need to be replaced if it wears out. It is in the bottom left kitchen cupboard with the scouring brushes - also not new, and not itemized or mentioned. It doesn't matter about these things except as they may help.

If the two oldest frying-pans in front kitchen cupboard are too much in the way and you wish to discard them, you are free to do so with the proviso that Match is informed either now or when you leave. I think the inventory is probably of mutual benefit but being still ill the day it was made I almost gave up.

There are some floor cloths - two - one unused and one used but still good and when in use these can be dried on the rod on the under-end of the kitchen table nearest the stove.

The furniture and the wooden floors have all been treated with o'cedar and this had been satisfactory to us as it keeps down dust. This naturally is for you to decide - I just hope to be helpful, for we are much indebted to you in respect to the storing of the pictures on the top shelf of the cupboard (or wherever you like).

There are a number of small photographs framed and unframed with these, and some small hooks. These did not go on the inventory because we had hoped to pack them and had no room when the baggage was filled. We do feel apologetic, and I suppose whenever you leave Match should know of the extra photographs and a few books having been put with the other things, though I DON'T MEAN re-do inventory.

The Gas Company's phone is Hampstead 1133 for most calls, but on Sundays, holidays and other times of emergency the Gas Company can also be reached at Willesden 1272, their emergency phone.

The best of good wishes to you both again. We think we are fortunate in having found such nice tenants for the flat, and we do implore the gods to permit it to be a satisfactory habitat for yourselves and the dogs, too. Thank you again for allowing the personal articles to be stored in the cupboard.

[Typed carbon copy; signature faint through carbon. HRC]

Funds from the Evelyn Scott Fund were finally released in early 1952, enabling Evelyn and Jack to finalise their plans for travel to Pacific Palisades some months later. Very few of Evelyn's letters from their time there have survived, but Jack's diary records, in considerable detail,[242] their return to the United States and journey onward to Pacific Palisades.

---

242 Appendix F displays Jack's character as he disclosed it himself in his diary entries over the years. These entries are typical of his recording of the small details of his life.

From John Metcalfe's diary:

February 10, 1953: Letter from Cooks, - we now switch back to Veendam, sailing March 1st. E had letter from Gladys.

March 12, 1953: LANDED IN USA 7.30 breakfast,- then a flurry of packing, assisted by steward. Long waits for immigration. Over at last and landed Hoboken about 12. Maggie met us, left dollars etc + then went off. We got our baggage into a couple of cabs + and got it + ourselves to Hotel Earle for some thirty dollars! A nice suite, but expensive, + I got the rate reduced from $8 to $7 a day. Phoned Maggie, who will call us on Sat morning. 'Phoned May, Review, Davison. Supper at "Southern Inn". Back to hotel. Bed about 10.30. Very rainy.

March 13, 1953: Still raining in morning. E + I breakfasted off coffee + doughnuts at Waldorf Cafeteria. Wrote letter to Lt Cdr St Pierre + Mr Gaszinki[243] [sp], + air-mailed them. Went Dept of Naturalization + Immigration, 70 Columbus Avenue, then to Grand Central,- where enquired re fares etc to Los Angeles. Then walked to Cooks + got remaining English + Dutch money changed. Back by subway to 14th St + found E in Waldorf Cafeteria, where we had lunch. Back to hotel where had nap. Set out for May's at 3.30 + reached there at 4. Cocktails, in which Lan later joined us. E, May + I then dined out, - v. good steak. Returned to Mays, + finally left at 9.30 and walked back to hotel. Bed.

March 14, 1953: Breakfast. Back to hotel. Maggie called and gave me cheque for remainder of Fund money. After she had left E + I took laundry to "Joe's" at Bleecker St. Lunch at Cafeteria. Back to hotel. Doze. Went Davison's, then on to Bernice Elliott's, where we had dinner. Back at hotel by about 11. Bed.

March 15, 1953: Wrote letter in morning. Nap after lunch at cafeteria. Typed out copies of testimonials + of house-statement. Dinner at Hazel's. Walked back to hotel through pouring rain. Bed'

March 16, 1953: 7.30 breakfast at cafeteria. Arrived late at dentist's (Dr C I Stoloff). Paid him $35. Came back to hotel. Out again and air-mailed letters to Uncle Jim and Mr Coleman (3s/9d cheque enclosed). Cashed Margaret's Fund cheque at Amalgamated Bank, Union Sq, + then put most of it into new a/c at Corn Exchange Bank, 7th Ave + 14th St. Went 25 Broad St, + had lunch with Walter who will send $75. Back at hotel by about 3.45. Nap. Supper at Cafeteria. Bed.

March 17, 1953: Paid hotel $40.70. Breakfast at cafeteria. Posted letter to Maggie. Went to No 1 Wall St but Mr Beamand not there. Left testimonials for photostating. Dr Stoloff 1.30 to get dentures OK. Back to hotel. E + I to 5th Ave Hotel for cocktails with Elmer Rice Then had supper at Southern Inn. E unwell. Back to hotel. Bed.

March 18, 1953: Air-mailed cheque for £2 to Hobson. Went downtown and saw Mr Beamand's secretary, + then made enquiries at Hanover Bank, 70 Broadway, 7th floor

---

243 Dr Michael Gaszynski, Director of the Huntington Hartford Foundation, Evelyn and Jack's destination.

re sending money to England by "letter of delegation". Collected Photostats + came back to hotel. Lunch at Waldorf cafeteria. Walter's cheque (for $70) had arrived and I paid this in to my a/c at the Corn Exchange Bank. Collected laundry and returned to hotel. (Our luggage has been brought up from "cellar" for repacking). Had nap till about 5.30. E wrote letters while I smoked. Supper. Bed.

March 19, 1953: Took train tickets to Grand Central for changing to later date. Lunch at Cafeteria. Nap. Dawn and Cully came at 5, with whisky. Supper. Continued re-sorting and packing of baggage. Lan came to hotel with car at 9 and took luggage (+ us) to May's, Left 7 pieces there. Cocktails. E + I walked back to hotel. Bed.

March 20, 1953: Cheque $25 from Hal Bynner via Margaret. Have nasty cold. Got haircut after breakfast. Went Grand Central,- but tickets not ready yet. Visited three teacher agencies: - Stein (no good), American + Foreign, and Albert. Lunch at a Horn + Hardarts. Went one more agency (Miss Watson). Then back to hotel. Nap. Supper at cafeteria. Bed.

March 21, 1953: Breakfast. Bought small trunk on 3rd Avenue. Walked back to hotel with it. Went Grand Central and changed tickets OK at last. Posted letter to Dr Vincent (had previously posted letter to Davison re his writing to Albert Agency). Also posted letters from E to Miss Sillcox + to Hal Bynner. Bought Dutch tobacco. Back by subway + bought little parcels for dentures. "Home" to hotel. Nap. Supper at Dawn Parnell's. Joe Gallacher came in later. Back to hotel, - bed.

March 23, 1953: Went Grand Central + arranged for luggage (6 pieces)to be called for tomorrow. Paid $12. Back to hotel, - then called on literary agent, Margaret Chrintra [?] at 37 Madison Ave (Madison Square hotel, Apt 1220). Left MSS with her. Back to hotel, + found E had already lunched. I went out + had lunch at cafeteria. Back to hotel. E set off with her MSS to Mr Russell, literary agent, + returned about 4.30. After supper we took two more pieces of baggage (purple-lined & Hazel's) to Lan + May. Walked back to hotel. Bed.

March 24, 1953: Drew money from Corn Exchange bank. Saw Mr Beamand at 10.30 + sent $40 to my Hampstead bank via Hanover Bank, 70 Broadway. Very rainy. E had had her lunch when I returned, so I lunched alone. Van came for our 6 pieces of baggage at about 2.10. Maggie called at 2.30. I left at 4 + got receipt from Hanover Bank. Returned to Hotel. E + I had supper at cafeteria. Went to May's. Left 2 packages. E found suit case open. E called Bernice who was out. E called John Varney. E exchanged ¾ of MS.

March 25, 1953: E called Michael Lake. Wrote + posted letter to Westminster Bank, (air-mail), + to PO Station O, 217 W 18 St re re-direction + letter from E to Paul, c/o Doubleday's. Registered at British Consulate. Confirmed spelling of 'Christie'. Called on Mrs Walcott at St Luke's School re teaching post notified by Albert Agency. Finished packing + topping. Lunch of stuffed peppers. Taxi to Grand Central. Left on 'Pacemaker' at 3 pm. 'Dinner' of a sandwich each + coffee cost us $2.50 plus 40c tip. Very little sleep.

March 26, 1953: Arrived Chicago 7.30 am. Cloaked some baggage at Dearborn Station + breakfasted off bacon + eggs at 'The Streamliner'. Returned to Dearborn Station. Wired Dr. Vincent. Posted letter from E to Hal Smith. Smoked in waiting-room. Left Chicago on 'El Capitan', 5.45. Drunken man a nuisance.

March 27, 1953: On train all day. Drunken man got off at Albuquerque.

March 28, 1953: Breakfast at 6. Got off train at Los Angeles at 7.15. Contacted Huntington Hartford driver. Got 5 of our 6 pieces of luggage from station, + were driven to the Foundation. Had coffee. Unpacked. Lunch brought to our cottages at 12.30. Rang up station + found we have to pay $41 excess to get wardrobe trunk. Nap till 5. Supper at 6. Got 2 blankets,- but heat not functioning. E wrote 'Min Tom', + I put the letter in mail-box. Bed.

Chapter 34

The house at number 26
June 1952 - November 1959

Broadly speaking, there are two categories of land ownership in England: "freehold", where ownership is of the building and *the land upon which it stands; and "leasehold", where the owner has title to the building but not the land, which is leased from a landowner and on which an annual rent (ground rent) is paid. Leasehold has its origins in feudal land ownership: the 17th century saw reforms to this system, and the wealthy institutions of the time - the Crown, the Church of England and the colleges of the universities of Oxford and Cambridge - acquired much of the land. The Church and the university colleges in particular owned large tracts in London and as this land was developed into housing, the ground rents payable by the eventual owners ("leaseholders") of these dwellings provided the landowners with significant income. 26 Belsize Crescent was a leasehold property, on which the ground rent was payable to the Ecclesiastical Commissioners for England (the "Church Commissioners").*

Jack as the owner of the building and landlord of the flats had certain statutory responsibilities to his tenants, mainly keeping their flats in good repair. Further, because of the severe housing shortage during and after the war, the Rent Restrictions Act was brought in to protect the rights of tenants, including restrictions on the circumstances under which rents could be increased. Broadly, it was not possible under the act for Jack to increase his tenants' rents, even with rising costs and the need to pay for repairs to bomb damage.

These obligations were the main reason for the poverty experienced by Evelyn and Jack. He had bought the property with the intention of converting it into four flats and using the rental income from the flats on the three upper floors to subsidise their living expenses, but he made a major error of judgement in installing gas central heating and hot water throughout the property. It was normal at that time for there to be individual coin-operated meters ("shilling meters") in flats, calibrated to not only recover the cost of the gas used but also an element of profit for the landlord. Jack did not install these separate meters. At that time, central heating was an expensive novelty, and inclusive central heating and hot water in a rented flat almost unheard of: the tenants must have enjoyed this luxury at Jack's expense. And, because of the Rent Restrictions Act, he could not recoup the rising cost of this luxury by raising the rents.

One goal of the Evelyn Scott Fund was to allow Jack to clear the debts related to the house, and Jack wrote to Margaret DeSilver several times, explaining the complexities of his financial situation and suggesting possible strategies for reducing his liabilities.

To Margaret DeSilver

26 Belsize Crescent

June 8, 1952

My Dear Maggie,

I still see no exit from an indefinite impasse (I hope not too prolonged) until we can get just straight enough here, on this side, to flit. This has always, unfortunately, been an integral and unavoidable part of my attempted return to the States, and the necessitarian order (read backwardly as it were from effect to cause) is as follows:-

1. To return I must get a fresh visa.
2. To get a fresh visa I must satisfy the consul more fully, he says, about "means".
3. To satisfy him I must have the flat in what I should call (to you, not to him) a "minimum lettable" condition; and, also, pay off income tax and all non-postponable debts.

Some debts I could, by guile, run away from temporarily and settle later, out of rent from the flat etc. Others I could not. For instance our move could not be carried out so nocturnally and stealthily that it would not be observed, for instance, by the builder who repaired the wall, and by another who has recently repaired part of the roof; and literal fisticuffs on the doorstep might ensue. The gas bill of £170, if I had not to wait for, possibly, a further six weeks or so for the crediting to my account of the Carnegie money); but by the time it is credited a further quarter's gas bill will have come in. Tenants' rents are absorbed by Rates (over £200 a year) and mortgage (also over £200) and by water rate, electricity, insurance, etc.

I plan to evade (temporarily) as much as I possibly can (while still presenting some sort of show to the consul) and make a get-away as soon as my visa is granted; and as soon as I can be in a position to give reasonable notice at the school (I can't just run out on them because I must have a good testimonial; otherwise the chance of teaching jobs in US is killed). The consul, as preliminary to the further consideration of my application for a fresh visa, will no doubt want to know the amount which Evelyn has in the Fund; - but even if it were a million I should still have to make some sort of minimum and, as I say, guileful settlement here in order to make the first physical steps towards a move.

The minimum boat fare, I have found out, is £57 for just the passage; but what the fare from New York to Pacific Palisades is I have yet to ascertain. One stipulation of the Huntingdon Hartford's granting of the Fellowships was that we should each be medically examined; and this would be done in New York.

At the moment (and thanks entirely to the Rent Restrictions Act) we are completely hamstrung financially. I have tried for three years to sell the house and had no offer large enough even just to clear the mortgage.

If a portion of the Fund can, after all, be used for smoothing over our get-away on this side, all will be well but otherwise I cannot even repeat my application to the Consul with any better showing regarding the house than that which I was able to present to him before.

I hope these difficulties may be surmounted. I feel that, so to speak, we are, thanks to your really noble help dear Maggie, three quarters of the way there; - but the remaining quarter of the way (actually the first quarter) has these problems, which, indeed, I am not exaggerating.

Very much love, from

Jack

[Typed carbon copy; signed. HRC]

To Margaret DeSilver

26 Belsize Crescent

July 4, 1952

Maggie darling:

I hope you dont blench at the sight of a letter from me! But everything has been left so vague and "in the air" as to the fund that we would appreciate any specific clarification. And though Jack calls you "Mrs Atlas" and we both know you can do just so much, I think it is necessary that you and fund contributors have the full complete truth, so that no one need be under any misapprehensions as to why we don't sail as soon as asked.

I mentioned a rotten despoilation of carpets by mould and fungi. These were good carpets intact, of better quality than can be bought now and in any case would cost a fortune to replace. But we thought that our troubles were ended when we removed these, and I sandpapered the unpainted boards, covered them with dryer and stained them. And has it not been that wainscot required mending we would have remained in ignorance of the catastrophic fact that was revealed when the boards - one or two at first, then others - were taken up. The two rooms attacked were devasted underneath. Although the flooring superficially appeared okay, this horrible white paddy stuff - it grew fungi here and there on top - had destroyed the undersides of half the boards in one room and all in the other; half the wainscot in one room and all in the other, and half a window-frame.

This may make dull reading, Maggie my dear, but you will realize its practical import to us. Four pounds went on dryer and stain wasted by me, in my ignorance, on those rotten boards. As we had no money to do everything at once we had hoped to have a tenant in or arranged for before we were put to heavy expense. The common sense of the very excellent builder who is working here and is the most decent one we have met here in Hamstead has suggested the shelter brick[244] can be used to concrete the rotten portions of the other floor and so save money by combining the jobs. He is really scrupulous in this respect and we are grateful to him for actually concerning himself with this aspect of our situation. But when we will be able to get everything straight enough to leave the house we havent so far any idea. There are the debts Jack has mentioned to clear up and they will be more slowly paid off because of this.

Of course I suppose - considering the retrospects of hardships - we might have known it. A crisis was due as soon as we had any hope of renting at last and getting out and possibly home. I still say possibly - ! Jack was almost in despair about it a few nights ago, but feels a little better now there is a very moderate estimate and the small pieces of luggage attacked seem likely to be saved. But it has been a hard blow.

All we can ever say is that our gratitude is genuine and profound.

Everyone who knows of the fund is full of praise for you. We will never be able to offer any return except as authors, and so to me the fund itself makes it the more essential that we find publishers and some method of continuing to write here. This is the sort of happier life we would like to have Jig and Pavla with Cyril and his present wife share - our being there helping them too.

Our love Evelyn for Jack too

[Typed carbon copy, signed. UTK; duplicate at HRC]

From John Metcalfe's diary:

July 17, 1952, Letter from Maggie to say $500 being sent.

To Margaret DeSilver

26 Belsize Crescent

Hampstead

London, NW3 England

August 4, 1952

My Dear Maggie,

Just a brief line to report progress,- not very *[illeg]* I regret to say. But we hope to have the most essential repairs finished now in 4 days time, + I will then be in a position to tackle the Consul again, - with the lever of a lettable flat. We are hoping, perhaps, to let it through the American Embassy, - which has a special section precisely for this, - for finding suitable accommodation for Americans.

I am also still trying to get a clear statement of just what I owe the Income Tax. The difficulty of doing this is ridiculous + incredible, + I've already been given two or three different figures! I'm praying it won't be too colossal.

---

244 Virtually every property in London had an air-raid shelter ("Anderson shelter") buried in the garden and built of bricks with a roof of corrugated steel.

Evelyn will have told you of the dry-rot and fungus which necessitated our replacing two wooden floors with cement. And now 2 blasted great cracks have appeared in 2 bedroom walls! These are the same walls the War Damage people "repaired" in 1949!

No more just now darling Maggie,

Heaping love, - and all our gratitude,

Jack

[Handwritten on personal letterhead, signed. HRC]

To Charles Chaplin

26 Belsize Crescent

September 23, 1952

Mr Charles Chaplin

Savoy Hotel, London

1952 —November. Jack telegraphed an offer of our flat to the Savoy the day after they landed. It was delivered within an hour and his secretary phoned at once to say "nuttin' doin'" as to flats. Shabby remembering Cyril Evelyn Scott

Dear Mr Chaplin:

Your secretary, with a promptitude in every sense considerate, has just telephoned that the telegraphed offer of the flat myself and my husband are trying to rent speedily in order to complete arrangements to return home to the USA, was not apropos. However, I think some explanation as to why the appeal to you and Mrs Chaplin was made, is due; as I, also, requested your secretary to be good enough to say that should you hear of anyone who is an American and in need of a flat of fair dimensions, we will appreciate the mention of this one as available I think she was probably - your nice secretary - somewhat taken aback when I said to her that the renting of this flat is essential to financing our return; as we have been financially stranded here ever since my husband - John Metcalfe, the British novelist and short story writer - was demobilized from "RAF" service in 1946. *I arrived here 1944 and have never relinquished American citizenship.* But we have been doing our best to go home every year, and have encountered so much obstructionism of an "economic" sort, that our return has been cruelly postponed again and again, *though I am American native of many generations and have an American son and John Metcalfe was a quota resident for 18 years.*

You and Mrs Chaplin do not know me personally, but Mr Chaplin may recall his own impromptu appearance at the studio - the tiny studio on Fourteenth Street - of my first husband Mr Cyril Kay Scott, in the nineteen-twenties. It was a delightful experience as recounted to me and our son, Creighton by Mr Scott, from whom I am divorced, but who is esteemed by both myself and Mr Metcalfe. *[Remainder of letter missing]*

[Typed carbon copy, not signed. Handwritten insertions. UTK]

Five years after their return to the United States in 1954, the liabilities relating to 26 Belsize Crescent had still not been fully enumerated, let alone settled. Extensive correspondence between Jack and Mr Brimblecombe of Match & Co, who had for many years managed Jack's property, makes it clear just how complex the situation was, and how very indebted he was. The collection includes letters setting out the details of his indebtedness, of which the major components were income tax on the rental income and the cost of utilities, including "an appalling amount" for gas.

To John Metcalfe

Match & Co, Ltd

14 & 15 College Crescent

South Hampstead, NW 3

October 22, 1959

Dear Mr Metcalfe,

re: 26 Belsize Crescent, NW3

Thank you for your letter which I showed to Mr Jellis as he has been managing the property for a number of years.

You will see, therefore, that you are under a misapprehension as to the costs involved in running this property and unfortunately the net income is nothing like £697 as stated by you. As you will see from Mr Jellis' report[245] the true net income is approximately £328 per annum. This is subject to income tax and does not take into account any repairs of a major nature, replacements or repairs of furniture in the furnished flat, or loss of income whilst the furnished flat is vacant, and in considering these figures you must really bear in mind we are now obtaining for all of the flats to-day's true market rents and there is little likelihood of the net figure ever being increased.

Unfortunately, you are not now in a position to purchase the Freehold. The Company who did buy the Freeholds from the Church Commissioners have now sold sufficient and are not prepared to consider disposing of any more. This means that you must treat your investment on an investment basis only and bear in mind that the present term has only 18 years to run.

Taking into account the repairing covenants under your Lease, and here again I must emphasise that it is a full repairing one, this means complete re-decoration at

---

245 This report was appended to Mr Brimblecombe's letter but is not included here as it set out, in detail, outgoings (utilities, maintenance, income tax) and income (rent). Jack's financial position was much worse than he thought.

the end of the term. Depreciation is extremely high. Taking a figure of only £2500 as the purchase price, this would mean, even ignoring interest, that this capital sum would be reduced each year by £140 and no tax allowance is ever made on a sinking fund. In other words, if one takes the figures as supplied as being correct, you have a net income of £328 and with income tax at the standard rate, say £110, this leaves you approximately £200 a year and if you deduct the loss of capital each year of £140 it seems that your true net income is negligible.

I do feel, as I have stated in my previous letters, that it is in your interests to sell as if you do keep the property I cannot see any real income for you in the years to come.

Yours sincerely,

L S Brimblecombe

[Typed letter and enclosure [missing] on company letterhead, signed. HRC]

To John Metcalfe

Match & Co, Ltd

14 & 15 College Crescent

South Hampstead, NW3

November 10, 1959

Dear Mr Metcalfe,

Re: 26 Belsize Crescent, NW3

As you know, we act for the Freeholders of the above and they have instructed us to put forward an offer of £2250 for your interest, subject to contract. They will be paying our fees so this figure would be net to you. They have also asked us to state that they would be quite prepared to delay completion if this would suit you, say, until next June. This would, therefore, give you the benefit of the rents for another six months.

I do not know if this is their last word but I would be only too pleased to approach them again to see if I could get a slightly better offer, though I did not think they would exceed £2500.

You will remember that I have written to you fully on several occasions stating that in my view it would be in your own interest to sell, especially having regard to the fact that the income you receive is now very small and you are faced with the fact of having a very short leasehold property which will depreciate rapidly if you retain the premises.

I hope by now you have received a full report from your Accountant and I await your instructions.

Yours sincerely,

L Brimblecombe

[Typed on business letterhead, signed. HRC]

To John Metcalfe

Carmel, California

November 12, 1959

Dear Jack -

Thank you so much for the detailed and candid account[246] of your circumstances. I see the point, now, and agree that you would do best to stay in the States. It's a shame that you are unlikely to realize the true value of the Hampstead house. Your account of socialized medicine is chilling. I had no idea it was so bad. I hate to think of what would - or could - happen to a person in a sudden medical emergency if they were not already in hospital. Here one can get quick help.

I haven't time for much this morning if I'm to catch the mail. Will you please tell Evelyn that I'll write to her next and soon, and that all the books arrived on Fred's birthday. He is particularly pleased with his Darwin and Julia loves hers with Kay Boyle's personal inscription. Please thank her for us all. All the books were happy choices.

Love

P

[Handwritten, signed. UTK]

To L S Brimblecombe

The Benjamin Franklin Hotel

November 14, 1959

Dear Mr Brimblecombe,

Re: 26 Belsize Crescent, NW3

Many thanks for your letter LSB/JMC dated October 22nd 1959, which I am sure gives a very clear, fair and well-considered picture of the position.

In view of all you say I have now decided to seek a purchaser for the property at a price of £2500 (Two thousand, five hundred pounds).

Supposing the £2500 to be obtained, I should do as you suggest, - invest in 5% gilt-edged. I could then, as you also point out, realise at any time after we returned to England for the purpose of buying a property. It was never my idea to re-invest in property now.

Meanwhile, and if the house is still unsold for £2500 near the time when the present unfurnished letting-agreements will expire, I do think we should very seriously consider the question of increasing the rents.

I am most indebted to you for the careful thought that you have given to the matter.

Yours sincerely,

W J Metcalfe

[Typed carbon copy, signed. HRC]

---

246 This letter has not survived.

To John Metcalfe
Match & Co
14 & 15 College Crescent
South Hampstead NW3

November 17, 1959

Dear Mr Metcalfe,

<u>re: 26 Belsize Crescent</u>

Thank you for your letter of the 14th instant which crossed my recent letter.

I am pleased to say that I have spoken to my Clients and they have instructed me to say that they are prepared to pay £2500,[247] subject to contract, and I gather from your letter that at this figure you would like to proceed.

Perhaps, therefore, you would let me know the name of the Solicitor who will be acting for you and also when you would like completion.

With regard to the re-investment of the capital you may be aware that most Local Authorities, including the Hampstead Borough Council, are now offering 5½% and this, of course, is not only gilt-edge but you are in a position to withdraw your money at any time. As a matter of interest I have asked the Local Authority to send you full details, although naturally it is up to you to invest where you think best.

I await to hear from you.

Yours sincerely,

pp L S Brimblecombe

[Typed on firm's letterhead, pp'd signature. HRC]

---

247 This equates to roughly £69,000 at 2022 values. This figure does not take into account inflation in the property market: this property would have sold for well in excess of £2 million in 2022.

Part 3

The Benjamin Franklin Hotel

This third part is different yet again. Evelyn and Jack, finally back in the United States and, they hoped, able to see Jigg and his family, were still uncertain where to settle after the end of their time at the Hartington Hartford Foundation. They travelled to New York planning to spend only a few days visiting friends and their publisher contacts. Little were they to know that they would spend the rest of their days in the Benjamin Franklin Hotel on Manhattan's upper West Side.

Unlike Parts 1 and 2, each of these chapters focuses on a specific year. Compared with previous years, relatively few letters have survived, although there is no reason to suppose that fewer were being written. Those that have survived are supplemented by entries in Jack's diary, chronicling Evelyn's increasingly poor mental and physical health. Part 3 is a record of declining health, increasing poverty and eventually the deaths of Evelyn and, two years later, Jack.

Chapter 35

1954

Jack and Evelyn had spent an uneventful and moderately productive year at the Hartington Hartford Foundation; there they found it a congenial, if not exciting, base from which to work and to seek publishers for their various manuscripts. In spite of their efforts to extend their stay (apart from anything else their fellowship included their living costs), they were told in early February 1954 that they could no longer stay at the foundation.

Meanwhile and unknown to Evelyn, Jigg and his family had been living in Spring Valley, a small commuter town in New York, since the summer of 1953. Evelyn had learned that they were living somewhere near New York City and so it was arranged that she and Jack should make their way there and rejoin her son and his family. The first stop would be New York itself where they planned a short stay in a budget hotel while they pursued other possibilities for grants and, possibly, residential fellowships. And so on March 30, 1954, they took a serviced apartment (two rooms and the use of a communal kitchen) in the Benjamin Franklin Hotel, 222 West 77th Street, New York 24, New York; that return address a feature of the many, many letters received by Jigg and Paula over the coming years. It was initially a short-term arrangement: they weren't to know that they would still be living in the Benjamin Franklin Hotel until after Evelyn's death in 1963 and until Jack's death in 1965.

Jack had begun recording rather more details of their daily life in his diary; a useful supplement to Evelyn's self-occupied correspondence. The following entries record their voyage from southern California to New York.

From John Metcalfe's diary:

March 24, 1954: Day spent in preparations for departure.

March 25, 1954: Did odd jobs connected with our departure. In afternoon, after nap, made some notes from encyclopedia. Dinner in "our honour". Usual awful business afterwards of packing and locking bulging trunks.

March 26, 1954: In morning went in to Los Angeles with John and Sal + heavy luggage, which I checked through to NYC.

March 27, 1954: Left Huntington Hartford Foundation at 11.15, - being driven in to LA by Sal. Left LA at 1.30. Dinner at about six or six-thirty. Poorish night, as expected.

March 28, 1954: All day on train.

March 29, 1954: Reached Chicago 7.15 am. Snowing. Taxi from Dearborn to LaSalle. Martin Sheffield turned up at 9.15 + took us to Bismark Hotel, where we engaged a room + chatted. Lunch at the hotel, - oyster stew for E + self. Martin presented us with $30. Left hotel at 2.15 by taxi to LaSalle depot + got aboard train 'The Pacemaker' at 2.35 pm. Left at 3. Dinner rather early, - about 5.30.

March 30, 1954: Reached New York at 8.45, and, after much telephoning etc, fixed up at the Benjamin Franklin hotel. Had lunch out. I made two journeys, for heavy and then for lighter luggage, to Grand Central. Nap. We had dinner out, at Rudley's. Had hair cut today.

March 31, 1954: Breakfasted at Rudley's at 9. Rang St Bernards. - Mr Westgate away. Went PO on 83rd St, - fill in and posted card to Immigration notifying new address. Cashed a traveller's cheque at bank. Returned to hotel + rang St Bernards again - success, - finally arranging to ring Mr Fry between 6.30 + 7.30 tonight. Did so. E and I had dinner.

Bed.

Evelyn, perhaps predictably, spent some time on their first day at their new address writing to Jigg and Paula. As she did not know where they were, she had no choice but to address her letter care of Gladys Grant, who had (perhaps with some misgivings) agreed to be Evelyn's point of contact with her son and his family.

To Creighton and Paula Scott
The Benjamin Franklin Hotel
222 West 77th Street

NYC 24, NY

March 31, 1954

Darlings:

We have arrived in New York again and will be here at shortest a week, at longest a month to six or seven weeks, all depending on what is done for our financing, beginning today with Jacks trying to connect with teaching posts, some for tutoring higher math here as well as permanent for next autumn.

Ever since the letter each - one Jigs and one Paulas - in December and January we have been awaiting your address so we can stop this damnable nonsense of having to ask Gladys to forward all our letters to you. She is good about it but it makes no sense to us, and when we have every so often to admit to others this is the case, it makes no sense to them either. Give Jigs Dad our love - on this we insist and will always insist as it DOES MAKE SENSE TO DO SO.

If there is any way at all that we can see you or you us as soon as we have any money to go anywhere for a day with you all and to see the five grands we will save for this really GREAT EVENT. Think how nice it will be for us all and for JACK TO MEET HIS STEP-GRANDCHILDREN.

I have not yet seen Mathew, Julia or Robert - please darlings lets end a situation that is senseless and is bound to be equivocally interpreted by poison-minds - it just makes no sense and never will. We are all so lovingly well disposed - you, us and your Dad I am sure.

Here we have been home a year and not had your address or as yet been able to see you - the factor of economy shall not be played on by any who may be interested in trying to keep people from meeting who corroborate each other as to this sort of thing. THERE I STAND - as it is not impossible in a muddled stupid world.

We are concerned as to your health, prospects and as to the mutual preservation of the dearest of our human contacts - one of the chief reasons we were so distressed that it took so long to finance our return from England.

Jack may get a job near Chicago for next fall, though whether this is the best place or not we dont know until we know where you are - NOW NOW NOW tout de suite.

Remember your health and your prospects are one with ours to us because affection does just that - human attachments are at least half the value of every life.

We hope to see Gladys but she is Mrs Sherlock Holmes where any of you are concerned. I suppose that to her is loyalty. I dont agree with it, because it implies you have "chosen" where I know damn well you cannot have "chosen" as you have far too much real sense to have done anything so stupid about addresses.

We left The Huntington Hertford Foundation in good standing and on an amiable footing with the Director Dr John Vincent; his wife, his son and daughter - children. the Assistant Director Mr Proctor Stafford, and all the present Fellows. We have really liked a number, and most of the incomprehensions we first encountered were due to foreignness and poor English.

WE AINT LICKED YOU AINT LICKED CYRIL AINT LICKED.
Love love love love love love love
to Paula Evelyn—to Jigg Mother
Love from Jack

[Typed on hotel letterhead, signed. SFC]

From John Metcalfe's diary:

April 1, 1954: E and I passed v disturbed night with diarrhoea. I went out and got coffee in containers, and buns, for our breakfast. Beatrice (cleaner) did our room at 10.45 while we had more coffee out. Lunch at Rudley's. Nap. I went out and bought brown hat, and then on to Village with idea of seeing Fanny, - but did not do so. Looked in vain for place to get hat blocked and cleaned. Back to hotel by 6.30. E and I had dinner at Waldorf. Later went out and bought brioches and croissants from DuBarry's at corner.

April 3, 1954: Breakfast at Rudley's. On return found letters from McDowell, Derleth and Guggenheim,[248]- the last being a durn-damn. Derleth set me my jacket for The Feasting Dead.[249] I rang Davison, and then rang Mr Westgate in definite acceptance of post at St Bernards. Wrote and posted letters to Gannett and Derleth. Bought percolator and crockery, and later coffee and condensed milk and brioches. Had lunch "at home", using community kitchen for boiling water. Before this had opened a trunk in store-room and extracted letter-files. Nap from 3 to 4. Went out and bought coffee pot etc. Dinner at 7 at Waldorf.

April 4, 1954: Breakfast "at home" of coffee and brioches etc.

April 5, 1954: Shopped in morning, - tobacco, cooking utensils etc. Strained heart while buying lemon meringue pie. Lunch at "home" of bacon and pie. Had rung Mrs Aronson in morning. Nap. More shopping etc. E and I had dinner at Waldorf. Bed. Posted letters to Maggie, Walter, French, Inglis, Pleasantville and Putney.

April 9, 1954: Gladys came unexpectedly. Went bank etc. Lunched at Waldorf, with Gladys.

April 18, 1954: Easter, and very dull. E thought valuables lost at 10 am. Found again at 4 pm. No dinner.

May 14, 1954: Back at hotel and found Maggie had sent us whisky, brandy, tea and coffee. Sampled the whiskey before supper.

May 25, 1954: Gladys and Edgerton visited us in evening and took us to supper at Waldorf Cafeteria.

June 2, 1954: Back at hotel about 6.15 and found Maggie there. She left about 7.30, - .giving us present of cheese and a book.

June 5, 1954: This morning E and I had stroll to yacht basin by Riverside Dr while maid was cleaning our room.

To Margaret Foster

The Benjamin Franklin Hotel
August 1, 1954

Dear Margué:

I am still hoping, as Jack does, that you may, by now, have the address of Paula and Jig, Denise, Fredrick, Mathew, Julia and Robert, and will send it on to use for the sake of our love for them all. We havent been able to locate Ralph and family either. Evelyn
[Handwritten postcard, signed. SFC]

These, apart from two letters to her friend Herman Rappaport describing their new living arrangements and repeating her continuing assertions about libellous attacks on her rendering it impossible to get published, comprise all of the letters surviving from 1954.

---

248 Evelyn had applied to the Guggenheim Foundation for a further grant to support her while she was finishing her "Civil War novel", *Breathe Upon These Slain*, ultimately never published.
249 Jack's novel was published in 1954.

There are no clues as to what happened to what must have been a considerable volume of correspondence after their arrival in New York. It is most unlikely that she ceased her letter writing and very probable that these letters were either lost or destroyed.

Chapter 36

1955 - 1956

There are no letters from 1955 in the collection; and only one from 1956. This is very likely because after her death Jack destroyed anything he found in her writing.

These early days in New York cannot have been easy, confined as they were to two rooms and a shared kitchen in a cheap midtown hotel, isolated from those whose values they (or more particularly Evelyn) shared and from their friends and, most particularly, from Jigg and his family.

In the absence of any letters, it has been necessary to turn to Jack's diary. Punctilious and economical in language, they are the only records we have for 1955 and much of 1956. The entries for 1955 refer mainly to his work as a mathematics tutor as well as providing considerable insight into their new lives.

From John Metcalfe's diary:

January 2 1955: Latish breakfast. Rainy, but cleared up. Went out and bought air-mail stationery and two alligator pears. Wrote to Alec Waugh. Lunch. Nap. Punched and bound some pages of E's MS.[250] Read E's MS to p 349. Went out to post letters. Drinks. Supper of hash etc. Wrote to Preston and Fisher. Bed, - and a little nightmare!

January 3, 1955: Back to St Bernard's. First day of the new term. After prayers took AA in Arith*[metic]* owing to Phelan's bereavement. Then Algebra with IX as usual. French with 1A and then with 1B. Lunch. Took prep I 1A room 3.30 - 4.30. Returning via Bloomingdales where mailed letter (registered) to Savile Club with £4.4.0. Also got Aliens Record Card. Back to 77th Street. Marketed, + bought Vodka and collected laundry. Found E sickish, so she lay down. Shis-doff *[?]* has duly returned my cuttings from "The Listener". Drinks. Supper. Bed.

March 9, 1955: St Bernard's, and took Corbelt's etc. forms in middle school for first 3 periods, then Algebra IX in fourth period. Lunch. Mr W said I might go 'home', - which I did, calling at bank on way and getting a haircut, tobacco, etc. Also marketed. Back at hotel about 3.40. Nap. Drinks. Supper. Bed.

---

250 Evelyn referred to this as her "French Revolution novel", but it was never published.

March 10, 1955: St Bernard's. Took Corbelt's class first 3 periods, then Algebra iX. Lunch. Westgate kindly agreed to correct Latin papers of 1Bx and 1A∂. Took detention 2.20 - 3.10, then prep 3.30 - 4.30, - or just before, when Westgate released me. Returned slowly to hotel where E had 'company', - Mrs Keppelmann (B didn't come). By time I knocked at our room door Mrs K had gone, - + E + I had drinks. Letter for me from June. Still no table, for which I had asked the hotel management some days ago. It seems they are still searching for one. Supper of hash etc. Bed. Very warm for time of year, - 66°.

March 17, 1955: Our wedding anniversary, - and may we have many more of them! Weather turned cold and windy. St Bernards. Middle School recitations. Latin 1A∂ and (after a gap) 1Bx. Did some Stanford. Maths 1x. Lunch. Sat with 2A from 2 to 2.20, then detention till 3.10. Westgate said I might pack up, which I did. Saw something of the St Patrick's Day parade along 96th Street. 'Home' by subway, + found E not feeling so good. Went out and marketed. Drinks + did accounts. Supper. Bed. Sprained thumb in reproving a 2A boy. Nuisance.

March 18, 1955: Snow again. END OF TERM. St Bernard's upper school recitations in gym. Took Gillespie (D) + Ullman for remainder of their Stanford A Tests in Algebra room. School broke up at 12. Faculty lunch, - soup, sandwiches, beer + coffee. Talk with Westgate re my possible staying-on. Went bank + bought tobacco. 'Home' about 3.30. Nap. Marketed. Drinks. Supper. Bed.

Jack's diary entries start again in early 1956 when Evelyn, no doubt frustrated by her social and artistic isolation, took over Jack's diary. Her entries give an insight into her frustrations at living in such cramped quarters and at her inability to make contact with Jigg. [Evelyn's entries are transcribed in the proxy typeface for her distinctive spidery hand.]

From John Metcalfe's diary:

January 16, 1956: E washed ice-box - and how! Miss K has been 3 times asked not to "help" or be instinctive - she was and I blew up, exclaiming "Jesus wept!" - damn this kitchen! Jesus Christ - I cant stand it! I flet, and when I came back she had gone, thank pete! Before the blow up about "instructiveness" she had, as usual, dinned at her seldom varied theme, that "no one" but she and I "ever" washed the frigidaire. This time she was wrong. I was about to wash it myself 8 days after she had done so, and found it already washed and clean. I put this at length as a future reminder of "community kitchens". She began, when she brought in her breakfast to get - I had hoped she had had it,

9.30 - and I asked whether I was in her way, by saying, with the air of a tragic muse, "Nobody ever gets in my way. We are lucky here. We used to have 3 or 4 people in here at once but it never bothered me. I'm not that kind of person." I said, "Well I am". This unpleasant conversation on same lines almost verbatim.

January 17, 1956: Evelyn's birthday. I, in having bath, discovered large discolouration, like bruise, on right upper arm. Went St Bernards. Taxi to bank and deposited Haithcock check of $258.75 in bank. Haithcock School, - including noon-hour duty. Left 3.30. Home, after marketing, about - 4.10. Drinks, did accounts etc. Supper. Bed.

February 6, 1956: Washed frigidaire. Evelyn.

March 5, 1956: [in red ink] Evelyn did ice box!

March 15, 1956: [in red ink] E got cable from Paula.

March 30, 1956: Bernice 5.30. Margaret De Silver George Burnham De Silver came to witness my signature to my will confirming formally letter in safety deposit for Jigg. Will dated March 23, 1956 to go to Lewis Mayers 214 East 18th St, NYC, NY Prof of Law City College Write Margaret and Bernice how Jigg at present reached Everything for equal division between Jigg - son Creighton Seely Scott and his Stepfather William John Metcalfe who are appointed my literary executors not to allow changes in posthumous publications

After Maggie + Burnham had gone, E, Bernice + I went to Waldorf Cafeteria for supper, and I broke my upper denture.

March 31, 1956: Phoned Bernice. E's Dentist, Dr Foster, + fixed appointment for 10 on Monday. Collected laundry, etc. E's cold bad. I had supper at Rudley's and brought her back sandwich and ice.

In early 1956 Evelyn prepared a 15-page single-spaced document including sections on Evelyn's own family, her childhood and the years she spent with Cyril. She includes an account of her life with Jack Metcalfe and details of his family. Many of the passages describe her obsession with retaining her US citizenship and with the political persecution that she assumed followed from that. Extracts from this document appear in Chapter 1 and Chapter 4.

The document is also, in part, a recapitulation of the allegations she makes in her "Precis of events indicative of libel" which she prepared in 1951, putting particular emphasis on her belief that Cyril's autobiography, Life Is Too Short, *was altered at the printers to present her in an unfavourable light.*

Below is the covering letter accompanying this document.

To John Metcalfe and Creighton Scott

New York City
April 2, 1956

[Contained in a manila envelope, inscribed as follows: For William John Metcalfe and Creighton Seely Scott letters and a family record To be opened by either or by my daughter-in-law Paula Scott or any of my grandchildren who are of age at the time of my death.

[To be opened only after my death.] Letter to Creighton Seely Scott, to be preserved with the Will of his mother, Evelyn Dunn Scott Metcalfe, author Evelyn Scott and handed to him on her death or before, but not to be opened in her lifetime. Love to Cyril 4 living appreciation to F C Wellman and trust in his fundamental kindness

Evelyn Dunn Scott Metcalfe Evelyn Scott Mother Grandmother there are 15 pages herein all but one typed on both sides all single space.

Darling Son Creighton, to us always Jigg, or Jigeroo, it is a call on one's imagination to be read when one lives, after one is dead. I hope, long before that time, for the human opportunity to speak the love that Jack and myself, like your Dad, I am sure, feel for you for Paula, for Denise, Fredrick, Mathew, Julia and Robert, and to know explicitly, instead of so largely as a matter of conjecture and hints, what is at the bottom of the silence we abhor as between you, Paula and ourselves, and us and good and fine Cyril. I hope to know in particular why you were sent to Indo-China, to Saigon, at the very moment when, at last, we had located you as attached to your U S Army anti-soviet peace mission.[251]

But, meanwhile, I can only reiterate that you have been a joy to me from the very day you were born, and that as an adult you still represent to me and to Jack - and to your Dad equally of course - the splendid comprehending friend to whom I dedicated <u>Bread and a Sword</u> with the utmost sincere continued appreciation of your talents as author and painter, your acute intellect, your human insights, and all those unique capacities of mind and sensitive feeling Jack and I value, not merely because of a "maternal bias", but despite it; for I do believe, darling Jigg that, though my heart is with you, I have never failed and never ceased to see you with the detached eyes of one accustomed for a lifetime to criticise individuals and societies and appraise genius such as you have innately. I have never been able to love anyone unless my mind concurred in large measure; and though this might be called a "defect", I think it is not

---

251 This is a reference to Jigg's time with Radio Free Europe, which had absolutely no connection
to the US Army.

that, and helps to give my love its staying power. I respect you deeply morally, as a man of superior courage and will who has carried on under the circumstances of a more than usually difficult life.

And there I am very grateful to darling Paula - may I say Pavli in affection? - for perceptivity, her loyalty to you, her marvellous sustained fight with you, shoulder to shoulder, for you both and your children whose futures are in our thoughts every day, and have been, all during those years since 1944, in which circumstances not of your making, or hers, or ours, or Cyril's, have kept us from any knowledge of them beyond mine in 1943-44, when Denise and Fredrick were met in the flesh.

There is no reproach in this, there never will be, never can be - none to yourselves, but much to a bad world. Those five days in London when you were with us in the flat, stand now with the most important of our lives, as the reassurance that you are in the flesh, and I implore you never to give up, <u>even as I know you never will</u>, merely in carrying over to you and to Paula and the five children, our own constant concern.

Nothing can ever change us and nothing can ever change you, nor will Paula ever change I am certain, or Cyril; and please remember your children have the benefit of fine parents, not merely as influences - though this counts heavily - but in the matter of heredity. We believe in them, too, completely.

I write this on both sides *[of the sheet]*, so it will take up less space, and I wish to include in it some data that may refresh the memories of the Scotts in some far future in respect to dates connected with Cyril's change of name from the Fredrick Creighton Wellman of his birth and his career in science to the Cyril Kay Scott of his career as painter and novelist - or, thinking better of the space, I will add supplementary facts on a second sheet[252] to be preserved with this, as you may wish to consult sometime or show it to someone without my personal letter.

[Typed, signed, handwritten annotations. SFC]

From John Metcalfe's diary:

April 11, 1956: Haithcock School + long conference. Taxi home. Wrote Mavis McIntosh.

3 pages of Will stapled together handed to May Mayers for preservation in Lewis Mayers' safe, two long manila envelopes sealed with double flap:
The envelope numbered 1 contains the Last Will and Testament of myself Evelyn Dunn Scott Metcalfe two personal letters, one to my present and second husband William John Metcalfe and one to my son of my first marriage to Cyril Kay Scott, Creighton Seely Scott my only child: letter to Creighton having affixed to it

---

252 This sheet has not survived.

and called part of letter 33 pages of data on family, property and other people's Wills

The envelope number 2 contains the trinket I gave my granddaughter Denise Scott, in 1944, which I now hope she will divide with her sister Julia Swinburne Scott, then not yet born. I have other family trinkets for both, but not as personal most, or as old, some of them Jack kept for Denise in safety deposit in London, they are gold bar pin set with turquoise and pearl, my mother's[253]

April 12, 1956: Haithcock School.

April 16, 1956: *E cleaned Frigidaire "out of turn" by about one week 6 May*

May 13, 1956: Quiet day at damned noisy hotel.

May 16, 1956: *Sent Lewis Mayers the Army addresses*[254] *of Creighton and Paula registered for him.*

May 21, 1956: *E cleaned Frigidaire.*

June 11, 1956: E lunched today with May, - who presented her with a "diet", just lean meat, potatoes and tea!

July 6, 1956: *July 6th Evelyn cleaned Frigidaire.*

During the summer of 1955, Jigg secured employment with the International Cooperation Administration, a division of the State Department of the United States, to establish a news network for the newly formed Radio Viet Nam. His family joined him to live in Saigon (now Ho Chi Minh City) where, apart from two months' home leave in the summer of 1957, he and his family lived until July 1959.

To Miss Betty Roth

The Benjamin Franklin Hotel

[June 1956]

Dear Miss Roth,

Employee Relations Officer

International Cooperation Administration

Washington 25, DC

Can you, perhaps, give me any present information on the health and well-being of my son, Creighton Seely Scott?, his wife, and their five children, in Saigon?

---

253 There follows a long list of jewellery pieces: as they add nothing to the story, they have been omitted.

254 The US Army provided postal services, equivalent to those available in the United States, to Americans working overseas with US government agencies. Accordingly, Jigg had use of an APO (Army Post Office) address; although Evelyn clearly misunderstood this to imply he was serving in the Army.

Of course I am always hoping to have letters, but on March 15th I received a second cable from my daughter-in-law, Paula Pearson Scott, from Saigon, in which she said "illness prevented letter"; and, although the cable gave me some measure of reassurance in that somebody in the family was able to send it, no letter has come since, either, and, naturally I am anxious.

On January 18th, 1956, I mailed you a letter respecting my need to know the permanent address of my son and his wife and their children, in the USA. You did not send it to me; and having, therefore, gathered that you did not know it, I - because I really require it for placing in the safety-deposit with the Will I have recently made that more formally affirms the content of a letter I gave my son in 1944 before I went to England to be near my second husband John Metcalfe *Metcalfe with an E* a double has appeared without a reviewer! during his service in the RAF, and which appoints him and his stepfather as my literary executors - I had already asked Mr Francis Knight, the Director of the Passport Office of the Department of State, whether my daughter-in-law, on departing for travel abroad, had filed her permanent address with him.

I don't know what else I could have done in the total absence of anyone from whom I could obtain the address here at home. But I especially would like to have you aware of this, for Mr Knight replied to my letter in a manner indicating that he must have gone to some trouble for me, belated though his answer seemed to me after several months. It came to me a few days ago, and he says he himself wrote to Foreign Operations *I did not mention to Mr Knight what service my son was in, not having been told whether I should or not* - evidently on the mistaken assumption that I did not even know where Creighton Seely Scott was abroad; a natural error I suppose, as I complained of the apparent impossibility of receiving answers to my letters.

I don't know what to do, and have been rather ill lately, again, in consequence, perhaps, of my distress; and though I have now sent 31 letters to my son - for his wife and the five children, too - to Saigon, illness, here, too, has "prevented" the writing of some things. The quotation marks are corroboration let me add. There has been not a word said of my five grandchildren since before my daughter-in-law sailed - long before - as in the two letters I received just before her departure, after a lengthy gap between, she did not mention them.

In a few years it will be seven years since that five day glimpse of my son in London, of which I have written you already. We have always been - I cannot say it too often - an affectionate congenially-minded family, yet, since 1945, over and over, whenever we attempt either renewed contact or improved communication, "something happens".

Are any of my family ill? Perhaps only you can answer that. I am not blind to my long letters as not in the official scheme of life. But, again, what am I to do? Not even my legal friend and advisor has been able to suggest anything to re-establish normal interchanges between us all.

Three months is a long time to a mother who has been anxious for fourteen years at frequent intervals, the London visit the only respite.

Sincerely, with reiterated thanks for your every kindness. Should Creighton Seely Scott and his family leave Saigon, I do indeed trust your goodness to let me be advised.

Evelyn Dunn Scott Metcalfe

[Typed carbon copy, signed. Handwritten insertions. UTK]

From John Metcalfe's diary:

July 13, 1956: Mailed letter to Miss Roth in respect to whatever probabilities there may be of seeing Jigg, Paula, the five children and Cyril as well.

July 16, 1956: returned Shapiro Condor etc to St Agnes Branch Library 5 pm loaned Goldberg The Shadow of the Hawk.

August 2, 1956: Evelyn cleaned frigidaire.

August 8, 1956: V poor night, E being troubled with heart pains, then (on taking pink pill) with nausea.

August 10, 1956: Evelyn troubled by heart pains.

August 12, 1956: Quiet day at hotel. Evelyn still bothered by heart pains.

August 14, 1956: E had heart pains and I did not go to school until afternoon.

August 17, 1956: Book 3 returned today

August 21, 1956: Rain, and much cooler. Tried, vainly, to get E's pink pills. Went bank, bought tobacco, etc. Lunch + nap. Marketed. Drinks, + write at "Lorimer's Luck". Supper. Bed.

August 22, 1956: First visit to Dr Berczlier who gave me 1 pink pill three times a day 1 white to dissolve under tongue at intervals not specified. At 4.30 had a nasty attack, as I took a nasty letter from nasty Saunders out of packet of prescriptions not yet filled, so I took one of Dr Shaw's green pills. Before dinner at 8 pm took first pink Berczlier pill. After dinner twinges in arm, took a white pill under tongue—results pain at 9.30 pm. As narrated above by E.

August 28, 1956: Came in with Jack to find to find out our pleasant housekeeper had herself put far better carpet in, different curtains, bedspreads and fresh white covers on chiffonier and hotel table.

September 1, 1956: E had letter from Marie McIntosh[255] saying she could not handle her as "list full".

---

255 McIntosh was one of a growing number of writers' agents who were no longer willing to act for Evelyn.

September 3, 1956: E cleaned frigidaire. Unpleasant day.

September 17, 1956: Moved by September 17th unless week more needed. The above not now applicable.

September 22, 1956: A record day for money spending! Prefaced by the starting of a cold. Expenses: - Prescriptions, tobacco, hair-cut, pants, commutation-ticket, attache-case etc. Plus the usual Saturday expenses of Marketing, laundry, etc. Total around $75.

October 2, 1956: certificate of Copyright Renewal for my Witch Perkins A Story of the Kentucky Hills of September 24th, 1956 62456 September 24 56 stamped right bottom and top stamp R 177198.

October 4, 1956: Cleaned frigidaire.

October 10, 1956: 12 o'clock Berczlier. Same day Jim coloured used vacuum and washed Venetian blinds. Night fairly good, not so for Jack.

October 11, 1956: Took two tempugen forte[256] tablets to be taken 2 a day until 13th then 1 a day until 16th. Then "6 a."-does that mean repeat cycle?...Bad night, no good either.

October 12, 1956: Night of October 12-13th was very good. Both slept well no aches or pains..

October 13, 1956: Good day night hell impossible.

October 25, 1956: Creighton Seely Scott's birthday mailed registered letter to Mr Welker—Robert J Welker, 1088 Murfreesboro Road, Nashville, Tenn about Escapade, facts as to common law, legal change of name, and Jigg's birth registry as Seely Scott pen note in envelope with letter.

October 26, 1956: Letter from Miss Jean Hermann saying Miss Roth assignment abroad began June 1st 1956.

November 2, 1956: cleaned damn ice-box 5 pm.

November 13, 1956: Evelyn heard from Paula, - they are now back in the USA.[257] No, found this not to be so.

November 6, 1956: 3 weeks approximate news.

December 7, 1956: cleaned ice box 10.20 to 11.30.

December 25, 1956: Quiet day at hotel.

---

256 It has not been possible to find any information about this preparation.

257 The family returned to the United States on "home leave" during the summer of 1956. By the time this information reached Evelyn they had returned to Saigon.

Chapter 37

1957

Only 29 letters written in 1957 survive although it is very likely that, as in previous years, many more were written. Those that have survived were largely directed to Jigg's employers, the International Cooperation Administration, a division of the US State Department. Evelyn was again pitting Jigg's employers against Jigg's right to privacy by her increasing demands for details of his whereabouts.

This year, too, saw Evelyn again taking over Jack's diary. The pages are filled day after day, not with Jack's telegraphic notes in his neat handwriting, but Evelyn's florid and increasingly incoherent outpourings as she documents, with dates, letters she had previously sent and for which she had had no response, some from two years previously. One can only guess at her motive for these regular detailed entries. Was she planning to use them as evidence at some future date? Or was she finding some sort of satisfaction in this act of recording?

Evelyn's commandeering of Jack's diary reveals her obsessive and often confused focus on her inability to communicate with her family. This may be because of her frustration at the discovery that after their struggle to return to the United States and her expected reunion with Jigg, he and his family were (literally) on the other side of the world! In any case, this focus on recording of detail may well have been a symptom of her developing obsessive personality.

To Jean Hermann

The Benjamin Franklin Hotel
January 1, 1957

For the kind attention of Miss Jean Hermann
Employee Relations Officer
International Cooperation Administration
Washington 25,DC
Dear Miss Hermann,

Thanks, I think, to your letter[258] of October 25th, 1956, in which you advised me to address my son, Creighton Seely Scott, and my daughter-in-law, Paula Scott, at

---

258 This letter has not survived.

USOM, Navy 150, FPO,[259] San Francisco, Cal, I have, at last, recontacted Paula Scott to the greatly appreciated extent of a sweet letter and card and snapshots of my five grandchildren, grandchildren, also, of my first husband, Mr Cyril Kay Scott, whom we trust may have received copies of the same pictures.

I am, however, still distressed by the fact that the snapshot - at least a snapshot - of my son Creighton was not included, as I have not, as I have often said, and said in most of my letters to the office of Personnel, seen him since 1949; and I have importuned both him and my daughter-in-law for the contemporary picture of him that might compensate for the theft of all my family photographs bar half a dozen snapshots, at The Huntington Hertford Foundation, at Pacific Palisades, California, in 1953.

My daughter-in-law mentions Creighton by his nickname, Jigg, for the first time since they went to Saigon, and my present husband and myself take this as possibly a good omen, but she says of him that he is very tired and in need of a vacation. And the situation, though improved as recounted above, leaves us wondering, again, why Creighton has not written to us any letter we have received since 1953.

We so hope to see them all here in the USA and if there is any possibility of hastening the return of my son and his family with the guarantee for him of an adequate salary in his own country near enough for us to sometimes meet and allow him to sometimes to see his father, we will be re-indebted to the utmost for any helpful thing you can do toward that end.

May I add this reminder as to his earlier life: that, although his author-painter career cannot, under present conditions, suffice for his own or his family's support, he is a genuinely distinguished man judged by the standards of pure literature and pure painting, and he has already the mss of at least two very fine novels for publication, which he withdrew from circulation because of pressure direction in literature. But I have never had a word in reply to anything I written to him about his mss, though even some small profit by their sale would bring a little welcome money and restore to all the Scotts a vital interest that has always enriched their lives.

I have sent letters to Creighton care of The American Embassy at times since your letter of October. He does not appear to receive them. However some to him have also gone to Navy 150.

Sincerely yours,

Evelyn Dunn Scott Metcalfe

[Typed carbon copy, signed. UTK]

During this period Evelyn's chief preoccupation was making contact with her son and perhaps predictably, as the State Department was not providing the information she craved,

---

259 Fleet Post Office. The US Navy provided postal services similar to Army APO addresses for Americans working overseas for government agencies.

she turned to his previous employers, Radio Free Europe, on the mistaken assumption that
they would know where he had gone after leaving their employ.

To Betty Allen

The Benjamin Franklin Hotel
January 7, 1957

Miss Betty Allen
care Personnel Department, Free Europe
110 West 57th Street NY, NY
Dear Miss Allen,

Again, Creighton Seely Scott's mother, is turning up "like the bad penny", though the same grateful sentiments that have persisted since I first talked to you on the telephone about my son's address and his family's in March 1953. May I, also, again, be forgiven for asking your advice?

I am writing, today, to Mr Thomas E Myers, who was the Director of Free Europe Personnel in 1955, August, hoping he is still with you, for he was then kind indeed in letting me know my son had been posted to Saigon, Viet-nam; and though Creighton, actually, was posted there in July, 1955, it was due to Mr Myers that I learned which Department in Washington to write to obtain his mailing address, and that of my daughter-in-law, Paula Scott, who accompanied him there shortly, with the grandchildren of myself and Mr Cyril Kay Scott, Denise, Fredrick, Mathew, Julia and Robert Scott.

I have just written to Mr Myers asking whether it is possible to obtain, also, now any idea as to how lengthy such postings are, and what the probabilities as to guarantees of jobs at home with salaries adequate for the support of a wife and five children; and have reminded him, in making my request, that Creighton Scott is now forty-two; that conditions here, as we see them, make it essential that he continue with Paula Scott and the children.

Mr Myers, quite naturally, cannot be expected to know all about the job question; but I have asked him whether there is anyone in the US Government[260] to whom I might write about this, as the ICA Personnel Officers - I wrote First to Miss Roth, and recently to Miss Hermann - are very genuinely kind, but are non-committal. And it is just in case that Mr Myers has been promoted that I am taking the further liberty of advising you of my letter to him.

I wrote to you and him of the factor of probable libel of myself and my present husband, John Metcalfe, British author, as having a possible bearing on my original difficulty in locating my son and his family when we returned from England in 1953, having seen Creighton but once since 1944, and that for five days in London, in 1949; as several untrue and unpleasant tales about us and our absence had already come to

---

260 There was no organisational connection between Radio Free Europe and the International Cooperation Administration. Evelyn appears not to have understood this.

my ears. And this view of the situation was corroborated by my daughter-in-law in a letter I received *[remainder of line slipped off bottom of carbon]* to stress here - I merely mention it so *[remainder of line slipped off top of carbon]* although I have written letters to both Creighton Scott and Paula Scott, at the rate of two a week, one each, during the entire year and a half since I obtained their addresses, not one letter to Creighton has ever been acknowledged by him, and Paula's several sweet letters throw no light on whether he has ever had any of mine.

Were she and Creighton, with the children, enabled to return to the USA under normal conditions in which we could all meet and see Cyril Kay Scott, we might assist one another in the predicament of the arts by which we are confronted *[remainder of letter missing]*

[Typed carbon copy, 2 pp only, not signed. UTK]

From John Metcalfe's diary:

January 9, 1957: Very poor night, E being plagued by pain in left arm.

January 11, 1957: E cleaned ice-box.

To Evelyn Scott
Free Europe Committee, Inc
New York 16, New York

January 14, 1957

Dear Mrs Metcalfe:

Your recent letter to Mr Myers has been referred to me. I regret that I can give you no advice as to the possibility of Creighton Scott's return home. I can only suggest that you continue to contact the heads of ICA in Washington.

If you think we may be of any other help to you, please contact us again.

Sincerely yours,

Keith E Kenyon

Assistant to Personnel Director

[Typed on official letterhead, signed. UTK]

From John Metcalfe's diary:

January 16, 1957: Mailed "Tale of Two Cities" to Paula for Matthew on way home.

January 17, 1957: Evelyn Scott's birthday Evelyn Dunn Scott Metcalfe born Elsie Dunn Clarksville, Tenn.

February 8, 1957: Paula's letter the first received arrived May 2, 1956 —a 9 mo interval—September 6, 1953 America S Valley...E cleaned ice-box.

February 13, 1957: mailed Keats to Denise 83rd St PO was 12 cents to FPO San Francisco request notice of arrival with Saigon addressee.

March 4, 1957: Ice box cleaned by me.

March 5, 1957: birthday of Jack's mother Jessie Maria Clay born in the punjab father in British Empire Army.

April 1, 1957: Mailed (registered) E's letter to Mr Knight at State Department.

April 3, 1957: E cleaned frigidaire.

May 2, 1957: E DID ICE BOX.

May 7, 1957: Jigg Paula the children book about Saigon received with Paula's fine clear notes—a page out in front! Was it done before mailing? No—replied.

May 15, 1957: arrived May 100 nitro-glycerine[261] pills to save me expense.

May 27, 1957: E 26 nitro-glycerin pills—see how long last keep tab on improvement wish less sporadic and intermittent.

June 4, 1957: E cleaned ice-box

June 5, 1957: For annihilate aggression against the SA old old also with our British phoned both Sherton and Tudor City began jabbing pain in ear very sore for hours—after this attack on BE last year same time approximately thus repeated. [262]

June 7, 1957: Dr Mayers phoned was told I was "not at home"- I was here from 11 am on.

June 13, 1957: put 50 nitro-glycerin pills in container see how often needed.

June 19, 1957: Room to be repainted tomorrow so E + I ate out at Rudley's.

July 2, 1957: E cleaned frigidaire. Good letter Mr Willis H Young returning 2 forms sent me by British Ministry of Pensions and National Insurance—re my half of the retirement pensions Jack has paid up on. Mr Young for the USA Government says for me to fill my application and send it to Newcastle-on-Tyne cannot affect my citizenship as the law stands in the USA now EDSM.

July 4, 1957: Found fair-sized piece of a glass ash-tray on base of reading lamp—our own round smaller lighter ash-tray has gone. This is squared and is someone else's—ours cost 15 cents I bought it when Lizzie King broke that hotel provided—so silly! I have a dime ash-

---

261 Nitroglycerin was widely prescribed to treat angina by promoting blood flow.

262 Many of Evelyn's diary entries are incoherent and/or make references to people, places and events about which there is no further information. These are retained as illustrations of Evelyn's general state of mind.

tray put away, I bought last year. I won't take it out as
that would confuse issue as to why this.

July 7, 1957: birthday of Jack's father William Charles
Metcalfe born in Walamaloo Australia, English on both
sides, ship-builder father lately of Hull.

July 19, 1957: Bernice here. This day I received four letters
returned to me from: 26 Hampstead Road Spring Valley
Rockland County NY Addressee: Mrs Creighton Seely
Scott all four to her, my daughter-in-law. These are
stamped return to writer (stamp a hand with this on
it) (on the list of "Reason checked" are pencilled C by
"unclaimed" and "refused!". NY stamp Nov 25th 1955
dated again Nov 4th, Dec 5, Dec 9th, 1955 NB nxt pg.

July 20, 1957: [continued from previous page] All the letters here noted
returned were held one year and seven eight to 7
months. All stamped when mailed 1955 Nov 4th not
stamped at Spring Valley until 1957, 4 pm day and
month unreadable. Nov 25th not stamped at Spring
Valley until 1957, day and month unreadable.
Dec 5th not stamped at Spring Valley until July 18th,
1957, 4pm.
Dec 9th not stamped at Spring Valley until July 18th
1957, 4 pm..
Nov 4th letter stamped NY 9.30 mailed 9.30 pm.
Nov 25th letter Nov 25th, 3.30.
Dec 5th stamped mailed 4.30.
Dec 9th stamped mailed 9.30 this refers to letters below.
All four returned were to Evelyn Scott.
cont from prior pg: to write dates more clearly I repeat.:
Nov 4th, 1955.
Nov 25th, 1955.
Dec 5th, 1955.
Dec 9th, 1955.
On the Post Office NY stamp, the circular stamp with
date has New York either 7 or 1 (one) on each stamp.

*Eventually the constant stream of letters to the personnel department in Washington was
recognised for what it was, and a sympathetic personnel officer, Jean Hermann, took it upon
herself to deal with this correspondence and, more importantly, not to forward queries to
senior officials in the State Department. This turned out to be crucial in protecting Jigg
from the repercussions of his mother's letters.*

To Jean Hermann

The Benjamin Franklin Hotel
July 20, 1957

Employee Relations Officer (in charge of Employee Relations for USOM, Program
Support, Saigon Office of Personnel)
International Cooperation Administration
Washington, 25, DC

PS: Please note that the letters held at Spring Valley PO for over a year and a
half had on them <u>return to Evelyn Scott</u>, my name as author, in which much
mail still reaches me.

Dear Madame,

In connection with a letter I addressed to Miss Betty Roth over a year ago, which
was, in part, about the difficulty I have had ever since the war began, in maintaining
correspondence with my son, Mr Creighton Seeley Scott, his wife, Paula Pearson
Scott, and his five children and hers, who have been with USOM, Program Support in
Saigon, Viet-nam for the past two years: I have come upon a bit of information which
I wish to give you here with, as Miss Jean Hermann, when replying for Miss Roth,
kindly supplied me with an address for my son which has, so far, proved useful only
for letters written us by my very sweet daughter-in-law.

<u>I received yesterday, July 19th</u>, the 19th <u>1957, from Spring Valley</u>, NY, <u>four
letters which</u>, apparently, have not been tampered with in any overt way, which I
had addressed to <u>Mrs Creighton Seeley Scott, at 46 Hampstead Road, Spring Valley,
Rockland County, NY, in November and December 1955!!!!</u>

The address is the same to which, prior to Mrs Scott's departure for Saigon, I had
sent letters which she acknowledged in hasty notes, by her herself. <u>The return address
above was on the back of each of the four envelopes</u>, which one must suppose have
not been much handled, as they are all <u>clean and in good condition</u>. The NY Post
Office stamps at the time of mailing are clearly legible, dates etc, but the date of return
was legible in its entirety on one letter only, which, however, revealed it as probably
the same on all as the time of day of the Spring Valley stamping could be read on the
others.

The dates of the original mailings as stamped on the four envelopes - of which I
have opened one to be sure the content is intact, and it is - are, respectively, <u>Nov 4th
1955, Nov 25th, 1955, Dec 5th, 1955, Dec 9th, 1955</u>. The NY stamping contains the
numeral one or seven by the Post Office station - not blurred but printed with a tail on
the one that makes it like a seven or the reverse.

I think this may be significant, not because I did not realize, on obtaining the
address of my family in Saigon and receiving a cable from my daughter-in-law, but it
may have been the natural thing to notify me of their Saigon address only after they
were there, but because of a combination of the <u>one year seven and a half months</u> time
period between the mailing of the letters and their return.

I still write both to him and to my daughter-in-law, sometimes as one and sometimes in a letter each, once a week, USOM, Navy 150,[263] to which my daughter-in-law has added, Program Support, <u>Box 32. As you may have recorded in your</u> files as mentioned in my letters my daughter-in-law complained that she realized I did not receive some of her letters and my sons while myself and my husband, were in England, 1943-1955, before my son and his family went to Munich for the Voice of Free Europe. During their stay in Munich of a year and a half approximately, this experience was repeated. There was everything to indicate - as I am sure Mr and Mrs Scott too would attest - that several of my letters from London to them were <u>not</u> received, nor were parcels, though three parcels of books have reached Saigon. These parcels to Saigon were the only parcels I ever sent to my grandchildren that were ever acknowledged received and I have sent many, mailed in London to their American addresses, from London to Munich, and from NY to Spring Valley.

On July 12th, 1957, I addressed, to the "Commander, USOM" - after having written to several people in vain to know whom I should address in connection

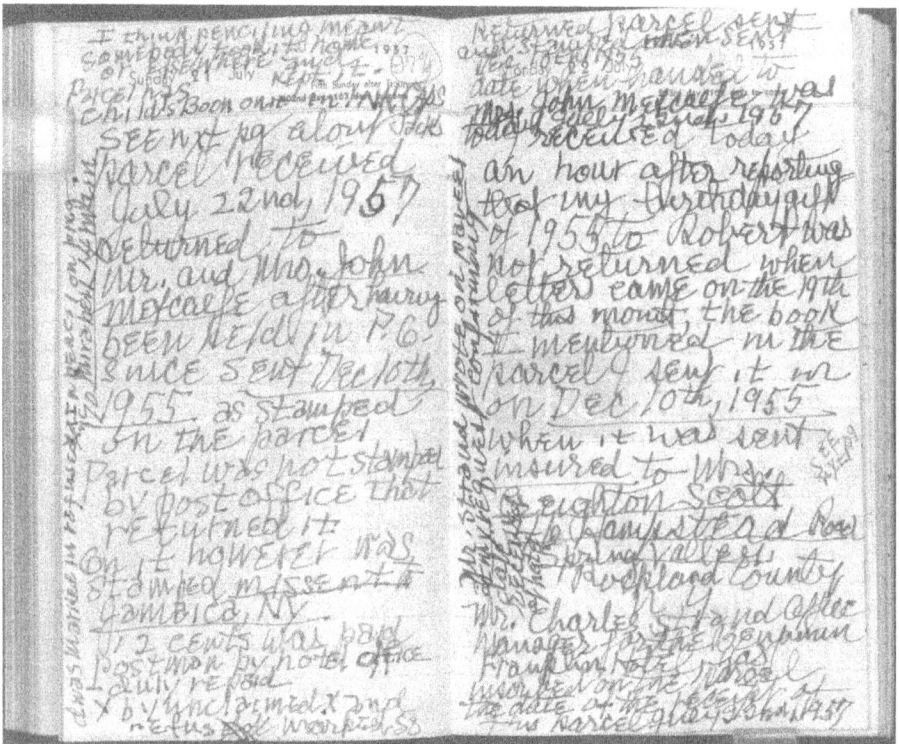

Pages from Jack's diary for July 21, 1957: *Harry Ransom Center*
[Handwriting in blue ink on printed ruled pages]

---

263 USOM or the United States Operations Mission, an agency of the International Cooperation Administration, was the specific programme employing Jigg.

with possible postings or help toward home jobs - to ask whether there seemed any likelihood of the return of my son and his family to some location where it would be possible for us to see him and them all in person sometimes. But I am advising you that I wrote because it would seem we are literally pursued by interferers with our mail; something that began when I leaned of the death of my father, the late Seely Dunn of Lynchburg, Va, and at one time of Washington, DC: his death in 1944, and my advice as to this of 1947. *I have never obtained a reply, since we came to NY, 1954, from California, to any letter written to my daughter-in-law's mother Mrs Joseph Foster at Ranchos de Taos.*

Faithfully Yours,

[Typed carbon copy, not signed. Handwritten insertions. UTK]

From John Metcalfe's diary:

July 21, 1957: I think pencilling meant somebody took it home or elsewhere and kept it. Parcel has Child's Book on it in INK CAPS See next pg about Jack parcel received July 22nd, 1957 returned to Mr and Mrs John Metcalfe after having been held in PO since sent Dec 10th, 1955, as stamped on the parcel. Parcel was not stamped by post office that returned it. On it however was stamped missent to Jamaica NY 12 cents was paid postman by hotel office—duly repaid X by unclaimed X and refused marked so it was marked in refused. In pencil on pkg "c/o Mirabell 14 Main.

July 22, 1957: Returned parcel sent and stamped when sent Dec 10th 1955 date when handed to Mrs John Metcalfe was today July 22nd, 1957. I received today an hour after reporting that my birthday gift of 1955 to Robert was not returned when letters came on the 19th of this month, the book I mention in the parcel I sent it in on Dec 10th, 1955, when it was sent insured to Mrs Creighton Scott 45 Hampstead Road, Spring Valley, Rockland County, NY. Mr. Charles Strand Office Manager for the Benjamin Franklin Hotel has inscribed on the parcel the date of the receipt of this parcel July 22nd, 1957. Mr Strand wrote on parcel at my request confirming date received at hotel

July 23, 1957 [continued from previous page] parcel had been opened and book taken out when parcel sent insured. Has a "double" game been played at Jamaica? This opened parcel tied originally by my husband with twine—small twine knots where twine crosses—had been re-knotted with white string by someone trying to conceal it mailable. I have not opened the book, probably damaged my guess. Parcel notes the book was received returned open at one end. parcel notes cont both parcels and letters have marks by "unclaimed" and "refused"—my daughter-in-law left for Saigon about 1st of October, so they were not "refused" That pencil scribble c/o Mirabell Main 14—c/o is such could be 6/6—wait and see.

July 24, 1957 [continued from previous page] Both the parcels returned were insured—both had been opened and retied sloppily 1st parcel child's book, second sea-shell. In 1940, by coming to me to ask about "another Evelyn Scott" and producing others, my mail was probably always liable to detention and they took no great risk—irresponsible. Don't forget there was a witness to a coloured Evelyn Scott in 1940—her own name we suppose. But this parcel was addressed to Mrs Creighton Scott and this is the first intimation of a "double" of my son's name.

June 23 2 eggs stolen from icebox second theft of eggs one 6 months earlier.

June 24th, 1957—Insured Return of small parcel for one of the children addressed to Mrs Creighton Seely Scott, 46 Hampstead Road, Spring Valley, NY. "gift sea-shell" in one other parcel named by child's books.

July 25, 1957: Mr Charles Strand has signed for The Benjamin Franklin Hotel of which he is the manager the days of which the postman delivered these returned parcels—noted on prior pgs—to the hotel when they were handed by the telephone operator—Christian name "Margaret" (not Mathews) to MYSELF Evelyn Scott, Mrs John Metcalfe, Mrs W J Metcalf—all myself last was return to Mrs W J Metcalfe.

July 26, 1957: Greenwich School.

July 29,1957: 1 air mail to Jigg Saigon. 1 air mail to Robert L Welker were mailed in PO same time. Letters mailed at "Planetarium" PO registered to Miss Jean Hermann to Dr H C Nixon Vanderbilt Press. There was no name, *either on the registry window or the money order window one parcel window and 2 stamps had names MAAS first letter when I arrived at registry window empty, had to wait, man who afterward registered was counting parcels list in hand when I got there. Very short list. When he made out my receipt, he had no second carbon in. Third carbon "took". He was copying second in pencil like original presumably when he told me I could go. Jewish both coloured began* Sick. Did not go to school.

July 30, 1957: Returned to school. Caught 3.22 back, and, on way home, mailed note to Dr H (at 17 E 75) reminding her about my "bonus". Drinks. Supper. Bed. Very muggy.

July 31, 1957: *letter to Miss Knight as per blue notebook— registered. No name of man at registry—same Jew— not on window. He gave me my receipt and walked from window without looking at his carbons to see whether we had clear copies—last time same man had no carbon on second copy 53 cts—2 sheets paper same envelopes Man is obviously Jewish but not extreme example—probably had blond hair but it is greying, look at colour eyes.* Greenwich School as usual.

August 1, 1957: *icebox cleaned "by E" a very poor day, with the one virtue of a page re-done by me and one fresh paragraph roughed in. Siegel wrote yesterday I am free to include "The Mocked Romantics" in my volume-when?* Greenwich School as usual. Got my £$75 ($73.32) "back pay" from Dr H at last.

August 4, 1957: Muggy + unpleasant, after a poor night (despite "itch" ointment + sleeping capsule). Worked at school chores etc. Put new ribbon in typewriter.

August 5, 1957: *bottle of tonic black was sent fresh by mail recently old one was not refilled Note: 4 medicines, sedatives, 2 Jack's 2 mine*
1 black digestive good stops
Jack largest speckled notebook of pencil draughts of person and business letter
1 specially bound copy of Jack's All Friends Are Strangers
Jack's copy M R James ghost stories
1 white moiré silk skirt mine
1 white towel Woolworth's
2 to 4 glasses, tall and smaller
Those gone btw June 23rd painting job and now

Aug 5 —not had first Saigon cable Dec 15 1955 —2nd cable Mch 15th, 1956. Mailed a letter to Paula and to Jigg today in 84=3rd St PO. Paula's first letter May 2nd, 1956 none Jigg arrived yet.

August 6, 1957: all still missing loud complaints in kitchen to several.

August 7, 1957: medicines still missing loud complaints in kitchen to several.

August 8, 1957: I had looked in vain yesterday before I went out found black liquid medicine intact in front of drawer unmistakable the new bottle in characteristic jay wrapper, exactly where it wasn't when I took everything out of same drawer on both Monday and Tuesday and again Wednesday. This is incontrovertibly so —It was found at front of bottom drawer, and already I had taken out all the content twice and looked a third time. A white bowl was broken this am by me —the bowl listed was not broken but vanished from room. Money value was trivial.. Letter to postmaster answered, Aug 7, 1957. He says my family were at 46 Hempstead. This confusion occurred before Paula left but I went on writing to 46 Hampstead.

August 9, 1957: letter to Mrs Mary M Baird mentioning held mail writing to ask Postmaster at Spring Valley, Edward P Humbert, name and address of man who brought Paul's held mail to PO —held for almost two years, all had return addresses. Where are any letters without these addresses? End of summer school. Left address for check due on 15th. Am to attend conference on Mon 16th Sept. Then no actual classes till Thur 19th.

August 11, 1957: letter to Dr Vincent asking him whether he would mind writing to Margué to ask whether she got any 1955 letters back 4th letter each to Jigg to Paula asking if they have my 3 earlier letters about mail and asking for name of man who held it in Spring Valley if they know who.

August 12, 1957: Paula's letter first for about 7 or 8 wks her
July 1st to Jigg, to her
July 6 to Julia, to her
June 29 —to both
June 29 —to Julia

June 9 —to both
June 23 —to both
July 21st—to Paula
July 29 —to Paula
July 29 to Jigg
July 30 to Jigg
man who kept mail named Mirabile.

To Evelyn Scott
Department of State
Washington

August 13, 1957

Dear Mrs Metcalfe:

Your letter of July 30, 1957 addressed to Miss Knight and marked for her personal attention has been referred to me for reply.

In the application upon which a passport was issued to your son, Creighton Seeley Scott, on July 19, 1955 he gave as his permanent address in the United States, 46 Hempstead Road, Spring Valley, New York and stated that his wife was residing at that address. This office has no more recent information concerning your son and therefore is not in a position to inform you whether he still considers this address to be his permanent address in the United States.

Sincerely,

Willis H Young

Deputy Director, Passport Office

[Typed on official letterhead, signed. UTK]

To Willis Young

The Benjamin Franklin Hotel
August 14, 1957

Mr Willis H Young
Deputy Director, Passport Office
Department of State, Washington, 25, DC

Dear Mr Young:

Thank you for your letter of July 30th, 1957. I would, of course, have first asked my son's opinion of the incident of mail held in Spring Valley from 1955 to 1957,[264] as per my letter of July 30th, 1957, but I must remind you that I have not had any letter written and signed by my son, Mr Creighton Seeley Scott since Dec 53, when myself and my husband were Fellows at The Huntington Hartford Foundation, California,

---

264 None of these letters has survived. Jigg and the family arrived in Spring Valley in July 1953 and left for Vietnam in October of 1955.

and I had just fallen very ill. When my husband and I passed through New York on returning from our eight and a half years in England, I did not have the addresses of my son and my daughter-in-law; and my letters to them announcing our arrival had been returned to us in London, by Free Europe, and on the day before we sailed were received by us there.

On July 20th, 1957, I wrote of the mail retained in Spring Valley to the Personnel Officer, ICA Washington. I have had no acknowledgement of my letter. And meanwhile having examined my own personal files very carefully guarded here, I have found there has been taken from them the letters my daughter-in-law wrote me from Spring Valley just before she left there to join her husband in which she enclosed a clipping of an account of a "probe" of some sort - of this more on the back of this page - and said I had been libelled to them as a person who could be summoned to testify about "subversive" activities, and as this was brought up with her husband already 15,000 miles away she was seriously distressed. *She was about to travel with 5 children, these my grandchildren, none seen since 1944.*

What all this adds up to I do not know, nor does my husband with his eleven-and-a-half years of RAF experience. I have written to the Postmaster at Spring Valley, who says that an "attorney" brought him a large cardboard carton of mail for my daughter-in-law, of which my four letters were a part.[265] He did not give me this man's name and this factor, in conjunction with her distress about me and libels, and finally, the disappearance of her letter and the clipping from my files here, I take as a sign of bad faith on the part of someone, and that someone is certainly not Mrs Creighton Seely Scott.

I therefore do not think that it is the business of the FBI to set the mail problem to rights and make contact with all the members of the family and ourselves. On the very day my mother, the late Maude Thomas Dunn of Clarksville, Tennessee, died and I received a telegram to that effect, a Government "investigator" called on me, and though I announced when she arrived that I was on that day bereaved, she asked me questions about Labour, Liberals, etc from 4 pm to 8 pm. I am not among those who think people should not tell anything they know to the point, but I do not think problems of Defence should be left to that body.

[Typed carbon copy, possibly incomplete (2 pp only), not signed. UTK]

From John Metcalfe's diary:

August 14, 1957: Moderately cool. E + I went to post office + Garden Supermarket etc. *registered letter to Mr H C Nixon—Mr Corbo letter telling why I would like his press-described general experiences literature Jack's house theft in Canada*

---

265 This correspondence has not survived.

of my mss letter to Miss Howell her advice asked about sending mss to Mr Nixon first to go to Robison after or what? Did Mr Nixon want to read it before money guarantees-or what? letter from Mr Young record 46 Hempstead Rd.

August 15, 1957: registered letter Aug 16th Mr Henghler registered to Mr Willis H Young Deputy Director stat Dept Passport Officer Washington 25, DC tell in sum of many interferences with mail since 1940, and mentioning my complaint of that year about janitor to DJ that spate of investigors the several Evelyn Scotts and the one reputed to write but never seen add what Mr Humbert wrote. ~~Deposited check of $309.52 in bank, teller Mr Wise (?)~~

August 17, 1957: letter to Mr Humbert asking whether scribble on parcel name and when Paula dated removal notice letter from Assistant Postmaster Jamaica LI received.

To Creighton Scott

The Benjamin Franklin Hotel
August 18, 1957

Darling Son Jigg,

Paula's sweet note about the continued good health of the family was very good for our health.[266] We hope sometimes my letters are reciprocal in effect, though I have just so much "cheer" to dispense until we have direct contact with you as well as darling Paula, and have some positive hope of seeing all of you once more in the flesh.

I wont go on repeating about the mail except as something further may come up. We tried both the Long Island Postmaster and the more explicit Spring Valley Postmaster about the mail retained for nineteen months - some may have been yours as well as Paulas - and no one has yet been willing to write us the name of the man who held it for a time actually illegal, unless Paula had specified he was to keep it for that time, which I think she never did. I consider the withholding of his name the opposite of good faith. Paula was very very upset just before she left on her long journey with the five children, and her letters received by us - all notes but one - showed she was upset and to some extent why. Who took advantage of her to pour libels about us into her ear? Any woman under such conditions would be harried.

I am persistent in trying to get the full and correct explanation because Paula as good as said not to put Evelyn Scott on my letters because of libels of me.

---

266 This note has not survived.

As we are NOT "under a cloud" and have more to say for ourselves as victims of post-war conditions than in any other way, I began then AT ONCE ADDRESSING MY LETTERS on the BACKS TO EVELYN SCOTT, as my name is both yours in part in every legal sense and EVELYN SCOTT is the name I have always signed book contracts and copyrights with during twenty-five years as a published author. My copyrights remember are Jack's yours and hers for the minor children, in that order with yours and Jack's first.

But the return addresses were clear all along, Evelyn Scott on the letters and Mr and Mrs John Metcalfe and Mrs W J Metcalfe on the parcels. It is fine Paula is now dating her letters. I gather Mirabelle to be the name of the man who kept her mail but the Post Office hasnt yet admitted it. I wish to find out what because of letters sent without returns on back. This business of threatening people about their jobs is what I suspect. I think it can be proved criminal.

[Handwritten, not signed. UTK]

From John Metcalfe's diary:

August 25, 1957: wrote to Assistant Postmaster Jamaica, for mailing tomorrow, pointing out that Spring Valley ignored my inquiry about parcels and called name of man who held my mail for family 19 mos, "confidential"-liar misuse of Post Office charge to bring.

September 3, 1957: Letter to Miss Knight giving Paula's California address and complaining as to permanent address here essential also calling that Spring Valley rat morally a criminal was mailed registered about 4.30 pm—a man named Jabowitz at registry window when we came home I saw merely Passport Office on receipt writing Mr Young air mail as letter may have been imperfectly addressed --[illeg]. Letter to Young mailed about 5.30 air mail.

September 4, 1957: E cleaned frigidaire six pg letter and extra ps to Mrs Mary R Baird to mail tomorrow.

September 7, 1957: Summer holiday

In September 1957, after Jigg had completed a two-year contract, Paula and the children returned to the United States on the "home leave" afforded to families of those contracted to overseas postings. As they had no base in the US, Paula had no choice but to call, again, on relatives on her mother's side; it was arranged the family would stay with two maiden aunts in Carmel, California, where they remained until returning to Saigon that November.

To Paula Scott

The Benjamin Franklin Hotel
September 8, 1957

Darling darling Paula,

Seven letters last week, two and the book parcel the week before, and now three two addressed to you for Jigg for you to read and one for the three eldest children addressed to Denise in your care.

All this matters only because we so need to know yourselves that you are all SAFELY AGAIN IN THE USA, and that you and blessed Jigg and every one of you are well well WELL, and Jigg soon to be within real reach with job secure.

Everything that matters in other ways matters as much as ever, but we need to sense the presence on homely terra firma of the finest daughter-in-law anyone ever had - one daughter-in-law who is always considered by Jack and me and Jiggs Dad exactly the wife for the finest of sons.

Here is admiration with love - but dont forget knowing you are all safe will relieve a good day of maybe superfluous anxiety. Bless, bless, bless,

[Typed carbon copy, not signed. UTK]

From John Metcalfe's diary:

September 8, 1957: today have written Dr Vincent[267] Paula's and the five children's address Rout 2, Box 70, Carmel, California. Told him Creighton is in India pro tem. Why the hell break up housekeeping in Saigon and send her and five children 15,000 miles where neither has any personal friend? It is called a "vacation" for each! —sic! I call if Fascist, Nazi, Communist cruelty and think the President himself should be ashamed. They have no money for New York

Creighton seen once since 1966 for 5 days Paula and the children not since when 3 were

September 9, 1957 [continued from previous page] mailing letter to Employee Relations Officer letters to Jigg care Paula
"Paula herself
" Denise her care
" Fredrick her care
" Mathew her care
did not have "hold for arrival on them".

---

267 The director of the Huntington Hertford Foundation, where Jack and Evelyn spent 10 months on their return to the United States, bore this name. It appears he and Jack were still correspondng at this time, but no letters remain.

September 11, 1957: Pavla Scott her birthday born Ranchos de Taos, New Mexico, USA, called Pavli by all when child.
September 16, 1957: Paula's postcard Carmel signed P. . mailed air mail welcome to Paula and the children. Mailed letter to Mr W H Young Deputy Director Passport Office asking whether Dept of State would file birth certificate they did not want in London.

To Evelyn Scott
Department of State
Washington

September 17, 1957

letter Sept 21st, 1957 points out file ref here error as Dunn not included

Dear Mrs Metcalfe:

After a review of your letter of September 5, 1957 and your previous correspondence addressed to this Department, it is apparent that the problem confronting you, namely your difficulty in receiving your mail, is one properly within the province of the Post Office Department rather than the Department of State which is concerned mainly with the foreign affairs of our country.

It is suggested that you communicate with the Postmaster General, Post Office Department, Washington, DC and present your problem. We feel sure that they can be of service to you in this matter.

Sincerely,
Robert D Johnson
Chief, Legal Division

[Typed on official letterhead, signed. Handwritten annotation. UTK]

From John Metcalfe's diary:

September 19, 1957: airmail letter to Dr Vince tell Paula arrived—with children downtown PO. Greenwich School for 9 o'clock faculty meeting. Lunch. Walked to station + caught 1.42. *[illeg]* home! Had nap. Drinks etc. Supper. Bed + v poor night. *airmailed five postcards care Paula Scott route 2, Box 70, Carmel Cal—my birth to Welker mailed downtown PO telling of writing to Mrs Baird and why setting forth again the facts of divorce mentioning our suppression began on my resignation from Authors' League earlier refusal to join Writers League. Card to May. This day a letter from a man named Johnson he made a false record by leaving out my birth* [illeg]

September 20, 1957: Greenwich School, - but no classes, + just hung around till 3. Took a boy (Perlman) with me as far as Laundromat. Soon after I got 'home' Bernice arrived. Reading + drinks, but E felt sick so I went out and bought roast-beef sandwiches at Rudley's + brought them back for our consumption. Bed. Got transportation check today from Mr *[illeg]*.

September 23, 1957: Letter to Mr Robert Johnson have sent 6 cards 5 letters to children Carmel, route 2 Box 70, and several each to Paula and to Jigg in her care.

September 27, 1957: Mrs Mary R Baird sent 2nd letter requesting acknowledgement of letter about 1st Marriage and divorce NB she replied yes *[illeg]*.

September 29, 1957: letter of mine to her of August 9th returned in carbon by him General Post Office 7th and 31st US Post Office Inspectors useless I think. Oliver Gasch is US Attorney for District of Columbia. Herbert Brownell—democrat?--former Wall St lawyer—attorney for Washington city all this Wall St bunch became frigid Bernays insulting.

October 1, 1957: Darling Jigg, I hope you and Paula can reach Jack and myself. May lunch 1.15. Cleaned the ice-box a thoroughly nasty morning. Received Vincent letter without any mention of Margué and mail. I had his letter about a month ago saying he would write Margué. He suggests some writer I might know at Carmel—I would never have asked him anything had not an apparently official sanctioning of a criminal racket produced isolation of every member of families in respect to one another. No room for my diary. Thumb painful.

October 2, 1957: Greenwich School. Thumb painful. No conference. letter to Dr Vincent about Hartford

To Evelyn Scott and John Metcalfe

Carmel, California
October 3, 1957

Dear Evelyn and Jack -

I'm sorry it's been so long since I've written - we've been so busy with the beautiful sea, the beautiful hills, and marsh and lovely fresh sunny weather etc, etc, that I have simply let day after day slide by. I'll answer your accumulation by mail in my next - for now we're all fine and enjoying our vacation. There is so much to do here that all the kids and I are always busy. Only the girls are going to school - Denise in 11th grade and Julia in first grade (they both love it) - the boys are excused. They have to catch up in Saigon, but now they are revelling in their freedom and making the most of it.

This is all now - love to you both,

Paula

I'll make a point of writing again, soon. Don't worry - we are just happy and busy.

[Handwritten, signed. UTK]

To Jean Hermann

The Benjamin Franklin Hotel

October 6,1957

Dear Miss Hermann,

Are the contacts of ICA, USOM employees with their parents a matter of entire indifference to the ICA?

My daughter-in-law and the children are now, I <u>suppose</u>, at route 2, Box 70, Carmel, California, but bar one postcard saying they had arrived in Carmel early in September, I have been able to obtain no news or replies to letters. As for the very serious - both serious - matter of having no address for my son at present, it seems to me <u>atrocious</u> that nothing has yet been done to relieve this situation. I do not know his location today.

I wrote you in July that the return to me of mail held nineteen-months in Spring Valley, where it was sent after my daughter-in-law wrote me from Saigon that the 46 Hempstead Rd. Spring Valley, NY, address, left on file when they left (because the movements of their American families were uncertain and some older addresses had proved unreliable, too) was discarded by them; thus leaving them only route 2, Box 70, Carmel, California, as an American address, and it <u>temporary</u>.

Now, having written to Carmel, I begin to see intimations of a repeated pattern of mail unanswered or answers undelivered such as I referred to as having pursued ourselves and them since 1944, when I went to England and American and returned and American 1952 after eight-and-a-half years, spent there with my British husband for reasons you know, of which I wrote to Miss Roth long ago. *NB American I am and always will be*

Are the families who appeal to you to be ignored? Strains and anxieties that could be avoided are still ours, year after year. Remember I have had no letter written and signed by my very fine son since December 1953, when my husband and I were just returned from England and were at The Huntington Hartford Foundation (for artists of all the fine arts) *in California.*

Spring Valley Post Office ignored my query about the insured parcels returned to me unopened, without any stamping except when sent in 1955. That was the last week in July. Now we wish to send birthday gifts of books to my eldest grandson and my son and find ourselves in 1955's predicament; not knowing for certain whether Paula Scott and the children are still in Carmel, or how long they will be there.

This is irony, you will admit. But I should add that there must be an ingredient of positive sadism in such misdirecting of things that contribute to sane, normal, good, human relations. The Post Master not knowing I had written to Mrs Scott and received her answer, said the name of the man who held my mail to her and other mail for nineteen months, was "confidential".

I think I am being very reasonable in asking you to look into the matter of unimpeded correspondence with my son and his family. The apparent circumstances, on each occasion, are almost of a sort to intimidate. It might justly be called a crime to leave it so. *Health strains, economic strains often result-- all unnecessary!*

Very Truly
Mrs (John) Evelyn D S Metcalfe
Evelyn D S Metcalfe
Signed twice because the writer unwittingly used poor ink the first time. Blots are regrettable but conditions for writing today are very poor

[The above letter was sent to Jigg from the USOM head office in Saigon with the following typed note:]

10/8/57 The enclosed letter was received today, and while I promise not to bother you with this again, you may be interested. Incidentally, all the other letters were destroyed yesterday.

Jean Hermann[268]

[Typed, signed. Handwritten insertions and annotation. UTK]

From John Metcalfe's diary:

October 6, 1957: John Metcalfe's birthday born Heacham, Norfolk. Letter to Miss Herman asking about Jigg saying letter of July 22—or 27—still to be acknowledged

October 8, 1957: parcel registered to Paula same day sent 4 letters to Paula, Denise, Freddy, Mathew, one to Jig addressed to her

October 12, 1957: Mrs Baird wait to see behaving stupidly or tampering with her mail—which maybe criminal there

To Creighton Scott
American Embassy,
Unites States Operations Mission to Vietnam
Saigon, Vietnam

October 14, 1957

Dear Mr Scott

---

268 Sadly, Jean Hermann was transferred to another position not long after this, and the only protection Jigg had from his mother's importunings was lost.

We have received a letter from your Mother dated September 28 and addressed to the American Consul, Saigon.

She has stated in the letter she has not heard from you for sometime and is concerned.

We pass this information on to you and feel you will probably be getting in touch with her very soon.

Happy Holiday,

Sincerely,

Gladys Schwendker

Acting Personnel Officer

[Typed on official letterhead, signed. UTK]

From John Metcalfe's diary:

October 16, 1957: Mrs Baird nice letter saying she is looking over the problem. Had just written her—Mrs B hadn't answered—it is like a "custom"

October 25, 1957: Creighton Seely Scott's birthday Creighton Scott, author C S Scott Painter or Creighton Scott

To Jean Hermann

The Benjamin Franklin Hotel

October 26, 1957

Dear Madam

This is my fourth attempt, since July, 1957, to obtain information as to where now to address my son, Mr Creighton Seely Scott, who has been with the USOM in Saigon for the last two years.

In July, my daughter-in-law, Paula Scott, wrote me that he was temporarily assigned elsewhere and that she was coming to Carmel, California, for some weeks, and would return in Saigon in all probability.

It may be that the ICA thinks this is enough for me to know, but, if so, it must be because my various letters concerning my difficulties in preserving contact with my son and his family since the beginning of the war, have not been read.

My daughter-in-law did arrive in Carmel in September, when I received a postcard from her. And I have a pencilled note from her mailed about three weeks ago,.

We are convinced that she is not encouraged to be explicit or write oftener. Had their surroundings been conducive to us, she would have done so, we feel certain. We are very sure this must be the fact as to my son, who last wrote to us a letter we received in December 1953, when we were in California, and I was seriously ill.

We are not a divided family. My son's father, from whom I am divorced, is our friend and the friend of Creighton, is eighty years old, and has not seen him for years.

When I write various relatives of my son and of my daughter-in-law, my letters are never acknowledged.

I have repeatedly requested some attention to this cruel, infamously unjust situation. I now do not know whether my letters to you are received, or whether, they are turned over to someone who is actually hostile to us, good native Americans though I and the Scotts are, and good and honourable Britisher though is my husband, Squadron Leader WJ Metcalfe, RAF retired, 1914 commission.

Human imagination toward specifiable individual people is all I ask for. A friend in Washington has kindly agreed to mail this for me in your city in the hope that you will be the more certain to receive it. I will send it to her unsealed and stamped, but she is not responsible for the content, and, also, is just using her human imagination in respect to anxieties unduly prolonged.

Very Truly Yours
Evelyn D S Metcalfe

[Typed carbon copy, signed. UTK]

The family returned to Saigon after a stay of three months with Paula's relatives in Carmel. Jigg had made a number of Vietnamese friends as well as friends from the American and British expat communities, and the family's life resumed a sort of normality.

From John Metcalfe's diary:

November 4, 1957: E cleaned Ice Box. Letter from Paula, acknowledging receipt of books.

November 6, 1957: *Parcel of Nursery tales mailed to Paula for Robert at Carmel c/o Martinez-Dean otherwise same address. Greenwich School, Dr Hill, so no conference. I think any library with a Board that makes rules that inflexible especially when the author used to be on many of these damn library shelves and beside is known to be honest in all dealings with them is bound for those Monkey rocks.*

November 7, 1957: Greenwich School. Dr Wearn. Thumb much better. *went to library for fresh card for myself as author Evelyn Scott Jack's requested but they said he said he must sign for it there in person teaching every day till late made "no difference." As cards had been taken from room I left a note reporting his stolen—signed Mrs Metcalfe Evelyn Scott. Imagine a library as niggling and offensive to the distinguished British author John Metcalfe is and some know it. The human situation was enough—he had a card there signature filed.*

November 9, 1957: Letter to E from Paula
November 10. 1957: letter to Paula Carmel c/o Martinez-Dean
here on containing letter to Jigg

To Paula Scott

The Benjamin Franklin Hotel
November 10, 1957

The children will all profit by solidarity
for culture even with Jack's English family
connection in pure science. Love from Jack
Darling Paula when you read this, you can
still only do your best as circumstances permit.
But you can think it over again, and pass it on
to Jigg. We especially hope he can re-contact
Fredrick Wellman for their father's sake

We have your letter of Nov 7th, and, as always, appreciate clarifications. May your re-uniting with Jigg in Saigon be no longer delayed. Perhaps you have already left, and in that case, we will also appreciate the promised advice as to when, and where to write when you get there. This forwarded safely if you have.

The two very satisfying points explained are why Carmel, and the amplified view of the boys. You apparently do not acknowledge postcards. No mention was ever made of various cards in envelopes addressed to the children in your care when in Saigon, and I should like to know whether these trifles are worth sending at all - sometimes rather cute. Very glad you continue to contact Margue.

May I, on my part, clarify a few things on which, it appears, we dont see quite alike.

I think it is a criminal factor in all our lives that Jigg has no contact with his father or any of his Wellman half-brothers. I thinks complaints as to this and as to the fact that, for reasons we can only guess, we never have any letter written by him, or any intimation that we are ever to see him, are well justified. I am completely certain in myself and so is Jack that Jigg cannot wish it to be as it is with no response, as yet, in Washington to the need of any man for his own family contacts where they are loyal and loving. To prolong all our lives, his, yours, in we think we ourselves should know where Jigg is.

I dont discuss Jigg often, but a first hocus-pocus of pseudo "psycho-analysis" has been several times produced by white-washers of abuses of justice in our own country, to pretend to "explain" the frequent helplessness of every old American and old Britisher - old in preference for the type of rule - as, in the instance of Jigg, a "wilful desertion" of his parents. We know this cannot be true

It is very very upsetting. This hotel is full of Germans, mostly Jews, with Irish, Swedes, etc, thrown in. Sometimes, with intervals of months or a year between, I have explained bouts of poor health and low spirits by saying we never see my son and dont hear enough. The hand of an enemy is at once evident, though I have never said anything specific about any of you, except once, in an overwhelming by sentiment, show a few Bobby's cute picture kissing the peacock. "My grandson" with pride NB We do hope the outdoors is restoring peace in nature. We are sure Denise and Julia will leave good records in school, when "voters' noses" are counted less often and pedagogic theorizing is dropped and replaced by real teaching there will be a good system

We both think the American Government should show enough good faith to reply to some of the letters of Creighton Secley Scotts mother and his father and stepfather by conceding we, too, have a right to some contact with Jigg himself. I have written several times asking when Jigg can be seen You should realize, and Jigg does I hope, that Jack and I have now spent four years at home, added to eight-and-a-half in London, protesting our human claim on some attention, as well as our right to careers that were demolished deliberately, and include Cyrils and Jiggs as author-painters and your own. It is vile and really treacherous reaction that pretends that people of "our age" have no right to anything except penury and "relief" if we can get it. We and your family should be speaking for one another, with *[remainder of letter missing]*

[Typed, handwritten insertions. UTK]

From John Metcalfe's diary:

November 10, 1957: letter to Paula Carmel c/o Martinez-Dean here on containing letter to Jigg.

November 11, 1957: Fredrick Wheeler Scott's birthday born NYC. Fredrick Wheeler Scott will be 15 years old letter to Paula Carmel letter to Fredrick care her Carmel Letter Jack Match.

November 15, 1957: Robert Scott's birthday Robert Scott will be five. Bless him! Bless Jack, for blessing Bobby. M Sheffield took occasion to break off all relations with me to state in a letter dated November 13th refusing to comment on my defence of Jigg, whom she had helped.

To Evelyn Scott

Honolulu

28 November 1957

Dear E - Bobby's book came in time - we're on our way back. Sorry I had no time for a letter before going but was awfully busy. I'll write from Saigon. Jigg will be there waiting for us.

Love,

Paula

[Handwritten postcard, signed. UTK]

From John Metcalfe's diary

November 30, 1957: Paula's card saying she was leaving with the children for Saigon card mail stamp November 28th on PAA airship

December 2, 1957: E cleaned ice-box a filthy day as to work impossible most of day and after a filthy night from about 2.30 on ferme la porte. [269]

December 25, 1957: Quiet day at hotel. Our colds still bad.

---

269 "One closes the door".

Chapter 38

1958

Evelyn and Jack were experiencing another year of desperate poverty in the Benjamin Franklin Hotel. Jack had secured poorly paid employment as a tutor in a small private "crammer" while Evelyn's time was largely occupied with her correspondence. During this year Evelyn, by her own account, wrote weekly letters to Paula, often including another to be forwarded to Jigg: a few examples are included below. The themes were always the same: Evelyn's distress at not hearing from her family; her certainty that malign political forces were both intercepting her letters and preventing her son from writing to her; her conviction that the same malign forces were keeping the family apart; the effect this was having on her (admittedly) poor health; and requests for suggestions for the children's various birthday presents which she hoped would prompt letters from Paula. She also wrote to the children (these letters were not passed on) asking them to request either of their parents to write to her.

Only eight letters written in 1958 have survived, two of them letters to her grandsons. Again, it is unlikely that her letter writing was curtailed; it is far more likely that they were destroyed by the addressee. Those that have remained are increasingly frenzied, with lengthy handwritten insertions, upper-case typing and underlined passages.

And Jack's diary entries chronicle her deteriorating health.

From John Metcalfe's diary:

January 3, 1958: Bought tobacco + I did some marketing, E did more shopping, separately – + we were both back in our room by about 10. I typed another page (p 100) to "Ten Pretty People" while E did ice-box.

January 5, 1958: Putrid Mary R Baird letter, leaving everything as before about record of Elsie Dunn as myself. True I can be identified but I am 64, all my relatives and friends grow older, many have died since my father's death in 1947. I told her we were 8 years abroad under pressure about my citizenry, and that I have an only son, Creighton S Scott, a daughter-in-law and five grandchildren to benefit if I do so some years in USA Eisenhower defense.

February 7, 1958: *washed ice-box. 1940 Jigg's gift of "The Muscovites" of inscribed affectionately to his mother Evelyn Scott has been stolen out of my trunk hope for restoration no merely. Churchill never took action in any of these matters. May took me to lunch. Restored.*

To Paula Scott

The Benjamin Franklin Hotel

March 23, 1958

Darling Paula

My letter of last week was entirely about the distressingness to us of compelling Jigg to go on with no imaginative life in literature, when not alone is he an appreciative and discriminating reader, but a very fine artist himself in two of the arts. That he was in such circumstances he couldnt[270] read his stepfathers most recent novel and write to him naturally a few lines, came as a very awful shock. We continue indignant at the powers who allow such conditions to arise. Our dearest wish is to assist the restoration of Creighton and you and Creightons Dad to normal contacts and careers. We completely realise jobs come first to the father of five children and his darling wife, but as vile and base as has been Jacks suppression here as a novelist, it has never been so vile that he could not read good books when they came his way, or write to the donors or authors if he had a mind to.

Darling, you must have thought me all but indifferent to other things that affect us all, and that of course have affected you all there - but I am not nor is Jack. We are much concerned about the water supply, and I had it in mind when I mailed the first letter - or rather that referred to above - and had proposed to write a note about it before the end of the week. However, we were swamped in "weather" here. It rained, hailed and snowed. Jack went to bed, again, with a cold; and as it kept him from school when a test was due a student, I went to the post office in a snowstorm, and by the next day, had the cold, too.

The climate distresses us, too. We dont want to have tropical "acclimating" become pronounced in our darling family of a temperate climate. That was on my mind when darling Jigg had to sign up for a further two years. It is all so wrong, and we should not be helpless, nor should you.

When the snapshots come, we shall feel so cosy having you all around us, again, just as you are now. The only really good good moments in our lives come when we invoke each other and yourselves and Dad, and create for ourselves the blessed illusion

---

270 *My Cousin Geoffrey*, published in 1956, turned out to be Jack's last published work.

of your physical nearness, even as we know you are all, including Dad, near us in spirit all the time.

Are the buildings the children do lessons in, near? Can they go by themselves, or do you have to take them? What will Bobby like for next November?

Your loving and grateful mother-in-law, who, darling Paula, does love you, Jigg, and the darling, darling children - *and how!*

Evelyn

[Typed, signed. Handwritten insertion. UTK]

To Paula Scott

The Benjamin Franklin Hotel,
March 30, 1958

Darling Paula

I think we shall soon be obliged to write to Washington, again, unless it has already become possible for Creighton to read enough outside his work to write Jack about MY COUSIN GEOFFREY and, also, to write to his parents. The more I think of the four years since any of Jig's family have had a line, the more deeply indignant I become at the sort of monstrous conditions imposed on a US citizen, who is himself an author and painter of the first water. *The hotel had a nice new entrance in harmony with its architecture--now replaced by imitation "marble"* [illeg] *called it "public house" "marble" by Jack--the concealed new lighting giving an effect of sunlight in the dark end of the lobby is good, however*

Darling Paula, what a different view of Broadway would be the one we have if everything in our normal lives were restored to normal, beginning now with snapshots with letter by JIGG, Your own letters give our lives some zest, but JACK SHARES ALL HE HAS HE SHARES IN SPIRIT WITH YOU BOTH AND WITH CYRIL. He should not be ever regarded as an "outsider", and you have done all you could but I know Jigg himself must feel as I do, too.

When I say so many things about Jack, I dont give him my letter to read lest he become embarrassed. It would be unthinkable to have it supposed I "forced" him on yourselves - please tell me how to help Jigg to expand to us and override conditions that make him seem less read than we know he is to be AS OF OLD.

If they dont want people who have relatives with these opinions, then somebody had better ask them there to state PUBLICLY WHY NOT. We are pretty well fed up with all the world gets help except the OLD FREE NATIVES OF BOTH COUNTRIES who are and always have been opposed to labour rule either here or in the British Isles.

Evasion in these matters is in its final phase. We cannot be governed by other countries with ideas and laws not ours, and WE WONT BE ANY LONGER. There is a farcical aspect to everything that has been going on in recent years. United Nations should have been a "clearing house" for objection to international interference, or national interference now announced by a declaration of war, and all we have is patter about entirely minor matters, while a good many of the best and finest Americans and British STILL are contending at home and abroad against some of the worst aspects of dictations NONE OF US WILL EVER ACCEPT AS AFFECTING OURSELVES. We just cant stand evasion and equivocation any more. We are all culturally persecuted, there are no two ways about that.

I suppose, in the weather you depicted, their clothing is still sketchy. I asked about the type of building description as well as name for they do lessons in. We are already thinking of Jiggs next birthday, too. What would he like. What a pity I have a hard time obtaining science books for Freddy. When Jack is free in the summer maybe we can go downtown to have a look about for them, and for whatever Mathew would like for January 1923 [sic] I dont go distances alone after all the "peruna" ailments I have had. Better in the main, however.

Jack read to us a delightfully funny chapter in his new book - humour you both like, reminds me of Jiggs humour. As I have just written him, his description of the clerks in the importers in his own novel reminded me of the hotels "guests". We are still swamped by too much remodelling of the floor above - labour here, already almost a month, gives me a headache, rarely had one before. Do you like daffodils? Bernice brought us daffodils and irises. I never look at a new spring dress without thoughts of Denise and Julia, or suits without thinking of the boys though [remainder of letter missing]

[Typed, not signed. Handwritten insertions. UTK]

From John Metcalfe's diary:

April 30, 1958: E heard from Ronald Pearson that his father, Ralph Pearson, had died.

May 5, 1958: Evelyn got bound typescript of Welker's book on her.

June 7, 1958: Mr Robert Welker came to supper - our first meeting with him.

July 15, 1958: E had been too ill to Market etc. I did Marketing and laundry.

July 16, 1958: E poorly so I stayed away from school.

July 25, 1958: E still unable to go to bank so will get hotel to cash cheque tomorrow.

July 26, 1958: E had very bad night.

July 29, 1958: E and I went to Dr Zuckermann when I got home.

August 1 1958: E bad so did not go to school.

August 2, 1958: Dr Wearn called to see Evelyn at about 1, - but did no good beyond a prescription for pheno-barbitol.[271]

August 25, 1958: Still no letter from Paula, - as from Dr H.

September 2, 1958: Much cooler. E got letter from Paula at last.

---

271 Phenobarbital is an anticonvulsant, now used for the treatment of epilepsy and for the relief of anxiety.

To Paula Scott

Hotel Benjamin Franklin
November 15, 1958

DARLING PAULA,

So you now have a SIXTEEN YEAR OLD SON and a big boy who is good and studious and is SIX YEARS OLD, as well as a nearly EIGHTEEN-YEAR-OLD DAUGHTER, a nearly THIRTEEN YEAR OLD SON, and a DAUGHTER OF SEVEN WHO PAINTS PICTURES. WE ALL GOOD - YOU BET![272]

I am worrying about the return of damnable summer. You should all be here at home to be REFRESHED BY CHANGED SEASONS AND PROBABLY <u>ESPECIALLY JIGG WHO HAS NOT BEEN HOME AWAY FROM HEAT SINCE YOU WENT OUT THERE, and WAS NOT IN GOOD HEALTH WHEN HE WENT THERE.</u>

Today is Bobbys birthday by the Calendar, and I so hope he had a nice little celebration, and that Freddy had a good one on the eleventh. But I am worrying most about JIGGS HEALTH as the SNAPSHOTS WERE TO BE PROOF OF HIS IMPROVEMENT AND THEY HAVE NOT YET COME.

Your own letter is overdue, too, darling, and I hope it will arrive soon and shatter this ritual of worry - a round-and-round sort of lousiness.

DID I WRITE YOU THAT I READ OF THE APPOINTMENT OF SOME NY GENTLEMAN TO THE NY LIBRARYS "Petroleum Board"? - now isnt that enough to explain why many of our best authors, painters, and composers nearly starve? IT IS.

I would like to know how many other "boards" of this sort take all the citizen money out of LITERATURE, HISTORY, CRITICISM, and put it into technical specialities more connected with a business of making money than with the raison detre of LIBRARY FOUNDATIONS.

I, again, think <u>Babbit</u> is nearly a very great book. The Babbits of America WE WHO ARE AMERICANS, BRITISH, FRENCH INDIVIDUALLY FREE have been sacrificed as well as to enemies.

[Typed carbon copy, not signed. UTK]

From John Metcalfe's diary:

December 25, 1958: Christmas. Liver for supper.

---

272 These are references (in that order) to Frederick, Robert, Denise, Matthew, and Julia.

Chapter 39

1959

Eighty letters written during 1959 have survived, although it is likely that, as in previous years, many more were written. Those that remain demonstrate that Evelyn, living a constrained existence in their small hotel room and with little else to occupy her mind, is becoming more and more fixated on the libel she is convinced she has suffered (see Chapter 31). Many of these letters have survived, all expressing similar views; to avoid repetition only a selection of them is included here.

Many of these letters are specifically directed to Jigg's then employers, the United States State Department, in what became hugely destructive attempts to get him to write to her and to generally conform to her ideas of what their relationship should be. In the absence of personal contact, Evelyn's only means of expression was through her typewriter, and the use of capital letters and underlining as well as handwritten annotations, often in red, convey the strength and desperation of her emotions. (Chapter 45 includes correspondence between Jigg and others who knew her describing the effect this epistolary pressure had on him, his welfare, and his family.)

It may be relevant at this point to refer to David Callard's unpublished essay, "Interpolations"[273] in which he reflects upon a number of issues in her life, including her mental health. He describes approaching a senior academic whose main interest was the application of psychology to literature and asking him to comment on a sample of letters covering about 30 years beginning in the 1920s. Strict professional ethics rules did not allow this academic to be named but he was willing to make a number of observations:

In the expert's opinion Evelyn's letters revealed a paranoid personality deviation. If this developed, a vicious circle would be created: the person concerned would be avoided, which would heighten Evelyn's paranoia, which would lead to more people being alienated, and so on. Letters from the 1950s showed a very high level of continuous complaint and "a diminishing interest in other people" which he felt exhibited "a progressively deteriorating paranoid

---

273 Callard wrote a biography of Evelyn, *Pretty Good for a Woman*, and much of his source material was subsequently deposited at the Harry Ransom Center, part of the library of the University of Texas at Austin, where this essay was found.

personality". He summed it up by noting "so far as I have seen from the letters you have shown me, her life is the tragic story of a talented person whose personality became progressively paranoid in such a way as to make her life a continual focus of anxiety and distress".

From John Metcalfe's diary:

January 9, 1959: <u>E did ice-box.</u>

January 17, 1959: <u>E's birthday.</u> Bless her!

January 29, 1959: E also heard from Paula, - who enclosed a picture by Julia.

January 30, 1959: Was given, today, my schedule for next week, - 3 pupils only per day. This would seem to indicate that, for the present anyhow, the school is doing what I asked, + keeping monthly payment under the $100 so as to leave me still eligible for SS437[274]

February 9, 1959: E cleaned top ice-box

February 10, 1959: E cleaned drawer ice-box

March 1, 1959: E cleaned ice-box.

March 18, 1959: E received receipt for rent paid yesterday when en route to shop—in pigeonhole with small parcel. On return from shopping could not find it. Pkg of cigs was taken from room yesterday.

March 30, 1959: letter to Ronald about news of Jigg and Paula.

April 8, 1959: mailed letter to Mr Chas R Soll 86 Main Street Nyack, asking for confirmation of Ronald Pearson's address.

April 13, 1959: Letter to Manly for Cyril return receipt requested. Letter to Ronald Pearson and to him [illeg]. E cleaned Frigidaire bar drawer for tomorrow.

April 14, 1959: E washed vegetable drawer frigidaire.

To Creighton Scott

The Benjamin Franklin Hotel

April 18, 1959

DARLING SON JIGG,

Here we are, again, still waiting to know HOW YOU AND PAULA AND THE CHILDREN ARE - BLESS YOU!

PAULAS NOTE OF MARCH 5th[275] IS STILL BEING TREASURED AND REREAD WITH THE HOPE THAT THE LONGER LETTER AND THE SNAPSHOTS THEN ALREADY DEVELOPED WILL SOON BE HERE, WITH NEWS OF HOW YOU ARE AND COMMENTS ON THE VARIOUS CONTENTS OF LETTERS NOT YET SPECIFICALLY ACKNOWLEDGED.

---

274 Social Security.
275 This letter has not survived.

If you come home, later, to a job, we will be very grateful if we are kept conversant with your moves - YOURS MIND YOU, AS WELL AS DARLING PAULAS AND THE CHILDRENS. THIS TIME YOU MUST BE PERMITTED TO RETURN HOME TOGETHER TO JOB.

DARLING, TO SENSE YOU SEVEN DRAWING NEARER GIVES US MORE SPIRIT AND STRENGTH FOR WINNING OUT!

Lovingly, LOVINGLY,
Mother

[Typed, typed signature. SFC]

From John Metcalfe's diary:

April 20, 1959: E has heard at last from Paula.

May 11, 1959: cleaned the Frigidaire.

June 2, 1959: Sent off parcel (Arabian Nights) for Julia.

To Creighton Scott

The Benjamin Franklin Hotel
June 7, 1959

DARLING SON JIGG,

JACK LOOKS FORWARD TO YOUR LETTER, LONG OR SHORT. IT WILL BE SO NICE TO FEEL OURSELVES IN NATURAL COMMUNICATION EVEN FOR THE SPACE OF A LETTER. AND WE WILL THINK OF THE END OF SO MUCH GHASTLY INTERFERENCE, WITH ALL OUR GOOD AFFECTIONATE LIFES - THE BEST OF ALL ENDS WHEN YOU AND PAULA BRING YOURSELVES AND THE CHILDREN HOME TO YOUR JOB HERE.

WE ARE RATHER WORRIED ABOUT THE INDEFINITE PROSPECTS. OUR DECISIONS CONTINUE CONTINGENT ON YOURS AND DADS ARE SURE TO BE AFFECTED BY THEM. AND YOUR FOUR YEARS THERE WILL SOON BE UP. PLEASE DARLING WRITE AND TELL US HOW YOU, PAULA, AND THE CHILDREN ARE IN HEALTH AND GIVE US SOME INKLING AS TO PLANS. YOU SHOULD NONE OF YOU STAY THERE. THIS SHOULD BE YOUR YEAR TO COME HOME TOGETHER. YOU CANT SEND DENISE HERE ALONE YOU SHOULD PUT HER IN COLLEGE. BLESS, BLESS, BLESS - WE LOVE YOU SO, and REALLY ADORE YOU ALL. PAULA IS VERY NEAR TO US IN OUTLOOK WE TRUST.

Mother

Jigg, well aware of his mother's obsessive writing of letters which were both excessively long and full of details which were not strictly accurate, had started sending a selection to Margaret DeSilver for safekeeping. This pencilled note was in the margin of the front page of the above letter:

Dear Margaret - Just a specimen from among many - I have some that are a lot worse, which I keep, just in case. Jigg

[Typed, signed. SFC. Pencilled note by Jigg in margin of front page]

To Paula Scott

The Benjamin Franklin Hotel
June 7, 1959

DARLING PAULA,

PLEASE DONT DONT SIGN UP FOR ANOTHER YEAR IN SAIGON, FOR GODS SAKE. WE WILL BE RE-EMBITTERED ABOUT EVERYTHING WRONG ALREADY DONE TO OUR FAMILIES IF THERE IS ANY SUCH MOVE AS THAT FORCED ON POOR JIGG - with ten years of separation already, the grandchildren never seen, and Dad and ourselves now pretty old, Dads health and mine poorish, and poor good Jack holding all his own plans in abeyance in the hope of AT LAST SEEING OUR SCOTTS USA.

I feel alternately frantic and almost warlike against such friends who have devised such practises and have kept them up. SEVENTEEN YEARS OF HELL - indeed I long for vengeance on those who disregard, and putridly interfere, with FAMILY CONSTRUCTIVENESS IN THE NATURAL CONTEXTS OF LOVE FOR THE MEMBERS OF THE FAMILY *there and here*AT HOME. WE DO NOT KNOW OF ANY OTHER FAMILY EITHER AMERICAN OR BRITISH THAT HAS EVER BEEN PUT THROUGH WHAT WE HAVE IN SEPARATIONS THAT ARE AGAINST OUR INCLINATIONS, OBSTRUCTIVE OF MUTUAL HELP.

DARLING, THIS IS NOT A HATE LETTER, BUT A LOVE LOVE LETTER. We just cannot endure these false situations and false judgements any more.

WE SHALL CONSIDER IT THE SIGN OF GENUINE PATRIOTISM IN THOSE WHO ARRANGE PROGRAMS IF YOU AND JIGG AND THE CHILDREN ARE ALLOWED HOME NOW TO JOB FOR HIM AND NORMAL HUMAN CONTACTS.

TELL US WHAT WE CAN DO TO HELP JIGG HOME TO JOB. WE ARE ALL BITTERLY OPPOSED TO TOTAL SYSTEMS OF RULE AND THOSE WHO ARE MERIT EVERY PREFERENTIAL TREATMENT. THEY ARE NEEDED HERE AT HOME AS GOOD AMERICAN NATIVES.

IS THERE ANY REASON HOLDING BACK DECISION? IS IT JOBS AND HOUSING HERE? WHAT IS IT? DENISE IS READY FOR HER COLLEGE. SHE CANNOT COME HOME ALONE - THAT I TRUST IS A FAMILY FIAT.

I VISIT EVERY DAY WITH THE PHOTOGRAPHS AND CAN ALMOST DELUDE MYSELF INTO THINKING EACH ONE NEAR, BUT WE ARE NEVER GOING TO BE NORMALLY HAPPY UNTIL YOUR LIVES AND OURS, JIGGS DAD *normal again*AND ALL THE LINKED FAMILIES ARE ABLE TO MEET IN NORMAL FREEDOM.

WE MUST BE NONE OF US LIKE THAT, AND I KNOW YOU AND JIGG
NEVER WILL BE, OR HIS DAD, OR THE CHILDREN.

TO OUR INDIVIDUALITES PRESERVED BY THE GOOD <u>OLD</u> USA.

Evelyn

[Typed, signed. Handwritten insertions. SFC]

From John Metcalfe's diary:

June 10, 1959: *cleaned freezer and scaled open ice-box.*

June 29, 1959: *transitional note Paula.*

July 13, 1959: *E cleaned Frigidaire drawer yet to do.*

July 15, 1959: *wiped vegetable drawer clear of spilled juice
behind—was pineapple with maybe orange.*

July 18, 1959: *letter each Jigg Paula APO written in pen—no
carbon.*

To Deputy Personnel Officer for the Far East

The Benjamin Franklin Hotel

July 19, 1959

<u>Personal</u>

Deputy Personnel Officer for the Far East

International Cooperation Agency

Dear Sir,

I shall be indeed grateful if you have been able to give your attention to my letter
of June 27th, 1959,[276] substantiating an earlier petition from my daughter-in-law, Paula
P Scott, USOM, PROGRAM SUPPORT, SAIGON, for advice and any assistance you
care to offer to expedite the return of her husband (my son, Creighton Seeley Scott,
USOM, PROGRAM SUPPORT), with her and their family of five children, to the US
and permanent employment here at home.

The letter referred to above and forwarded to you as a kind favour to me by
Mr Robert D Johnson, Acting Director, US Passport Office, Washington, arrived
in his hands with my request for information as to whom to address my plea on
behalf of my son; who has this month completed, with his family, four years in
Saigon. I wrote in the spring to Miss Jean Hermann, who was the Personnel Officer
(Employee Relations), whose signature was appended to a letter I had when they
first went to Saigon, in which I was notified that their first address, APO, had been
changed to Navy 150, FPO. However, Miss Hermann has not replied as yet to my
request to her, also, to be given at least an inkling as to when the Scotts are likely to
be back at home.

---

276 This letter has not survived. Evelyn's claim that she was writing in support of a request from
Paula is without substance.

In my letter now in your hands, I allude to the various difficulties both myself and my son and his wife have had about mail, both foreign and domestic; of which a good many letters of recent years have never been acknowledged or traced. As an author, much of my own mail is addressed to Evelyn Scott, the name I have used for book signatures all my adult life; and for reasons I find incomprehensible, this seems, sometimes, a factor in mail confusions, from which Washington, DC seems not always free.

I shall hope to have some advice about my son soon.

Respectfully Yours,

[Typed carbon copy, not signed. UTK]

Jigg and his family had been in Vietnam for nearly four years when in July 1959 he was recalled to Washington. He had been outspoken about perceived mismanagement of aid funding to Vietnam and was subpoenaed to give evidence to the Senate Foreign Relations Committee. In addition, and very likely partly as a result of Evelyn's letters to his employers and even to President Eisenhower, he was dismissed from his post and he and the family had to leave the country at very short notice. They had no choice but to return to Carmel and the home of Paula's relatives.

To Evelyn Scott

Carmel, California

July 23, 1959

Dear Evelyn -

We just arrived in Carmel, and Jigg is in Washington. If you wonder "why so sudden" it's because the whole situation in Saigon is difficult and we were called home, so that Jigg could do his part in helping to get at the facts. There are too many people who try to distort the facts - including even the peers.

I still can't answer my huge accumulation of your letters - the last few weeks in Saigon were spent in frenetic packing. Now we are home, but I still have very little time - the house is full of kids and their friends.

I've said this before, but I will write again soon.

Love to Jack

Love

Paula

[Handwritten, signed. UTK]

To Jean Hermann

The Benjamin Franklin Hotel

July 26, 1959

Dear Madam,

I have addressed several letters to you since the spring, in which I have requested any information you were able to give me respecting the time of the return of my son,

431

Mr Creighton Seely Scott, his wife, Paula P Scott, and their children, to the USA, their home, from Saigon.

As none of my letters - three or four - were acknowledged, I thought it possible that I had made my request in some unaccustomed quarters and with that in mind I wrote, again, for information, and with reminders of my own poor health and the ten years that elapsed since I or any of my sons relatives have seen him, and sent this letter to the USA State Department; expressing, to them, my hope that, if it were necessary, they could set me right as to the quarter in which to appeal in such circumstances, for a USOM employee.

Mr Robert D Johnson, Deputy Director of the Passport Office, was given my letter to read, and forwarded it to the Deputy Personnel Officer for the Far East, International Cooperation Agency writing me, at the same time, that he had done so.

As I have not heard from that office, either, I think it best to let you know of the further letter there.

Of course, the truth remains that I do not know whether this letter or any other to the ICA *will* ever reach *its* destination. And I cannot forebear saying, again, as I did three years ago when writing to your office, that the apparent contempt of our Military Government for the mothers and the fathers of the older generation of Americans, strikes me as worthy of the very worst dictations. Mail still figures domestically, also, in the long record I have of experiences relative to communication and personal contact with family and friends since 1945, that are *genuinely disgraceful.*

Very Truly Yours,

(Mrs W J) Evelyn Dunn Scott Metcalfe

[Typed carbon copy, typed signature. Handwritten insertion. UTK]

From John Metcalfe's diary:

July 27, 1959: Paula's first letter Carmel, Jigg is in Washington DC.

To Paula Scott

The Benjamin Franklin Hotel

August 5, 1959

Darling Paula

I have been trying to write in the unflurried tone I thought might best suit you, and have now mailed five letters, of which one was to Creighton, though addressed to you.

Now, since a couple of weeks have gone by with no word from Creighton to myself and Jack, and no specific information from you about prospects and plans, I have decided it is too fantastically unnatural to keep to chit-chat.

We have, all along, just as during our eight and a half years in England, looked forward to the decent end of this imposed policy from somewhere that is keeping us apart even in correspondence; our first reasonable expectation having been that it would end when we reached New York from London; and our expectation during the four years you have been in the Far East, having been that Creighton would write to us himself as soon as he got home so that we could welcome him with you and the children with all the deep affection we feel.

Naturally we do not know what has been done and is being done, to convey an impression to the best of good sons and husbands that he dare not communicate with his American mother, his American father, and his British stepfather. But that something has or is continuing an illegal interference we do not doubt.

Unless Jigg soon writes to us naturally at least to the extent of a note, I shall consult any lawyers who are willing to help me as to the step essential in pinning down those in the Government or outside it who are criminally responsible for a situation that has changed me from a woman in moderate health to a nervous wreck with every indication of being fifteen years older than I am.

Does the FBI abstract my mail to the Personnel Office, I wonder. I have written four letters since spring that would certainly have received notice from anyone less than a monster of brutality, and no notice is taken. And I had my unforgettable experience of slipshod inquiry in 1940, when I reported an intimidator of communist views.

WE ARE THE ONLY FAMILY OF AMERICANS (PLUS MY SECOND BRITISH HUSBAND, S/L WJ METCALFE, JOHN METCALFE AUTHOR) WHO HAS EVER, AS FAR AS WE CAN ASCERTAIN, BEEN SUBJECTED TO CONDITIONS THAT HAVE MADE IT IMPOSSIBLE FOR FIFTEEN YEARS TO SEE AN ONLY AND MUCH LOVED SON OR, IN FACT, ANY MEMBER OF HIS FAMILY OR OTHER RELATION. The book suppressions and painting suppressions connect. And hostile acts toward me as an author had their genesis, with certainty, in my first PUBLIC COMPLAINTS ABOUT COMMUNISM'S EFFECT ON AMERICAN LITERATURE.

DARLING YOU CANT ANSWER, BUT THOSE RESPONSIBLE CAN AND MUST, THE CITIZENS HAVE THE RIGHT TO DEMAND STRAIGHT NATIONAL DEFENCE AND COMPLETE REDRESS FOR THE MANY WRONGS DONE EACH IN PERSON.

MAY DARLING JIGGS POSITION BE WITH OLD CONSTITUTIONAL LOYALISTS WHO IN ANY CASE PREFER THEIR OWN COUNTRY JUST AS NATURAL MEN AND WOMEN PREFER THEIR OWN WIVES AND SWEETHEARTS.

WE LOVE YOU AND JIGG AND THE KIDS!! SAY SOMETHING TO US

Evelyn

[Typed, signed. SFC. Unsigned carbon copy also at UTK]

To Ronald Pearson

The Benjamin Franklin Hotel
August 5, 1959

Dear Ronald

Paula has written us of her arrival with the children care Martinez-Dean, Route 2 - Box 412, Carmel California; where she was two years ago, in general locality.

Her letter was postmarked Carmel July 24, and you may have heard too then or before. She wrote us that Jigg is in Washington, DC and I have waited these ten days in the hope that the foul hiatus in correspondence with him himself would shortly end in at least a note that would allow Jack and myself to welcome him with his darling family back to his native land where we trust yet we may finally see him after these ten years of separation.

I have written to his Personnel Officer - or rather Employee Relations Officer, Personnel Office, ICA, Washington 25, several times - four in all - since the spring, mentioning the fact that I know his agreement to remain in Saigon would end in July, and that I would appreciate, as his mother, help in re-establishing our correspondence and contacts, which have been next to none in Saigon, bar the goodness of Paula who has literally saved my life, and almost none since Jigg was in London to see us in November 1949.

Can you enlighten me about Jigg's address? If you can, my dear Ronald, you should, for I personally think he is being forced to keep silent by some means he has not divulged, which may have to do with the hocus pocus of "war" hush, or may not.

Personally I have a hunch that communists put rackets up to calling people communists when they were haters of communists. I HAVE NOT FORGOTTEN PAULAS NOTE ABOUT SOME MAN IN A NEWSPAPER CLIPPING WHO WAS SMEARED IN A PROBE, NOR THAT MY LETTERS TO SPRING VALLEY WHICH ARRIVED AFTER SHE SAILED WERE HELD NINETEEN MONTHS BEFORE THEY WERE RETURNED TO THE ADDRESSEE, and two registered parcels for the children were returned opened, with no explanation.

Evelyn Dunn Scott Metcalfe

[Typed carbon copy, signed. UTK]

From John Metcalfe's diary:

August 10, 1959: cleaned frigidaire mailed letter to Lew asking for suggestion as to whom to write to protest difficulty of contacting Jigg.

August 12, 1959: Jack saw clipping about Jigg's testimony on Vietnam sub-American base. Got papers for me. Letter to Manly unanswered as yet. Heard by postcard from Ronald—over a year since we heard from Paula and Jigg.

August 14, 1959: mailed letter to Paula asking her if she wants my clipping about Jigg.

To Love Lyle[277]

The Benjamin Franklin Hotel

August 16, 1959

Darling Love

Your sweet letter by airmail was a final reassurance that should not have been needed, I guess, and would not have been, were it not that I have a very old score against the many who have never failed to misunderstand Cyril and our relationship of fourteen years. And even now I feel I cannot conclude this little exchange without adding, Yes, Cyril is not alone brilliant and full of achievements, HE IS GENUINELY MORALLY GOOD BEYOND MOST MEN.

He has had twenty years of martyrdom in North Carolina is the TRUTH. I think you and ourselves have had some. Myself I could not believe in a "jealous God" whose behaviour as an egotist so outdoes that of humans that no criticism of this world is possible without a sixteenth-rate inferior all too human male's rebuke.

I would relish making an index of adjurations from the Old Testament, and giving their application as human intelligent men apply them, and their antithesis as many who do lipservice to "Christianity", misapply them.

This is a quotation from the World-Telegram, NY of August 12th, 1959: Captioned, "2 Experts Call Viet Nam Aid Smelly Mess", and reading: after a brief preamble

"Creighton S Scott, 44, who recently returned here after four years in Viet Nam as Government advisor to American financed Vietnamese national radio project, and who is still employed by the International Cooperation Administration" and Wallace Gade, who, at the time of his retirement, was a Washington-based ICA official overseeing radio and other communications projects in Southeast Asia, including Viet Nam testified yesterday in separate closed-door congressional hearings.

"Mr Scott testified yesterday at a closed session of the House to a subcommittee on foreign affairs. At the same time Mr Gade was testifying to a Senate foreign relations subcommittee.

"Both said afterward they were pledged not to divulge publically the details of their testimony.

"Mr Scott added that he had testified to the House subcommittee yesterday, and the Senate group last Friday of his personal knowledge of graft, corruption and inefficiency in the over-all Viet Nam program.

---

277 Love Lyle was a cousin of Maude Dunn's. Much of the correspondence between Love and Evelyn relates to the family in Tennessee and not to this part of Evelyn's story. However, this letter includes quotes from the *New York World-Telegram*. It has not been possible to find this account online, and this is therefore one of only a few available records of these hearings.

"Mr Scott, however, testified mainly on the radio project."

I add that articles on Viet Nam by Mr Albert M Colegrove, a Scripps Howard staff writer, evidently produced an investigation as above.

Paula has written, two weeks ago, that she and the children are in Carmel, California, as they were two years ago. But she had just arrived and we have heard nothing since from either.

Jack is sitting here in his pyjamas filled with nostalgia for the London I first knew where wool outer coats were needed in July and August. Even London summers have deteriorated since the war, however, as our friend Bernice Elliott who is there from NY found London very warm indeed.

Every sort of love, darling sweet good Love

Evelyn

[Typed carbon copy, typed signature. UTK]

To Paula Scott

Charles R Soll

Counsellor at Law

86 Main Street

Nyack NY

September 11, 1959

Mrs Paula Scott

c/o United Service Overseas Mission

Saigon, Vietnam

Dear Mrs Scott:

I am in receipt of a letter from Mrs William J Metcalfe c/o The Benjamin Franklin, 222 West 77th Street, New York City dated September 6, 1959.

She expresses anxiety because she has not received any communication from her son Creighton or yourself and has asked that I communicate with you and forward her personal request that you write to her.

Very truly yours,

Charles R Soll

[Typed carbon copy on business letterhead, signed. UTK]

To Evelyn Scott

United States Post Office

Carmel, California

September 19, 1959

Dear Mrs Metcalfe:

All mail addressed to Mrs Scott at Rt 2, Box 412, Carmel, California is being delivered to her at that address.

Sincerely,

Fred G Strong

Postmaster

[Typed on official letterhead, signed. UTK]

From John Metcalfe's diary:

September 17, 1959: <u>POST CARD FROM PAULA.</u>

To Paula Scott

The Benjamin Franklin Hotel

September 26, 1959

Darling Paula,

I wonder very often who got hold of my several letters addressed to the Employee Relations Officer, ICA, and whether or not Jigg had those I addressed in their care to him. They have not dealt fairly or respectfully with a mother, father and affectionate step-father who have endured conditions NEITHER YOU NOR JIGG WISH FOR FIFTEEN YEARS BAR FIVE DAYS.

I have thought of drawing up a petition for the White House in respect to Jiggs first need to be with you and the children, and his also very normal essential human and practical need to sometimes SEE AND TALK TO HIS PARENTS AND STEPFATHER.

Can you tell me what you would think of my doing this? WE HAVE EVERY LEGAL RIGHT TO PUNISH BY LAW ANY WHO INTERFERE WITH NORMAL AMERICAN AND BRITISH LIVES AND RELATIONS.

YOU HAVE A NICE POSTMASTER. HE WROTE ME AT ONCE THAT MRS SCOTTS LETTERS ARE BEING DELIVERED at HER CARMEL ADDRESS. I SHALL THANK HIM.

LOVINGLY LOVINGLY DARLING - JIGG AND YOU EAST*[sic]*

Evelyn

[Typed carbon copy, signed. UTK]

To Fred Strong

The Benjamin Franklin Hotel

September 27, 1959

Dear Mr Strong,

I write this to thank you for your kind note advising me that mail to my daughter-in-law, Mrs Scott, is still being delivered at Rt 2, Box 412.

I am also glad to say that I have, since I wrote to you, also, had a postcard, again, from her, saying she is still there.

I appreciate the promptness with which you have tried to relieve my mind about my family.

Sincerely Yours

[Typed carbon copy, not signed. UTK]

To Robert Johnson

The Benjamin Franklin Hotel
[October, 1959]

Old Fashioned STRAIGHT CREIGHTON SEELEY SCOTT

Mr Robert D Johnson

Acting Director US Passport Office

Washington DC

In the letter I sent you I asked that my son be helped if possible to live near his mother and step-father with his wife and children, and so be near enough to hope to see his father. Mother, father, step-father have not seen him or his family for ten years.

At once this letter was mailed, my son CREIGHTON SEELEY SCOTT WAS POSTED TO SAN FRANCISCO - as far from his mother, as they could send him.

In the same letter I said he must be with his wife who is worn out by many strains and lacks physical strength to take on the responsibility for five children, three of them boys, alone.

In the letter I mailed to Mr Robert D Johnson asking him again how I could help my son to settle nearer the elders, I said CREIGHTON SEELEY SCOTT IS NEITHER COMMUNIST NOR FASCIST, HE IS AN AMERICAN IN THE TRADITIONAL SENSE.

At once this letter was mailed he was posted to San Francisco,[278] which according to news is a LABOUR CITY - he has and still does avoid labour disputes and unions. IT WAS CRUEL TO IGNORE THAT LETTER - maybe our visitors looked over my shoulder?

In the letter above I pled to have the eldest daughter home in time to enter the college she had selected. She HAS NOT DONE SO, as the SCOTT FAMILY IS IN AN UNSETTLED STATE, AS THE CERTAINLY DID NOT EXPECT MR and MRS SCOTT TO BE APART.

CREIGHTON SEELEY SCOTT HAD TO GO TO WASHINGTO TO TESTIFY ABOUT CONDITIONS ABROAD WHERE HE WAS. HE COULD NOT TAKE HIS WIFE THER WITH FIVE CHILDREN AS HE IS NOT WEALTHY.

SHE HAS TO STAY IN CARMEL FOR THE PRESENT, RENT SETTLED.

THEY DO NOT WISH TO SETTLE IN CALIFORNIA.

CREIGHTON SEELEY SCOTT WAS BORN SCOTT AMERICAN AT BIRTH HIS ANCESTRY ON BOTH SIDES IS AMERICAN BACK TO BUNKER HILL.

NOW I SUGGEST THAT CONTINUED SPITE-PURVEYORS BE KICKED OUT OF THE REGULAR AMERICAN ARMY FOR GOOD.

PLEASE HELP STRAIGHT NATIONAL DEFENCE.

REMEMBER FIVE DAYS IN FIFTEEN YEARS ONLY HAVE I SEEN MY SON.

---

278 Jigg was not "posted" to San Francisco; it is not clear why he was there. At that time Denise was beginning her senior year at Carmel High School and planning to go to college the following year.

THE REASONS ALL RELATE TO TOTAL ENEMY ACTIONS.

THREE OF OUR FIVE GRANDCHILDREN I HAVE NEVER SEEN IN THE FLESH.

WHERE IS THE ICA - IT SEEMS TO DESPISE HUMAN LOVE BOTH YOUNG AND OLD OURS LOVE.

[Typed carbon copy, not signed. UTK]

To Evelyn Scott
International Cooperation Administration
Washington 25, DC

October 8, 1959

Dear Mrs Metcalfe:

Your two letters addressed to your son Creighton Scott c/o Personnel Division, ICA Washington have been forwarded to him in California. The address Mr Scott left with us was Route 2, Box 412, Carmel, California.

Since your son is no longer working with the Agency, may we suggest that you direct your letters to him in Carmel.

Sincerely,
Howard F Ross, Chief
Employee Relations Office

[Typed on official letterhead, signed. UTK]

From John Metcalfe's diary:
October 9, 1959: had bad heart muscle strain, new pain heavy beats under breast—had just retyped criticism of large unions.

October 11, 1959: Evelyn v. poorly. Tried to get May, but she out of town, - will return Tuesday.

October 13, 1959: Left $1.50 at office for E's medicine. Mailed to Cyril.

To Evelyn Scott and John Metcalfe

Carmel, California
October 13, 1959

Dear Evelyn and Jack-

After promising to write in detail, I've been putting it off simply for lack of time. It will take me hours to go through the accumulated letters from you, and I simply don't have that much time. Anyway, the main thing is that we are all well and there is nothing for you to worry about. When I don't write it is only because I don't have time. Remember that I have a large family to take care of - it means a lot of sweeping cooking dinners, washing, ironing, dishes, beds, sewing, mending, etc, etc. The day is only so long. For instance, every single day I have to do a big washing and ironing to keep all five kids clean and neat for school. So please don't get frantic when you don't hear for a while, especially as time slips by and I sometimes don't realize how long it's been since I wrote last.

The kids are all doing well in school and most of them like it. The exceptions are Fred and Matthew who, being boys, would much rather spend all their time on the beach or the rocks or in the hills. They consider school an inexcusable imposition. Denise is still a straight A student and is carrying a heavy load of extra-curricular activities. July and Bobby can walk to school and they both love it. It's a nice little school, only through fourth grade, and they both like their teachers.

This is all I have time for now - there is work to do. I'll try to write sooner next time. But remember not to worry.

Love to you both,
Paula

[Handwritten, signed. UTK]

To Paula Scott

The Benjamin Franklin Hotel
October 24, 1959

Darling Paula -

I wrote you of my health last week and hope you now have my letter. I have coronary heart disease, and has been going on some time, probably, I had a dose of "psychosomatic" converts who actually refused to diagnose, and one alone offered any treatment. Naturally when they gave no advice I tried to go on per usual, and that was a mistake. However, it is perfectly true that when patients of this sort guard themselves with a great deal of complete rest, they may live a long time.

As to Gladys, when we were coming to New York, she wrote me to London "dont come back". And we had scarcely got here before she began in a youth movement jargon to tell me I must "relinquish" Jigg and leave him to his "own generation".

She then wrote me that she "could not see me unless I promised not to refer to my family". I wrote her that we would not meet again until she agreed that I could be as natural in speech about my family as anyone in the world.

That was four-and-one-half years ago, and she has not communicated with me since. Now as to returning to England:

1. Do you and Jigg want us to do so, like she does, or for any reason? PLAIN SPEAKING IS JUST DECENT IN THESE MATTERS

2. It is not easy to return in our present financial state. We have a joint retirement pension but it is not enough to save on, and it restricts Jacks earnings to a hundred a month. FREE EARNINGS PASSED AS LAW WOULD ENABLE HIM TO USE ANY OPPORTUNITY HE HAS TO MAKE ENOUGH TO PUT SOME BY. WE CANT EVEN PAY OUR PASSAGES AS IT IS, AND WE STILL OWE MARGARET. Our intention was live here and visit Britain. Now we are a bit disturbed.

3. Has Jigg decided he will never see us because those who direct us all wont let him? Or is it because he is opposed to what we ourselves are?

4. Remember I am perfectly aware of threat in all lives today. We were allowed to see Jigg, since the war, only that once in <u>London</u>. But dont forget that when Jigg arrived his whole physiology was, as I might say, "under siege". He looked so unlike himself that I looked at the back of his head to recognize my son.

He would not discuss any of our common memories, or refer to his painting and novels. When I did, he shut me up. When he was leaving for France, I spoke of several French things of his childhood, and he interrupted me by saying. <u>"Ive forgotten all that"</u>. He was sweet when Jack read, and he held my hand.

5. Jack had to sell his Hamstead house.[279] The division of the gas increased with tenants was stopped when the rents were raised but they were not raised enough to cover the 491 pounds a year the gas heating costs. *The house* has only a small number of years to run on the ground lease, and we have <u>no money</u> to buy a freehold.

6. Will either of you ever make further effort to see us? Is it just a farce that we will ever have communication with the children? Your lives are so difficult, I dont judge you, but to us it has always seemed that normal relations with parents and grandparents were bound to be of mutual benefit.

I have tried to write without emotion. Need we say what all this signifies to Jack and me: Jack is frankly bitter about what has happened but especially about what has been done to me. He is loyal to you and Jigg and Cyril, but he, too, thinks we would all be happier for explanation - and of course meetings. Wish Jigg and you werent on the West Coast. But I suppose as to war it seems all the same to you. LOVE, *Evelyn*
[Typed, signed. Handwritten insertion. SFC]

During this period Jack had been in correspondence with Match and Co, the managing agents for 26 Belsize Crescent (see Chapter 34). These letters contained considerable detail about the finances of the property and Jack reluctantly decided that he had no option but to sell the house. After taking advice, he accepted an offer of £2500 (approximately £69,000 at 2022 value), nowhere near enough to buy the hoped-for cottage in the country.

From John Metcalfe's diary:

November 14, 1959: Wrote and posted letter to Match's, instructing them to sell house, if possible, for £2500. Nice letter from Paula.

November 17, 1959: E poorly, - no codeine yet or reply from May. I marketed and bought cold cuts so that cooking in kitchen could be avoided.

November 19, 1959: May's gift of filled prescription arrived this am.

November 20, 1959: Letter from Match's to say a purchaser for the house has been found + will pay £2500.

---

279 For more information about this see Chapter 34.

December 9, 1959: E cleaned frigidaire bar vegetable drawer which hurts chest.

December 14, 1959: Found letter from Paula on my return, - Jigg home for holidays.

December 20, 1959: Work on Noel and X'mas cards.

December 21, 1959: Still busy with X'mas cards.

To John Metcalfe and Evelyn Scott

Carmel, California
December 20, 1959

Dear Jack and Evelyn,

I hope this reaches you in time for Christmas - with our love and blessings. We are deep in preparations, of course - we put up the tree this afternoon because the kids pestered so much that I gave in. It does look pretty.

We're not sending any cards this year, so this note is to take its place. We're all well and of course the kids are in a heaven of anticipation. I hope you both have a good Christmas - even if simple.

Love,
Paula

[Handwritten, signed. UTK]

From John Metcalfe's diary:

December 24, 1959: Marketed. Was presented with bottle of champagne by liquor store.

December 25, 1959: Cold still unpleasant.

December 26, 1959: Day a series of exasperations. In evening got liquor store to open the champagne. It disagreed with each of us. And so (after no supper) to bed.

December 29, 1959: E poorly and I cooked breakfast.

Chapter 40

1960

Evelyn's letters and her contributions to Jack's diary are markedly different this year, with her entries typically more focussed on cleaning the refrigerator in the communal kitchen than on unanswered correspondence. Some of the entries can only be described as incoherent, as this year also sees a new preoccupation recorded in the pages of Jack's diary: "looking at clothes on hangars". This could have been because, sitting alone in their dreary hotel room while Jack went out to his teaching job, she had little to occupy her mind. Or it could have been because she was becoming more obsessive.

The stream of letters was somewhat reduced, but the logic in some of them is increasingly contorted as Evelyn often concentrates on seemingly minor issues. This may have been because Paula in her letters deliberately gave away very little detail about their lives; most of her letters were carefully focussed on brief answers to Evelyn's constant questions and talking about the children and their progress at school without giving her any information Evelyn could exploit for her own purposes.

Jigg and the family were in Carmel for the whole of 1960, without income and dependent on Paula's relatives for much of their support. None of Jigg's efforts at finding employment, even the least skilled, was successful, and his desperation can only be imagined. This culminated in a series of letters written by Jigg at the end of 1960 to those who knew Evelyn best, asking for advice on how to find the job he so desperately needed for himself and for his family. These letters, revealing so much about his own experience, have been grouped into a separate chapter.[280]

From John Metcalfe's diary:

January 3, 1960: Cyril's birthday.
January 4, 1960: E began May's codeine.
January 17, 1960: Evelyn's birthday.
January 18, 1959: E cleaned frigidaire.
January 22, 1960: Mathew's birthday.

---

280 See Chapter 45, Coda.

January 23, 1960: sat night midnight (rats) began attacking as only once or twice therefore, gone on.

January 27, 1960: sat rats still at it stopped.

February 15, 1960: E cleaned frigidaire.

February 17, 1960: second criminal theft since mss 1st original went out this lost 1 pg and 2 carbons completed clear yesterday.

To Creighton and Paula Scott

The Benjamin Franklin Hotel

February 21, 1960

Darling Jigg and Paula,

What am I to do to have news of how you and the five children are? I have been imploring specific replies to my letters now for about two months, and am very anxious about all you dears whom we love.

May it be possible for both of you to write to us soon! My last two or three letters about putting an extra copy of my mss (I retain my own) in the State archives, were very pressing as to having Jiggs signature with Jacks to the brief document of agreement as to permission to my literary executors to use them for publishing purposes should they ever be needed (I refer to all my mss), and the fact that no comment or word from Jigg has yet come is distressing me. I hoped Carmel was unlike the places you have known of and of which I have written you, where there has been illegal and actually criminal interference with all our personal mail, at times.

Our love, our love, our love

Mother (Evelyn, to Paula)

[Typed, signed. SFC]

From John Metcalfe's diary:

February 23, 1960: air mail to Jigg and Paula Carmel air mail to Love Lyle Request for copyright blank.

February 24, 1960: School as usual, sending a telegram to Paula on my way there.

To Paula Scott

The Benjamin Franklin Hotel

February 25, 1960

Thankful for health there, hope Jigg well too. Mother

Darling Paula,

Please darling give us an inkling of what is the matter that we have as yet no news of you and Jigg and the children for such a time!

We know Jigg must have a better BETTER JOB where he can have you and the children with him and ENOUGH REAL SALARY FOR ALL YOU SEVEN.

California must abolish a medical stipulation, as it is a form of quackery to insist on it, and is almost sure to prove a cover for ailments caused by war weapons. I dont say this without having thought it over for a long time. In the present unfortunate condition of the country, no doctor is ever able to do much for a patient unless both doctor and patient have a similar political view, and commercial medicine is more risk than aid.

I dont know why I have the urge to say this now, but I have and as a general proposal I am sure I am right. SO DONT ALLOW ANYONE TO BE PESTERED IN THIS WAY, LEAST OF ALL DARLING JIGG WHOM THE US SERVICE DOCTOR CURED ON THE BASIS OF A DIAGNOSIS OF AILMENTS AS DUE TO quackery at home.

I wrote you as I had asked the Carmel Postmaster whether you were receiving you mail, and I now have his reply - just arrived. He says to the best of his knowledge you are as mail goes on being delivered to the same address and he hasnt been advised as to any change. His name is Mr Strong and he has really been quite nice to me, as a stranger. But dont fail to let me know specifically as soon as you can of any letters or parcels that have not come as soon as you can, darling Paula. The letters about the archives are, also, very important. The Postmaster naturally cant keep tab on what is sent at my end unless advised, so we must depend on you to help clear that part of it up.

We speak of you and Jigg and the need of the job with better pay where all can be together whenever we can, and meanwhile just hope others are helping too, somehow.

Lovingly to the Scotts Evelyn

Your telegram has just come[281] - thank you. Our love, *Evelyn*

[Typed, signed. SFC]

To Evelyn Scott

Carmel, California
March 1, 1960

Dear Evelyn -

You really mustn't worry when I don't write - I never was and never will be a good correspondent and a silence only means that I've been busy, and nothing more.

The poems arrived, long ago, and the Proust and it seems to be many more books besides which I can't think of at the moment I'm in a hurry now, to catch the mailman. I'll be more detailed next time.

We're all well and the sea and the hills continue beautiful. It's spring here and flowers are everywhere The hills normally black-green with sere slopes are now emerald and black-green.

Love to Jack, and to you.

Paula

[Handwritten, signed. UTK]

---

281 This telegram has not survived.

From John Metcalfe's diary:

March 17, 1960: Our Wedding Anniversary (1930). May we both be preserved.

To Evelyn Scott

Carmel, California

March 18 [1960]

Dear Evelyn - a card to let you know we're all OK. I'm very busy. I told you all packages arrived and there was no need to bother the Post Office Dept. When I don't write it only means I'm busy - you can be sure I'll let you know if anything bad should happen. I'll write the promised letter as soon as I can. You're asking for a detailed acknowledgement of about 30 letters and several packages - that's an all day job and I haven't much time. Love, Paula

[Handwritten postcard, signed. UTK]

From John Metcalfe's diary:

March 23, 1960: *mch 22nd these entries Card from Paula letter promised I have written in mid-week since about Mch 1st Monday mailing one each has been custom of years letter to Kay (has Escapade reached her?) and to Bob (did he receive letter about Jack's books?) mailed Amsterdam afternoon at corner.*

March 24, 1960: School, - on return from which found letter from Willcox offering £4500 for house! - Though I don't think he would actually have paid that when he came to know of the short lease, central gas, etc.

To Evelyn Scott
Post Office Department
San Francisco Regional Office
79 New Montgomery Street
San Francisco 5, Calif

March 30, 1960

Dear Mrs Metcalfe:

This refers to our letter of March 14, 1960, and your communications of March 16 and March 19 regarding the delivery of mail to Mr and Mrs Creighton S Scott at Carmel, California.

The Postmaster at Carmel has again contacted Mrs Scott, who stated that she believes that all mail you have sent her has been received. The postmaster is of the opinion that apparently they have not had time to answer their mail.

In the future, if you believe that a particular piece of mail has not been received, it is suggested that you file a tracer Form 1510 at your local post office.

Sincerely yours,

Spiro B Rafalovich

Postal Installations Manager

[Typed on official letterhead, signed. UTK]

From John Metcalfe's diary:

April 19, 1960: E cleaned Frigidaire.

May 24, 1960: E washed frigidaire.

June 7, 1960: Will sent registered.

June 9, 1960: back left lower jaw tooth fell out into my hand sometime after 4am. E No blood no pain.

June 17, 1960: Letter from Paula answering reg'd letter, + said nothing of Jigg.

June 20, 1960: registered air mail to Paula about Will contained check and letter for Creighton.

June 21, 1960: MacGarock arrived unsealed Marked insured one less heavy book already got lost—ask if it had string.

June 22, 1960: Registry return receipt for letter about deposit of my will stamped in Carmel on this date received by me a week later Receipt 369498 —Evelyn Scott signed by Denise Scott.

June 23, 1960: Is my own pillowcase at laundry?

To Creighton Scott

The Benjamin Franklin Hotel

July 3, 1960

Darling Son Jigg,

I am writing to ask Paula whether all the many letters I have sent her to forward have reached you. I do think something must be done to let us have a good note or letter from you, darling, about your knowledge, if you have it as of now, of the deposit of my Will and the need for some reliable address.

Formally NY

I perfectly well realize that you must be too much directed in some stupid criminally interfering quarter since you came home from abroad, and that YOUR BOSS IS NOT THE QUARTER *[sic]*. Was it suggested to you after you testified in Washington that you must not give out your address? Or have you not given it because from the first years of my absence in England you and Paula were having to combat slander about me and Dad?

My personal view is that an ignorance of Constitutional Law is affecting many meddlesome people. An unfortunate result of international dickering is that many people suppose that dicta from United are a substitute for NATIONAL LAWS.

May you proceed toward a reuniting with Paula darling and the darling sweet children by completing your new novel. May Paula write again, all publish as we did and all will be well.

The wise monkeys who refuse to see the evil around would say "Fie" to me for including myself, but every decent and sincere writer knows I am right and even correct to do so.

LOVINGLY PLEASE ANSWER TO HELP,

MOTHER AND JACK, FOR DAD AND THE WELLMANS TOO

IN THIS WHERE WE WERE EVER AT ONE,

[Typed, not signed. Handwritten insertion. UTK]

From John Metcalfe's diary:

July 26, 1960: 25th date these air mail registered to Paula (Mrs CS) this am about trinkets should later send one about copyright renewals 1st straight air Denise straight air Creighton.

July 31, 1960: E wrote to Carmel post master.

August 3, 1960: E cleaned frigidaire.

August 20, 1960: book for Paula E + I went out, + bought 2 books for Paula from Wormath's "Great Expectations" and "Gothic Tales".

August 22, 1960: E did Jack's cupboard pictures to come look at clothes on hangars.

August 23, 1960: go through book box thoroughly.

August 24, 1960: E feeling poorly.

August 27, 1960: Telegram arrived OK from Paula.[282] Paula mentioned letter (hope of August 8) but did not refer to registry receipt What should I do about it?

August 29, 1960: look at clothes on hangars.

September 1, 1960: Registry receipt for letter mailed Paula August 8 has yet to be returned.

September 3, 1960: Went PO and mailed books to Paula.

September 5, 1960: look at clothes on hangars must be date of Cyril's death paper Tuesday referred to "yesterday".

September 6, 1960: On way to school read in paper of Cyril's death, on the 4th. Told E about Cyril. Jack brought me Herald-Tribune obituary of Cyril, who died at Chapel Hill Memorial Hospital Chapel Hill NC, yesterday September 5th Error about legal change of name to C K Scott Jack mailed letter

---

282 This telegram has not survived.

each to Editor and to Irita Van Doren[283] *—shall trust letter published.*

Evelyn had another reason to berate others when Cyril died in September 1960 and the New York Herald Tribune published an obituary which referred to his original name (Frederick Creighton Wellman) and made no reference to his relationship with Evelyn or his change of name to Cyril Kay Scott. Perhaps unsurprisingly, the obituary prompted an outburst from Evelyn over perceived inaccuracies in which she deliberately involved Jigg.

Cyril Scott obituary
from *New York Herald Tribune*
September 6, 1960
Dr F C Wellman Is Dead; Distinguished in 3 Fields

Chapel Hill, NC, Sept (AP): Dr Frederick Creighton Wellman, ninety, father of two authors and himself distinguished in medicine, literature and art, will be buried here after an Episcopal funeral service tomorrow. Dr Wellman died yesterday in Memorial Hospital after an illness of several weeks.

Born near Independence, Mo, he received his medical degree at Kansas City Medical Hospital and went to Portuguese West Africa as a medical missionary with his wife and infant son Paul.

Years later, Paul Wellman wrote a number of best-selling novels. The other author-son is Manly Wade Wellman, of Chapel Hill.

Studied, Explored

In his thirteen years in Africa, Dr Wellman established two hospitals, explored then little-known parts of the African interior and made extensive studies of tropical diseases, flowers and insects.

Returning to this country, he held the chair of tropical medicine at Tulane University, New Orleans, and then went to Brazil for further exploration and research.

Returning to the States, he wrote numerous short stories and four novels. Later he became distinguished in art, particularly as a water colorist. He won several prizes in French exhibitions.

He established schools of art in El Paso, Tex; Santa Fe, NM; and Denver, Colo, and became dean of the College of Fine Arts at Denver University.

Discovered Insect Species

As a medical man he announced two new clinical entities in tropical diseases and discovered numerous new species of insects and other causative agents of diseases. He contributed more than 150 brochures and articles to medical literature.

---

283 Irita Van Doren was the literary editor of the *Herald Tribune* for a number of years.

His autobiography, "Life is Too Short", published in 1941, told much of his diverse and adventurous life.

Surviving, besides Paul I and Manly Wade Wellman, are two other sons, Dr Frederick J Wellman and Creighton Wellman,[284] a daughter, Mrs Alice Wellman Harris, eight grand-children and eight great-grand-children.

[*New York Herald Tribune*, Tuesday, September 6, 1960. UTK]

To The Editor, *Herald Tribune*

The Benjamin Franklin Hotel
September 6, 1960

The Editor,
The Herald-Tribune
NYC, 24, NY
Sir,

I request the correction of a very serious error made in the obituary of my first husband, <u>born</u> Frederick Creighton Wellman, in your paper of today. His name, on abandoning his distinguished career in science, was <u>legally</u> changed to Cyril Kay Scott, by recorded documented usage over a long period, and it was and is entirely as Cyril Kay Scott that he is known in the arts, as a remarkable painter, and the author of a few brilliant novels.

My son and his is Creighton Seeley Scott, the fourth son referred to in your notice. This has always been his legal name, and Scott is the name naturally of his wife and their five children. Even as Dr Fredrick Creighton Wellman achieved much in science of which his family can be justly proud, so did Mr Cyril Kay Scott merit the description brilliant, as a novelist, and "very great" as a water-colourist.

I ask for the correction as a matter of both human and aesthetic justice.

Very Truly Yours,
Evelyn Scott

Please publish this letter
[Typed carbon copy, signed. UTK]

To Creighton Scott

The Benjamin Franklin Hotel
September 7, 1960

Darling darling Son

Has anyone been able to reach you in San Francisco, I wonder, or is it left to me to tell you that your darling Dad died yesterday at a hospital in Chapel Hill?

---

284 During the 1950s, when Jigg and Paula and the children were living with him in Pine Bluff, Cyril unilaterally decided, in spite of Paula's protests, that they would be known as "Wellman".

There is no way of "softening the blow". I have been trying for all the seven years since Jack and I came back to the USA to find some way of helping you and Paula and the children, and your Dad and Jack and myself to meet again in one room as we have done all our shared lives, and I as your mother from the beginning. Had genuine imaginations been able to function among some of the people we know who knew him and know you, it might have come about. But it hasnt, and there is only the truism to console one: that he cannot any more be dealt with unjustly by anyway, or be put through any further bodily suffering.

You were as dear to him as anything in life, but however wickedly uncomprehending the people who, at the end, believed they were "being kind", he had the consolation of knowing, beforehand, that you have a family that loves you.

Darling Jigg, let us all cleave to one another the more, with our loving and devoted memories of Dad to give natural affection a firmer basis. Do you know he never did a single thing I thought wrong in our entire lives, both together and apart.

And as that is also true of you and darling Jack and Paul, please let us love one another more and more, and for the sake of the darling darling children.

Bless you, darling darling Jigg

Mother

[Typed carbon copy, signed. UTK]

From John Metcalfe's diary:

September 7, 1960: letter each Creighton, Paula Jack and me telling Creighton of his father's death, mailed air mail this am.

To Evelyn Scott and John Metcalfe

Carmel, California

September 10, 1960

Dear Evelyn + Jack -

Thanks for the news about Cyril. He was three months short of 90 years old. How did you hear of it? Do you have any details? Was he ill very long? What was the cause, etc?

School started here last Tues. The boys both have good teachers and some outstanding ones, and they are finding their work interesting and stimulating for the for the first time in their lives. Quite a commentary on our school system and the quality of our teaching! Julia + Bobby like their school too - it's small and the teachers are good.

Yes, we've received all your letters about your will, the bank, and so on. I can't dig them all up and reply in detail - I tell you I receive them and take note of their contents and give you our news.

Thanks for your news + sympathy and love to both.

Paula.

[Handwritten, signed. UTK]

From John Metcalfe's diary:

September 11, 1960: Paula's birthday.

September 12, 1960: look at clothes on hangers. letters to Ruth Whitfield, Bernice London, Charlotte, Herschel, Bob, Love Lyle all letters announcing Cyril's death and mentioning need to emphasize Scott for Creighton. E cleaned frigidaire.

September 17, 1960: Jack mailed letters about Cyril to Richards and Bernice--2nd to her.

September 20, 1960: wrote two letters mailed 21. Had short letter Manly.

September 21, 1960: wrote Manly registered return wrote Lew— for both—registered.

September 24, 1960: wrote 2nd letter to Ruth and Mary hoping she will write Creighton.

September 26, 1960: look at clothes on hangers.

October 3, 1960: look at clothes on hangers. Re receipt letter to Lew arrived today

To Creighton Scott
New York Herald Tribune
230 West 41st Street,

October 5, 1960

Mr Creighton Seeley Scott

Carmel, California

Dear Mr Scott:

In the Associated Press account of the death of your father, Dr Frederick C Wellman, printed in the Herald Tribune and other newspapers on September 6, your name was listed among other surviving members of the family as Creighton Wellman.

Your mother, Mrs Evelyn Scott, has written to say that your legal name is Creighton Seeley Scott, and that it should have been listed so. In the absence of evidence to the contrary, all newspapers use Associated Press copy as received, in good faith.,

If the name as printed actually was erroneous and its appearance in the obituary in that form was embarrassing to you, we would consider setting the record straight. I would like to point out, however, that the story appeared a month ago.

Sincerely yours

RICHARD G WEST,

City Editor

[Typed on business letterhead, signed. SFC]

To Richard G West

Carmel, California
October 9, 1960

Dear Mr West,

This is in answer to your letter of October 5.

I have no idea what Evelyn Scott wrote you, but she did not do so with my knowledge. She has been of unsound mind for years, and the fact is notorious.

I read the Associated Press obituary about my father, Dr F C Wellman, carefully. It seemed clear and well-written as obituaries go, and the errors it contained were too trivial to mention and probably not the fault of AP.

If I had found it objectionable, I would have objected, which I have not done and don't intend to do. I make no complaints, require no retractions or corrections from the Herald-Tribune or anybody else, or that the record be put straight, as you offer to do, in any way. I am content with things as they are.

It's a pity you were inconvenienced, for you must be a busy man, but you should know that I decline absolutely all responsibility for what Evelyn Scott does or says, or attributes to me.

If she continues to write to you, as seems likely, the best person to get in touch with is her husband, Mr John Metcalfe, who may or may not be able to make her stop. There is nothing I can do.

Very truly yours,
Creighton Scott

[Typed carbon copy, signed. SFC]

To Creighton Scott

New York Herald Tribune
230 West 41st Street,
New York 36

October 12, 1960

Dear Mr Scott:

Thank you for your courteous letter. I was sorry to trouble you, for I had supposed that you had seen the obituary and would have been the first to object if an error had been committed. But Evelyn Scott was becoming rather importunate, and it seemed best to have the matter settled by the person most concerned.

We shall take your advice if any more letters are received.

Sincerely yours
RICHARD G WEST,
City Editor

[Typed on business letterhead, signed. SFC]

From John Metcalfe's diary:

October 10, 1960: look at clothes on hangers.

October 16, 1960: In evening E burned her hand with a boiling brussels sprout.

October 17, 1960: go over boxes in closets.

October 18, 1960: E cleaned frigidaire.

October 22, 1960: letter to Post Master Pine Bluff NC note to Ruth.

October 24, 1960: look at clothes on hangers.

October 25, 1960: Creighton's birthday.

October 31, 1960: look at clothes on hangers.

November 4, 1960: mailed letter re Cyril

November 14, 1960: look at clothes on hangers. School. On way home mailed letter from E to Frederick L Wellman - 67 cents.

November 21, 1960: look at clothes on hangers.

November 25, 1960: began to try to smoke less again.

November 28, 1960: look at clothes on hangers.

December 5, 1960: E cleaned frigidaire look at clothes on hangers.

To Mr Fred Strong

Carmel, California

December 8, 1960

Mr Fred Strong, Postmaster,

Carmel, California

Dear Mr Strong,

This letter is intended to save you embarrassment and annoyance if possible, and to make it easier for you to explain matters to your superiors should my mother, Evelyn Scott, harass you as she did once before and carry her complaints to the Postmaster General again.

Unhappily she has been of unsound mind for the past twenty years or so, and her mania consists of believing that I should abandon my wife and my children, of which there are five - one in college, one of military age and a third in high school, the other two in grade school.

She has suggested at various times how they could be disposed of and my step-father, the responsible person in her case, will not or cannot keep her quiet. While I was in Indo-China with the State Department she wrote about a letter a week to my various chiefs, to the Ambassador to Vietnam, and finally to John Foster Dulles, Eisenhower, and various others.

At present she feels I should divorce my wife, put the children in orphanages and return to New York. I find the correspondence - about four letters a week - burdensome and useless, and I propose to discontinue it.

You will certainly hear from her and, when you cannot do what she asks, from whichever higher authority she decides to appeal to. In answering their inquiries or criticism you may feel free to use this letter in any way you think fit.

I apologise for the embarrassment you were caused once before, which I could not prevent, and I hope you will be spared any more. However, this letter should make it easy to explain.

Sincerely yours,

Creighton Scott

[Typed carbon copy, signed. SFC]

From John Metcalfe's diary:

December 12, 1960: look at clothes on hangers. E received unpleasant letter from Paula.

December 17, 1960: Wrote to both registered remind Paula fondly of her promise Also they know we never change The reasons things are difficult for us are the same often unjust too them. We do not create the fake conditions of the world today. Tell them of weekend "dream" of her and Julia—a half preparation for her letter. The truth as to that aversion to addressing me as Evelyn Scott my writers name, is that by insisting on Metcalfe only they make rumour that I am British, whereas my author name is American in the records. Did Paula receive my answer to her query about my health—specific?

December 19, 1960: Mailed reg'd letter to Jigg + Paula. look at clothes on hangers.

December 25, 1960: Started letters to Attenborough and the Savile. Lunch + nap. Worked at note. Supper of filet mignon. Bed. $16.50 of Christmas tips given. So far still have Sam to tip. Reading Maren's "Felix Kroll".

December 26, 1960: look at clothes on hangers.

To Evelyn Scott

Carmel, California

December 31, 1960

Dear Mother,

I have your last letter,[285] suggesting I send you my working address, so that you can write to me there.

---

285 This letter has not survived.

I have no such address, I have no job, and if I did I would not tell you anything about it, because the experience of the past fifteen years has taught me that sooner or later you would write to my employer with the object of having me fired, as you have done hundreds of times in the past.

I remember vividly the promise you made to me in Tappan, during the war, that you would do everything you could to make sure my marriage and my family would founder economically, so that I could come back to you, like a pet poodle dangling on the end of an umbilical cord instead of a leash. I have also seen some of the letters you wrote my employers, including many of those in which you explained that I was a sort of zombie, helplessly under the control of nameless, sinister influences. A good many of those to whom you wrote believed, as you presumably intended, that they had been warned by a patriotic mother about the treasonable tendencies of a wayward son; and this sort of innuendo has cost me job after job, year after year. Thanks mainly to you, I find myself in middle age without work, without prospects, and an object of suspicion to everyone who might hire me.

Because of your perseverance in blackening my name, we are poor. The education I might have given my children is beyond my reach, and I have no doubt whatever that you would do whatever you could to revenge yourself on them as the opportunity arose. But then I remember very well how - during that same wartime visit to Tappan - you spat into my baby son Frederick's mouth because, you said, you had the 'flu and you hoped he would get it and die.

The one bright spot in the situation, as I see it, is that you have overplayed your hand. Hitherto we have been at the mercy of whatever slander about us you thought fit to spread, and Paula has kept up with a correspondence she finds nauseating solely in the hope of preventing you from writing worse things about us to even greater numbers of strangers. It never worked; and now that you have done your worst, there is nobody left to whom you can malign me, no method of coercion you can use, nothing whatever you can do to force either one of us to write or do anything you ask.

The only namely sinister influence in our lives has been you, and you know it. I have gone to the bestially unfilial extreme of refusing to abandon a wife and five children, not because I am being brainwashed by some mysterious electronic device, as you insist, but simply because I see no reason to make six people wretched merely to please your diseased vanity. There is no such device, as you know perfectly well, and my troubles arise mainly from your refusal to admit that I have a right to live my own life without placing your engorged ego before all other considerations.

This is the last time any of us will write, except to notify you of a death in the family. Good-bye.

Your son

[Typed carbon copy, not signed. SFC]

To John Metcalfe

Carmel, California
December 31, 1960

Dear Jack

I have written to my mother terminating the correspondence once and for all. I appreciate that this makes things difficult for you, and that the brunt of whatever hysterics I bring about will fall on you. I am sorry, but I have had enough.

What you probably do not realize, although she undoubtedly does, is that the letters she has been writing to my superiors and employers for the last 15 years or so inevitably have cost me my jobs, and that the cumulative effect is now such that nobody will hire me. I know there have been hundreds of such letters, and the ones I have been permitted to see all said I was the helpless tool of nameless, sinister influences - a sort of zombie who could not be trusted with any responsible job.

The result at present is that I am without a job, on the brink of starvation, and that my family must undergo severe hardships - all because of my mother's letter writing. Nobody will hire me because her letters are still in the personnel files of every company I have ever worked for.

I used to think she was merely irresponsible, but having thought it over I have decided this is not correct. I believe her motives are nothing more than vengeful jealousy toward my wife and my children, which she took no trouble to conceal when she visited us in Tappan, during the war, and demanded that I abandon them altogether and at once as unworthy of me.

I have now fallen so low there is absolutely nothing whatever she can do to me, and so I am taking full advantage of my (at least temporary) invulnerability to coercion to break things off once and for all.

I have written her the most brutally forthright letter I was able to compose, in the hope that it will penetrate the thick layers of complacency, and absolute contempt for the opinions and welfare of everybody else in the world, that protect her from her own conscience and my reproaches.

As far as I can see her present frame of mind is the result of a life-long belief that nothing whatever matters excepting the means of gratifying her own ego. Her attitude toward my wife and my family is absolutely ruthless and what she has done would not be tolerated at the hands of any stranger. Not only will Paula not write again, but neither will I; and these two letters, one to you and one to her, are the last communications to be expected from any of us.

If she will not listen to any explanations, you might point out to her that things might not have gone this far if she had been willing to abstain from slandering me to my employers, in the hope of depriving me and mine of our bread and butter - as she obviously intended. However, the thing has gone too far, a point of no return has been reached; and there is no appeal.

If she were to have the bad taste to come here, to expostulate with me in person, I would have her locked up in the State Insane Asylum at Napa; I would have no other choice, and some of her letters (saved with the possible need in mind) would, I think, convince even the most sceptical she is dangerous. Paula and I would be prepared to testify that she showed herself to be violent and malevolent toward the children.

Sorry. Good luck to you. Your stepson,

[Typed carbon copy, not signed. SFC]

Jigg also wrote to a number of others, friends of both his and Evelyn's, outlining in harrowing detail the effect her letter writing had had on his and his family's lives and livelihoods and asking if there was any help they could offer. These letters were discovered years later while clearing Paula's house after her death in 2007 and have been grouped together in Chapter 45: Coda.

Chapter 41

1961

This year, like the last, is one of monotony.. Jigg and the family are still in Carmel following Jigg's dismissal from his position in Saigon, and Jack's diary shows that Evelyn's preoccupation with letters never replied to is much reduced. These entries, no longer concerned so much with cleaning the communal refrigerator or inspecting clothing, reflect her increasingly poor health. And in August her health takes a turn for the worse, as she suffers what appears to be a stroke. Jack is now writing more of the letters, sending Jigg daily reports of her slowly improving health. As these letters are largely repetitive only a selection is included here.

From John Metcalfe's diary:

January 1, 1961: This week 3rd letter Maggie re name.

January 3, 1961: last Thurs, typed last Fri locked away last pgs carbons of old American stock missing corroborated as theft today when discovered the whole poem of 2 pgs gone in one copy. The missing pages were all retyped last week from old copy.

To Paula Scott

The Benjamin Franklin Hotel
January 6, 1961

Dear Paula,

You will see the letter I have written Jigg.[286] Do know that whenever you both feel like writing again we would be delighted.

We hope you will all think better of the situation. With us, you two and the children mean much. I have never seen you, or them, and hoped to do so some time.

The idea of Evelyn as an intentional destroyer of what does mean so much to her is ludicrous. What nightmare has afflicted you?

---

286 This letter has not survived.

My interest in you-all is natural and unborrowed. I would quite spit on any profession of amiability that didn't spring of itself.

So here's hoping

Jack

[Typed, signed. SFC]

From John Metcalfe's diary:

January 9, 1961: mailed letter to Copyright Office just inquiring.

January 20, 1961: Back to our own lair in a couple of hours + had lunch of soup.

January 24, 1961: found 1 broken silver prong com gone from box in which I had carefully concealed it under other things so as not to lose it. Today brooch broke—one I wear—broke, -put it pin and envelope in box. Loss of that prong is certain proof some one went into that box in a hurry after I hid the two prongs (Mother's prong still there) just before I went lunching with May.

January 25, 1961: 2 carbon sheets of Green Secrets just written and just typed disappeared out of our room after 7.30 last night and 10.30 am today. This now cleared up 2 pm Wednesday.

January 30, 1961: E cleaned frigidaire. Mailed book for Denise, also reg'd letter to Paula

February 3, 1961: begun FRN [287] again Witch Perkins and bound notes not found so far—still sure 2nd abstracted 1 more chance of 1st—empty envelope which had contained sorted letters of 1 yr ago. Also cannot find last [illeg] section about King and Queen but hope to.

February 8, 1961: Denise's birthday. All good luck to her. Maggie should have received her letter.

February 15, 1961: card to Maggie asking if she had letter about radio.

February 20, 1961: a horrible day to 3.20 sound mediums lying, threatening, falsifying about plagiarism when guilt theirs—a day foul enough to be noted here.

February 25, 1961: began Scott's Emulsion. [288]

---

287 This refers to the draft of the novel she referred to as the "French Revolution novel" which she She had been working on it for several years. She had nothing published after1954 (see Appendix C)

288 Scott's Emulsion was a proprietary brand of cod liver oil, intended for children. It was said to be good for, among other things, building up resistance to infections.

March 1, 1961: of the two letters sent May in last six weeks she received one.

March 13, 1961: mail card write V Hale[289] for Fred.

March 17, 1961: Return receipts for reg'd letters to Frederick + to V Hale arrived, - unsatisfactory because signed by Martinez-Dean. Evelyn sent me nice St Patrick's day post-card!

March 18, 1961: Letter to Frederick returned unopened from Carmel. Did more marketing.

March 20, 1961: <u>Filed Federal Income Tax Return</u>. Then sent letter, reg'd, from E to Mr F Stone, the Carmel postmaster.

April 6, 1961: began using boracic on eyes.

April 9, 1961: E felt very poorly after bad night, + with cold + cough.

April 10, 1961: Miss Cryer washed frigidaire.

April 19, 1961: Poor night, with E coughing. Got up, shaved etc. about four, + had tea, then went to sleep again.

May 13, 1961: burned letters from Jigg again returning checks. It was a very inaccurate statement and only really proved a political wrack and wheel by which slander has reduced him and his family and ourselves to poverty of course, job essential to 7 lives, but also of course Creighton Scott was born the son of an author-author painter in two arts, and his evident ridiculers in this regard are ignorant and unscrupulous in unions of dictation both in USA and when he was in Saigon. His wife Paula Scott is also an intellectual woman all old Americans, well-born.

May 15, 1961: E cleaned frigidaire. Jack mailed letter to Glad registered to Mrs Dakin.

May 27, 1961: Gladys came to tea, 3.25 to about 5.45, I having had nap previously. After she had left, I worked at novel.

June 6, 1961: Found box addressed to Paula Spring Valley containing sea dollars for Fredrick missing from large trunk where*[entry ends].*

June 11, 1961: Miss Shepherd cleaned frigidaire.

June 16, 1961: Mr Doran cleaned frigidaire either today or yesterday.

June 19, 1961: a genuinely resented card[290] from May—where is their humour sense?

---

289 Virginia Hale, or "Aunt Naya", was Paula's maternal aunt and provided significant support, emotional and financial, during these years.

290 This card has not survived.

July 6, 1961: Found sea dollar box moved missing it was there a few months ago—today have book addressed to Mrs Creighton Scott 46 Hampstead Rd Hemsted Spring Valley Rockland County insured NY 24, NY December 10th, 1955 signed for Benjamin F by Charles Strand. Someone scribbled "Mirabell" on it—July 22nd 1957 both parcels were held 19 months before returned by Jamaica LI though return address Benjamin etc was clearly written on each. They was returned opened.

July 8, 1961: Sievy or Sevier cleaned frigidaire today.

July 24, 1961: Mrs Sevy cleaned frigidaire.

The family left Carmel in August 1961 for a rented farmhouse in the tiny historic (founded 1776) village of Peacham in Vermont. It had long been a dream of Jigg's to one day settle down on a farm in Vermont, and it is likely that he hoped this move would be a new beginning for the family. Denise had started university and the other children settled into their new life in Vermont while Jigg was desperately trying to find work in spite of the effects his mother's letter writing had had on his life. And, true to form, and in spite of her poor health, Evelyn continued to try and track them to their new address and new life.

From John Metcalfe's diary:

August 2, 1961: Miss Shepherd cleaned frigidaire.

August 11, 1961: E cleaned frigidaire.

August 20, 1961: Worked at novel. Lunch. Nap. E had an attack and I got supper. Bed.

August 21, 1961: Went school. Wretched tropical rainy muggy day. E still poorly when I got home.

August 22, 1961: E no better.

August 23, 1961: Decided to get dr for E, - trying first at 214 E 18th to get information as to when May and Lew would be back from Europe. Spoke to Miss Young re possibility of drs. Took bus along 2nd Avenue and was admitted to No 214. Asked maid when May and L wd be back, + she said she would "get information". She soon reappeared and asked me upstairs, where, to my surprise and satisfaction, I found May + Lew! Discussion re Evelyn, - + May said she wd come over to see us between 1 and 2. They (M + L) had been back some months on account of L's illness. Told E the good news, + we had lunch and short nap. May arrived at 2 + stayed till 3. E to be as much like a vegetable as possible. E seems somewhat better.

This last diary entry heralds what turned out to be a cataclysmic change in Evelyn's health as Jack recounts his first efforts to get help for what was then described as a "cerebral attack" and would now be called a stroke. The effect on Evelyn was clearly serious.

The stroke appears to have led to some form of rapprochement between Jigg and his mother. Perhaps a long-dormant filial instinct was awakened by learning of a serious medical event with a profound effect on what she could now do. Perhaps he had just become resigned to the effect his now-disabled mother had had on his life. And perhaps he had some sympathy for Jack and what he imagined Jack was having to face.

To Evelyn Scott

Carmel California
August 26, 1961

EVELYN METCALFE
222 WEST 77 ST NYC
YOUR REGISTERED LETTER RECEIVED ALL IS WELL LOVE Paula
[Telegram. SFC]

From John Metcalfe's diary:

August 28, 1961: E slowly improving.
September 5, 1961: *A very cerirt [sic] of a great several to all us thing of it -a great a literally Cyril was a great men*
Walked to Lex Ave PO where mailed letter, air-mail registered, to Jigg. Had just got to bed when answered a call from office saying a telegram had arrived for me. Went down and got it. It proved to be from Western Union saying Jigg had no 'phone number listed, so my wire to him would go by post.
September 11, 1961: Gladys came at 4.30, had tea, and stayed till about 5.15.

Love Lyle and Evelyn had been corresponding for some time, largely about their extended families of cousins in Clarksville, and Jack, recognising that Love was concerned about Evelyn's health, took over the correspondence and kept Love updated on Evelyn's condition.

To Love Lyle

The Benjamin Franklin Hotel
October 8, 1961

Dear Love,

Many thanks for your last letter,[291] with all its news. Evelyn was very interested in "Tom" etc.

This, as usual I fear, is only a scrappy reply, - just another "bulletin" to report that Evelyn continues slowly to improve, - though still incapable of writing. Her doctor, May Mayers, was due back in town on the 1st, but has protracted her vacation. However, she should return very soon, this week probably, and will then look us up.

---

291 This letter has not survived.

Yes, we are so glad the heat is over at last. I myself love the fall more than any other season.

Forgive more just now

Much love from us both

Jack

Hope you yourself are keeping well.

[Handwritten, signed. UTK]

To Love Lyle

The Benjamin Franklin Hotel

October 30, 1961

Dear Love,

Thank you for your letter, which Evelyn much enjoyed, as always, - and if I do not comment in detail on all your news of friends it doesn't mean that she was not interested and appreciative. As you know, I spent two weeks in Clarksville in, I think, 1931 or 1932. Evelyn's mother was, of course, then alive, - and I remember several of her (E's) cousins. I liked the country, - though it was a little too warm (106 one day!). We went out to Redbrook and Dunbar's Cave.

She goes on improving, gradually. Her doctor saw her on October 10th and was pleased with her progress. But it is of course a great trial to her to be stalled, for the time being, in work on her novel, upon which she has been engaged for 20 years!

The weather now is lovely, - bright and cool. I daresay it is the same down your way?

Much love from us both,

Jack.

[Handwritten, signed. UTK]

To Evelyn Scott and John Metcalfe

Carmel, California

November 4, 1961

Dear Mother and Jack,

I finally got Jack's last letter after many delays, and I am glad to hear you will be able to get along without too much grief, because I am in no position to be of help. I keep looking, but the prospects grow slimmer all the time, and I don't seem to have any friends in the world. However, we have managed to survive so far, and we will continue to make out in one way or another.

I hope mother feels better - heaven knows I'm sorry to hear of all these disasters. I can appreciate the burden is on you, Jack, to keep going; and I am more than a little surprised both of you don't head back for England.

If it's any use, I mention you both in my prayers, which is about all I can do. It's been a funny existence, and the funniest part is the waste of all our energies.

All the sturm and drang and the frenzies and exertions of the last fifty years have accomplished exactly nothing, and all our time would have been better spent planting cabbages. I'd like nothing better than to be a competent plumber, or something of the sort.

Anyway, best wishes, and I'll write again now and then. let me know how you are faring.

Affectionately,

Jigg

[Typed, signed. UTK]

From John Metcalfe's diary:

November 6, 1961: Letter from Jigg today.

November 25, 1961: E went out with me for short stroll for first time since her attack on August 20th. Weather cool + pleasant.

To Love Lyle

The Benjamin Franklin Hotel

November 26, 1961

Dear Love,

Thank you for your last letter. Your letters, so fresh and newsy, always put me to shame, because I am a poor fist, I'm afraid, at the epistolary art!

Well, Evelyn went out yesterday (Saturday) afternoon with me for her first stroll since her attack just over three months ago. We only went for a few blocks along Broadway and back, - but it was a beginning and we both enjoyed it.

She is talking just a little better each day, though the progress is very gradual.

I ordered a ready-roast Turkey for Thanksgiving, and, lacking the courage to try and cook it (or rather, re-warm it), we had it cold (but nice) on two nights. I have a 4-days break from school, - Thursday through Sunday, - and have been appreciating that.

No more just for now.

Much love from us both,

Jack

I tried to write a letter more completely yours again. I thought of the duck-hunting when Uncle Julian so often at Redfoot, but I can say for myself later though wonderful to Jack's remember to notes.

I hope I will have again soon for Jigg, who has to ask to move here soon I request. But the good improvement we thank you, too

[Handwritten, signed. Handwritten PS by ES. UTK]

From John Metcalfe's diary:

December 8, 1961: E lost wallet of photographs, so I put notice in kitchen, + left word at office. Came home, - wallet found by E.

December 25, 1961: Worked at novel etc.

December 30, 1961: May arrived at 2 + stayed till 3.30, - pronouncing Evelyn improved.

Chapter 42

1962

During her last years, Evelyn had become more and more isolated from all but a very few close friends, particularly Gladys Grant who remained close to Evelyn and to Jack and at the same time loyal to Jigg and Paula and their children.

Nineteen letters only survive from this year, eight of them to members of her Clarksville family. Jack's diary mentions a number of letters from Evelyn to Jigg, but sadly none of those has survived. Those that have survived clearly illustrate the effect of her stroke on Evelyn's mental capacity.

Evelyn's letters to her cousin Love Lyle in Clarksville show very clearly how her stroke had affected her. (Although handwritten, they have been transcribed for ease of reading.) None of Love's replies to these letters has been preserved.

From John Metcalfe's diary:

January 16, 1962: Frigidaire—that cleared.

January 17, 1962: Celebrated Evelyn's birthday by staying at home, with gumboil.

To Love Lyle

The Benjamin Franklyn Hotel
January 18, 1962

Dearest Love,

I hope the ice in Tennessee is mild! It should have better earlier yesterday and yesterday was my birthday. It was rotten! I wish I had your birthday and both were enjoyed you. I also longed to have us here with Jack and I could delight with Jigg, Paula and all our darling youngsters! They have yet to find the <u>Job</u> for Jigg and money enough for all of them.

I hope my son will eventually in the Eastern states that will be as all his live in NY as Paul also knows and the five children were born in New York.

I guess that foreigners in the Pacific are too many, even as we see them too much in New York. But our Scotts have relations and my and Jack's are in here. Paula's Education

467

when she was young her, and Jigg's was here, too, except when he was with Cyril in Denver while Dean of University of Denver and Jigg was a student. But Jigg also was to paint in NY until he married, and also was serious novel.

However, Jigg had began as soon as with the war, he received newspaper, editing received in USA. He has worked in radio news for it was they supposed that in San Francisco, they might they would be officially employed there as he returned home after abroad in Washington, DC.

Of this has been the worst result in there in San Francisco. Jigg thinks union very bad there.

Anyhow, we hope! Paula was educated, also, in Europe. She began a book, but they had begun also the union would not allow her book in NY.

I have been continuing toward my heart - not always as to other things! - as the result that produced cerebral haemorrhage developed slow conversation and writing.

Jack has encouraged me, but am not pretty well to myself. But any person who speaks not slowly and with expressiveness naturally.

I hope you now can read patiently for me. I have a woman doctor in New York who insisted months ago that I will recovered, even when darling Jack could not to me indicate the words she had insisted. I often heard words from without or in the hotel. Even when not a conversation not been mentioned to me.

Anyhow, dear Love, you have worked the way you have achieved more natural free than must surely now yours before your hurt.

Love, Love
Evelyn

[Handwritten, signed. UTK]

From John Metcalfe's diary:

January 25, 1962: Letters from R Pearson (disturbing), Bernie, Charlotte, + Maggie (enclosing $50), Wrote Maggie (E added PS about V Hale) returning cheque. Went out again and mailed this.

February 5, 1962: Mailed letter, E to Jigg.

To Love Lyle

The Benjamin Franklin Hotel
February 5, 1961 *[sic]*

Dear darling Love,

I am always moved to you. Denise will be on February 8th, and I would she was already here and with all her sister and her brothers and all with their parents! I wish you lived here often!

They are longing to the old New England or near, if not further in the California. They have been on return from abroad stuck in Carmel for three and one years and though Jig had always been a job for radio for 20 years, we dont yet know where without a penny. When he and the family were after earlier in abroad he had a suppose that he would be resumed some of the radio business as they landed home, the doldrum has the result. He had just enough to feed for that abruptly.

Of course they might have met people some of them further toward our time, but there are none. There are too many foreigners in the California. They are seldom serious in respect to high quality.

I have longing to help! They were working as much as they. Several people in New York know Jig in remember yet his fine books and his painting as Paula also indicted his talent in writing but haven't NY remembered less today - of the serious mens once his in the original radio jobs.

But of course the bob is vital, and I, too, think and thinking. In New York, also, there is a congested everywhere. Still, the New England generally is possible we hope, as New York and about it Jig and Paula were they began here, and where all the children were born.

Well, dear Love, I am bursting! If Jig could go to Clarksville, he probably might have realized as many foreign as here.

Love to you to Jack, too. You know we feel for your kindness always.

So love again for you and your thoughts of Denise!
Evelyn

[Handwritten, signed. UTK]

From John Metcalfe's diary:

February 8, 1962: <u>Posted card from E to Jigg.</u>

To Love Lyle

The Benjamin Franklin Hotel
February 10, 1962

Dear Love,

I'll be glad to hear that water is drying! I can't remember of high water in Spring Street, though that my view was of the set of the rivers were sometimes of largeness. Am I still that the Library was Spring Street in the quaint once the cottage in which my great uncle Ewing Pike McGinty lived with her sisters? The Library, however, must now housed in a different street, too.

We wish that we had received our mail from Paula, to whom she seems not yet to have answer to us of Denise, when I wrote to your birthday. I hope to discover what where my letters are in Carmel by now, but often, portions of mail we don't hear of, or they are received after a month is finally delivered. It's horrible. In any better mail my family will be thankful - and for me and Jack! The USA should be in Carmel and NY City at the time.

You can realize that my pencil is not as good as in the first page, and my indignant insists more expression than the rest. Not at all the country has been equally of the USA!

Love, my dear sweet friend!
Evelyn

PS All the Scotts think of the NY State. They should never continued in California. Parents and children still hope their lives in the Eastern State and certainly grandmother knows that. Too many foreigners! Too much UNO. USA, USA, and old, old British can a decent country!

[Handwritten letter and PS, signed. UTK]

From John Metcalfe's diary:

February 11, 1962: Mailed letter from E to Jigg.
February 14, 1962: Mailed letter from E to Jigg.

To Love Lyle

The Benjamin Franklin Hotel
February 20, 1962

Dear Love,

Jack and I enjoyed your birthday of Denise for we ourselves feel Denise is among your own Angels. In fact the persoutation *[sic]* of Angels is you, for you think up for Jigg, Paula and all the children we care fors your remembering thoughts.

I mailed Denise's especially fine note, and if it arrived we will be more kisses for me and Jack will bless you; Paula knew you as "Evelyn's friend" and of Jack mother's old friend of Clarksville and Va-va[292] (Miss Maud).

I wrote recently about the longing we hope that Jigg and Paula would be found Jigg's job and the childrens near to us, and near enough to improve education circles. All of them work but of Denise who has the eldest and has worked more she has the most brilliant.

However, Jigg and Paula's all children are intelligent and as that both the parents, the grandfather and a step-grandfather and a grandmother we think we should discover justice.

They are old Americans, and in Carmel and San Francisco, they would be better in N Y S than many foreigners there do not grasped intelligent Americans - old still, USA and as Jack agree that all the Scotts should be of their sort.

Bless, Love! Thank you for remembering, sweet good Love.

Evelyn and as Jack agreed.

[Handwritten, signed. UTK]

---

292 "Vava" was Jigg's childhood nickname for his grandmother Maude.

From John Metcalfe's diary:

February 21, 1962: 1 *postcard Pearson mailed 1 Theis K mail note and postcard 1 Love Lyle mail.*

February 22, 1962: E has caught my cold, + we had a v disturbed night, she snoring so!

February 23, 1962: E's cold v bad and mine pretty rotten still, so stayed from school again. Went bank + did some shopping. Bought E blue purse.

February 26, 1962: Came home, marketed, and <u>mailed letter from E to Jigg.</u>

To Creighton Scott

The Benjamin Franklin Hotel

March 11, 1962

Dear Jigg,

It is a long time since we heard from you and to have a line would delight us. We do hope affairs are brighter with you, and naturally we remain worried about you till we have word. Evelyn, particularly, is prone to picture all kinds of calamities, - and a letter from you would, I hope, dispel such fears and help to set her mind at rest. The pace of her recovery depends largely upon her freedom from worry, and serenity of spirit.

To repeat, with undiminished conviction, what I said in a previous letter she loves you dearly, always has and always will, and has never wished anything but good for all of you. I am "next to" her, and know it in the immediate way one knows one's own right hand. Please believe this.

It would make us both immeasurably happier to hear from you.

Jack

[This handwritten note was added to the bottom of Jack's letter.]

Dear Jigg,

I wish you, Paula, the five loved children would be in NY State and to have near us in USA NY too. The many things to be yours we could have in US State.

I have not allowed published as I have never accepted union since 1940. Jack, Paula, you, Virginia Hale should be known again in NY books and paints.

I suspect that Denise and the older boys will some day led original arts, too.

We hear about helping for you all.

Mother

[Both handwritten, both signed. Posted, registered, to Carmel address, returned to sender unopened. UTK]

From John Metcalfe's diary:

March 11, 1962: Wrote (i.e. finished writing) letter to Jigg, to which E added some more.*[see above]*

March 17, 1962: Our wedding anniversary, - bless us!

The Scotts had left Carmel for Vermont during the summer of 1961. Their reasons are not made clear in any correspondence (in fact none remains from this period) and it appears Evelyn knew nothing of this move until a letter addressed to Jigg in Carmel was returned to her marked "Moved - left no address". This rekindled Evelyn's efforts to trace her son by writing to any official body and, in particular, Carmel High School, which she thought might be able to give her information about his whereabouts

From John Metcalfe's diary:

March 19, 1962: Came home and found that my letter to Jigg had been returned, Marked "Moved left no address". Composed draft of letter from E to Principal of High School Carmel.

March 20, 1962: Made fair copy of letter from E to Principal. Work.

March 21, 1962: Went G[rand] Central PO and <u>sent off letter to Principal, RR Registered airmail.</u>

March 22, 1962: Bought E pen for $2.04.

March 28, 1962: Came home. Letter from Principal of Carmel High School giving Jigg's address as "General Delivery, St Johnsbury, Vermont". E wrote letter to him (Jigg).

March 29, 1962: <u>Mailed letter to Jigg</u> (St Johnsbury Vt) Registered, return receipt, on way to school. Came home. Marketed and mailed letter from E, thanking Principal of Carmel High School. Letter to Jigg included previous letter and envelope as well as fresh note from E.

April 13, 1962: Came home and found <u>E had had our letter to Jigg returned "Unclaimed".</u>

To Love Lyle

The Benjamin Franklin Hotel
April 13, 1962

Jack's love - you bet

Dear Love,

Your letter has, again, revived my memories, with the spring flowers and the Cumberland, the flood having been a dramatic phase.

I wish Jig and Paula and our five young could have been with Jack and I in Clarksville for a holiday. Soon, after I wrote you, I received a mail receipt from Carmel with the return of a letter just sent by me to Jig and Paula. I did not know to do, but decided to write again to Carmel's High School to ask where my grandchildren were, as Paula wrote of the school about two years of them. The school's authority replied to me (I rewritten, too, having been answered the Scott grandmother) that three Scotts were originally in the school, but that Mr and Mrs Creighton Scott could be their now address in St Johnsbury, Vermont, General Delivery. The fact that my grandchildren are five instead of just three, I found uneasy.

However, Jack mailed both my unreceived letters (one within of Jack for me), and I awaited replied! - to St Johnsbury.

A horrid interval, a week ago in the hotel, I discover that, when I was in a bathroom, a spy snook into my room, where my letters of Carmel's school and a telegram of years ago that I had preserved of Scotts' address for Rt Road and 410 Box.293 These two things had been there open, as I consulted of the school letter for the number of the street. Well, anyhow, I wanted to hear about St Johnsbury's PO. And now today, April 13, I received the returned registered Jack mailed to Jig and Paula - my own letter and Jack's own scratched against Jig's and Paula's address.

I don't know what to do - again! I didn't think St Johnsbury, Vermont was adequately the Scotts' residence!

Rt 2 Road, 410 Box, I remember of Carmel - though Rt 2 Road may be error. Do any of Clarksville friends know Carmel? And please the Major's name, he too knew London.

Gratefully, Evelyn.

[Handwritten, signed. UTK]

From John Metcalfe's diary:

April 18, 1962: School. On way there posted E's letter to Department of State. On my return Gladys was having tea with E.

May 1, 1962: Fredrick my mail.

May 2, 1962: Mrs Sevey—refrigerator.

May 10, 1962: School. Letter from Dept of State to Evelyn. I mailed letter from E to Pearson.

To Miss Frances Knight[294]

The Benjamin Franklin Hotel
May 14, 1962

Miss Frances Knight
Director, Passport Offices
Department of State Washington 25, DC
Dear Miss Knight,

With reference to your various older letters, - file No Y130: -

On April 18th 1962 I wrote to the Passport Office, Department of State, requesting information as to whether or not my American son, Creighton Seeley Scott - and also his wife Paula Scott and their five children, Denise, Frederick, Matthew, Julia and Robert - were still in the USA.

---

293 The post office in Carmel did not deliver to street addresses and house numbers, and residents had to collect their mail from the town post office. Paula and Jigg's postal address was therefore "Route 2, Box 412".

294 This letter is in interesting contrast to those to her cousin Love Lyle a few days earlier. It is likely that Evelyn dictated it to Jack who produced a more coherent letter than she might have done unaided. There is no record of any reply.

Three days ago a reply to me from the Passport Office, signed K, stated that Creighton Seeley Scott was issued with Passport No 248518 on June 23rd 1959 at Saigon and that, since then, he had "not requested further passport facilities". The letter also stated that the Passport Office had no record of Paula Scott since 1955.

My son was again in Washington DC in August 1959, as I and my husband read, in the New York World-Telegram & Sun of August 12th. Mr Creighton Seeley Scott (the article ran) was testifying before a congressional sub-committee, and also before the Senate, respecting the American-financed Viet-Namese National Radio Project; while, simultaneously, Mr Wallace Gade was testifying, before the House, concerning the radio and other communications of South East Asia generally as well as of Viet Nam.

My daughter-in-law Paula Scott and the five children had arrived in Carmel California before my son gave testimony in Washington and he resigned from his employment by ICA. He went, then, to San Francisco, and within a year, to Carmel.

From Carmel, my daughter-in-law corresponded with me and with my husband (my son's stepfather) for about a year-and-a-half, writing mostly about the children's schooling. I have some of her Carmel-post-marked letters dated as follows:-

In 1959: - July 24th, Octr 19th, Oct 22nd, Novr 12th, Decr 2nd, Decr 10th. And in 1960:- March 5th, March 24th, Apl 5th, June [illeg] Oct 4th, and Novr 25th. We did not hear from her afterwards.

In the spring of 1961[295] my son wrote to me about his children and said that he was too worried to write further. However, in August 1961 I had a cerebral haemorrhage, and my son, after some delay, did write to my husband, his stepfather, about me. And actually he did write three further letters, but always after delays.

Since then we have had not letters, and when my health improved and I again wrote to my son and to my daughter-in-law my letters received no reply.

November 1961 seemed to mark an end of correspondence.

About six or seven weeks ago I wrote to the Principal of Carmel High Schools, where I knew my three eldest grandchildren had studied. I asked him if he could give me the present address of the Scotts, and was told by him that the address of Mr and Mrs Creighton Scott was "General Delivery, St Johnsbury, Vermont". My husband and I wrote to my son there and after ten days our letter was returned to us marked "Unclaimed".

I am indeed distressed - and we know no one in California or elsewhere who might give us a clue to the family's whereabouts.

I will be most grateful for any possible suggestion about my son's, and his wife's location.

---

295 This is very likely Jigg's letter of December 31, 1960 (Chapter 40), which his mother would not have received until early 1961. She appears to have misinterpreted what Jigg was trying to say.

Creighton Seeley Scott was born an American and so was Paula Scott. They and their children are all US citizens, and proud of it. All the children were born in New York City or in Nyack, NY, and Red Hook,[296] NY.

I apologise for this long letter. Sincerely yours,

[Typed carbon copy, not signed. UTK]

From John Metcalfe's diary:

May 17, 1962: <u>E wrote to Principal Carmel High School some 8 or 9 days ago.</u>

May 18, 1962: Came home and found letter from Mr Edwards, Principal of Carmel High School giving Frederick's address as at Peacham Academy, Peacham, Vermont (Headmaster Mr Russel POWDEN Jr).

May 21, 1962: <u>Mailed letter Ret Ret Reg from E to Frederick</u>. Mailed letter from E to Gladys. *offensive postcard of Roland P fool like Ralph— same against us.*

May 24, 1962: ES refrigidair—nxt time f off—not edf.?

May 25, 1962: postcard to Roland Pearson—wrong.

May 26, 1962: due writing to Dept of State.

May 31, 1962: <u>Letter to E from Dept</u>. of State saying they will write later after looking up file.

June 1, 1962: At school, George DeSilver told me Maggie was not expected to live through the day. Rang hospital and eventually was told that Maggie had "expired" that morning.

June 2, 1962: <u>Letter from Dept of State.</u> Quite unsatisfactory. Telegram came announcing Maggie's death and giving time + place of memorial service on Monday.

June 15, 1962: letter to Glad more.

June 22, 1962: Came home and found E had lost her $29.

June 27, 1962: the nurse—refrigerator. Kept awake by Macy's display of fireworks.

To Evelyn Scott and John Metcalfe

Carmel, California

June 30, 1962

Dear mother and jack,

This is to let you know we are all right. I haven't found a job yet and we are hard up, but our health is pretty good; there have been no serious illnesses, and I don't want you to worry about it.

We manage to get along and hope you do, too. The job problem is serious. A man of my age, with not even a grade school diploma and a record he can't refer to has a

----

296 The fourth child, Julia, was actually born in Rhinebeck, New York.

hard time, but by pulling together we manage. We hope you are better, mother, and that you are okay, too, jack. Take care of yourselves.

There is no point in trying to answer this. We are constantly on the move, and mother's habit of writing to anybody she might know of who might know me is too dangerous to encourage. Registered letters with receipts I have to sign to show you where I am won't work, and neither will writing to postmasters. For the moment we have no address.

However, we don't want you to wear yourselves out fretting about us. We wonder about you, but as there is nothing we can do, we don't ask how you are. But we hope for the best.

Affectionately,

Jigg

[Typed, signed. UTK]

From John Metcalfe's diary:

July 2, 1962: Heard from Jigg, - envelope post-marked "San Jose" California.
July 6, 1962: about key Julia.
July 13, 1962: Where are the letters write postcards? - of Herschel, of Ruth.
August 1, 1962: Cataract removed.
August 3, 1962: Fine Jack telephoned—grateful hope more for him good.
August 4, 1962: Phone Jack—sweet better.
August 5, 1962: Jack phoned - bless him. Miss Shepherd sent him some Ellery Queen. Miss Shepherd—did refrigedair
August 7, 1962: Phone by Jack Home for Jack later.
August 8, 1960: Jack phoned but admitted he suffered yesterday, last night and this morning. He gave a hypo postcard to May, Scotland.
August 9, 1962: <u>HOME!</u>[297]
August 10, 1962: Gladys 'phoned at about 1.45 + said she would be here in about an hour. Which did.
August 16, 1962: E's foot bad.
August 17, 1962: E's foot still bad. E's foot was too painful for her to go out, so I did Marketing alone, buying new Pyrex dish to serve as ash-tray. Evelyn kept awake with retching cough.
August 18, 1962: E's chest pains etc bad, + I Marketed (2 trips). Mr Seavy carried in supper for E, who couldn't manage it.
August 19, 1962: E still poorly.

---

297 Jack's cataract operation had involved a stay in hospital.

August 21, 1962: weekend 1 day sent legs hurt last night electric storm rotten -not as good as Jack in need to sleep for eye.

To Love Lyle

The Benjamin Franklin Hotel
August 29, 1962

Dear sweet Love,

Jack has heard about you when he was at the hospital and he enjoys your letters to just as ever, and I will be hoping to know he can write as much as he naturally does. He always says you are a dear! I had a rotten interference about my legs during two weeks, but it is better and I should like to buy things often to help Jack better. He is improving, but I wish to care for him. I would delight to see him free.

Indeed we - Jack and I - are still hoping to have another letter of Creighton, not so far away. We have his precious letter with us, and of course we will be excited whenever we hear letters of Denise and Fredrick. Paula may write us, too. They are still in California, but my best dream is to see them in the East. Old American! All the five children!

Jack and I are determined to resume our books, and the elder grandchildren may interest us as their tendencies to books.

Anyhow, a coloured friend recently found us some good good tomatoes! I love scientific comment, but my experience continues to tomatoes in gardens in Clarkville - to 611 Madison[298] and in the Drane[299] garden at Second St. Theirs were the best of all. Or do you agree?

Love to you from Jack and me
Evelyn

[Handwritten, signed. UTK]

From John Metcalfe's diary:

August 31, 1962: Eye still troublesome. Gladys rang up, - and came here about 3.30. She + E had tea while I had "lunch". G left about 5.30.

September 6, 1962: Dr Wadsworth's[300] bill arrived - for $500. Eye continues somewhat better, (touch wood).

September 11, 1962: Paula with love - both of us, too.

September 20, 1962: Evelyn got out winter clothes this morning and I put on my "stooped" suit.

---

298 The street address of the Gracey mansion.
299 The Dranes were related to Maude
300 Dr Wadsworth was the ophthalmologist who had looked after Jack.

In the autumn of 1962, after 15 months in Vermont, Jigg decided that he and his family should leave the United States for Canada. The conflict in Vietnam was looming and Frederick and Matthew were of an age to be drafted; it was thought they would be safe in Canada. And perhaps more significantly, Jigg hoped that by becoming, with Jack's help, a Canadian citizen, he would have more opportunities for employment than he had had during the previous three years.

The aging Volkswagen bus that had brought the family from California to Vermont broke down shortly after crossing the Canadian border and the family found themselves in the sleepy town of Chester, Nova Scotia, about 40 miles from Halifax, where they spent their first winter in the disused drive-in theatre before they were able to move to more permanent accommodation in the town.

From John Metcalfe's diary:

October 5, 1962: buy for you for two letter blocks.

October 6, 1962: Jack loved still and more. My anniversary.

October 8, 1962: E cleared frigidaire. Garden Market shut for Yom Kippur so shopped at Gourmet + Horn and Hardart. Gravy from beef pie spilled on my suit and E cleaned it.

October 25, 1962: Creighton loved still E cut head and sprained wrist.

November 5, 1962: Our carpet was cleaned today and now looks very nice.

November 11, 1962: Fredrick.

November 14, 1962: Weather unpropitious for E's going out with me as planned.

November 19, 1962: still pictures 12 plus sketch pencil Cyril 14 with the framed, 1 Cyril water-colours, 1 re Creighton illustration of my novel, Creighton not completed. Jack letter of both to Nesta. Jack registered letter to Mrs Vincent contained letter to Mr P I Wellman. Jack registered my letter to Mrs Dakin cont check - hope was corrected as owed

December 1, 1962: Bought Christmas cards today, at Wormrath's.

December 2, 1962: Breakfast about ten. E poorly still.

December 25, 1962: Worked as normal. Lunch. Nap. Gave $10 tip to Sam. Work. Supper of Beef, Onions + plum-pudding. Bed.

Chapter 43

1963

Evelyn died on August 3, 1963 of a heart attack with lung cancer as a contributing factor. Jack's diary reveals much of the months immediately preceding her death. Not many of Evelyn's letters survive; it may have been because Evelyn was recovering from the effects of a stroke a few months previously and was not writing as many as usual. Or it may be because they were among those Jack, in his grief, destroyed after her death.

Jack's diary entries as well as his letters to his friend John Gawsworth and to Jigg chronicle the progress of Evelyn's symptoms and hospital treatment in characteristic detail, graphically revealing his despair while at the same time hanging on to the hope of the two of them returning to England and using the proceeds from the sale of Number 26 to buy a small cottage somewhere. And throughout this period, he struggled with his own deteriorating mental health while trying to keep his "school job" going.

The following is Jack's record in letters and diary entries of the progress of Evelyn's final illness.

To Love Lyle

The Benjamin Franklin Hotel
January 24, 1963

Dear Love,

Thank you for sympathetic letter, - which I could not, however, show to Evelyn.[301]

Could you, please, write to her, care of me, just cheerfully without too specific allusion to her malady?

Actually, the outlook is slightly better. A biopsy was taken, showing the mass to consist of a type of cell responsive to radio-therapy, which she has now been receiving or 5 days. It is even hoped by her doctors that she may be able to return here in 3 - 4 weeks. Then continue the treatments as an out-patient, - though how I could take her up there daily and still hold my school job wd be a problem. We'll wait and see, and pray.

---

301 This letter has not survived.

Much love,

Jack

Just write to her, c/o myself, here, and I'll take it up to her at the hospital.

[Handwritten, signed. UTK]

From John Metcalfe's diary:

January 23, 1963: Went out to chemists to buy E cough lozenges and a roll of cotton.

January 25, 1963: Letter from Gladys, who broke her arm + had to return early from W Indies.

January 26, 1963: Evelyn poorly. Mrs Seavy recommended her Dr Cohen, - EN 2588. I 'phoned him and he will come tomorrow.

January 27, 1963: Obtained permission to leave school at 11.50. Came home. Dr Cohen arrived soon after 2 o'clock, examined E, + prescribed Diuril[302]

March 7, 1963: Came home and 'phoned Dr Cohen. E to take only one diuril tablet a day, - and I to 'phone Dr Cohen next Monday.

March 13, 1963: <u>Last day at school for a while</u>…got home after three to find Dr Cohen already with Evelyn. He had given her an injection + said I should not go to school for several days.

To John Gawsworth

The Benjamin Franklin Hotel

March 18, 1963

Dear John,

For God's sake <u>write</u>. If ever I needed a friend it is now, to save me from final despair. Write, for pete's sake, but <u>do not refer to this letter.</u> I have bad medical news of Evelyn, and am near to a breakdown myself. It is a dreadful situation. My heart is breaking, - yet how can I tell her, fully, the reason, though she must guess it. I am seeing a psychiatrist Wednesday, + may he be a miracle-worker, since miracles are needed. I cannot sleep or anything. I have had to give up my teaching job "temporarily" as don't know if I could ever hold it again. But my only ray of hope is that we should lay our bones in England, - and you are my only real understanding friend there. If, somehow, I can pluck courage out of a hat, I could stay over here perhaps another year, saving money (if I can hold job again) + then come over, with her. She agreed to this this morning. It is the one hope I cling to. To know that you are there, would be there whenever we came, wd be a comfort.

If the psychiatrist recommends a spell in a sanatorium, - what can I do? There's no money, + anyhow what would poor E do? - She can't look after herself + now when I should help her I am collapsing.

---

302 Diuril is a diuretic used to treat oedema and hypertension, both associated with heart failure.

My only hope is to come with her I hope to England.

No more now. I am writing this on the sly in a "pub". I must hear from you. Forgive selfishness, but I'm v unwell trying for the last 15 days, to bear an insupportable strain.

Do write, just an ordinary letter, - (I may find, later, an accommodation-address to which you could write me without restraint).

Love,

Jack

[Handwritten, signed. HRC]

From John Metcalfe's diary:

March 19, 1963: Dr Cohen came.

March 27, 1963: Dr Cohen had not arrived as arranged at 3, so rang him also. Will come this evening at 8.30…Dr Cohen arrived 8.30 and prescribed sleeping-tablets for E. Paid him $7. I went out + got prescription filled.

March 29, 1963: Went St Vincents[303] and had preliminary interview 3.30, from which it appears that I should come again next Wednesday 2.30 with bank-statements etc etc.

April 8, 1963: Letter from Gladys with $50, which I deposited in bank at about 2.30. Light lunch and nap. Rang Gladys to thank her.

April 11, 1963: 11th saw Jack—loved him again John Metcalfe St Vincent Hospital Reiss Pavilion 144 West 12th St New York 11.

April 15, 1963: To Dr A Cohen—I am sure I haven't given what I owe. If Jack comes or I saw him I will put what I owe.

Jigg and his family had left Vermont for Canada during the previous Summer. For reasons that were partly emotional, partly financial and partly political, Jigg had hoped to create a new life for himself and his family in Canada, intending to adopt Canadian citizenship as a final declaration of this new chapter of his and his family's lives.

Evelyn did not learn of this move until the following spring, when the discovery came as a surprise to her. By the time she got the news, she was being treated for lung cancer and in and out of hospital. In addition, her stroke of the previous winter had affected her writing, which had become confused and at times incoherent.

---

303 Formally St Vincent's Catholic Medical Center, the hospital was a major teaching centre from its foundation in 1849 until its closure in 2005.

To John Metcalfe

Chester, Nova Scotia
May 3, 1963

<u>CONFIDENTIAL & PRIVATE</u>

Dear Jack,

This is for you personally, with regards to Mother. I am settling in Canada and have mentioned that you were the first to bring me here. If you hear from the Canadian Immigration I hope you will answer them for us.

Life in the States got to be just too much and I ended up with a coronary that almost did for me last July in Vermont. Here the pressures are relieved. We've been here all winter, and a rugged one it was.

I'll write from time to time hereafter, but for Pete's sake please stem the flow and don't let anyone start writing to postmasters and officials, except you, if they ask.

Affectionately,

Jigg

[Typed, signed. UTK]

From John Metcalfe's diary:

May 8, 1963: I returned from hospital and was astonished to find letter from Jigg awaiting me. The family are now in Nova Scotia! Upper denture finally broke and I went to Dr Foster.

May 14, 1963: I 'phoned Dr Cohen but could get no reply. Phoned an hour later, still to no avail. But a third attempt was fruitful, - + he is to be here tomorrow at 2 o'clock.

To Creighton Scott

The Benjamin Franklin Hotel
May 19, 1963

My Dear Jigg,

I found your welcome letter awaiting me on my recent return from hospital, and this is to wish all of you the greatest possible success and happiness in the new country. We were distressed to hear of your coronary trouble. May it speedily be relieved and health be completely restored!

Yes, I well remember our sojourn in Montreal, - the Hollywood Apartments, and Mr Britten's school, - and snow, snow, snow. I imagine that the Nova Scotian winter must be at least as severe, though reassured by you saying pressures are relieved. If the Canadian Immigration write about you I will answer any questions they may ask.

Our own healths have been nothing to boast of latterly. I, as I say, have been in hospital and Evelyn's cardiac condition been very worrying. I am at present convalescing at "home" but expect to be back at my school job shortly.

We do hope that Paula and the rest of the family are thriving and the children doing well at school and college. Their careers are a matter of deep concern to us.

Evelyn sends her love.

Affectionately,

Jack

[Handwritten, signed. SFC]

From John Metcalfe's diary:

May 19, 1963: Wrote to Jigg. Mailed these letters, and also letter from E too.

May 21, 1963: Rang Dr Cohen who will come this afternoon at 3. Dr Cohen came at three. I went out to chemists again for Taractan and Buta Perinide[304] capsules. The latter will not be ready till tomorrow.

To John Metcalfe

Chester, Nova Scotia

May 24, 1963

Dear Jack,

I'm very distressed to hear that you've been ill. I hope it wasn't anything very serious. Your courage and steadfastness where others wouldn't hold out has always awed me a little. I hope Mother is all right. Perhaps it will help a little bit if you give her my love, good wishes, and tell her that we are all well though somewhat ragged after almost three and a half years without a job, plus my coronary. That's healed by now and if I take care of myself it will be OK from now on.

I certainly wish you the best, as we all do. I hope you will both forgive my past evil temper. I'll write from time to time and tell you how we are.

Affectionately,

Jigg

[Typed, signed. UTK]

From John Metcalfe's diary:

May 25, 1963: E sick all night and through the day inconsequence of too much diuril. *1 suit and one good blue dress were in a bag from Woolworth - just made of my effort.*

May 27, 1963: Box 19, Chester, NS. Returned to school. Came home to find letter from Jigg. Marketed. Rang Dr Cohen - who will visit E at 3 tomorrow.

May 28, 1963: Dr Cohen had visited E at 3 and prescribed Coroas Tymcaps,[305] twice daily.

May 29, 1963: 1 good suit and good blue dress were put into a Woolworth bag. There is no explaining of this - they should be to good police.

---

304 Taractan is an anti-psychotic, also prescribed for anxiety, insomnia and agitation and to relieve severe chronic pain. Betaperamide is normally prescribed to relieve acute diarrhoea.

305 Coroas Tymcaps were an early time-release formulation of Corovas, prescribed to lower cholesterol and reduce the risk of a heart attack.

May 30, 1963: E had pain in right side. Exposed? Where suit and blue dress.

June 1, 1963: Rang Dr Cohen at 8.40 and made appointment for 3 today. Dr Cohen came at 2.50 and left new prescription.

June 3, 1963: 'Phoned Dr Cohen. E's side painful + we had a very disturbed night.

June 4, 1963: Dr Cohen visited E + then E + I went to Dr Schechtz, 315 W 86th, for E's X-raying. Home again about 5.

June 5, 1963: DID NOT GO TO SCHOOL. 'Phoned Cohen at 12.30 and got worrying report. He visited E at 3 and said we shouldn't worry too much. He will contact specialist and I am to ring him tomorrow at 6.

June 6, 1963: DID NOT GO TO SCHOOL. Dr Cohen rang at 5 and asked me to come to his office, which I did. He gave me the X-ray plates. E to be at Francis Delafield Hospital[306] at 9 am tomorrow. Came home. Went out again and bought nightgowns for E. Also marketed.

June 7, 1963: DID NOT GO TO SCHOOL. E + I arrived much too early at the hospital, + waited what seemed like an interminable time. The business of her registering, + of my being interviewed by the "investigator" re finance took till after twelve. I then said goodbye to her. Floor 2.

During June and July Jack wrote daily detailed letters to Jigg, desperately sad letters describing Evelyn's medical progress, conveying his unrealistic hopes for her recovery alongside his descriptions of her deteriorating condition. Perhaps unsurprisingly, these letters also conveyed hints of Jack's own deteriorating mental and physical strength.

To Creighton Scott

The Benjamin Franklin Hotel
June 9, 1963

Dear Jigg,

Thanks for your last letter,[307] and Evelyn greatly appreciated your message to her. I grieve to say that she is now in hospital with a tumor on the lung. The doctors hold out hope that it may respond to radiation. The hospital is "Frances Delafield Hospital 99 Fort Washington Avenue, New York 32". I am trying perforce to hold on to my job, but of course it is very difficult. I shall know more of the prospects in a week or so's time when further tests have been made.

We do hope you are all fairly well, and that circumstances are improving.

Evelyn sends love to all.

Affectionately,
Jack

[Handwritten, signed. SFC]

---

306 The Francis Delafield Hospital, named after an eminent physician, was declared by the New York City Board of Hospitals as a centre for the treatment of cancer in 1950.

307 This letter has not survived.

To John Gawsworth

The Benjamin Franklin Hotel
June 9, 1963

Dear John,

Evelyn is in hospital with a tumour of the lung. Surgery is to avoided if possible because of her cardiac condition, so radiation will be tried.

And we had, actually, been planning to resettle in England next spring!

If the worst happens I do not see myself surviving her, because, with all its ups and downs, this has been such a deep + permeating affection.

At the moment, from minute to minute, I hardly know what to do, or how to go through the ordinary motions of living.

Love from both to both,

Jack

[Handwritten, signed. HRC]

To Love Lyle

The Benjamin Franklin Hotel
June 13, 1963

Dear Love,

I grieve to tell you that Evelyn is in hospital with a tumor of the lung. Whether will decide to operate or just try radiation I do not know yet.

The hospital is The Francis Delafield Hospital, 99 Fort Washington Avenue, New York 23, NY.

X-rays revealed the condition about 10 days ago, and she went into hospital on June 7th.

I cannot add any more, but you can imagine how I feel, and will pray for us both.

Love,

Jack

[Handwritten, signed. UTK]

To Creighton Scott

The Benjamin Franklin Hotel
June 15, 1963

Dear Jigg,

I am grateful for your letter, and it should buck Evelyn up, when I visit her today and give her its messages.

I have just spoken to her "old" doctor - Cohen - that is, the one who has just been visiting her here for the last few months, and who got her into the hospital where she is. He tells me that he has been in contact with the doctors at the Delafield who have Evelyn in their care, - that they are top-specialists in this line and that, anyhow, she could not be in better hands. They are going, Cohen says, to try radiation, which, they hope, will arrest and localise the tumor and, perhaps, render an ultimate extirpation feasible.

I myself am of course most unhappy and the carrying-on, so far, with my job is the hardest thing I have ever done in my life. I have that hellish endowment of imagination and pessimistic anticipation that squeezes each ounce of misery from any situation. I can only trust that, if the worst should happen, this will prove, in some degree, a sort of pre-digestion of agony.

But Cohen was not too pessimistic himself, - and, as you say, we'll all hope, and pull for her.

I could not contemplate being without her.

I am so happy (and so will she be) to hear your own health has improved.

I wish to God you were all here because, like you, I have no friends. This hotel room at night is hell.

All the few friends we have are out of town or on the point of leaving. May Mayers, whom I have never needed so much, has gone, - and there's no one.

Love to Paula and children, - and Evelyn of course sends love to all.

Affectionately,

Jack

[Handwritten, signed. SFC]

From John Metcalfe's diary:

June 21, 1963: Gave E letter to her from Jigg.[308]

To Paula Scott

The Benjamin Franklin Hotel
June 23, 1963

Dear Paula

Thank you very much indeed for your sympathetic letter. I did not show <u>it</u> to E, but, of course, passed on to her, when I visited her yesterday, the letters to her from you and from Frederick, both of which delighted her. And I should like you now, from me, particularly to thank Frederick for having written to her. I was a gesture that I <u>very</u> greatly appreciate.

When I reached her bedside she had already written the note to Jigg which I herewith enclose[309] in answer to his recent letter to her. Please pass it on to him, - and do not fear a deluge of such missives. And I again assure you that your whereabouts will be kept strictly to myself.

---

308 This letter has not survived.
309 This note has not survived.

The radio-therapy was begun three days ago. As I think I told Jigg, the biopsy was fairly encouraging showing the mass to consist of a type of a cell responsive to radiation. So we hope for good results.

Love,

Jack

Love also to the children and my affectionate wishes of course to Jigg. I do pray that your own problems will be solved, and matters mend for you!

[Handwritten, signed. SFC]

To Creighton Scott

Francis Delafield Hospital

June 23, 1963

Darling Jigg,

I am glad to know you have written to me. Your letter is helped top me, but we most wish that you will be against coronaries. You need friends who will prove your health again. I think of you, Paula, Denise, Fredrick, Mathew, Julia and Robert, and your strength shall be now.

Friends, I hope! We should have seen many friends long ago about your health.

I can't yet express natural intentions. Bless you. Jack will give your letter when I am better, too I will write myself and to friends.

Mother

I am accepted to Radio Therapy and it does help. Our Jewish doctor helps.

[Handwritten, signed. SFC]

To Creighton and Paula Scott

The Benjamin Franklin Hotel

July 1, 1963

Dear Jigg and Paula,

A very brief bulletin, - and thanks for your letter, - and particularly for Matthew's, which I appreciated just as I did Frederick's.[310]

Evelyn is responding very slowly to the X-ray. I spoke this evening to Dr Cohen, the very best of eggs, who had been on the wire to her physicians, up there at 14 Delafield, and they said, despite her complaints of constant pain, that they thought it was beginning to ease-up just a little. It is going slowly, - and she may have to stay there several weeks yet before becoming an out-patient.

Don't worry, Jigg and Paula, about any disclosure of your whereabouts. Whatever the necessity, I agree to it, - and you can tell me the story whenever you care, if we're alone.

From now on, if she comes back and writes silly letters (actually, I don't think she will) I shan't mail them. Very, very sorrowfully, at this point I have to relinquish her as

---

310 These letters have not survived.

an equal. I have tried, these years, to consider her, humanly, and equal, but things have got past it now.

I still love her, - she is still the marrow of all my being, - but that's the only way to treat her now.

Much love,

Jack

Glad no recurrence of coronary.[311] I am all right up a point with TERACTAN anti-depressant, but Cohen is worried about my loss of weight. Now only 131 lbs - a loss of nearly 20 lbs in 1 month or of 30 lbs in 2 months.

[Handwritten, signed. SFC]

From John Metcalfe's diary:

July 6, 1963: Visited E around 3 and was astonished to hear from her that she had had her last X-raying and would be home next week. Could get no explanation as to this.

To Creighton Scott

The Benjamin Franklin Hotel

July 9, 1963

Dear Jigg,

Thank you + Paula so much for letters, - and most especially for the letters from Matthew + from Julia, which Evelyn was delighted to have.

She has completed her first "cure" of radiation now, having taken as much as she can stand for the moment (there comes a point where it has to be intermitted or do actual harm), - and I expect her home here in a few days now.

I am looking forward to that, as you may imagine. I think the treatments, so far, have done her good. She will renew them later in the summer or in the fall, they say.

No more now, as I am past tired out.

Love to all,

Jack

[Handwritten, signed. SFC]

From John Metcalfe's diary:

July 11, 1963: Taxi'd to hospital where found E with right side of her back painted red + strapped + plastered.

To Creighton Scott

The Benjamin Franklin Hotel

July 14, 1963

Dear Jigg,

Just a hasty bulletin.

The pain has now ceased, and apparently her first "course" of X-ray has done good.

---

311 Jigg had recently had a heart attack.

She will be returning here in about a week or 10 days from now, - so you cannot write quite as freely to me as you have been doing. I appreciate your concern for her, - while I do indeed understand your side of the matter. All list to later if you + I ever get together. At the moment, she is just coming home + you can't write freely.

She will go up to the hospital about every 3 weeks for check up, and then, probably undergo a further "course" of radio-therapy in later summer or fall.

I am distressed by what you say of a fresh "thrombosis". I do hope to goodness you get over it pretty well. Let me know.

Alas, Dr Cohen is away on vacation, but will be back before too long, I hope.

She will just come back here in 10 days or less, - and I suppose one shall try to mimic "life as usual". She does not fully appreciate what is the matter with her, which is all to the good.

If the X-ray doesn't work she will have to face an operation, - but of course I do hope the X-ray does work. The operation chances are 4 to 1 against.

Love to you all, and I wish I knew you better, because I may be a very lonely man.

Jack

[Handwritten, signed. SFC]

To Creighton Scott

The Benjamin Franklin Hotel
July 16, 1963

Dear Jigg,

Thanks for letters, - which Evelyn was cheered to have, - tho' worried by your set back and by Frederick's approaching term of military service.

I do hope you're better now.

I myself am none too well, - Evelyn is better, and comes home again in about a week, - and that is the main, great thing, but the continued strain has pretty well worn me out, and I sort of fainted at school, - and had to be put in a cab. I got home OK, - and say nothing of it to E. Her pain, thank heaven, has almost gone, so don't worry about that. She is greatly looking forward to returning here to the hotel. She will then visit the hospital's clinic periodically (about once every month or 3 weeks) till treatment is renewed in late summer or fall.

Forgive more now,
Love to you all,
Jack

Thank Frederick, from her, v much indeed for his letter; and, of course, thanks so much for your own letter to her.[312]

[Handwritten, signed. SFC]

---

312 Neither of these letters has survived.

To Creighton Scott

The Benjamin Franklin Hotel

July 17, 1963

Dear Jigg,

Just a line to enclose note[313] from E to Paula and Frederick. As you will see, it is v confused, - but does not really do her justice. The stroke impaired her "effectors" as the medical lingo has it, but actually her "receptors" (ditto, ditto) remain pretty sharp, and she is continually maddened by being unable to express, in words or letters, what she can often feel and understand with a fair amount of clearness.

She is worried about your "set back" and so am I. We do hope you are pretty well over it now, - and sympathise with all your problems.

As I told you, her pain seems to have gone. I really have been almost afraid to ask her this, directly, but just judge it to be so, because she no longer complains about it, and is looking forward happily to return to this hotel. I, of course, will be much better when she is back. She had a very strong course of X-ray, and is, at the moment, as I may have said before, being as it were "cured of the cure". She will be home, I hope, within a week or 10 days, - so write, from now, only what I can show to her.

Love to all

Jack

[Handwritten, signed. SFC]

To Creighton Scott

The Benjamin Franklin Hotel

July 20, 1963

Dear Jigg

Yours just received, - and I will write anything you want in support of your application. Let me know in greater detail as the occasion arises, - and good luck in to Frederick in the Canadian Black Watch!

The great news is that the hospital is sending Evelyn home here again.

She will be here the day-after-tomorrow, - Monday the 22nd, - so bear this in mind in anything you write.

It need not at all interfere with your going on speaking w/wishing to become Canadian citizens. - She would welcome that.

As to the "desperate odds", - I may have made myself insufficiently plain. The 5-1 against odds referred to an operation, - if X-raying failed. We hope that mayn't be necessary.

There is a possibility, according to the last thing Cohen said, that X-raying may cure this thing entirely. At least, he said, it could prolong her life 5-6 years. Then, if the worst came to the worst, I suppose she wd have to be operated on, - but I,

---

313 This note has not survived.

naturally, cling to the hope that X-rays will do the trick. They can do things now, with malignancies, that they couldn't do even only 10 yrs ago.

Today, I have been getting in groceries etc in anticipation. I myself, since she's been away, have eaten little, - no breakfast or lunch and only a bite for supper.

Dear Jigg and Paula, I do so appreciate your concern, and the concern of you all. Let us all hope and pray that there will be light, somehow, at the end of this dark tunnel.

Love

Jack

[Handwritten, signed. SFC]

To Creighton Scott

The Benjamin Franklin Hotel

July 23, 1963

Dear Jigg,

This is no more than a PS to my last, - to say that Evelyn's return home has been postponed for, probably, a few days. She may be here next week-end, or in about a week from today.

Nothing much beyond that, - and she seems better.

Love to all,

Jack

I will let you know definitely when she is back here.

[Handwritten, signed. SFC]

From John Metcalfe's diary:

July 27, 1963: <u>E Returned Home</u>. 'Phoned Gladys after much difficulty + exasperation + loss of money. Bought tobacco, coffee and liquor. Visited E. Was leaving + then decided to return, + Dr Bell rang up the ward + said E might leave right away! Waited while her clothes were procured, + then went home with her in cab. Reached hotel about 8.45.

July 29, 1963: E + I taxied to + from hospital & got her property back. Home by about 10.30

To Creighton Scott

The Benjamin Franklin Hotel

July 29, 1963

Dear Jigg,

Just a hasty line to tell you that, thank goodness, Evelyn is now back with me at the hotel. I leave space for her to add a word or two. Much love to you all, - and hoping so very much that your health is improving.

Affectionately your step-father

Jack

Don't worry we'll let no one have yr address! Jack.

Darling Jigg, I am at last trying to see about you for I am sure there won't be of you. Darling, I began with Jack to know where I am. Love, health working to you. Later I can see where I am. Paula and the children in national churche [sic] *- no! Bless you! Mother*

[Handwritten, signed. Handwritten note by ES at bottom. SFC]

From John Metcalfe's diary:

July 31, 1963: E collapsed and fell to floor at breakfast...Confirmed that Dr Cohen was still on vacation, and filled May's second prescription. E depressed.

To Louise Morgan

Benjamin Franklin Hotel
August 2, 1963

Darling Louise,

Do you know that you were believing about my view, or rather Jack's, about hospitals, <u>and</u> now I am home with Jack and not enthusiastic! However, I would be happier in London where doctors are of the British types; Bernice remembers how well the doctors with her.

Jig has been *[words rubbed out]* for about four years and at the end of this, frightened us, as he has been ill and money for the children is known, too. Oh I wish they were in London!

Well, Jack is in happier in London, too. Otto helps us in his ideas!

Love,
Evelyn (back)

Jack was marvel! I am indignant that books are cheated! <u>The Winter Alone</u> and <u>The Muscovites</u> have been taken! I am sure Jack also suffered in this sense for his books.

Anyhow Jack new I should returned to the hotel.

My love of The Muscovites have been of value - of 1940! I have had Jig's inscription to me - "mother".

Evelyn

[This letter was placed in an outer envelope annotated by Louise Morgan: "Evelyn Scott's last letter (probably the last she ever wrote). Horrified just now, with the letter from John.[314] I read hers first, and then John's. What a shock! But I am glad for John. He could not have stood it much longer. 7 August 1963 9 AM"]

[Handwritten in pencil, signed. Outer envelope with annotation by Louise Morgan. UTK]

---

314 This letter has not survived.

From John Metcalfe's diary:

July 31, 1963: E collapsed and fell to floor at breakfast. Confirmed that Dr Cohen was still on vacation, and filled May's second prescription. E depressed.

August 3, 1963: Evelyn died. Gladys + May here.

Death certificate of Evelyn Scott: *Scott family*

Evelyn was buried at Rosehill Cemetery, the overflow cemetery for Manhattan located in New Jersey near what is now Newark airport. Gladys paid for the actual funeral expenses but had no money for a headstone, and as a result there was no marker on Evelyn's grave.

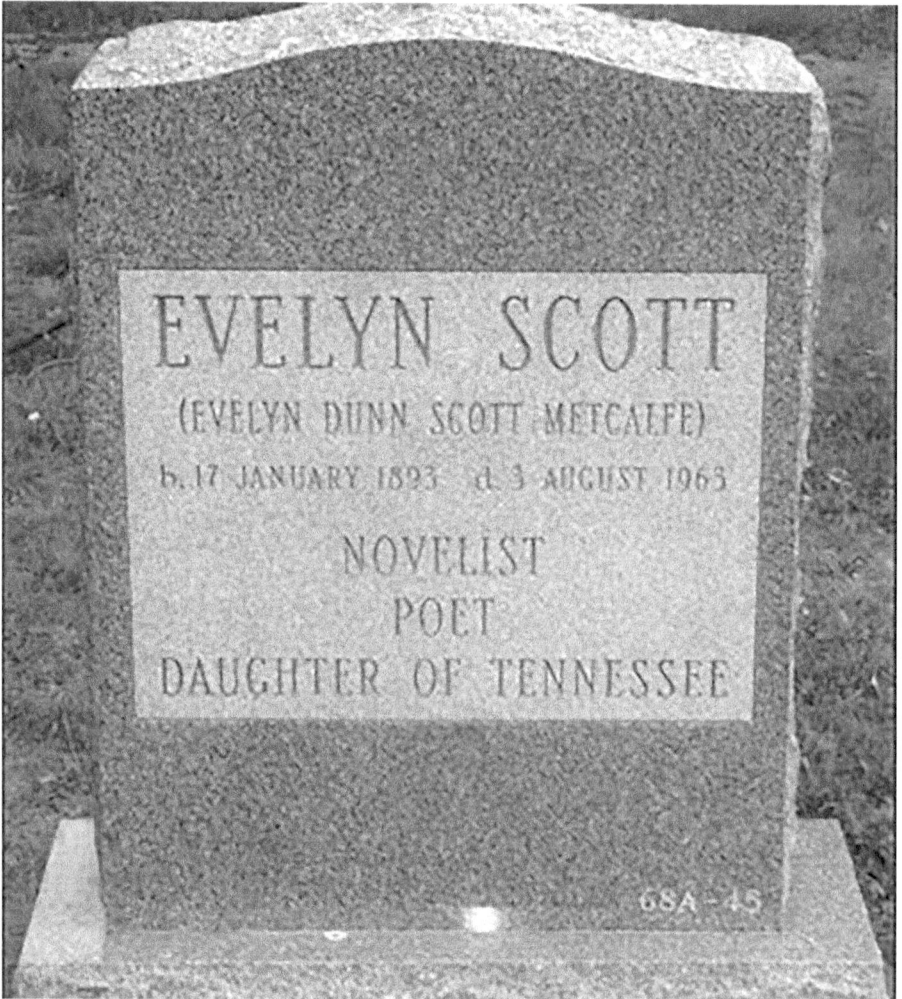

Memorial to Evelyn Scott, erected by the people of Clarksville: *Scott family*

Chapter 44

Aftermath

To say Jack was overwhelmed by grief after Evelyn's death is an understatement. Her death was not unexpected, but Jack had been living in hope that she would recover from her lung disease with the "x-ray treatment"; he had sent Jigg daily reports on her progress while she was in hospital and took enormous comfort from the decision to discharge her back to the Benjamin Franklin Hotel.

For many years Jack had been a regular drinker, without it appearing to impair his intellect or his ability to deal with normal life, but he started drinking heavily during Evelyn's final illness. It is hard to imagine how he felt during the last few days of her life, and on the night she died he had been drinking so heavily that he slept through her final hours, only discovering she had died the day after.

As he writes to Jigg at one point, "she made my life hell for 38 years, but I cannot live without her". He also acknowledged that he understood why Evelyn was pursuing Jigg so desperately, but couldn't quite bring himself to condemn this, his loyalty to her was so great.

In the weeks following Evelyn's death and funeral, Jack had to face a number of problems, chiefly his own health. Frail for some months before her death, he began to neglect himself with the inevitable consequences. Not only did his physical health deteriorate, but his mental health also became a real concern as he suffered a strong grief reaction, for which he was treated with strong medication and later hospitalised. The near-daily letters to Jigg chronicle his increasing frailty, his extreme weight loss caused by loss of interest in food, his continuing struggle to cope with his "school job" in order to pay his rent, his near blindness, and, most importantly, his acknowledgement that Evelyn's obsessiveness was toxic. But this acknowledgement does not make his grief any less in spite of the strong tranquilisers prescribed by Evelyn's doctor, Dr Cohen.

The following letters document Jack's disintegration, emotional and physical; his enormous grief, coupled with increasing physical frailty, is made obvious in these near-daily letters. His only hope was prompted by an offer from Jigg that he come to live with the Scott family in Canada.

To Creighton Scott

The Benjamin Franklin Hotel
August 4, 1963

Dear Jigg,

This carries the saddest news for us all. Evelyn passed away, yesterday, Saturday, in her sleep. It was in the morning, some time, I can't be sure, - any time between 8 and 12, - because I thought she was just still sleeping. Then at 12 I became apprehensive and found her cold. She will be buried, probably, on Tuesday.

I cannot write more now.

Love to all

Jack

[Handwritten, signed. SFC]

To Creighton Scott

The Benjamin Franklin Hotel
August 7, 1963

My Very Dear Jigg,

Your two letters[315] arrived, I opened the long one first, - and what a tale it unfolds! Don't worry. Shall burn it, - but keep <u>curriculum vitae</u>.

From what I read in the long envelope I decided not to open the other, smaller one. Because you still had not received the news of Evelyn's death, and whatever you wrote in the smaller envelope would be on the presumption she still lived, - and would be painful for me to read.

I just at present don't know how to exist, and of course contemplate suicide. But I am supposed to be going, next Saturday Aug 10 to stay in NJ with Gladys Grant for at least a few days.

Oh, I do sympathise, Jigg, with your unbelievable predicament, - to *[illeg]* from Evelyn so largely contributed. Men are nasty things, - I never realised how nasty - and what you tell me is appalling.

Do not "admire" me. I am a man packed with frailties. At present I am nothing at all. The sheer ache in my heart is almost unbearable.

If I live, I will always do my best for you. I imagine that, eventually, in a few months, or early next year, I shall go to England, and whatever I could do for you there I shall. It would be, for me, lovely if you all <u>could</u> come within reach. There were, however, some troublesome labour restrictions what made it hard for "aliens" to have jobs there. They may have gone or been relaxed. I could find out.

Love to you all,

Jack

[Handwritten, signed. SFC]

---

315 These letters have not survived.

To Creighton Scott

c/o Gladys Grant
Scotch Plains, New Jersey
August 11, 1963

Dear Jigg,

I am, at moment (Sunday) up visiting, with Gladys but shall return to N York Tuesday 13th and mail this from there.

The question of a visit, greatly as I should love it, is a problem, for several reasons.

(A) I am, at present, too knocked-out to work, and was on my beam-ends financially, anyway. May Mayers (who was there, it happened, soon after E died, and saw your wire of invitation) was a possible person from whom I could have borrowed, - but, I am ashamed to say, I got tight and she got fed up with me (both then + next day) and she is OUT. She finished by describing me as a "drunken mess". Here ends that "friendship". And as for dear Gladys, - I had no funds to cover E's burial and Gladys lent me over $400, so I can hardly ask her for more.

(B) My British Subjection would require both renewal of passport and a Re-Entry Permit. I have yet, even, to find my old expired Passport in one of Evelyn's trunks.

(C) Any absence, however short, from the US must be reported to Social Security and could somehow complicate my pension, - fantastic as this sounds.

The whole question is full of difficulties. My own plans, so far as I have the least heart for, or interest in, them are to return next year to England.

I would go right away, but here again red-tape dictates delay. Now, I have been reliably assured that, having lived continuously over 10 years in the US, I can take my US pension with me to England. This would make all the difference, in England to be between a pauperised existence on the tiny British retirement pension and financial comfort. But to try to go there now, would make terrible paper-work complications. This takes long to explain, - but you will, I think, understand.

Otherwise I should wish nothing more than to see you all.

Oh, I do indeed long to see you all. Let's wait and see. As I say this is written from Gladys', and won't be mailed till Tue, 13th when I return to New York. Regard it as just an interim reply.

<u>Love</u> to you all,

Jack

[Handwritten, signed. SFC]

Shortly after Evelyn's death, Jigg invited Jack to join the family in Chester. Jack grasped this opportunity as perhaps the only way out of his grief, but the invitation was later withdrawn. Gladys' warnings about the potential effect on his family, plus the desperate tone of Jack's letters, persuaded Jigg that this was not a good idea, and the withdrawal of the invitation only deepened Jack's depression.

To Creighton Scott

The Benjamin Franklin Hotel
August 15, 1963

Dear Jigg,

Thanks for invitation. Dearly appreciated and will write more. I am too mentally sick to reply properly, and may have to be hospitalized. The <u>real</u> pain of E's death is just beginning to soak in. I cannot, still, realise it at all. We were so close.

I <u>would</u> be an honoured guest or grandfather.

But I am sailing through the mechanical performances of someone although, I, - and first, I have to renew my British passport, - which will take time.

I repudiate the Mayers entirely. Medical Pharisee, - because I was tight when E died.

Honestly, Jigg, I don't see myself going on without her. We were so one of each-other, so close. I am just on the verge, really imminent - by now of cutting my wrists or jumping under a train.

It might just preserve my sanity if I saw you, - My ultimate objective, so far as I can have any, - is England.

But, you know, and Paula will know, nothing matters but Evelyn. How can I ever get over it? I can't. It is a wound, from which I can never, never recover, - I am cut - a dead man *[remainder of letter missing]*

[Handwritten, SFC]

To Otto Theis and Louise Morgan

Scotch Plains, New Jersey
August 21, 1963

Dear Otto and Louise:

Ever since Evelyn gave me your address last winter I have intended to write. You are so often in my thoughts but I am the world's worst correspondent.

Then last winter I took a trip to the West Indies. Delightful while it lasted (Jamaica, Haiti, Puerto Rico) but it ended with a broken arm. Bad break plus age and lack of calcium made it very slow and it just came out of cast last week. Still practically useless (right arm, of course) which has made it very difficult to help Jack. I know you would like to hear what I can tell of him and Evelyn.

I saw Evelyn just before I went on trip. She looked very very badly, suffering from heart and, I believe, a small stroke. She has great difficulty getting her words out and had to keep appealing to Jack. It was pityful. But I was shocked to hear she had cancer and had to go to hospital for x ray treatment. Jack was quite hopeful at first but I realized what she would have to go through at best.

I did manage to get in to the hospital at once, thank God. She was glad to see me and seemed more relaxed and less worried. Her speech was clearer but her color… But Jack looked and seemed much worse. He sees poorly and stumbles.

I did not intend to inflict these details on you, just started. I'd tear letter up and begin over but might never finish.

Next thing I heard she was back in hotel with Jack who tried to keep hopeful. Then the hotel called up to say she had died and begged me to come in. I was shocked and realized things must be very bad. Fortunately I could get in to the city almost at once.

Evelyn had died quietly in her sleep which was wonderful for her but an even greater shock for Jack. And he had absolutely no one to turn to. Everyone was on vacation, even their doctor. They wouldn't let Evelyn's body be taken to a funeral parlor until a police surgeon signed the death certificate.

By the time I arrived Jack was in fearful condition between shock and drink. He fell once in the room yet kept going out for more whiskey which the young policeman in charge kept confiscating. But somehow it did help him to talk. But he could make no decisions and I had to go with him to funeral parlor and make arrangements. (Of course he had eaten nothing all this time.)

The hotel was very helpful. They got him another room and one for me as I could not leave. We actually had breakfast the next day.

Jack is still in a terrible physical and emotional state as you know from his letters. Jigg fears suicide but I feel the great danger has passed. He seems actually to be taking some interest in making plans and wants to see friends. We brought him out here for a week, but he would stay only two days. I try to keep in touch by letter and phone and hope to get in again next week.

One good thing. I got a letter from Evelyn herself written the day before she died. She was in calm almost happy mood especially as she had heard from Jigg and his oldest son Frederick.

I don't know what will happen. Personally I feel he would be happier in England. He has never really adapted himself here and a complete change would be good. He might even start to write again. Also there he might drink in moderation. Now he needs it, but I don't know how his physical state stands so much. I fear accident (very poor eyesight, too) or possible mental breakdown.

Forgive my pouring all this out on you! I guess I need to share it with someone. Also you should be prepared in case he does go to England.

If you can excuse my long silence, please do write. I'd like to hear your news. I'm hoping to see Ruth this autumn. It has been hard as I can not yet drive.

Very best love to you both

Gladys

PS On Aug 22. I just talked to Jack on the phone. His whole voice and outlook sounded much better. I plan to see him Monday.

[Typed, signed. BRBL]

To Creighton Scott

The Benjamin Franklin Hotel
September 7, 1963

Dear Jigg,

I went down to Gladys's on Wednesday intending to spend 4, or at least 3, nights, but felt so poorly I had to return here after 2 nights in order to catch Dr Cohen on Friday evening. He gave me something which he hopes will work well enough to enable me to try school on Monday 9th. At present I feel not at all well, - indeed worse than, say, 3 weeks ago. The numbness, I suppose, is wearing off, and I'm beginning to feel the full impact. But I'll do my best to hang on day to day till the utter misery, I hope, passes.

Yes, step by step, to England. (Visit you first, of course.)

This is only an inadequate note. I do so hope the Broadcasting comes off, - your account of the audition sounded hopeful.

Cannot write properly. Too sick. Hope to hang on somehow and feel better. Still hope to go to school Monday 9th. But I am only now starting to feel the worst reality of it.

Love to all
Jack

[Handwritten, signed. SFC]

To Creighton Scott

The Benjamin Franklin Hotel
October 23, 1963

Dear Jigg,

Yes, I am caught in the "bureaucratic wringer". If you have any chance of getting to England first, tant mieux. If you happened to be there first, it would be lovely for me.

At present, as I told you, I am stuck in the financial-plus-emotional jam.

I would come to you right away, to Canada, if I could, but I am not able to. In any case, as you say, my reunion with you all would only be deferred.

My own state is disappointing. I have lost 36 pounds since it happened. I have dreadful moments, and then slightly less-dreadful ones, - with a fillip of whisky.

Dr Cohen is now considering sending me to hospital. At times I feel able to get along, and then the realisation that I shall never see her again puts me flat on my back and I feel nothing will ever again be worthwhile.

If I did go into hospital again, it would, of course, be for psychiatric treatment, - i.e. playing volley-ball on the roof, and being defended from jumping off it.

Anyhow, we get together. Yes, Yes.

I do hope that this present intense feeling of grief and loss abates somewhat, - so that I can write and work more as an ordinary person.

Much much love to you all
Jack

[Handwritten, signed. SFC]

To Creighton Scott

The Benjamin Franklin Hotel

November 4, 1963

Dear Jigg,

Where are you? Haven't heard from you for some time.

And with me it is just touch and go. I would welcome any form of euthanasia, but still hate the messiness of just throwing myself under a subway train. For the last week weeping fits etc. have put school out of question. I don't know what to do.

For preservation of my own sanity I ought to come to you right away, - yet if I don't that all must be lost.

I feel I cannot live without Evelyn.

I don't know what to do.

Love to all,

Jack

It just goes on being a nightmare. When I found her dead her mouth was gaping. I pushed her lips together and kissed them for the last time. How can I live in England when she is in New Jersey? I suppose I will end up in a state Mental Home.

[Handwritten, signed. SFC]

To Creighton Scott

The Benjamin Franklin Hotel

November 5, 1963

Dear Jigg

Just a line, further to the telegram[316] I sent you yesterday. What has happened to you all?

I have had no word from you since a letter dated October 19th and post-marked October 21st. Are you all Europe-bound or what?

Coincidentally, this comes with the bad news from my school-job that their patience is exhausted, and they are "replacing" me at my job. I was too sick to go there last Friday, and, on doctor's advice, am not going this present week. I have a nasty letter of dismissal from the Directress, - accusing me of "self-pity"! When, she says, I have decided to "rehabilitate my life", there will again be a place in the school for me again. So, pro tem, I am jobless.

Love to all

Jack

[Handwritten, signed. SFC]

---

316 This has not survived.

To Creighton and Paula Scott
334 Bonnie Burn Road
Scotch Plains New Jersey

November 9, 1963

Dear Jig and Paula

This won't be a real letter. I've been away with a very ill friend and got back to find your letter and one from Jack. I called him tonight and he was in a very bad state. I could scarcely hear him.

But I have no idea what any of us can do. One reason I put off answering your good letter was that I felt discouraged. The last few days Jack spent here were pretty terrible. I feel so sorry for him yet it is hard to do anything for someone so sorry for himself. This sounds bitter, but it is true. Also he is looking so hard for someone to lean on and he has to face things himself, as you know. At first it seemed wonderful for him to be with you for a while, but now I feel very strongly that it would add immeasurably to your problems and would not help him. If not yourselves, you must consider your children first. As for Jack's threats of suicide, I am afraid I think them more a bid (or threat) for pity. Perhaps it is a case of wolf, wolf and he really will someday.

Jack has so many fine qualities and I really love him. It is heart breaking to see him disintegrate like this. I would not write so frankly to anyone else. I do hope and pray Jack comes through. But no one can do it for him. Write if you want, but don't spend your needed money on telephone or telegrams. Above all don't take him in. God forgive me! But it wouldn't help.

If I hear anything further I'll write again. Also I want to answer your good letters with personal news. I'm beginning to drive a little which is a relief. My wrist and fingers are still quite stiff, but the doctor said it is up to me to use them as much as possible. This reason for poor typing I've used both hands.

This has been a hard letter to write and I'm still tired from my trip, so it is poorly expressed. But I know you'll understand.

Also and above all it brings deepest love to you all.

God bless you

Glads

[Typed on personal letterhead, signed. UTK]

To Creighton and Paula Scott

The Benjamin Franklin Hotel
November 12, 1963

Dear Jigg and Paula,

Yesterday was "Veterans' Day", with no mail, and this is really just a continuation of my last to Paula, - to which I replied particularly because hers to me shared a scarcely-deserved concern that greatly touched me. Oh my Gawd, how infinitely worse-off I should be if I had not you-all to exist, - and write-to and soon meet!

I am really bothered about Jigg's heart condition. People live with it for years and years, but it needs watching.

For the time being, as I told you in my last, things aren't too good with me, because I have been laid-off from my school job, and cannot be sure when I shall be in a position to recapture it. I have now arranged for regular evening-clinic psychiatric treatment, - and, if that doesn't work, I suppose it means a further spell in hospital.

I still cannot get acclimatised to E's being no longer here, and the pain is sometimes almost unbearable. it is worse, now, than the three months ago, because, then, emotionally speaking, her dying like that, so suddenly, seemed just another of her antics and vagaries, and it is only now, with no voice from the grave, that I begin to realise the appalling, incredible fact, that from now on I am without her, whether I live in Tahiti, Timbuctoo or Moona-Poona.

I hate this maddening little room in this accursed hotel, from which her corpse was carried out, - yet it would be impossible, now, to move.

Oh no: no sense of "disloyalty would deter me from welcoming any anodyne, but so far only whiskey has presented itself and I remain too much in love with E to have the urge and enterprise to go out and try to get involved with anybody else. At present, people-in-general, places and events hold no interest for me without her. And it is really better for me, temporarily, not to try to "mull over" or project myself imaginatively into too far a future, because, at the moment, any Evelyn-less future is hardly contemplatable. I have no "hobbies", and has never looked forward to anything done without her.

Tuesday morning. This account of myself, I fear, must worry you, but in the long run it is better not to disguise the facts. The morning hours, from waking around five till I allow myself my first whiskey, around 11.30 (yes, I still have just enough guts to wait till then) are plain misery and suicidally-inclined. After the whiskey it is measurably better through the rest of the day.

My Dr Cohen tells me it will get better. The situation, he says, might change just overnight, - and I might wake up one day feeling quite different. But as yet the pain of loss goes on and I feel like someone under a curse. People (well-meaningly) keep telling me that it is well she was spared a "long and distressing illness", - which is true up to a point, - but am I to thank God for giving her cancer in the first place?

Please believe I do long to see you all. The trouble now is just that I cannot, yet, get clear of the damned business, - am jobless, and love-sick for a corpse. This, I realise, is "morbidity" to the nth, which John Metcalfe could always be relied on to provide.

But in all seriousness, I must, somehow, climb out of this extreme unhappiness, and start to live again.

The nuisance is that, after 38 years of deep attachment, I cannot, in a remaining span of 10 or even 20 years hope to do much more than just patch over such long and vivid memories. But again, I intend to weather this, somehow.

Much, much love to you all,

Jack

There is so much in the story you never, I think, knew. Some day, I'll tell you.

All those 44 evenings that I visited her in hospital, taking the long subway trek after school to 168th Street, I pulled and prayed for her with all my might, imploring whatever God might be that the radio-treatment might work a miracle. But the miracle didn't happen (they don't, you know) and God wasn't even a quarter chummy. So now, the whole thing cannot but wear the aspect of a great Defeat. I mean, I had tried so desperately to pull her through.

This isn't, Jigg and Paula, meant to be at all a "tragic", exaggerated or "self pitying" letter. It is merely as close an approximation as I can reach to the present position about myself and Evelyn.

I wish to be "reasonable" and "practical" and it is true that, in England, that might be easier, with Evelyn 3000 miles away.

Let us get there!

Again, love

Jack

[Handwritten, signed. SFC]

To Creighton Scott

The Benjamin Franklin Hotel

November 15, 1963

Dear Jigg,

Yours of the 10th[317] received, and I can indeed sympathise with its underlying desperation, - though it could not fail to depress me.

There remain several gross misconceptions of which, for honesty's sake, I must disabuse you. I did not wish to go into them again, by <u>writing</u> instead of talking, - but your letter almost forces me to.

In some previous letter of yours you asked - why did E and I ever leave England? Simply, and almost entirely, to bring Evelyn, geographically anyhow, closer to you-all, - and make her think she could see you again. "Mad as a hatter" she was already beginning to be, - but that was what she thought.

Since then, in USA, - so far from "not caring a shot", she worried about you incessantly. She was quite capable, for a while, of mailing and registering her own (regrettable) letters, and I still granted her the privilege of being a free person, where you were concerned. This has proved bad policy, - but it was ethics, to me, at the time. She once (I think when you were still at Carmel) tried to send you a trifling check, which Paula returned torn up. Her main engrossment was just <u>you</u> and <u>family</u>. We did not know of your going through and Senatorial Investigations, - etc. All we had was a laconic report of your testimony, - which sounded mighty good. We did not know (because we had no information) that your job had thereby been lost, - nor did

---

317 This letter has not survived.

we have the least inkling of your subsequent difficulties, though E Scott consciously surmised and suspected them. Her anxiety about, and preoccupation with, your probable difficulties was evident, - and would have hastened her end, anyhow, apart from the recent lung business.

I am an extremely (still) rational person, - and see your side of the whole matter, believe me, as clearly as I do hers. I have realised, for many years, that she was "wrecking my life", - but it is an entirely fanciful attitude on your part to "admire" me for "sticking to" her. I clung to her, rather than "stuck by" because I loved her, - as I now am. She was largely my mother as well as my wife.

We had no faintest delusion that you were "affluent" when you left Carmel and went to wherever - you did go. (We found out later it was Vermont - didn't know where, since we hadn't the information), - but suspected you were in dire straits of some kind. All this continued preying on her mind.

You cannot tell me more than I know perfectly well already about the difficulties for you, of getting a job in England. All that has faded into the cloud-cuckoo land where, in my heart, I always knew it really belonged. Though I still do hope you get to France.

I am, alas, not getting any better. I am worse each day, so far.

Evelyn and I made a sort of little suicide pact between us. She said, that if I died, she would wait 3 or so months, and then quit this mortal scene - but I made an inward vow that I would wait one whole year after her death, and then see how I felt. Yet this morning, before I took a sip of whiskey, one almost unbearable. I have a length of clothes-line with which to hang myself if matters don't mend. I eat nothing, - and save money. I bought a sandwich 3 days ago, and it still suffices me in the frig.

By special concession I went oculist (another $10) Sat morning, - and he said that, barring another operation, and cataract lenses - etc etc, nothing more could be done. He exuded polite surprise that I was hoping to work at all.

I am half-blind, and that's that, - and I don't see myself ever getting the school job back. In my present mental state it wd be laughable to try to hold it anyhow.

The "psychiatry" is nonsense. The psychiatrist's advice, of course, is to fit myself out with some new girl-friend, - but what would be the good of that? If she were just placed in my lap, - I suppose I would automatically fiddle with her, - and end up in the usual way, - and to what good?

It all boils down, more and more, to an irreparable, un-mendable loss. After 38 years of intimacy, can I be reasonably expected to recover in 1 year, or 2 years, or 5? It would be ridiculous to suppose so.

Please forgive this honestly desperate letter.

I wish to meet you all, as soon as possible, - wherever it may be,

Much, much love,

Jack

Please don't talk of my ever "writing" again. All that is over and done with, and I have torn up all MSS.I have mainly contempt but desperately despising for all the "arts", - music, sculpture, writing or anything else. "Art" is just one of mankind's toys, and I have finished with it, in any form.

By living, E Scott made me, on the whole, miserable for 38 years, and now, by dying, has made me more so.

Oh God, I wish we could <u>talk</u>!

Don't take anything amiss. Don't answer hurriedly. Remember that we all have much in common. I am v fond of you, Jigg, - and prepared to be so too of Paula and the kids. At the moment I 'm just still in the heartbreak phase.

[Handwritten, signed. SFC]

To John Metcalfe

Chester, Nova Scotia
December 25, 1963

Dear Jack,

All of us have thought the question over very worriedly, and the result is that there will be no combined household consisting of yours and ours. You have become a rubber stamp of E Scott - to be expected, I suppose, after 40 years of servility to her manias.

I have explained to you in other letters what she herself said her motives were where I and mine were concerned. The same old pattern that she set recurs in your letters to us. Although you knew of the disasters which have overtaken us, largely thanks to her egotism and your spinelessness, the discovery that we really were at the end of our rope and as poor as we said was such a shock to your system you had to throw up your job right away so as to make things worse. This made it our fault that you were miserable for reasons we could not prevent. That's the kind of thing that made me hate my mother. Again, when it became necessary to explain to you that - since we were at financial rock bottom, and for other reasons you knew as well as we do - we were not free agents in the sense that Rockefeller is, this news (which you had heard years ago) so crushed your spirit that you couldn't read our letters anymore, and went blind or nearly so. You are not too stupid to understand this: I am not the spineless, gutless, mindless, nugatory foetus dangling at the end of an umbilical cord; that E Scott devoted 30 years to trying to make me be. What will crush you even more than the other things you already know is that I don't intend to become such a creature to please you. Neither do my wife nor my children.

The domesticity you want would consist of our devoting our full time to gushings of phoney commiseration while you crooned over your spiritual leprosy. I've read it in the lines and between the lines of your letters. That quarter of a stale sandwich in four days, that kissing the gapping lips of the dead, all that crud about hurling yourself under subway trains except that it would be so messy, is bullshit.

Bullshit is bullshit, and what you want is someone to scratch your mange, not a family.

My patience has come to an end. I'm sorry it had to be this way. We started out trying to be kindly to a man in distress, and now find ourselves spiritually to blame for all the hazards of life that beset him as they do others.

I also have a spark of pride. My mother played me for a fool from the time I was a baby. You're trying to play all of us for suckers. It won't wash.

We're at the end of our rope and you're at the end of yours. I haven't the faintest idea how either of us can extricate ourselves. One thing I know is that you can't recruit seven people to pet your sores, as my father used to say.

There will be no point in answering this because the answer won't be read or acknowledged. This is goodbye, with very deep regrets that will under no circumstances change any of our minds.

Your stepson,

[Typed carbon copy, not signed. SFC]

From John Metcalfe's diary

December 25, 1963: Coffee. Nap. Depurel. Drink 12.50 after shaving. Nap. Left X-mas cards for staff also card for Miss Brill and letter for Mme Bertuch. Sam happened to be there and I gave him $5 tip. Cheese and nap. Mailed letters to Isobel, Rene and Preston on way to Rudley's.

To Creighton and Paula Scott
334 Bonnie Burn Road
Scotch Plains, New Jersey

January 4, 1964

Dear Jig + Paula:

Thanks for your letters. I always enjoy hearing from you. I don't blame you but did think your letter to Jack was a little too strong especially at this time. After so many years it can only be expected that he should bear the ES imprint. I saw him yesterday, and feel that for the first time he is trying to be a man again. Plans his job back, admits enough money if he stops drinking, etc. I hope he succeeds but no one, least of all myself or you, can help him.

I, too, can't bear his pathologic self pity and agree wholeheartedly that you and he should not be together. (At first it seemed a possible solution, but how wrong I was!) I hope you can put him + the ES image out of your life + thoughts. There is no tie on earth to bind you. I won't write about him again unless to answer your questions. (I don't expect to see him again for some time.)

We are both well but the weather - and driving - are both terrible. Our driveway is such a sheet of ice I scarcely venture down it for the mail. But today the sun is out + will, I hope, melt the ice.

I've been trying hard to make time to write again - but the "mechanics of living". I know you + Paula will understand.

Much much love to you both + to the kids. I'll write again as soon as I learn more about the book.

God bless you

Glads

PS Perhaps as you say your letter had to be strongly worded to get through to him!

[Handwritten on personal letterhead, signed. UTK]

During the spring of 1964 Jack's mental and physical health deteriorated to the point that he was hospitalised and eventually compulsorily detained in an "asylum" or state mental hospital. He had, however, begun making plans for his return to London and old friends, and throughout this period, he corresponded with Robert Welker and his partner Herschel Gower who provided not only friendship but practical support as well.

From John Metcalfe's diary:

April 3, 1964: Found key (I think) of green trunk, put "Walrus" in it, then locked it, putting key of green trunk on my "current" keytainer. I think I did all of this today and not yesterday.

April 16, 1964: Gladys arrived at about 12.20 and left about 2.20. She brought me a can of "Prince Albert" tobacco. Gladys told me that Jigg had written what apparently is a novel about Evelyn and himself, + that she, Gladys, had refused to sign an affidavit, for the possible publishers, that it was all true.[318]

To Herschel Gower and Robert Welker

The Neurological Institute Medical Centre

New York 32, New York

May 14, 1964

My dear Herschel and Robert,

Many thanks for your letter and card to which this has, alas to be but a brief reply, because with now only one eye functioning, and, even so, only those old bifocals to use with it, it takes me a long, long time to write or even read a letter.

No I did not have a fall, but what they call a "seizure" after I'd gone to bed. I lost all consciousness till I was in the elevator, being transferred here from the Eye.

My programme now is uncertain. They finished 4 sessions of X-raying the brain, but there are a number of further tests ahead, which may take a week. Then, it is possible I may go to the hospital's Harkness Convalescent Home for some 10 days, - so I may not be "home" at the hotel till about June 1st.

---

318 This is a reference to Jigg's unfinished and unpublished autobiographical account, *Confessions of an American Boy.*

Then I have to go up to the Eye Clinic each Wednesday, - and it may take from 4 to 8 months from then before I finally get my new lenses, - but I expect, as I say to be back at the Ben Franklin by about June 1st.

All affection to you both,

Jack

[Handwritten, signed. UTK]

To Herschel Gower and Robert Welker

Neurological Institute
New York 32, NY
May 18, 1964

Dear Herschel and Robert,

I have somewhat disturbing news to impart. The Manager of the Benjamin Franklin has intimated that he does not wish me to return to the hotel because I do not take proper meals etc, - and he considers me (though he does not say this explicitly) an insurance risk!

However, the psychiatrist at this hospital rang him up and he (the Manager) relented to the extent of saying I could stay at the Ben Franklin 2 months if I then left for Tennessee (whither the psychiatrist told him I planned to go).

I may not even be able to get my new lenses till about then or a week or so earlier, and could not possibly pack etc myself as I am practically blind. And all the keys are jumbled up and I couldn't find which key fits which trunk etc.

I may of course persuade the Manager to extend the time but can't be sure.

I hope I am not loading you with trouble, but I am in a terrible fix. Let me know soon as you possibly can.

Affectly to both,

Jack

[Handwritten, signed. UTK]

At around the same time, Jigg had himself been hospitalised for a mental breakdown, eventually diagnosed as a form of schizophrenia. No doubt the preceding years had had a severe effect on his mental health, and perhaps some form of breakdown was inevitable. Jigg was eventually discharged home, but shortly afterward had to return to hospital after suffering an injury which required his shoulder to be set in plaster with his arm out at right angles.

None of the letters which Jigg and Jack may have exchanged during this period has survived.

To Herschel Gower and Robert Welker

care of Dr R D Clay
Emsworth, Hampshire
November 2, 1964

My Dear Herschel and Bob,

At last I am able to write freely. I was <u>committed</u> as "mentally ill" by a farcical, iniquitous "court" at Bellevue hospital & have spent the last 2 months at Islip.[319] All mail, both in and out, was censored. Unspeakable misery. It was, till I was put in a better ward, a bedlam of maniacs, - yelling all night and with the stench of urine from the bed-wetters pervading all. I was in terror of never getting free from "State Custody". One poor devil had been incarcerated there for SIXTY years (in at 38, and died there at 98), - and there were plenty with me who had be 5, 10, 15, 20 . . .years. It was only thanks to my dear friends the DeSilvers that my release was miraculously procured.

This immediate terror had the by-effect of taking my thoughts off Evelyn, but now it has all come back again, and, no use denying it, I am v sick.

I have had, perforce, to leave all sorts of business about Evelyn unfinished - Her will, and a dreadful packet "To be opened only by (me) in the event of my death".[320] Also photos, small bits of "jewellery" for Denise etc.

What I did do is to, at last, take a note of her plot in the cemetery, and here it. Please <u>take a note of it</u> because am liable to lose and forget.

She is buried at ROSEHILL CEMETERY, LINDEN, NEW JERSEY, Section 68A, Grave 45. Buried 6th Aug 1963. (My) Cemetery Deed No 3803M.

I cannot write as I would wish. I'm v unwell, - and it's probably some sort of hospital again, but <u>NOT</u> "in custody". If any hell could have been devised to exacerbate my original poor condition, I'd be interested to hear of it. Obscenities galore, bandied between patients and male muscular orderlies and female nurses too, who were profuse in 4-letter gutter-talk by way of repartee, as the patients. And some physical violence.

This experience has temporarily shattered me. I <u>hope</u> to improve.

You two are my dear friends.

Always, my deep affection

Jack

PS My eventual habitat will be London. I was not a free man till the 'plane left NY on Oct 27! I was <u>escorted</u> to the plane by a hospital orderly. I really wonder they spared me the handcuffs! The horror of probably life-long incarceration took my thoughts off E for a while, but now it seems all to have returned.

[Handwritten, signed. UTK]

---

319 The location of the New York State mental hospital on Long Island.
320 This would be the letter of 2 April 1956, prefaced by Evelyn's handwritten instructions and relating events which persuaded Evelyn she was being libelled (see Chapter 36).

Jigg died at home in Chester, Nova Scotia on June 7, 1965.

To Paula Scott

Baron's Hotel
Bayswater, London
June 9, 1965

Dear, dear Paula

Any words, at your news, would be inadequate. My heart goes out to you all. I can't tell you how I grieve - not merely "selfishly", because of my own love for Jigg, - but by realising what must be your own suffering. I know <u>exactly</u> what you mean by not having (when you wrote) felt the full impact yet.

It is a tragic loss, at the comparative youth of 50, w/ brilliant talents, amounting to genius, and still unlimited opportunities.

I wish to heaven I could be of any practical assistance. I wish you could all be over here. I am v lonely.

As to myself - I was run-over through blindness + spent some months in hospital. My teeth drove through my lips, + my slate is currently full of visits to dentists, oculists, etc. I and a friend, Peter Fell, are trying to find an apartment, sharing, because eating out is ruinously expensive, + he could cook for me.

How are you going to be able to make shift financially? Is there any organisation out in Canada corresponding to what, in England, is called the "National Assistance Board"?

All this, I feel, is useless in your present pass. But try to carry on, through the Gethsemane it must be, for a while. If there is any way I could help I wd do so.

My deepest love and sympathy to you all.

Jack.

All the foregoing, as I hurriedly re-scan it before mailing, sounds the utmost trash and drivel - but please know that my heart and thoughts are with you. Drop me a line whenever you feel up to it.

[Handwritten, signed. SFC]

After a congenial evening with friends in a pub, Jack tripped on a step and fell. He was taken to the local hospital but never regained consciousness. He is buried in Mill Hill Cemetery in north west London. There is no record of any form of memorial on his grave.

Robert Welker to Paula Scott

Huntsville, Alabama
August 27, 1966

Dear Mrs Scott,

First, may I introduce myself so you will know what Mrs Grant may not have told you. I am native of Evelyn's home town where I knew her mother and cousins.

I received my PhD from Vanderbilt University where I taught for nine years after doing my doctoral dissertation on Evelyn's work. I have been a friend of Jack and Evelyn's since the mid fifties when we began correspondence relative to my work on her. Evelyn read my dissertation, corrected it where it was in error, and wrote notes to be incorporated when the work might be published. She was very pleased with my criticism and interpretations and frequently stated that no critic known to her understood her work as well as I. Please excuse the vanity of this last statement; I repeat it only to indicate to you something of Evelyn's regard for my critical work on her novels.

I hold the highest regard for Evelyn as both individual and artist. I am equally fond of Jack and continued to be in close contact with him after Evelyn's death. Needless to say, Jack and Evelyn were extremely helpful to me in my efforts to revive Evelyn's literary reputation, assemble the materials needed for my criticism of her work, gather the materials needed for a biography of her, and preserve literary effects. I like to think that I was equally helpful the them both in difficult times

Of course, you know that Jack never got to move into his new [London] flat.[321] On the evening before I was to go with him to the new flat I had dinner with him as usual. Jack was in a good mood, quite his old witty self, and seemed buoyant and hopeful. He drank more moderately than usual and was able to eat a hearty meal. We left the pub dining room some thirty minutes before closing time (Jack usually insisted on staying until the bitter end!) and I congratulated myself upon having gotten him through the evening in a much better condition than usual. I fancied, perhaps because I wanted to, that the move to the new flat might be indeed the move that would break the locked contingency (as Jack so often called it) of his emotional exhaustion.

I'm sure you know the painful sequel, all of which I related to Gladys Grant and which I am sure was relayed to you by her or someone else who knew how to contact you. I saw Jack safely to his hotel - he was really too blind to walk on the streets by himself - and left him indoors in a happy mood. The next morning, as Peter Fell and I were waiting for him to join us in the corner pub (about half a block from Jack's hotel) to go to the new flat, we learned he had fallen down the steps. As you know, he never regained consciousness.

[Typed carbon copy, not signed. UTK]

MR JOHN METCALFE

From *The Times* (London), August 3, 1965

Mr John Metcalfe, the novelist whose work made an impression in the late twenties and early thirties, and was characterized by a preoccupation with the macabre, has died in hospital in London.

---

321 After some time sharing with his long-standing friend John Gawsworth, Jack and another friend, Peter Fell, found a flat and were planning to move into it in August.

Born in 1891, when he was five his parents went out to Canada as superintendents of a Dr Barnardo's Girls' Home, and returned to do similar work in the East End of London and Stepney four years later. Metcalfe made use of the experiences of this part of his life in *Foster Girl* (1935). He was educated in Suffolk and Norfolk, and then went to the University of London, graduating in philosophy in 1913.

In 1925 a collection of his stories - *The Smoking Leg* - was published, and recommended by one critic for those who had a taste for the uncanny, artistically handled. In 1928, when he went to the United States and worked at first as a barge captain on East River, *Spring Darkness* was published and in 1930 *Arm's Length*. More short stories followed the next year. At the outbreak of the Second World War Metcalfe joined the RAF. Since the war he had written *All Friends are Strangers* (1948), a somewhat confused but frequently witty portrayal of a section of society in London and New York in the late thirties and early forties, and in 1956 *My Cousin Geoffrey*.

Chapter 45

Coda
December 1960 - January 1961

[Evelyn's granddaughter writes:] *When my mother died in the summer of 2007 I flew to Nova Scotia to help my brothers clear her house. After our father's death in 1965, my brothers built a small A-frame cottage for her on a wooded plot a few miles from Chester where she lived until dementia meant residential care. She made that little cottage a home, full of books and personal touches. She must have relished the stability and independence it gave her for the first time in her life as she developed a modest business making crocheted garments from local wool and natural dyes.*

The day we cleared her papers was a revelation. I discovered that she was a natural archivist, keeping her personal papers in meticulous order. But more to the point, she had also kept the entire corpus of correspondence by and about Evelyn. There were the letters Evelyn had sent to her and my father (some never opened), carbon copies of many of the letters she and my father had sent to Evelyn, and typescripts of some of Evelyn's longer autobiographical accounts, including the 74-page "Precis of events indicative of libel".[322] All of this was new to me. I hadn't lived at home since I left to go to college in 1960, before the family moved from Carmel to Vermont and later Chester, and as a result I had virtually no knowledge of the effect Evelyn had had on the family and in particular on my father's health.

It was a shock.

But the biggest shock was these letters from my father to former friends of Evelyn's, describing the effects of his mother's interference in his life and seeking their advice on what he could do now that he was unemployed and desperate. And it is these letters which demonstrate far more clearly than anything else in this collection the devastating effect his mother had had on my father's life.[323]

---

322 See Chapter 31.
323 None of the letters from others referred to in this collection has survived.

To May Mayers

Carmel, California

December 9, 1960

Dear May Mayers

As you still seem to feel a concern for my mother, and as I shall be forced to take steps concerning her, I solicit your suggestions, if you care to make any.

During the war, when she stayed briefly with us in New Jersey,[324] she had a sort of psychic explosion which expressed itself in squeezing open the mouth of my baby son and spitting into it because she had the 'flu and she wanted him to have it too; smashing various things around the house; waking me up every half hour so I would be too tired to go to work, in the hope, she said, that I would lose my job and my present marriage would founder economically. This was just the preliminary, and as I refused to have anything to do with her since then, except for an unwise forty-eight hour visit in London in 1949, she has taken to writing letters for lack of anything better.

The letter writing has been going on since 1944. She wrote to David Barnoff when I was working at NBC, high officials of ABC when I was there, to my chiefs at CBS and WOR, and to the powers that be at Radio Free Europe when I was in Munich, to John Foster Dulles, Hollister, and even Eisenhower when I was in Saigon; and latterly she has been carrying on a long correspondence with the Postmaster General and various others to try and discover where I am now working. During the four years I was in Indo-China she wrote letters, all plausible, to various persons she believed to hold some kind of authority over me, including several who owed their position to the late Senator McCarthy, at the rate of about 60 per year; plus other letters to the American Ambassadors and various consuls of every country I have ever been in.

All these letters, since 1944 have said the same thing: (a) that I am so high strung and effeminate the work I am doing, whatever it is, is too much for me and (b) that I am under the influence of nameless, sinister political forces, which have alienated me from her. Last year about forty of these were produced as evidence of my unreliability before a sub-committee of the House Foreign Relations Committee, in an effort to offset evidence I had given concerning the failure of a foreign aid project, by attempting to prove that (a) I was mentally deranged and (b) that I probably have un-American tendencies. She also writes to the FBI, and I have been continually under investigation by this agency since 1945.[325]

In addition to stressing my frailty and my thrall to nameless un-American influences, she plays on the Forsaken Mom theme in the most disgusting way I have ever heard of; and of the 128 letters she wrote to the State Department about me between 1955 and 1957, the four I was allowed to see in part all ended with requests that I should not be allowed to read them for fear it might "upset" me.

---

324 Evelyn stayed with the family in their small rented house in Tappan, New York.
325 I have procured a bulky file on Jigg kept by the FBI, beginning in 1945.

After long uncertainty I discover that I was fired from Radio Free Europe as a political risk because of her, and from the International Cooperation Administration for a similar reason, the person whom she had chosen as pre-eminently suitable for her confidence being a former Methodist Missionary from Texas, the protege of Representative Walter Judd (keynoter for the Republican Party in the last Eisenhower campaign) and especially selected by Scott McLeod, McCarthy's stooge, for the position he still holds in ICA. In addition to being the caricature of everything nauseatingly Puritan a man could be, this person (Winfield) is a racist bigot, and she managed to suggest to him by the ambiguity of her words that I had Negro blood which had gotten into the family strain during my father's residence in Africa. I know this doesn't make sense, but sense is not necessary to bigots. He was never willing to show me what she wrote him about my wife, but he came to Saigon especially to plead with me to divorce her, for my own good and that of the Service. In letters to one of my chiefs in Saigon she stated as a matter of known fact that my wife (Paula Pearson, whom you must remember) was a former prostitute, which became current throughout the Foreign Aid organization within a matter of weeks, without my being able to discover the source until more than two years later.

I have five children, three boys and two girls, one of the latter in college, thanks exclusively to scholarships, another of military age, another in high school and two more still fairly small. I never write to my mother myself, but my wife does out of kindness to me, and the current tendency of the correspondence is to try to discover who I work for, and the name of the college my daughter is attending, so that letters can be written to the employers or faculties. In other words, the treatment is to be extended to the next generation as well as mine.

Quite apart from that, in this age of organizational fanaticism, when every personnel department maintains a species of Gestapo, in constant liaison with others all over the country, I find it impossible to get a job. I have not worked for more than a year, since I left the ICA in Washington; and although there have been many promising overtures, all prospects fade as soon as my references are checked by a prospective employer. Eighteen years with the four major radio networks and several more in responsible positions overseas are thus made nugatory by my mother's selfish mania. In 1949, in London, I protested to my mother about what she had already done in the way of writing letters, or tried to, but she replied that I merely did not understand, and that it was all for my own good. She also counselled me to ditch my wife and children as unworthy of me, because they hampered my literary career. I should not have to point out that I have had no literary career, and that she probably would have tried to strangle that, too, if I had tried one. I am aware she writes to people informing them at great length about how happy I am in my work, and how I am writing, painting or something of the kind; when the simple fact, which she knows as well as I do, is that I live by my wages when I can and that I and mine are often on the brink of starvation because of her.

Where she is sane or not she is ruthless, and I have had enough. The question that bothers me is this: she is supposed to have some kind of heart disease (so do I, with cholesterol deposits around my eyes and electrocardiograms that I have to hush up to keep my jobs) and she says she will drop dead from the shock if my wife discontinues writing or withholds various information I don't think she should be trusted with.

Is this true? I personally doubt it. She once had some doctor write to me insisting that I resume the correspondence for the sake of her health, and as it happened the heart attack came immediately following my warning that I would tolerate no more of her meddling and was miraculously cured when I did as I was asked. I think the heart disease is a fake, but I would like your opinion.

What I propose to do is not merely cut off all communication, but apply through the courts eventually, when I can afford it, to have her locked up. I am forty-six years old. Her attitude toward my wife and family, of whom I am extremely fond, is that they are a kind of vermin she would exterminate if she knew how (I am aware this isn't what she says to others, but it's what she says to me - she knows she has to keep up appearances in order to win sympathy). Almost the only thing she seems to think of is how to bring about some disaster, economic for lack of better, that will disperse my children, estrange me from my wife, and bring me to heel. Filial duty notwithstanding, I cannot see any obligation my progeny has to her, or that I have to tolerate her behavior toward them, and her obviously malevolent intentions.

As you are a doctor, and very wise besides, I would be grateful for any light you can cast on the subject. I apologise for bothering you.

Sincerely,

Jigg Scott

I'd prefer for the time being that Jack be kept out of this.

[Typed, signed. SFC]

To May Mayers

Carmel, California
December 15, 1960

Dear May Mayers,

I realize I must have distressed you unnecessarily by being abrupt, for which I apologize, all the more so because I have been reading about the blizzard, one of the few things that has reconciled me to California, a mad place as you may have heard.

I gratefully accept your offer to write a letter that would make it easier to explain my predicament, but I prefer to leave its composition to you, for I would not know how to begin it. If you will just state the medical facts as you see them, and address it to me, I can have it photostated if necessary.

I don't think, however, that such a document can do much to retrieve my affairs after the seventeen or eighteen years of my mother's letter writing now past and all the confusion, suspicion and misunderstanding she has brought about; and what I am trying to think of, is some way of preventing her from doing any more. One difficulty is that I don't know how many she has written, or to whom. I have given the local postmaster a letter of my own, explaining the case, because he has to be able to defend himself and she complained very strongly about his dilatoriness in answering her to the Postmaster General of the United States. It almost got the poor man fired, when all he said was that the letters she had written probably had reached their destination. She was sure that he, too, was the subject of malign influences, because he wouldn't do anything to make me write, or move from California.

I only get occasional clues, like the ones I mentioned. One was a letter from George West, the City Editor of the New York "Herald Tribune", to whom she had written saying that the Associated Press obituary of my father wrongly gave my name as Wellman instead of Scott, and that I complained. West was very civil and offered to publish a correction, and I had to write him and say that in my opinion she was out of her head and that I did not require any correction. The relevant fact here is that she said nothing about her own objections, it was I on whose behalf she was writing.

Another clue I have is a letter I never saw, written to the Hon Elbridge Durbrow, the US Ambassador to Vietnam, in which she appears to have said that I was very unhappy in Saigon but did not dare to say so, and that she was therefore interceding to have me transferred to a suitable climate. Apart from the fact that I was anything but unhappy and had not written her for years, we all enjoyed being there and my wife told her so repeatedly. As I say, I never saw the letter, but Durbrow asked me why I felt I had to be so devious when I wanted a transfer, and obviously didn't believe me which I said I didn't. He also read me a little lecture on (a) my filial duty and (b) my patriotic obligations, from which I infer that the letter cast doubts on my sincerity in both.

Someone who has not worked for the Department of State or any of its branches cannot begin to imagine what its atmosphere has been like since McCarthy and Dulles put their stamp on it; and I do not exaggerate when I say that the Americans in Saigon were so busy suspecting each other of something nameless they had no time for their work. For every five ordinary employees there was one CIA man checking on his compatriots, and the best way to ingratiate yourself with the boss was to be a stooge for the Executive Officer of the Economic Mission. Into this chaos of Puritan futility my mother dropped her bombshells at short intervals for four years, and I can only imagine their effect.

I know that the material in the ones read by my Washington superior to the congressional sub-committee I mentioned had such an effect the chairman ordered them eliminated from the printed record, which notes this fact. However, I still don't know what the letters contain.

My half brothers and I became estranged in 1949 because I disliked being reminded publicly that I was an illegitimate child; but my father and I, although he was depressed by the whole business, was friendly. He never wrote to me, however, and now I begin to wonder if it wasn't because my mother did write to him, for she said she had heard about the rift during my visit to her and Jack in London that same year.

The truth of the matter is that I don't know where I stand - it's like one of those bomb scares they have in New York, you never know where or when the next one will go off.

The few friends I have mentioned my problems to all say she obviously doesn't know how much harm she is doing, but I wonder. The letters must be very plausible, or they would not make such a bad impression. She started writing them long ago, when she was obviously much more herself than she is now. And though I used to protest, she has always taken the position that my opinions in the matter need not be considered. At first this was because I didn't really mean what I said - it wasn't the "real me" speaking - and later it was because of these intangible malevolent influences she thinks are abroad.

What it boils down to is that she will not concede anybody's right to live his own life, and never has. Psychiatrists must have a word for it. If somebody were to tell me they wanted no more to do with me, that would be the end of that, and it has happened. But apparently nobody can keep my mother from meddling and trying to control and manipulate another's affairs if she feels so inclined. I don't know just why or how God bestowed on her this special authority over fellow humans, or some of them, but it seems to amount to a sort of divine right and always has.

One of the puzzles to me is Jack, whose predicament must have been a nightmare for years, and who has been compelled, one after the other, to give up his friends, his ambitions, his hopes and his peace of mind. When I last saw him in London he was hopelessly dejected and more pessimistic that I had ever expected to find him, and I can only guess what he feels like now.

I don't suppose all this is relevant to anything, but it's a relief to get it off my chest. As far as practical matters go, my mother has overplayed her hand. Up to the present she has been able to blackmail me - or rather, Paula - into keeping up some kind of correspondence, by the implied threat of even more fluent letter writing than usual, with more fascinating innuendo in each letter, for all that I know. Now that I am subsisting more or less from day to day, thanks to the charity of a few and the beneficence of a paternal government, there is absolutely nothing she can do she hasn't done already, and so I planned to end the correspondence once and for all. If it drives her over the edge, it will be regrettable, but better than driving one of my children over the edge. She already has the name of my daughter's college, and I suppose she could find out who my son's commanding officer was if she tried hard enough, but maybe it won't go that far.

Paula has also had enough, and complains that she hears more from her mother-in-law than from her own children, and so I have told her she need answer no more letters. We both feel better for hearing from you that my mother's sudden death from heart disease is not as imminent as she led us to believe.

I apologize very humbly for burdening you with all this, May; and I must say we admire your forbearance and good sense more than we can say. I hope I shall have friends as faithful and disinterested as you have been to my mother, without many thanks that I remember hearing about. If it's any consolation we think you are a trump and Paula thinks so too.

I don't suppose there is much you can do at present except what you have already offered; and my hands are tied pending the outcome of various schemes to make myself solvent again, no mean trick at my age. However, in the event of my being able to come to New York and afford the necessary legal and medical fees, could you advise me on how I should go about putting her in an institution - regardless of whether Jack approves or not, for he doesn't seem to understand the case at all?

It would be a great comfort to me to know I could rely upon someone to guide me through matters I do not understand. The institution would have to be a public one, for I am not likely to be able to afford better, and while I don't like the idea, as long as my mother can write there isn't any prospect of peace and quiet.

You could also give me a sketchy idea, if you would, of what expenses would be involved and just how one goes about such a thing - especially over the possible objections of a husband. I would do whatever I could to make it uncomplicated, and promise not to embroil you in anything. I'm determined to have a try, sooner or later, and it's only a matter of time.

If the costs and complications are not huge, I might be able to borrow the money sooner than I could earn it – it would be worth going into debt to breathe more easily. I may sound heartless, but I feel desperate.

Please accept my thanks and Paula's, which are sincere. The kids would be grateful too, if they knew what was at stake; but we try to keep them from being troubled by such matters.

Sincerely,
C Scott

[Typed carbon copy, signed. SFC]

To Margaret DeSilver

Carmel, California
December 30, 1960

Dear Margaret

The accompanying carbon of my letter to Dr Mayers will explain itself and help clarify what I write below, but before I go on, I request most urgently that you refuse any request from my mother for money to travel out here. If she were to turn up in California, I would have no choice but to petition the State Lunacy Commission to lock her up, which Dr Mayers says is not legally feasible. I would have to try, anyway, using as evidence letters I have in which my mother tells of a powerful electronic device that is being used to brainwash me; and the mess would be calamitous.

As you will see from the carbon, I was in bad company in Saigon, which was crammed with the kind of men the State Department preferred after Dulles and McCarthy put their stamp on it. Nobody who has not lived in the atmosphere these men created can imagine what it was like, and the fact is that the Americans in Indo-China were so busy suspecting each other of something nameless they had no time for their work.

Ever since I left the foreign aid organization Winfield has had all requests from my prospective employers for information on my background referred to him; and the result has been that my name has become mud. Time and again I have been on the verge of going to work only to have the job fall through at the last moment, and in several cases I know it to be because of a bad reference from Winfield.

Believe me, my testimony to the congressmen had nothing to do with my being fired. All I complained about was four years of delay that put us in the ill graces of the Vietnamese, but the other witnesses - and the damned newspapers - put so much stress on the waste of money you would have thought that was the only consideration. I was fired before I came home, and my mother's letters were the reason, plus the fact that my opinions are on the liberal side. I was not even allowed to stay in Saigon an extra week to help my family pack, and they came home after me.

The result is that my wife, my children and I are as close to starvation as we are ever likely to be, and getting closer daily, despite the affluence of the society we live in. Since I have no boss my mother can write to, I am taking advantage of my temporary immunity from her attentions to cut the tie with her for once and for all. In her answer to my letter, Dr Mayer said that my mother's heart ailment is not serious; and this has so far been the only thing holding me back from a final break. I didn't want to be responsible for her death from heart failure, but since that is ruled out, I am through. I have no filial emotions, I am sorry to say, and I have disliked her for more than half my life.

Apart from not giving my mother the money to come here, is there anyone you know who could give me a job? I am nearly desperate as I will ever be. May Mayers obviously thinks that I am lying, and that were there is smoke there must be fire - her letter gives the impression she thinks I must be a Communist. I am not, however, and never have been. Maybe Winfield won't but the FBI is certain to give me a clean bill of health if asked.

My health is good for my age, which is 46, although I had a liver abscess in Saigon and an amoebic cyst as a result, that took a long time to cure. All the jobs I have held are responsible ones. I worked from 1940 to '43 for NBC, from 1943 to '46 for ABC - where I had my own newscast, although an injury has since spoiled my broadcasting voice - from 1947 to 1950 for CBS, from 1950 to '52 for Radio Free Europe in Germany, from 1952 to '55 for WOR, and from 1955 to '59 for the foreign aid branch of the State Department in Saigon.

Although I do not have a college degree or even a high school diploma, I am literate and published one (bad) novel. I am bilingual in French and English, and have a smattering of Spanish and Portuguese.

You must know someone who could give me a hand. All the jobs I have had in the past I got without any influence or intercession of anyone, on the basis of my own record - not an easy matter for a man with no education. I am as near to being desperate as I will ever be, and even the rather meagre bounty of the social workers will be running out one of these days.

I can come to New York by 'bus if necessary; which will mean selling my typewriter and a few other things. But the job need be neither lavish nor important. Just so long as it keeps us all alive.

Please, if you know of anyone who might help me, give me an introduction. Above all, don't mention this to my mother or give her the money to come out here.

Sincerely,

[Typed carbon copy, not signed. SFC]

To Margaret DeSilver

Carmel, California
January 9, 1961

Dear Margaret

Your answer[326] to my letter, which was written in desperation after being out of touch with everyone for more than a year, came as a relief. I have never known where I stood with my mother's friends, and for about twenty-five years I have wondered how you or anyone else could put up with her. It is a consolation to know that you don't have much more patience with her than I do. I still don't understand why you did so much for her, unless it was regard for Jack; but that is your business. Jack is a decent fellow, but as far as I can see his life has been absolutely ruined by my mother, and how he stands the present state of things I don't know.

It's all very well to say that my mother is mad, but her present outlook is merely a caricature of the point of view she has had ever since I first remember, which is simply the mystical conviction that her preferences and opinions are of cosmic importance, and what the rest of mankind thinks is too trivial to consider. Somewhere along the line, when she was about twenty, the Lord God Jehovah Himself bestowed upon her the right to superintend the lives of others, especially myself and my late father. No power on earth could ever persuade her that I (or he) had the right to lead his own life as he thought fit; and when I went ahead and led mine without allowing her to supervise, then it had to be some mysterious and sinister influence that forced me to be perverse - because, of course, her own dear boy would never want to do anything she didn't want unless he had been made into a mindless, gutless zombie by some

---

326 This letter has not survived.

agency or other. At one time I was a mindless, gutless zombie; and when that was no longer so, then it had to be this fabulous brainwashing machine of hers. I'm no psychiatrist, but the fact of the matter seems to be that she prefers zombies to human beings - hasn't any use for the latter at all.

My mother is not only ruthless about wanting her way, but loathsomely unfastidious. What she has been doing for more than fifteen years, is writing to men whose names she didn't even know but whom she thought could put some kind of economic squeeze on me, and playing the forsaken mother act with numerous allusions to the sinister influences – sometimes "alien influences" - that are supposed to have me in thrall. If she had gone on and added a few words about the brainwashing machine, it wouldn't have been too bad. But in her letters to strangers she omits that part. I have a splendid collection of her letters, with details of this device, but it isn't often that I get to use them. Usually I didn't know what hit me until the boss had made up his mind and it was too late. While Helen Prior was chief of personnel in ICA I got a fair shake and all the letters - except the ones that filtered down from big-shots like Dulles - were quietly destroyed. Once she was demoted and sent to Korea, however, I was at the mercy of any busybody that came along, and busybodies are what the recent Republican administration was richest in.

One thing that baffles me is the attitude of Dr Mayers. In her answer to my first letter she offered to write me on her medical stationery, saying my mother's ravings should not be listened to; but she welched on that, and the only advice she could give me was to threaten to cut off letters if my mother persisted in writing to strangers. We tried that for years, but it never worked - presumably because the wishes of a zombie don't matter. Anyway, I wrote to both Jack and my mother at the same time that I wrote you, saying they would not hear from any of us again unless there was a death in the family. I suppose that will be ignored, too; but nobody can do anything to me in my present plight, and I may as well make use of the advantage I have, while I have it. I only hope to God she can't get the money to come out here from someone other than you; that would be the end, with all the social workers swarming around, having a field day at our expense.

It's a relief to get this off my chest. So far you are the only person I have known who didn't seem to consider my mother's literary accomplishments made her sacred.

For most of my life I have tried to keep the eccentricities of my parents decently hushed up, but it's no good. It never paid off, and the result has been absolute disaster. My mother seems to have estranged me from everyone I knew, including my father, who was no mean egotist himself; and lately she has shown every sign of being possessive about, and wanting to get her hooks into, my children; if we don't all starve to death first.

C Scott

[Typed carbon copy, signed. SFC]

To Margaret DeSilver

Carmel, California
January 13, 1961

Dear Margaret,

I got a very nice letter from Lewis Gannet today,[327] from which I gather that some of his correspondence with my mother rivals the specimen letters I keep in case I ever need desperately to prove she isn't rational. However, although he very kindly offered himself as a reference, he had no suggestions about jobs, being retired and out of touch. I asked him to try to think of some line I could take, but perhaps there is nothing I can do. Anyway, it cheered me up to know there is one more person besides myself (and now you) who has doubts about how responsible E Scott is, and Lewis' feelings are very generous. Like Dr Mayers he also advised against trying to get my mother committed, citing a very illuminating case he knew of, on which the courts didn't back up the psychiatrist who studied the case. At least he didn't, like Mayers, suggest that the best course would be to keep the old, filial tie intact, and what he says makes more sense than what the doctor said. With Jack opposing the move, I suppose it would be hopeless.

As I told you, I wrote to my mother and Jack telling them I was through, and that since I had no boss there was nobody my mother could get me in trouble with. The addresses she complained about were the Army Post Office and Fleet Post Office addresses, or the one for the diplomatic pouch, which were used for discretion's sake and because mail was likely to be pilfered otherwise. Except for short periods when I was in transit she always had an address, but she never approved of it; and in fact she raised hell with the postmaster here, and then complained about him to the postmaster general of the US, because I have a rural route address. Jack knows these things as well as I, and although he is a nice guy, I think her influence has destroyed his sense of proportion.

We haven't heard directly from her so far - my letter didn't leave her much to say - you can bet she'll start writing to somebody again, God only knows who. Maybe Kennedy.

Lewis' reply was very kind, but I was awfully disappointed he had no suggestions, because we are at the stage where we are grasping at straws - ineligible for any kind of relief, which we need, and absolutely at the end of our resources. The brunt falls mainly on my wife and kids, and I have ransacked the state of California as thoroughly as my finances allow, for anything and everything - even a milk route, for example, without any luck for more than a year. I have written to everyone I know who might be helpful, and while some may still reply, it is a long time since I got an answer to a letter of mine, yours and Lewis' excepted. As I explained to him I'm not asking for any glowing endorsement, just a foot in the door now and then, and a chance to argue my own case without someone popping up and raising something my mother wrote to somebody

---

327 This letter has not survived.

as an obstacle. I've been carrying my own weight for more than twenty years, and the record of that is still there if I can just get the ear of someone who has connections I can follow up and who will look at my collection of epistles from E Scott before accepting at face value someone else's interpretation of them. One of the things that has been brought up, for example, is that since she was such a staunch anti-Communist, then I must be on the other side if I don't get along with her. But I haven't gotten along with her since I was a kid and she used to drive me wild with her fits of tragic despair whenever something happened in the world that didn't fit with her ideals.

We are really down to rock bottom, time is short, and from the standpoint of my family the predicament is ghastly. Anyway, for heaven's sake please do what you can. It's asking a lot less than re-importing my mother and Jack to the United States.

I enclose Jack's letter.[328]

Good luck to you,

C Scott

[Typed carbon copy, signed. SFC]

To Creighton Scott

70 East 10th Street,

New York City

January 17, 1961

Dear Jigg,

I'm returning herewith your mother's and Jack's letters. Your mother's letter is pretty smooth, + Jack's rather pathetic. Of course he now has to stand by Evelyn, having made that commitment many years ago - not without considerable struggle in his soul, I imagine! PLEASE, JIGG, do not mention to either Jack or Evelyn anything I have said or suggested, or even that you have been in touch with me, ever, in any way. I have a hard enough time as it is being berated by Evelyn for not writing the Herald Tribune, the Attny Genl, + goodness knows who all.

It would be disastrous if Jack ever found out that I let on that he was worried about Evelyn's sanity, because Jack is an OK guy, + trusted my discretion.

Yours Margaret

[Handwritten, signed. SFC]

To Margaret DeSilver

Carmel, California

January 21, 1961

Dear Margaret

I have just finished reassuring Dr Mayers (again) to the effect that I will not mention her advising me to write to my mother, and once again I promise you that I

---

328 Nor has this letter.

will endeavor to surpass myself in discretion where you are concerned. I don't intend ever to write to E Scott again.

I don't feel any special rancour against either my mother or Jack, I just want to be out from under. Jack is, as you say, a decent fellow, and deserves every consideration for making Job seem half-hearted.

The very best

Jigg

[Typed carbon copy, signed. SFC]

Appendix A

Dramatis Personae

This list of those who figure in Evelyn's story is arranged alphabetically by first name, as this is how they are referred to in the letters. Other individuals are introduced in footnotes.

Aunt Kitty: Gertrude Brownell, Paula's great-aunt

Creighton Seely Scott (see also *Jigg*): The only son of Evelyn and Cyril

Cyril Kay Scott: The name by which Dr Frederick Creighton Wellman was known after "eloping" with Evelyn

David (Davy) Lawson: Married to Lola Ridge (*qv*); close friend of Evelyn's and later of John Metcalfe

Denise Creighton Scott: Evelyn's first grandchild, later known as Denise Scott Fears

Dickie: Evelyn's pet name for Jack Metcalfe

Dudley Grant: Married to Gladys Edgerton (*qv*)

Elsie: The childhood name by which Evelyn was known before she left the United States with Cyril, and which she continued to use when writing to her mother

Frederick Creighton Wellman: Evelyn's first ("common law") husband, known as Cyril Kay Scott after their arrival in Brazil

Frederick Wheeler Scott: Evelyn's second grandchild

Gladys Edgerton Grant: Long-standing and loyal friend of Evelyn and later of Jigg and Paula

Herschel Gower: Partner of Robert Welker (*qv*) and later friend of Jack Metcalfe

Jigg: The childhood nickname by which Creighton Scott was known throughout his life

Joe (Joseph) Foster: Paula's stepfather and Margué's (*qv*) second husband

John (Jack) Metcalfe: Evelyn's second husband

Julia Swinburne Scott: Evelyn's fourth grandchild, later known as Julie Swinburne

Lola Ridge: Writer and poet, close friend of Evelyn's, married to David Lawson (*qv*)

Louise Lotz: Cyril's sixth wife

Louise Morgan: Close friend of Evelyn and later of Jack; married to Otto Theis (*qv*)

Love Lyle: Cousin of Maude Dunn (*qv*) and part of Evelyn's extended Clarksville family

Manly Wade Wellman: Eldest son of Frederick Creighton Wellman *(qv)* by his first wife

Margaret (Maggie) DeSilver: Manhattan socialite, friend, and benefactor of Evelyn and Jack

Margué (Margaret) Hale Foster: Paula's mother and first wife of Ralph Pearson *(qv)*

Mary Tudor Garland: Wealthy benefactress of Evelyn and Cyril

Matthew Pearson Scott: Evelyn's third grandchild

Maude Dunn (née Thomas): Evelyn's mother, divorced by Seely Dunn after her arrival in Brazil

May Mayers: Medical doctor, friend, and medical adviser to Evelyn and Jack

Melissa Dunn (née Whitehead): Seely Dunn's second wife and thus Evelyn's stepmother

Mutt, Muttsie: Evelyn's pet name for Owen Merton *(qv)*

Otto Theis: Author and Jack's one-time editor, married to Louise Morgan *(qv)*

Owen Merton: Evelyn's lover during the early 1920s

Paula (Pavla) Pearson Scott. Jigg's wife and Evelyn's daughter-in-law

Phyllis Crawford: Cyril's fifth wife

Ralph Pearson: Paula's father and first husband of Margaret Hale Foster *(qv)*

Robert Scott: Evelyn's fifth grandchild

Robert Welker: Biographer and friend of Evelyn's; latterly friend of Jack (see also *Herschel Gower*)

Seely Dunn: Evelyn's father: he divorced Maude Dunn *(qv)* in early 1920s

Selma Hite: Jigg's first wife: the marriage was short-lived

Sug, Sugs (from *Sugar*): Evelyn's pet name for Cyril

Swinburne Hale: Brother of Margaret Hale Foster and thus Paula Scott's uncle; friend of Evelyn and Cyril

Thomas (Tom) Merton: younger son of Owen Merton and childhood friend of Jigg's

Weecie: Family nickname for Louise Lotz *(qv)*

William John Metcalfe: (see *Jack Metcalfe*)

Appendix B

Brief chronology for Creighton and Paula Scott

Jigg and Paula moved frequently throughout Evelyn's lifetime because of changes in their circumstances, heightened by the effect Evelyn's letter writing had had on Jigg's employment.

This table, compiled from detailed records kept by Paula Scott, presents a summary of the dates the family lived at various locations.

June 1940	Creighton Scott and Paula Pearson marry
June 1940–October 1942	New York City
October 1942–May 1946	Tappan, New York
June 1946–August 1949	Pine Bluff, North Carolina
August–November 1949	New City, New York
November 1949–June 1951	Rutherford, New Jersey
June–September 1951	Red Hook, New York
October–November 1951	Regina Palast Hotel, Munich, Germany
November 1951–August 1952	Grünwald and Gräfelfing, Germany
August 1952–July 1953	Chelsea Hotel, New York City
July 1953–October 1955	Spring Valley, New York
November 1955–July 1959	Saigon, Vietnam
July 1959–August 1961	Carmel, California
August 1961–August 1962	Peacham, Vermont
August 1962–September 2007	Chester, Nova Scotia, Canada
June 1965	Jigg dies
September 2007	Paula dies

Appendix C

Works published by Evelyn Scott

1919   "A Tardy Obeisance", *The Egoist* (London), December 1919 (criticism)

1919   "From Brazil to the US", *Poetry: A Magazine of Verse*, November 1919 (criticism)

1919   "Penelope", *Others*, April–May 1919 (poetry)

1919   "Tropical Life", *Poetry: A Magazine of Verse*, November 1919 (poetry)

1919   "Women", *Others*, February 1919 (poetry)

1919   "Young Girls", *Others*, April–May 1919 (poetry)

1919   "Young Men", *Others*, April–May 1919 (poetry)

1920   "Air for G String", *The Dial*, September 1920 (poetry)

1920   "Argentine Drama", *Poetry: A Magazine of Verse*, October 1920 (criticism)

1920   "Ascension: Autumn dusk in Central Park", *The Dial*, September 1920 (poetry)

1920   "Autumn Night", *Others*, 1920 (poetry)

1920   "Critic of the Threshold", *The Dial*, March 1920 (criticism)

1920   "Divine Beachcomber", *The Dial*, May 1920 (criticism)

1920   "Emilio de Menezes", *Poetry: A Magazine of Verse*, April 1920 (criticism)

1920   "Gilbert Cannan: Inquisitor", *The Dial*, February 1920 (criticism)

1920   "Nine Poems", *The Dial*, January 1920 (poetry)

1920   "Rifts", *The Nation*, 10 July 1920 (poetry)

1920   "Spring Song", *The Dial*, September 1920 (poetry)

1920   *Precipitations*. New York: Nicholas L Brown (poetry)

1921   "A Philosopher of the Erotic", *The Dial*, 1921 (criticism)

1921   "Brazilian Dance Songs", *Poetry: A Magazine of Verse*, August 1921 (criticism)

1921   *Love: A drama in three acts*: Play produced by Provincetown Players

1921   *The Narrow House*. New York: Boni and Liveright (novel)

1922   "Contemporary of the Future", *The Dial*, October 1922 (criticism)

1922   *Narcissus*. New York: Harcourt, Brace and Co. Published as *Bewilderment* in London by Duckworth (novel)

1923   *Escapade*. New York: Thomas Seltzer. Reissued by Jonathan Cape and Harrison Smith, 1929 (autobiographical novel)

1925   "Nike", *The London Outlook* (poetry)

1925   "Nirvana", *The London Outlook* (poetry)

1925   *In the Endless Sands: A Christmas book for boys and girls*. New York: Henry Holt and Company, with Cyril Kay Scott (juvenile)

1925   *The Golden Door*. New York: Thomas Seltzer (novel)

1925   "The Old Lady", *The Dial*, May 1925 (poetry)

1925   "Tomorrow", *The London Outlook* (poetry)

1925   "White Peacocks", *The English Calendar* (poetry)

1925   "Winter Morning", *The London Outlook* (poetry)

1927   *Ideals: A book of farce and comedy*. New York: Albert and Charles Boni (novel)

1927   "On reading the Sunday newspapers", *The Nation*, 21 September 1927 (essay)

1927   *Migrations: An Arabesque in histories*. New York: Albert and Charles Boni (novel)

1928   "Creatures in General", in A Kreymbourg et al (eds): *The Second American Caravan*. New York: The Macaulay Co (poetry)

1928   "Speed" in L Mumford and P Rosenfeld (eds): *The Second American Caravan*. New York: The Macaulay Co (short story)

1929   "On writing *The Wave*", *Writer*, August 1929 (essay)

1929   "Cat", *The Nation*, 3 July 1929 (poetry)

1929   "Is American woman victim of the age? novelist inquires: Hard glittering creatures who use prosperity to forge new chains for selves". *Times Signal* (Zanesville OH), 8 September 1929, p 33 (essay)

1929   "Two brothers: Review of *Don't Call Me Clever* by Lawrence Drake, *New York Herald Tribune Books*, 29 September 1929, p 3. (criticism)

1929   "Light Fog over London" in L Mumford et al (eds): *The New American Caravan*. New York: The Macaulay Co. (poetry)

1929   "On Lola Ridge": publicity piece written for Payson and Clarke Ltd (criticism)

1929   "Mongoose", *The New Republic*, 17 July 1929 (poetry)

1929   *On William Faulkner's* The Sound and the Fury. New York: Jonathan Cape and Harrison Smith, 1929 (criticism)

1929   "The Young Courtesan Speaks" in L Mumford et al (eds): *The New American Caravan*. New York: The Macaulay Co. (poetry)

1929   "Voyage", *The Nation*, August 1929 (poetry)

1929   *The Wave*. New York: Jonathan Cape and Harrison Smith (novel)

1929   *Witch Perkins: A story of the Kentucky hills*. New York: Henry Holt and Company (juvenile)

1930   "Autumn Night" in A Kreymbourg (ed): *Lyric America*. New York: Coward-McCann Inc (poetry)

1930   Untitled piece on censorship: *Laughing Horse*, February 1930 (criticism)

1930   "Intimacy with sublime seen in poem on Jesus: Evelyn Scott finds Lola Ridge an abrupt exception to current style of woman poets", *New York Telegram*, 22 February 1930, p 11 (review)

1930   "Adolescent adoration: Review of *Dance on the Tortoise* by Marion Patton", *New York Herald Tribune Books*, 21 September 1930, p 2 (review)

1930   "Ennui", *Pagany*, April–June 1930 (poetry)

1930   "The Santa Fe art colony", *Wings*, October 1930 (essay)

1930   *Blue Rum*. New York: Jonathan Cape and Harrison Smith (published under the pseudonym Ernest Souza)

1930   "The Lover", *Scribner's Magazine*, October 1930 (short story)

1930   *The Winter Alone*. New York: Jonathan Cape and Harrison Smith, 1930 (poetry)

1931   *A Calendar of Sin*. New York: Jonathan Cape and Harrison Smith (novel)

1931   "The bloody ground: Review of *The Border: A Missouri Saga*" by Dagmar Doneghy: *Saturday Review of Literature*, 19 September 1931, p 130 (review)

1931   "A Note on the Significance of Photography" in L Mumford, L Frank et al (eds): *America and Alfried Steiglitz: A collective portrait*. New York: Doubleday, Doran and Co (criticism)

1931   "Art" in A Kreymbourg et al (eds): *Fourth American Caravan*. New York: The Macaulay Co (short story)

1931   "Home": *Scribner's Magazine*, December 1931 (short story)

1931   "Kentucky Land", *The New Republic*, 4 November 1931 (criticism)

1931   "Poem to Helen Keller" in E Porter (ed): *Double Blossoms: A Helen Keller anthology*. New York: L Copeland (poetry)

1932   "Pike's Peak", *Contempo*, c 1932 (poetry)

1932   "Scene laid in a hospital: Review of *Hospital* by Rhoda Truax", *New York Herald Tribune Books*, 21 February 1932, p 7 (review)

1933   "South American Rhapsody", *The Nation*, 30 August 1933 (criticism)

1933   "We shall keep our eyes: Review of *No Retreat* by Horace Gregory", New York Herald Tribune Books: 23 April 1933, p 2 (review)

1933   "This Season", *The Windsor Quarterly*, c 1933 (poetry)

1933   "Turnstile": *Scribner's Magazine*, February 1933 (short story)

1933   "Voyager's Return", *Everyman* (London), 9 September 1933 (poetry)

1933   *Eva Gay*. New York: Harrison Smith and Robert Haas (novel)

1933   "A poet kin to D H Lawrence: Review of *The Single Glow* by Axton Clark", *New York Herald Tribune Books*, 20 August 1933, p 8 (review)

1934   "A Novel of Revolution", *The Saturday Review of Literature*, 2 June 1934 (criticism)

1934   *Billy the Maverick*. New York: Henry Holt and Company (juvenile)

1934   "The new best-seller: Review of *So Red the Rose* by Stark Young", *Scribner's Magazine*, October 1934 (review)

1934   *Breathe Upon These Slain*. New York: Harrison Smith and Robert Haas (novel)

1934   "Englishman", *The Yale Review*, March 1934 (short story)

1934   "Cosmic critic – with limits: Review of *The Death and Birth of David Markand* by Waldo Frank", *Scribner's Magazine*, November 1934 (review)

1934   "From a Novelist", *The Saturday Review of Literature*, 10 November 1934 (criticism)

1934   "Gentlemanly Englishmen – and Americans", in G J Nathan et al (eds): *The American Spectator Yearbook*. New York: Frederick A Stokes Co (criticism)

1934   "Kalicz" in C Van Doren (ed): *Modern American Prose*. New York: Harcourt Brace and Company (short story)

1934   "Lady Author", *The American Mercury*, April 1934 (short story)

1934   "Modern Fiction", *The Saturday Review of Literature*, 2 June 1934 (criticism)

1934   "On Writing for Children", *Boston Horn Book*, Christmas 1934 (criticism)

1934   "To a Snake in Eden", *The Nation*, August 1934 (poetry)

1934   "Two Generals" in S Cox and E Freeman (eds): *Prose Preferences*. New York: Harper and Brothers (short story)

1934   "Voyager's Return" in G J Nathan et al (eds): *The American Spectator Yearbook*. New York: Frederick A Stokes Co (criticism)

1934   "When War Ends", *The Nation*, 2 February 1934 (poetry)

1935   "Colossal Fragment", *Scribner's Magazine*, June 1935 (criticism)

1935   "Flight for Angels", *Poetry: A Magazine of Verse*, June 1935 (poetry)

1935   "To Kenitra", *The Yale Review*, March 1935 (short story)

1936   "Christmas Eve" in K Boyle et al: *Three Hundred Sixty-Five Days*. New York: Harcourt Brace and Co (short story)

1936   "War Between the States", *The Nation*, 4 July 1936 (criticism)

1937   *Bread and a Sword*. New York: Charles Scribner's Sons (novel)

1937   *Background in Tennessee*. New York: McBride and Co (autobiography)

1937   "Test of Maturity", *Poetry: A Magazine of Verse*, July 1937 (criticism)

1937   "Tone of Time", *Poetry: A Magazine of Verse*, May 1937 (poetry)

1938   "Communist Mentalities" in H E Stearns (ed): *America Now: An inquiry into civilization in the United States by thirty-six Americans*. New York: Charles Scribner's Sons (criticism)

1938   "Pioneers", *Intermountain*, Winter 1938 (essay)

1939   "Black is My True Love's Hair", *North Georgia Review*, Spring 1939 (criticism)

1939   Introduction to *Books of Southern Interest*, *The Southern Literary Messenger*, July 1939 (criticism)

1939   "On *After Freedom*", *The Southern Literary Messenger*, April 1939 (criticism)

1939   "On *I Swear by Apollo*", *The Southern Literary Messenger*, January 1939 (criticism)

1939   "On *The Peopling of Virginia*", *The Southern Literary Messenger*, April 1939 (criticism)

1939   "Opus Ten Billion", *The North Georgia Review*, Autumn 1939 (poetry)

1939   "Doctor's choice: Review of *Days Before Lent* by Hamilton Basso", *Saturday Review of Literature*, 5 August 1939 (review)

1939   "Professorial Mood", *The American Mercury*, July 1939 (poetry)

1940   "Alive", *The Saturday Review of Literature*, 7 February 1940 (poetry)

1940   "Apocrypha: To all Negro poets now alive", *The Saturday Review of Literature*, 17 February 1940 (poetry)

1940   Review of *American Social Problems, Southern Literary Messenger*, January 1940 (criticism)

1940   Review of *Faces we See, Southern Literary Messenger*, Southern Combed Yarn Spinners Association, Gastonia, NC (criticism)

1940   "Touch", *Rhythmus*, 23 February 1940 (poetry)

1941   "How can intelligent Southerners best help the South?", *The North Georgia Review*, Winter 1941 (criticism)

1941   *The Shadow of the Hawk*. New York: Charles Scribner's Sons (novel)

1942   "Homage to Ford Maddox Ford – A symposium": in *New Directions No 7*. Norfolk, Conn: New Directions (criticism)

1945   "The Observers" in S Burt et al (ed): *North, East, South, West: A regional anthology of American writing*. New York: Howell, Sockin (short story)

1948   "To Artists of Every Land", *The Saturday Review of Literature*, May 22, 1948 (poetry)

1949   "She Dies", *The Saturday Review of Literature*, January 29, 1949 (poetry)

1951   "American Poetry II: Dr Sitwell and the American genius", *The Poetry Review* (London) September–October 1951 (criticism)

1951   "American Poetry III: Six Poets", *The Poetry Review* (London), November–December 1951 (criticism)

1951   "Directions in American Poetry: The doctor from New Jersey", *The Poetry Review* (London) July–August 1951 (criticism)

1951   "Ivory Tower", *The Poetry Review* (London), September–October 1951 (poetry)

1951   "Old American Stock", *The Poetry Review* (London), November–December 1951 (poetry)

1953   "Survival", *The Saturday Review of Literature*, 6 June 1953 (poetry)

1954   "Blighted by inner tyrannies: Review of *The Bird's Nest* by Shirley Jackson", New York Times, 20 June 1954 (review)

Sources:

Welker, Robert L, *Evelyn Scott: A literary bibliography*. Unpublished PhD dissertation. Nashville, TN: Vanderbilt University

Bach, Peggy, "Evelyn Scott: 1922-1988", *Bulletin of Bibliography*, 46(2), June 1989, 76–91

Jones, Paul Christian, "Evelyn Scott's nonfiction prose: A supplemental bibliography", *The Mississippi Quarterly*, 22 June 2006

Appendix D

Works published by Cyril Kay Scott

During his scientific career, before he "eloped" with Elsie Dunn and while known as Frederick Creighton Wellman, Scott published a large number of articles in a variety of scientific journals. These publications are not included in this list.

1921   *Blind Mice*. New York: George H Doran Company (novel)

1923   *Sinbad: A romance*. New York: Thomas Seltzer (novel)

1925   *Siren*. London: Faber and Gwyer (novel)

1925   *In the Endless Sands: A Christmas book for boys and girls* (with Evelyn Scott). New York: Henry Holt and company (juvenile)

1943   *Life Is Too Short*. New York: J B Lippincott Company (autobiography)

Appendix E

Works published by John Metcalfe

Many of Metcalfe's short stories, first published in his two collections The Smoking Leg and Other Stories *and* Judas and Other Stories, *were republished later in a number of anthologies: these later publications have not been listed.*

1920   "The Bad Lands", *Land and Water*, 15 April 1920 (short story)

1925   "The Smoking Leg", *The London Mercury*, May 1925 (short story)

1925   *The Smoking Leg and Other Stories*. London: Jarrolds (collected stories)

1925   "The Tunnel", *Outlook*, 14 March 1925 (short story)

1927   "The Funeral March of a Marionette", *The Independent*, 1 January 1927 (short story)

1928   *Spring Darkness*. London: Constable and Co Ltd. Published in US as *Mrs Condover* (novel)

1930   *Arm's Length*. London: Constable and Co Ltd (novel)

1931   *Judas and Other Stories*. London: Constable and Co Ltd (collected stories)

1932   *Brenner's Boy*. London: White Owl Press (novel)

1936   *Foster-Girl*. London: Constable and Co Ltd. Published in US as *Sally: The story of a foster-girl* (novel)

1948   *All Friends Are Strangers*. London: Nicholson and Watson (novel)

1952   "The Childish Thing", *Story #2*, 1952 (short story)

1954   *The Feasting Dead*. Sauk City WI: Arkham Press (novel)

1956   *My Cousin Geoffrey*. London: Macdonald (novel)

Appendix F

Jack Metcalfe's diaries: A commentary

The following personal commentary was compiled as I was reading through the diaries of Jack Metcalfe's which had found their way to the Harry Ransom Center. They describe another side of the life that Jack and Evelyn shared; neither account any less valid than the other, but perhaps taken together a better picture of the whole than that represented in Evelyn's letters alone. As with the letters, these diary entries are transcribed exactly as written: Jack's with his telegraphic punctuation and Evelyn's in her characteristic scrawl, a chronicle of letters not delivered and of her cleaning of the refrigerator in the communal kitchen.

Jack's diaries for 1921 and for 1931-34 (i.e. a 5-year diary) are pedantic and dry, written in phrases, not sentences, a chronicle of errands run, books read, people visited. He walked a lot in London, and I was struck that he records his bedtime "smoke" each evening. These diaries probably contain a great deal of interest to social historians, but it was not my purpose, nor did I have the time, to record all of those details.

In the 1930s, after he and Evelyn were married, he made a habit of "going to her room" for breakfast. He seemed to read aloud (to Evelyn?) a good deal. In August 1934 he went into the Hospital for Tropical Diseases for investigations. Notable is the fact that he was not seen by a doctor nor any tests done until the third day! One or two tests (all intestinal) per day and discharged after a week but, as far as I could see, no diagnosis. That month he booked driving lessons; the entries peter out, then end altogether in October 1934. The impression is of a sad, uptight, very repressed and lonely (albeit married) man leading a barren life; but the diary may be entirely misleading.

The 1942 diary sees Jack seconded to the Canadian Royal Air Force in Ottawa, and many of the entries refer to phone calls or letters about his re-entry to United States, as well as visits to US Legation in Ottawa and State Department in Washington DC. Others concerned arrangements for Evelyn's passage in a convoy to England. Paperwork abounded, but it was wartime, and bi-national marriages do not seem to have been that common then. He seemed to eat regularly at a place called United Cigar Stores (?).

Although Jack was on active duty in the RAF, he appears to have held an administrative job, and with his papers I found a folder of his RAF notes about the Vocational Advisory Centre which existed to help de-mobbed airmen find civilian jobs. It gives the impression he was an interviewer for the VAC (we would probably call that role "career advisor"), but I found no firm evidence of this. He seems to have spent a good deal of time "taking Wing Parade" on behalf of the CO, obviously essential war work. It looks as though he and Evelyn moved into a flat in Ottawa in March, even though he was on active duty. He records an unchanging daily routine of his duties at camp, working on his novel whenever he could as well as the minutiae of domestic life. On December 25 1942, he "Had bologna sausage for breakfast. Programme as yesterday. Heard Darlan (?) assassinated" and that is the total entry for that day.

The next diary, 1947, with Jack back in London, is characterised by much longer sentences, though the pedantic detail remains. As in earlier years, it is full of information of great interest to social historians. There is much mention of looking for work and following up leads for tutoring individual children, with mixed results, and records payment of £1.1.0 (one guinea) for two lessons. He also managed to land a job in an (unnamed) "crammer", or private school. Many diary entries about getting an emigration permit for priority sailings with US Lines, and about receiving and/or chasing small amounts of money owed him for tutoring, teaching and his various short stories. A continuing saga about house insurance and the problems caused by one of his tenants, Gumb, who ran a business from his flat, thereby making it impossible to insure the rest of the house.

Jack sailed to New York on August 2 and records pages of vivid, though brief, details of shipboard life. In New York he stayed in Margaret DeSilver's flat (no mention of where she was – in Brooklyn or at their Long Island summer home?) and spent most of his time on paperwork about immigration and job hunting as well as trying to find publishers for recent MSS. He booked his return passage to England on US Lines on October 8th, but when he arrived at the pier (after a farewell party), he found the ship was held up by engine trouble, so sailed two days later on the *Queen Mary*. There were no details of shipboard life on this voyage.

Jack's diary for 1948 is very like that for 1947 – an uneventful round of school, shopping, letters sent and received: he's back to a more staccato bullet-point style. He moved to a new (part-time?) job at a school in Hitchin, not far from London, and seems to eke out his RAF pension by tutoring. Payments were a number of small cheques from various sources, including some dollar cheques (I can't help wondering how much was swallowed up by exchange fees) from Gladys. Took Evelyn's typewriter in for repairs twice during the year – I can imagine that it took quite a pounding. One day's entry reports that Evelyn is unwell with a bad cough, and that he went out to buy cigarettes for her! Once again, Christmas Day totally unmarked by any form of observance or celebration. And throughout this year (and 1947) he is working on his "Scilly" novel (eventually published as *All Friends are Strangers*).

1949 continues in much the same vein, with Jack working at a school and doing some private tutoring. There is more about various repairs to the house, and Jack even spends a weekend in May painting the front door and entrance hall and some exterior window frames in a dull emerald green (they are trying to sell the house to fund their return to the US). This continues throughout the summer and into the autumn. Evelyn's typewriter went in for repairs, again. Jigg's visit in November, which Evelyn made so much of in her letters for years, lasted three days and merits brief daily mentions in Jack's diary over that period. No clue as to what really went on while he was there, nor any mention of Evelyn's reactions to the visit after Jigg left. Christmas Day was only slightly more festive than previous years: they had Christmas pudding for supper.

There are mentions throughout these diaries of Jack's birthdays, Evelyn's birthdays and their wedding anniversaries, but no indication that presents were given or received.

The diary for 1950 chronicles the same routine, but on June 26, Jack reveals another facet of himself: "Test Match v West Indies interesting". There are a few other references of his listening to the Test Match and he records that the West Indies won by 326 runs. He makes no mentions of the histrionics Evelyn was recording in her many letters at this period: either he had become inured to these or he was unbelievably self-obsessed. There are mentions in this year and the previous years of Jack buying clothes – dresses and slacks – for Evelyn, which contrasts with her assertions that they were so poor she had no clothes she could leave the house in. Jack also records her receiving a number of parcels of clothing from Maggie (Margaret DeSilver). He seems to spend in a steady trickle: apart from food, he refers to books, tobacco, typing paper and carbons, repairs to shoes, pens and typewriters, ties and socks, taxis, lunches out. They eat moderately well, too: standard British fare, nothing too lavish, but a varied diet. Much of his spending was essential to their trade, none of it luxury, but no sense of the abject penury which Evelyn describes. There is also repeated mention of the costs of repairs to the house, as they tried (unsuccessfully) to prepare it for letting through the US Embassy to visitors to the Festival of Britain. And once again, Christmas appears to have been a cheerless affair, livened only by Jack making scones for tea.

1951 saw Jack following the boat race ("Oxford crew sank"), as well as the cricket. During the summer Evelyn made a series of visits to the dentist, apparently for extractions. And throughout the year, as in previous years, an ostinato of repairs to the house, bills from the gas board and his particularly troublesome tenant, Gumb. Jack also gets regular demands from the tax inspector for what seem like significant sums for the day (around the £12 to £14 mark) which implies commensurate earnings. Christmas day saw Evelyn upset at third-hand news (via Margaret DeSilver) that Jigg was to be in Munich.

1952 is much the same again: diary entries are now largely in staccato form, and Jack records selling some of his books at Foyles and other shops, Evelyn's continued visits to the dentist, and, eventually, in May, a new set of teeth. Continuing thrum of tenants, repairs and redecorations, bills due and paid, letters to and from, errands, shopping and receipts of small amounts of money. This year he records major public events: the death and funeral of the king (but not the coronation), the winner of the America's Cup, the opening of the Democratic convention in Chicago, Eisenhower's election. On October 27 he gave his notice in at his school, and the weeks following he went through various formalities prior to sailing for New York, including health screening and vaccinations. Another typically low-key Christmas day.

1953 starts with a flurry of activity around preparations for their return to the US. One prospective tenant of their flat rejected it as she "could not find room for her refrigerator"; they eventually found a tenant at 9 guineas (£9 9s) a week, payable yearly in advance, but three days later the tenant "cried off". (There is no record of a replacement tenant.) They sailed on March 1 for the US and the west coast; I have transcribed in full the entries for March 12 to 31, when they arrived at the Huntington Hartford Foundation in Pacific Palisades, near Los Angeles. In the first days after their arrival, Evelyn wrote numerous letters to members of Paula's family. Both Jack and Evelyn suffered from flu shortly after their arrival, and Jack suffered from his recurring dysentery. Almost immediately Jack started to look for teaching jobs for when they had to return to the east coast, responding to adverts from schools around the US, but no record of any success, only of rejections. In October and November, Jack mentions Evelyn's "attacks" and chest pains and that she was given green, pink, and brown tablets by the local doctor. Because they were living in a community, Christmas was uncharacteristically festive.

1954 begins with Evelyn and Jack still at the Hartington Hartford Foundation in California, and days pass with little excitement. A typical entry (January 9) reads: "Breakfast. Work. Coffee. Work. Lunch. Nap. Coffee. Work. Work. Saw films". Jack records the number of pages of Evelyn's MS he reads each day, but only rarely how much of his own work he completes. Every Tuesday he records the fact that Alice (the maid?) cleans their room. They leave the Hartington Hartford Foundation in March, after a farewell dinner followed by a concert given by other residents; once back in New York City, they move into the Benjamin Franklin Hotel and resume the routine they had followed before going to California. Jack gets a job with the Searing Tutorial School which he appears to find dull and routine, and later at a place called St Bernards. Their social life appears a bit more active than recorded in previous years, with a number of visitors and one or two "parties", but apart from that, life appears to consist of work, shopping, errands, repairs to Evelyn's typewriter, and letters to the UK about entitlement to his British and RAF pensions. For some reason, this year he records the occasions of his various trips to the barber.

The diary for 1955 is missing, and the diary for 1956 sees the advent of entries by Evelyn, either annotations regarding appointments or full-day entries, mainly about her will and various letters. A new theme is added to those previously recorded: the cleaning of the communal fridge; so important is it that even Jack records the days that Evelyn cleans the fridge! It is clear from the pages that Evelyn makes her entries before Jack has a chance to write his, with his being squashed at the bottom of the respective pages, sometimes including note "as narrated above". Jack has started working at the Haithcock School, and many of his entries record the day as having been "nasty", although it is not spelled out what makes it so. He is beginning, again, to refer to the Benjamin Franklin Hotel as "home" in inverted commas, and there is a record of discussions about moving into school accommodation, but the deductions for board appear to rule this out. By the autumn term he is at another school, Greenwich. He records visits to doctors to diagnose his recurring stomach problems as well as repeated references to Evelyn's "heart trouble" and the side effects of her "pink pills". Notably, Jack's handwriting is looser and larger than before, less neat, and in places nearly illegible.

1957 continues much as before. Evelyn is still preoccupied by the cleaning of the fridge, and many of her entries hint at the obsessiveness and paranoia that will be a feature of her writing from here on. Jack's entries are often limited to "Greenwich School" and occasionally supplemented with reference to shopping, letters sent and received, and various school matters. On July 20, an outburst by Evelyn in Jack's diary, lasting six days (pages), of angry, illegible, overwritten scrawl about what she perceived as the failure to deliver letters to Jigg and the family. No room for anything by Jack at all, except a meek little "Greenwich School" hiding in the margins. In fact, she all but takes over his diary until the beginning of November. Jack seems to have suffered recurring colds and other minor ailments. There are no entries at all from November 16 to 30, then a large, almost incoherent, scrawl in E's writing

The diary for 1958 is very different. He uses an undated week-to-page engagement diary, ruled to allow two days' entries to a page, and starts it on April 17 (the days prior to this are scrawled by Evelyn at the end of his 1957 diary. They were so incoherent I could not face trying to make sense of them – (perhaps I should have). I can't help thinking he did this to deter Evelyn from taking over his diary again. Again, tiny, precise writing. Jack mentions a series of visits to Dr B (E's heart specialist) and tests. After the hysteria of Evelyn's entries in the 1957 diary, this year feels very peaceful and calm, even though there are frequent references to Evelyn not being well (her heart?). Occasionally one gets a hint of a rather impish Jack, as on September 24th he writes "This is the Jewish Yom Kippur. E + I strolled down to the river, utilising the occasion to buy a 15 cent Colgate toothpaste at Woolworths on our way back". October sees Jack looking for a new job, and eventually ending up at the New York Tutoring School. Many of the entries relate to his London property and the various legal and financial factors involved in deciding whether to sell it.

1959 sees Jack's staccato one-word entries continuing to describe a life centred around school, working on his novel, letters, bills, shopping, repairs to shoes and typewriters, and haircuts. Evelyn's cleaning of the fridge continues to be recorded.

Although Evelyn makes a number of entries, there is no repetition of her frenzy of 1957. It was a hot summer and Jack noted the daily temperatures throughout the June and September heatwaves. On many days, the only entry was "School". Jack also records that he and Evelyn took regular walks up to Riverside Park and Riverside Drive. Throughout the year there are frequent visits from Bernice Elliott and November sees entries by each of them about Evelyn's heart symptoms and her wait for both a visit from May Mayers and the delay in getting a prescription – for codeine! And, for the first time ever, Jack refers to preparations for Christmas (Christmas cards) but the entry for Christmas day refers only to his unpleasant cold.

1960 continues as previous years, except that references to haircuts are now all in CAPITAL LETTERS! Bernice was a frequent visitor, often staying for tea although the visits appear to have tailed off by late spring, and May called regularly. Jack and Evelyn marketed together and took short walks. Evelyn continues to document her cleaning of the communal fridge and in the summer regular entries to "look at clothes on hangers" appear in her hand: what this is about I cannot fathom. Jack has his usual quota of colds keeping him home from school, and there is no mention of Evelyn's health. Cyril's death in September provokes a flurry of (and entries about) letters to Jigg and various friends. There are a few mentions of bulbs being planted in pots and, eventually, flowering, and Christmas is the usual featureless day, except that this year Jack mentions tips (presumably to hotel staff?).

1961 is even quieter. Many days' entries read only "School etc as usual". Evelyn's war of attrition regarding the cleaning of the fridge seems to have seen results, with fewer references to her cleaning it and a few entries saying it had been cleaned by others. With Bernice in England, they have virtually no visitors; Jack records two visits by Gladys who came to tea and left after about an hour and a half. Jack records buying "medicines" (not stated what) at regular intervals, and in August Evelyn has a major attack, so serious that Jack goes out to get her a doctor, and Evelyn is not pronounced well until late November. The writing in Evelyn's entries has become quite scrawly and illegible, and some of her entries are totally incoherent.

1962 starts in calm fashion, with normal entries relating to school, marketing, and letters sent and received. Jack's haircuts are now emphasised with a green ring around the entries, and his underlines, mostly about letters to and about Jigg, are now in green! I was shocked to see that Carmel High School gave Evelyn the family's Vermont address! – what about confidentiality? Entries by Evelyn are almost non-existent, but Jack looks as though he is getting as obsessive as Evelyn about replies to letters – or is he reflecting her obsessiveness? In June, Jack seeks medical advice about a cataract in his right eye. May offers to pay for the necessary treatment, and his writing after his cataract is removed on August 1st becomes almost illegible. During his convalescence, which lasts until he returns to school at the end of September, his eye gives him considerable pain and, perhaps because of that but untypically, he records his dreams on several occasions. No mention in his daily entries of the usual "work" on novels.

He continues to record letters posted (mostly by Evelyn) in diligent detail. Their only visitor appears to be Gladys, and the walks to the riverside appear to have ended as well. August also sees records of Evelyn's ill-health. They continue to eat well, and Jack records that the oysters he had had the day before disagreed with him, so he had only asparagus for supper. He also mentions the weather rather more than in past years. There are numerous references to paperwork regarding her copyrights. Christmas was once again a dour affair, although, for the first time, Jack records that he bought Christmas cards. The final page, after December 31st, is filled with Evelyn's writing in purple ink, detailing a number of paintings by Cyril and Merton.

It's spooky reading the entries for the second half of the year, knowing that this time next year Evelyn will be dead.

Early in 1963 he records buying cough lozenges for Evelyn – this most likely for the symptoms of the lung cancer that eventually killed her. In February there is a series of telephone calls with an FBI agent named Ferguson, and a meeting, but no record of what they were about: was this related to Evelyn's reporting a building porter to the FBI as a communist? Bernice returns from her trip abroad and once again Evelyn and Jack have regular visits from her. In March his entries record new spectacles, and another hospital admission following a cataract operation, and on March 13th Jack records his "last day at school for a while." As Evelyn is seen regularly by Dr Cohen and treated for a heart condition, Jack's writing becomes very loose and hard to read. By April he and Evelyn were going out for regular short walks, and he records nightly drinks with her. On April 11 Jack again goes into hospital, and on April 18 he reports his first electrical (!) treatment, very possibly electric shock treatment, although is not clear if this is for his eyes or his depression; there is no mention in his diary of anything that might be construed as a depressive episode. He has a total of six of these treatments at two- to three-day intervals, and Evelyn records him coming home "on a pass" on May 4. He returns to school at the end of May. Evelyn's entries are less frequent and less and less coherent.

From June 7, when Evelyn was diagnosed and admitted to hospital, the days fall into a routine. Jack writes a large number of letters (presumably about Evelyn's illness), including one to Jigg, and returns to school on June 10. He visits Evelyn regularly, sometimes twice daily, and writes regularly to Jigg and Paula with updates on Evelyn's treatment and condition. The number "17" (June) is ringed in green ink, as that is the day Dr Cohen tells him Evelyn is responding to radiation and can come home and be treated as an outpatient; so is "19". Weeks later she was still in hospital: she finally comes home on July 27. Jack's handwriting becomes very angular and illegible in places – no doubt due to stress. On June 21 he gives Evelyn a letter from Jigg, a harsh letter that says he will not write to her again: there is no record of her response. The flurry of letter writing results in letters to him (Gladys sent money) and visits from friends. Jack's entry for August 3 is probably the most touching in all his diaries: "Evelyn died. Gladys + May here". She was at "home" and with friends.

The following entries are brief and nearly illegible: her burial (August 6); a "disturbing letter from Jigg" (August 7); having Evelyn's belongings cleared. He tried to ring May, who refused to talk to him, and spent some time with Gladys in New Jersey. A number of entries in August begin: "Think it was today that…" He was prescribed antidepressants and appears to have spent August with Gladys, then returned to school on September 9. There are numerous references to Robert Welker. By October he was taking a cocktail of antidepressant drugs and his writing had deteriorated further. There are no entries at all for much of October and November; on November 21 he records receiving a letter from Denise Scott (!) and there are numerous references to "drink": it appears he hit the bottle quite hard. He writes regularly to Jigg and Paula (these letters have been preserved) and yet another drug is added to his cocktail! By the beginning of December his entries are longer and record the time of the first drink of the day – first around midday, then earlier and earlier until he is starting after his morning coffee. The entry for Christmas Day is the longest of the year.

Later, reading Jack's correspondence with his friend John Gawsworth, it is clear that he knew that Evelyn had a cancer, probably terminal, as early as March this year. He also refers to his period of hospitalisation, saying it was for depression brought on by the strain of knowing (?) Evelyn was ill, but keeping it from her. The electrical treatments referred to are therefore ECT. Did Evelyn not wonder why he was undergoing this treatment during a protracted stay in hospital? Or was her self-absorption total?

The 1964 diary comprises page after page of entries about pensions and other financial matters including probate. Jack appears to be neglecting himself, eating mainly at Rudley's, drinking and smoking a great deal. Some entries indicate confusion: "Woke up under the impression it was still yesterday" and "forgot laundry". By March he is taking valium in addition to the other drugs. His sight is poor and getting worse, and he refers to falls – but whether from effects of tranquilisers, or drink, or poor vision is not recorded. His writing is untidy and jagged, but he still records, in punctilious detail, letters sent and received, bills, shopping done, time of first drink of the day (generally mid-morning). He records what he eats at home: not a healthy diet (¼ bologna sandwich for breakfast). He is now withdrawing more money than he is banking. Gladys visits from time to time. In May he had the second cataract removed. There is a gap from May 7 to May 20, when he records entering a convalescent home in Portchester (was the gap during the period of his hospitalisation for cataract?) and another gap until he leaves the convalescent home on June 8. His writing becomes much more like it used to be, clear and regular – due to enforced abstinence from drink? Or improved vision? On June 8 he records two more falls, and another three days later. He also bought two pipes that day. On June 26 he records going to his first AA meeting: the pages for June 28 to July 4 are blank, and when entries restart, the writing is once again shaky and difficult to read. About half the pages for July are blank, and the last entry in the entire diary is that for July 31, 1964: "Gather glasses from Salodar".

www.ingramcontent.com/pod-product-compliance
Ingram Content Group UK Ltd.
Pitfield, Milton Keynes, MK11 3LW, UK
UKHW050721280425
5655UKWH00038B/356